ORTHOPEDIC ASSESSMENT AND TREATMENT OF THE GERIATRIC PATIENT

Orthopedic Assessment and Treatment of the Geriatric Patient

CAROLE B. LEWIS, P.T., PH.D.
Director
Physical Therapy Services of Washington D.C., Inc.
Washington, D.C.

KAREN A. KNORTZ, P.T., PH.D.
Co-owner
Knortz/Snyder Physical Therapy, P.C.
Lincoln, Nebraska

Mosby

St. Louis Baltimore Boston Chicago London Philadelphia Sydney Toronto

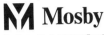
Mosby
Dedicated to Publishing Excellence

Sponsoring Editor: David K. Marshall/Martha Sasser
Associate Managing Editor, Manuscript Services: Deborah Thorp
Production Supervisor: Carol A. Reynolds
Proofroom Manager: Barbara M. Kelly

1 2 3 4 5 6 7 8 9 0 CL/MV 97 96 95 94 93

Library of Congress Cataloging-in-Publication Data
Orthopedic assessment and treatment of the geriatric patient / [edited
  by] Carole Lewis, Karen Knortz.
      p.   cm.
    Includes bibliographical references and index.
    ISBN 0-8016-6512-4
    1. Geriatric orthopedics.   2. Musculoskeletal system—Wounds and
injuries—Treatment.   I. Lewis, Carole Bernstein.   II. Knortz,
Karen.
    [DNLM: 1. Bone and Bones—injuries.   2. Exercise—in old age.
3. Joint Diseases—in old age.   4. Orthopedics—in old age.   WE 168
07624]
RD732.3.A4408   1992
617.3′0084′6—dc20
DNLM/DLC   92-48210
for Library of Congress   CIP

DEDICATION

One of the most exciting aspects of my work in the area of geriatrics is the tremendous amount of advice, guidance, and tales of life experiences that I gather from my patients. Nevertheless, this dedication is not to someone older, but rather younger: someone who has provided an enormous amount to my personal growth. She has worked very hard to teach me a balance between work and play. As a matter of fact, our first opportunity to really talk occurred when I was persuaded to miss a local meeting of the American Geriatric Society for a much-needed night out.

Therese McNerney, my business partner, is one of the most fun but hardest-working people I know. I want to thank her for providing me with the support and encouragement that I needed to prepare this text. I also would like to thank her for providing me with a great deal of clinical information in the area of orthopedics. I am so glad that we are friends, colleagues, and business partners. I couldn't have done it without her. Therese, may you always have your joy for life. It will suit you well when you finally do grow old.—C.B.L.

I would like to dedicate this book to the most special people in my life: my parents, Edward and Sudie Knortz. They have taught me the most important things that they have learned in life, supported my educational and professional growth, and motivated me through example.

My father has been a healthy, extremely productive individual most of his life, but recently suffered a stroke with profound neurological effects. Though he was critically ill, my father refused to give up. At a time when he was exhausted from the effort required for every breath, my father chose life, struggling through the crisis with the support of a very loving family. I will always be grateful for my father's extraordinary effort at a time when he had every right to give up. He demonstrates the same tenacity toward his goal of recovery, and although I've never thought of my father as a patient, I must say that he is the type of patient a health care provider loves to work with: someone who is dedicated to success.

My mother, a woman of great strength and love, steadfastly serves as his health care advocate. She, like my father never gives up. Her actions are true to her integrity. My mother is the epitome of the adjective "considerate". She gives unselfishly of herself to let people know how much she cares. She taught me that people don't care how much you know until they know how much you care. I remember that often in my clinical practice, and I thank her for teaching me how to care.

I know that I would not be in a position to offer professional contributions, such as my efforts toward this book, were it not for my parents. Their example inspired me to believe that nothing is impossible as long as you are persistent in your efforts.—K.A.K.

FOREWORD

The recognition that no one practitioner or a given health care discipline has the breadth of knowledge and skills to provide comprehensive care to our elders is one of the basic tenets of geriatrics and gerontology. The basis for this belief is our growing understanding of the complex interaction of disease and the aging process, and of the physical, psychological, and social factors that contribute to the loss of function and consequent disabilities that are common in old age. Nowhere is this complexity more evident than in the area of musculoskeletal problems. An injury such as a rotator cuff tear, which might be merely an inconvenience for a young person, may precipitate nursing home admission in an older woman who has preceding functional loss in dexterity and mobility from osteoarthritis and osteoporosis. Moreover, underlying conditions, such as cardiovascular disease or dementia, which may shift the balance of risks and benefits between surgical, drug, and other therapeutic modalities, are the rule rather than the exception. Thus, it is just as important for the clinician, regardless of her own professional discipline, to bring to the clinical encounter a broad understanding of the possible approaches to a given problem as it is to have the indepth knowledge and skills needed to provide a specific intervention.

While many of us who care for elderly persons have come to recognize this imperative, it has been difficult to put into practice. Few of us have the time to read the many textbooks and journals that would be required to gain such a perspective. Moreover, very few of us were exposed to this spectrum of knowledge during our initial education and training. *Orthopedic Assessment and Treatment of the Geriatric Patient,* edited by Carole Lewis P.T., Ph.D., and Karen Knortz, P.T., Ph.D., uniquely provides the practitioner or student with this crucial, multidisciplinary approach to musculoskeletal problems of older persons. It brings together in one volume the perspectives of highly regarded clinicians with differing disciplinary backgrounds to help solve a variety of difficult clinical problems. Using the information contained in this book, our ability to provide older patients with an intervention that will maximally improve function is substantially enhanced.

L. GREGORY PAWLSON, M.D., M.P.H.
Professor and Chairman
Department of Health Care Sciences
George Washington University Medical Center
Former President of the American
  Geriatrics Society

CONTRIBUTORS

ARI BEN-YISHAY, M.D.
Senior Resident, Orthopedic Surgery
Hospital for Joint Diseases
Orthopedic Institute
New York, New York

JENNIFER M. BOTTOMLEY, M.S., P.T.
Area Rehabilitation Coordinator
Medicare and Rehabilitation Specialists
Wayland, Massachusetts

CHRISTOPHER A. DESOUZA, M.A.
Doctoral Student
Department of Kinesiology
University of Maryland
College Park, Maryland

SAM DOVELLE, O.T.R.
Hand Rehabilitation Services
Gaithersburg, Maryland

PERRY S. ESTERSON, M.S., P.T., Sc.S., A.T.,C.
Director
Center for Orthopedic and Sports Physical Therapy
Vienna, Virginia

WILLIAM F. GARVIN, M.D.
Assistant Clinical Professor
Department of Orthopedics and Rehabilitation
University of Nebraska Medical Center
Lincoln, Nebraska

CATHERINE GILLIGAN, B.A.
Associate Researcher
Biogerontology Laboratory
Department of Preventive Medicine
University of Wisconsin—Madison
Madison, Wisconsin

PATRICIA K. HEETER, M.S., O.T.R.
Chief, Deparment of Occupational Therapy
U.S. Army 130th Station Hospital
Heidelberg, Germany

HOLLIS HERMAN, M.S., P.T.
Co-owner
Cambridge Physical Therapy Maternal and Child Health Center
Cambridge, Massachusetts
Clinical Supervisor
Women's Physical Therapy Center
Braintree Hospital
Weymouth, Massachusetts

JANET JENSEN, B.S., M.S., P.T.
Physical Therapist
Independent Contractor and Private Practice
New York City/Long Island, New York

KATHY KAMPA-HUDSON, B.S., M.S., P.T.
Rehabilitation Coordinator
Functional Abilities, Inc.
Fort Myers, Florida

ROBERT R. KARPMAN, M.D., M.B.A.
Chief of Orthopedics
Maricopa Medical Center
Phoenix, Arizona

KAREN A. KNORTZ, P.T., PH. D.
Co-owner
Knortz/Snyder Physical Therapy
Lincoln, Nebraska

BETH SPELLBERG KWIATKOWSKI, B.A.
Director
Neuromuscular Retraining Clinic
University of Wisconsin Hospitals and
   clinics
Madison, Wisconsin

CAROLE B. LEWIS, P.T., PH.D.
Director
Physical Therapy Services of
   Washington, D.C., Inc.
Washington, D.C.

THERESE MCNERNEY, P.T.
Vice President
Physical Therapy Services of Washington, D.C.
Washington, D.C.

MARC O. MEADOWS, P.T., A.T.,C.
Clinical Director
Center for Orthopedic and Sports Physical Therapy
Sterling, Virginia

DARRELL C. MENARD, M.D.
Health Promotion Coordinator
Directorate of Health Protection and Promotion
National Defense Headquarters
Ottawa, Ontario, Canada

RICHARD J. NASCA, M.D.
Associate Clinical Professor of Orthopedic Surgery
Tulane University School of Medicine
New Orleans, Louisiana

TERI NISHIMOTO, B.S., P.T.
Physical Therapist
Associated Healthfocus
Portland, Oregon

LEO M. ROZMARYN, M.D.
Attending Head Surgeon
Department of Orthopedics
Shady Grove Adventist Hospital
Rockville, Maryland
Suburban Hospital
Bethesda, Maryland

DANIEL W. SCHMOLL, M.D.
Trinity Lutheran Family Practice
Kansas City, Missouri

CAROL SCHUNK, P.T., PSY.D.
Regional Director
Medicare and Rehabilitation Specialists
Portland, Oregon

EVERETT L. SMITH, PH.D.
Associate Professor
Director, Biogerontology Laboratory
Department of Preventive Medicine
University of Wisconsin-Madison
Madison, Wisconsin

STEPHEN H. SMITH, M.D.
Quakertown Orthopedics
Quakertown, Pennsylvania

JANET SOBEL, P.T.
Clinical Director
Virginia Sports Medicine Institute
Arlington, Virginia

IRVING E. WESTON, M.D.
Practicing Family Physician
Phoenix, Arizona

JOHN G. YOST, JR., M.D.
Chief of Surgery
Research Medical Center
Kansas City, Missouri

JOSEPH D. ZUCKERMAN, M.D.
Vice Chairman
Department of Orthopedic Surgery
Hospital for Joint Diseases
New York, New York

PREFACE

At a recent dinner, one of my ex-patients asked me about the book that Karen Knortz and I were writing. I informed him that the book was based on an interdisciplinary approach to the management of orthopedic rehabilitation, presenting alternate viewpoints from the perspective of physicians and therapists. My patient was very excited about the approach, as he currently is attempting to determine the best options for management of recently diagnosed prostate cancer. He had been in contact with numerous physicians and health care professionals, many of whom presented contradictory advice.

In his quest for information in relation to his illness, he was confronted by numerous medical professionals who believed that their approach was the only way of treating the problem. Being a well-educated person, he was not satisfied with this type of response and continued to seek information. Finally, he came across the *Consensus Development Statement on Prostate Cancer*, published by the National Institutes of Health.[1]

This document gave him tremendous insight into the method by which the evaluation and management of prostate cancer should be investigated. Based on the approach and list of available treatment strategies presented in the consensus statement, he felt that his interactions with various health professionals and the advice they gave were so biased in one direction or another as to be almost worthless. None of the health professionals he consulted took into account the six criteria outlined in the consensus development statement. This is a particularly alarming revelation considering that he consulted some of the areas finest urologists and oncologists.

Because of the single-minded focus of each practitioner, alternative approaches (i.e., different than their preferred approach) to management of the problem were not considered viable. In my estimation, this lack of objectivity transformed otherwise outstanding health professionals into substandard zealots.

This type of bias in health care was the major reason for our deciding to write a book. We believe that the purpose of this textbook is to present physicians, physical therapists, and occupational therapists with objective strategies for and alternate approaches to the management of health care conditions.

For example, when a person with a rotator cuff tear presents to the various health care professionals, what are the alternatives for evaluation and treatment? Surgery may not be the only option. Exercise may not be the modality of choice. This text presents different views to treatment, with the goal to provide the best care with the most favorable outcome for the patient. It is our opinion that this can only be achieved through teamwork.

In the clinical setting, the geriatric patient often is overlooked or inadequately treated. Although, according to Felsenthal, 30% of older patients' visits to their physician are as a result of complaints regarding musculoskeletal conditions.[2] Considering the large proportion of physician visits for which these conditions account, it is remarkable that their treatment receives so little attention.

Another study, prepared by Rodecki et al.,[3] showed that physicians spend less time with their older patients than they do with younger patients who exhibit similar symptoms. A review of the treatment practices of internists, cardiologists, and other specialists revealed that the amount of time spent with patients was significantly less for older compared to younger patients.

This is distressing, considering that older patients often have multiple, interactive, and synergistic disease processes at work, use medications at a higher rate, and may experience psychological trauma and other complications to a greater degree than younger patients. These factors tend to complicate the diagnosis, treatment, and outcome of patient conditions, indicating that older patients should receive more, not less, care. Although we are not aware of a similar study tracking the behavior of rehabilitation personnel with regard to older patient care time, it seems likely that the results of such a study would indicate less time spent with older patients.

We believe, therefore, that it is imperative for all health care professionals to refocus their attention on this rapidly growing segment of the population. It is our hope that our book will provide practitioners with new approaches for solving problems and will help them to focus on appropriate treatment strategies for older persons with these conditions.

Frequently, therapists read only textbooks, journals, and reports by therapists, and orthopedic surgeons read only periodicals, articles, and texts by orthopedic surgeons. The menu of alternatives for the patient is limited or biased, therefore, by the scope of the material familiar to the practitioner in question.

I believe that the authors who have contributed the chapters that follow are the finest authors in their particular areas of orthopedic intervention and have provided both the rehabilitative and orthopedic surgery communities with an excellent overview of approaches for management of every major joint condition and complication.

It is our hope that this text will be used as a working handbook for professionals dealing with orthopedic conditions. We also hope that the material presented will be updated and improved by the orthopedic surgeons and physical and occupational therapists who have contributed to it as developments in the interactive approach are realized. We thank each of them for taking so much time to provide current insights and concepts that will enable the practitioner to gain perspective on the proper management of their older patients.

Carole B. Lewis, P.T., Ph.D.

REFERENCES

1. National Institutes of Health: National Institutes of Health Consensus Development Conference Statement. *The Management of Clinically Localized Prostate Cancer.* Vol. 6, No. 10. June 15–17, 1987.
2. Steinberg F: Principles of geriatric rehabilitation. *Arch Phys Med Rehabil* January 1989; 70:68–69.
3. Rodecki S, Kane R, Solomon D, et al: Do physicians spend less time with older patients? *J Am Geriatr Soc* 1988; 36:713–718.

ACKNOWLEDGMENTS

We would like to extend our sincere appreciation and respect to the authors who have contributed to this book; their combined efforts will help to improve orthopedics and rehabilitation for the older person. We are very grateful to all of the authors who have generously given their expertise to make this text as clinical as possible for both orthopedic surgeons and therapists.

We sincerely thank David K. Marshall, Mosby–Year Book, for his encouragement to publish and for taking us by the hand and walking us through the process. Frequently, publishing can be very painful; we thank David for making it painless, and for his belief in and commitment to our text.

We would also like to thank our business partners, Therese McNerney and Jayne Snyder, for allowing us the freedom to be able to accomplish this rather overwhelming task and for being encouraging and supporting of our efforts.

Special thanks to the staff of Mosby–Year Book for assisting in the production of this book, especially Julie Tryboski and Wendi Sweetland.

Many thanks also to Terry Scanlin for all her valued organizational abilities and for communicating so beautifully with the authors; her time, effort, and thoroughness are very much appreciated.

Carole B. Lewis, P.T., Ph.D.
Karen A. Knortz, P.T., Ph.D.

CONTENTS

Chapter 1

Cardiovascular Benefits of Exercise

Christopher A. DeSouza, M.A.

With advancing age the cardiovascular system undergoes changes in both structure and function. These changes can occur independent of pathologic processes but due to the prevalence of coronary artery disease it is often difficult to differentiate between the effects of aging per se and the changes that result from the interaction of disease and age. It is important that orthopedic surgeons, physiotherapists, and other members of the orthopedic rehabilitation team be aware of the cardiovascular capabilities and limitations of older patients. Rehabilitation modalities should enhance the patient's cardiovascular system as well as musculoskeletal system in order to restore and maximize the patient's physical capabilities. If the cardiovascular system is ignored during the rehabilitative process progress may be slowed and compromised. Patients recovering the use of their lower limbs may have difficulty progressing through the rehabilitation regimen of parallel bars, walking frames, crutches, and sticks to independence[1] because they have cardiovascular limitations. Older patients can improve their functional capacity through daily physical activity and where appropriate should be encouraged to do so during and after the rehabilitation process. This chapter will focus on the age-related structural and functional alterations that affect the cardiovascular system and the role that exercise can play in diminishing these deleterious effects.

AGE-RELATED STRUCTURAL CHANGES

Heart Size

It was originally believed that with increasing age the myocardium atrophied due to reduction in demand caused by lower daily activity levels.[35] This hypothesis, however, has been rejected as a result of studies employing both invasive and noninvasive techniques. Linzbach and Akuamoa-Boateng reviewed the autopsy records of 7,112 human hearts and reported an average increase in heart mass of 1 to 1.5 g/year in persons between the ages of 30 and 90 years. Specific cases of cardiac atrophy were not found. This investigation involved both healthy and diseased hearts; therefore, the reported increase in heart mass may have been due at least in part to the prevalence of disease in older hearts.[21]

Using M-mode echocardiography, Sjorgen[62] noted a progressive increase in left ventricular (LV) posterior wall thickness from the second to the seventh decade. Gerstenblith et al[26] also demonstrated an increase in LV wall thickness in healthy subjects between the ages of 25 to 84 years (Fig 1–1). Although increases in LV wall thickness were noted in these and other studies, the LV cavity size at diastole and systole was not affected. These findings imply that age-related LV hypertrophy is the product of pressure overload resulting from a normal age-related increase in systolic blood pressure (Fig 1–2) and greater LV impedance caused by changes in aging blood vessels.

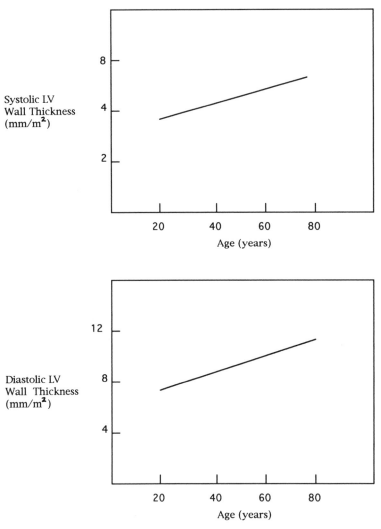

FIG 1–1.
Linear regression plot depicting the relationship between age and systolic and diastolic LV wall thickness per square meter. (From Gerstenblith G, et al: Echocardiographic assessment of a normal adult aging population. *Circulation* 1977; 56:273–277. Used by permission.)

Vascular System

When evaluating the influence of age on structural changes of the myocardium it is important to consider the effects of age on the properties of the vascular system. As previously mentioned, alterations in senescent blood vessels influence not only LV hypertrophy but also LV function. Each vessel is composed of three basic layers: the intima, media, and adventitia. Advancing age adversely affects both the intima and media while changes in the adventia are less specific and not clearly understood.

Histologic studies in humans have demonstrated that with advancing age there is an increase in intima thickness resulting from the accumulation of connective tissue.[36, 67, 72] Intima thickening has been found to take place at varying times in different coronary arteries; for example, the posterior descending arteries are affected only after the fifth decade. The media thickens via elastic fragmentation and calcification. Medial calcification is a progressive process and has been shown to be significant by the fourth decade.[41] These alterations in the structure of aging arteries results in a reduction in compliance and distensibility causing a twofold increase in pulse wave velocity between the ages of 20 and 60 years.[36] Similar histologic, mechanical and functional changes occur in the veins with age.[67] These changes include intima thickening, progressive fibrosis of the tunica media, loss of elasticity, and the occurrence of varicose veins in areas of high pressure.[36] These

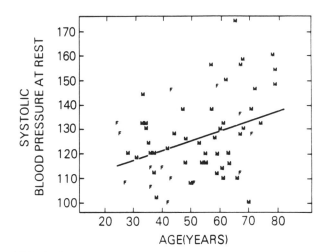

FIG 1–2.
Normal rise in resting systolic blood pressure with age. (From Rodeheffer RJ et al: Exercise cardiac output is maintained with advancing age in healthy human subjects: Cardiac dilatation and increased stroke volume compensate for a diminished heart rate. *Circulation* 1984; 69:203–212. Used by permission.)

changes put additional stress on the aging heart to meet the body's oxygen demands. Figures 1–3 and 1–4 illustrate the major structural features of a mature (25 to 65 years) and aged (more than 65 years) artery.

Valves

Changes in cardiac valves with age are generally the result of disease. In the absence of disease cardiac valves remain thin, delicate, and functional. If valve thickening does occur it is attributed to injury and repair, a process accentuated by abnormal mechanics. A common byproduct of minute valve injury is the formation of a thrombus on the valve's line of closure.[34] In a study conducted by Sell and Scully,[57] the age-related changes in 100 aortic and 200 mitral valves were evaluated. The investigators reported that with advancing age both valves showed similar decreases in size and number of nuclei in the leaflets, increases in fibrous tissue and fragmentation of collagen, and increases in lipid buildup and calcification. When calcification occurred the fibrous tissue of the aortic valve was affected, while in the mitral valve the annulus was the

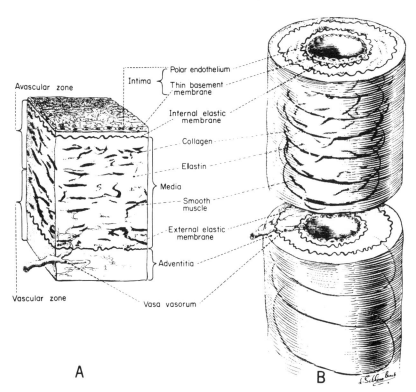

A

B

FIG 1–3.
Major structural features of a mature artery. **A,** cross-sectional view of wall. **B,** longitudinal view of vessel. (From Yin CP: The aging vasculature and its effect on the heart, in

Weisfeldt ML, (ed): *The Aging Heart: Its Function and Response to Stress.* New York, Raven Press, 1980. Used by permission.)

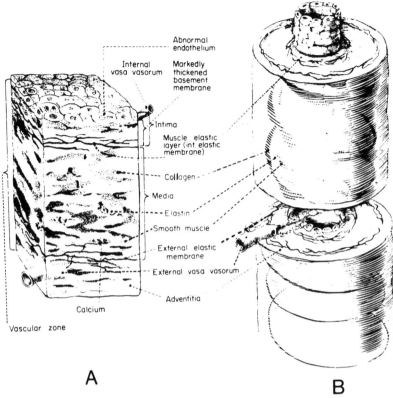

A   B

FIG 1–4.
Major structural features of an old artery. **A,** cross-sectional view of wall. **B,** longitudinal view of vessel. (From Yin CP: The aging vasculature and its effect on the heart, in Weis-

feldt ML (eds): *The Aging Heart: Its Function and Response to Stress.* New York, Raven Press, 1980, pp . Used by permission.)

location of calcification. Valve calcification is generally preceded by changes in collagen, ground substances, and lipids.[34]

EFFECTS OF AGE ON CARDIOVASCULAR FUNCTION AT REST

Heart Rate

Resting heart rate does not significantly change with age.[68] There is, however, a reduction in both sinus rate variation with respiration and spontaneous heart rate variations over a 24-hour period in healthy older men.[12, 37]

Preload

Studies utilizing M-mode echocardiography, two-dimensional echocardiography, and gated blood pool scans have shown no age-related changes in resting LV end-diastolic area, diameter, or volume.[26, 53] However, preloading of the ventricles is affected with age.[59] During early diastole there is a reduction in blood flow from the left atrium to the left ventricle. In order to compensate for the reduction in early filling, atrial contraction is enhanced in older hearts.[38] In young, healthy hearts atrial contraction is not essential for ventricular filling but with advancing age it is relied upon to maintain adequate filling volume. The reduction in early diastolic filling may be the result of one or a combination of the following age-related myocardial changes: progressive thickening of the mitral valve, decreased LV compliance, longer isovolumic relaxation time, varicose veins, or a general loss of physical condition.[4, 38, 59]

Afterload

Structural changes in the aorta and other major arteries occurring with age include increased stiffness and reduced diastolic recoil. These changes, coupled with a normal age-related rise in systolic blood pressure, increase afterload in elderly persons. The augmented volume of blood in the aorta, a result in part of an age-related 6% increase in aortic root dilation between the ages of 40 and 80 years, creates greater impedance against which the left ventricle must contract. Thus, an increase in afterload is considered to be the stimulus for the LV hypertrophy observed in older hearts.[36, 38, 59, 67]

Cardiac Output

By definition, cardiac output is the product of heart rate and stroke volume and it represents the ability of the myocardium to meet the body's oxygen requirements both at rest and exercise.[21, 38] The effect of advancing age on resting cardiac output has been investigated in many cross-sectional studies. In an early study conducted by Brandfonbrener et al,[8] cardiac output was reported to decline by approximately 50% from 6.5 L/min to 3.9 L/min with a concomitant decrease in stroke volume between the ages of 20 and 80 years. The study involved 67 male inpatients of a community hospital who were reportedly free of cardiovascular disease. It is important to note, however, that many of these patients were suffering from respiratory infections or orthopedic problems.

Rodeheffer et al[53] reported strikingly different results in 61 persons who participated in the Baltimore Longitudinal Study of Aging (BLSA). Forty-seven men and 14 women ranging in age from 25 to 79 years were examined using radionucleotide scintigraphy. All subjects underwent rigid cardiovascular disease screening, which included both resting and stress electrocardiograms (ECGs). In addition, all subjects 40 years of age and older underwent an exercise thallium test. All subjects were described as being active members of the community who maintained moderate levels of physical activity. The authors found no significant age-related decline in cardiac output in this group. Table 1–1 shows the resting hemodynamic variables that were measured in both studies. The decrease in stroke volume and increase in peripheral vascular resistance noted in population A was likely attributable to undiagnosed coronary disease. The findings of Rodeheffer et al[53] suggest that in the absence of disease a decrease in cardiac output may not always occur.

Kenney,[36] however, has indicated that cardiac output does decrease with age by approximately 1% per year with a concomitant fall in stroke volume of approximately 0.7% per year between the ages of 20 and 80 years (Fig 1–5). Given the components of cardiac output, other investigators have suggested that an unchanged or reduced resting heart rate coupled with a reduced stroke volume results in a lower resting cardiac output in many older persons.[33, 50, 59] The lack of consistency across studies is likely a result of variations in study populations with regard to overall physical condition and the presence of latent coronary artery disease.

Contractility

The primary function of the myocardium is to pump blood continuously throughout the circulatory system. Although it is difficult to assess the contractile state of the intact cardiac muscle, studies utilizing isolated cardiac muscle preparations have provided valuable insight regarding the effects of age

TABLE 1–1.

Effect of Adult Age on Resting Cardiac Function*

	Population A†	Population B‡
	Institutionalized, Unscreened for Occult Coronary Artery Disease (CAD) (2nd–9th Decade)	Active in Community, Screened for Occult CAD With Cardiovascular Stress (3rd–8th Decade)
Heart rate	Slight decrease	No effect
Systolic blood pressure (BP)	Increase	Increase
Stroke volume	Decrease	Slight increase
Diastolic BP	No effect	No effect
Cardiac output	Decrease	No effect
Cardiac index	Decrease	No effect
Peripheral vascular resistance	Increase	No effect

*From Fleg JL: Alterations in cardiovascular structure and function with advancing age. *Am J Cardiol* 1986; 57:33C–44C. Used by permission.
†Data from Brandfonbrener et al.[8]
‡Data from Rodeheffer et al.[53]

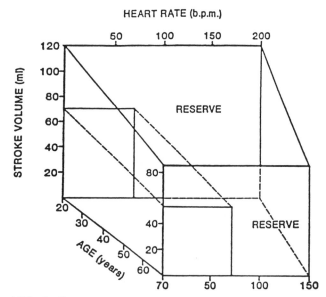

FIG 1–5.
Changes in resting cardiac output and reserve of output between 20 and 70 years of age. (From Kenney RA: *Clin Geriatr Med* 1985; 1:37–59. Used by permission.)

on myocardial contractility. A consistent finding is a 20% prolongation of contraction resulting from an increase in both time to peak force and relaxation time. Prolonged contraction may be indicative of an age-related increase in time of contractile activation or in the excitation-contraction process.[40] Age-related changes in the vasculature, specifically viscoelastic properties, may also affect the duration of contraction. In order to test the relationship between prolonged contraction and prolongation in the excitation-contraction cycle, Lakatta et al[39] conducted a study involving a series of progressively premature electrical stimuli in both adult and older hearts. The senescent heart consistently had a greater restitution interval as compared with younger adult cardiac muscle. This indicates that the electromechanical restitution in older hearts is delayed and is manifested as prolonged time to peak force.[39, 67] Prolonged activation in older hearts may be the consequence of both a lower rate of calcium uptake by the sarcoplasmic reticulum and changes in the transmembrane action potential.[40, 69]

It is of interest to note that the sinoatrial (SA) node (the heart's pacemaker) begins to lose cells early in adulthood and continues to do so until the age of 60 years. The SA node is also affected by the formation of fibrous tissue. In aged hearts, over 90% of the original cell population may already be lost. Surprisingly, the function of the SA node is not critically impaired by these changes. There is also cell

loss in the bundle of His and in the bundle branches. The atrioventricular (AV) node is the last to show cell loss, remaining unaffected up to the seventh decade.[36]

EFFECTS OF AGE ON CARDIOVASCULAR FUNCTION DURING EXERCISE

Maximal Oxygen Consumption

Many longitudinal and cross-sectional studies have shown that aerobic capacity reflected by maximal oxygen consumption ($\dot{V}O_2$max) declines with age by approximately 0.45 mL/kg/min/year.[9, 14, 17, 32, 52] This rate of decline amounts to a 9% reduction in aerobic capacity per decade after the age of 25 in sedentary healthy men. This decline, however, is not exclusively attributable to the aging process but also to other factors such as genetic endowment, physical inactivity, gender, changes in body weight and composition, disability, and disease.[9] After an extensive review of cross-sectional and longitudinal studies, Buskirk and Hodgson[9] suggested that the rate of decline of $\dot{V}O_2$max with age may be curvilinear instead of linear. The authors based their suggestion on the disparity of results between the two types of studies, differences caused by factors such as life-style, physical inactivity, and weight gain.

Maximal oxygen consumption is composed of both a central component (cardiac output) and a peripheral component (arteriovenous oxygen difference). Both components are adversely affected by age, causing a decline in $\dot{V}O_2$max.

$$\dot{V}O_2max = Qmax \times (A - V)O_2 \text{ difference}$$

$$\dot{V}O_2max = (HRmax \times SVmax) \times (AV)O_2 \text{ difference}$$

$$\dot{V}O_2max = (HRmax \times [EDVmax - ESVmax]) \times (A - V)O_2 \text{ difference}$$

where Qmax = maximal cardiac output; $(A - V)O_2$ = maximal arteriovenous oxygen difference; EDVmax = maximal end diastolic volume; and ESVmax = maximal end systolic volume.

Maximal Heart Rate

Maximal heart rate decreases in a linear fashion with age at a rate of 0.4 to 0.95 beats/min/year.[64]

Various studies have reported a decline in maximum heart rate from 195 beats/min at the age of 20 to 150 to 160 beats/min at 60 years of age.[51] Considering that heart rate decreases with age at the same rate in both athletically trained and untrained persons, one may predict maximum heart rate from the following equation[35]:

$$\text{Maximum HR} = 220 - \text{age (years)}$$

The mechanisms behind the decline in maximum heart rate with age are currently unknown. Possible explanations include a reduced drive to the sympathetic pacemaker or a reduced sensitivity to catecholamines.[59]

Stroke Volume

Research has indicated that stroke volume decreases with age as work rates approach maximum.[45, 55] The diminution in stroke volume may be related to higher systolic pressure, increased afterload, changes in myocardial compliance, and diminished myocardial contractility.[59] However, interesting results concerning stroke volume have been documented by Rodeheffer et al.[53] The authors reported that in their healthy BLSA subjects, end-diastolic volume (EDV) increased during exercise and stroke volume was therefore maintained or increased via the Frank-Starling mechanism. The study also indicated that end-systolic volume (ESV) increased and ejection fraction decreased compared with those of younger adults. These changes were considered to result from the age-related increase in aortic impedance, larger preload, or diminished myocardial contractile function. Nevertheless, the authors concluded that cardiac output can be maintained during exercise in healthy older people. They hypothesized that this increase reflected a shift from a catecholamine-mediated increase in heart rate and a reduction in end systolic volume to the utilization of the Frank-Starling mechanism. It is important to note both the highly selective study population and that neither $\dot{V}O_2$max nor maximal cardiac output was measured in this study. It is possible that if the subjects in this study exercised maximally a reduction in cardiac output would have been noticed.

Arteriovenous Oxygen Difference

Maximal arteriovenous oxygen difference tends to decrease with age, meaning less oxygen is being extracted by the exercising muscles. This may be caused by several factors—physical inactivity, lower hemoglobin levels and oxygen saturation, reduction in aerobic enzyme activity, or increased vascular stiffness—which could prevent blood redistribution and increased blood flow to the skin.[59, 64]

CARDIOVASCULAR BENEFITS OF EXERCISE

Contrary to what previous investigations have shown, recent studies have shown that persons older than 60 years can increase $\dot{V}O_2$max through endurance exercise. Thomas et al[64] reported a 12% increase in $\dot{V}O_2$max in men in their mid-60s after completing a 1-year training protocol consisting of walking or jogging three times per week. In shorter-duration studies, DeVries[16] and Haber et al[28] documented increases in $\dot{V}O_2$max of 8% in men 52 to 88 years of age and 12% in men 67 to 76 years of age, respectively. Perhaps the best study that demonstrates $\dot{V}O_2$max can be increased in an older population was conducted by Seals et al.[56] The study involved 24 healthy, sedentary men and women between the ages of 60 and 69 years. The exercise group comprised 14 subjects while the remaining 8 acted as the nonexercising control group. Training involved two 6-month training protocols. The first 6 months involved low-intensity exercise such as walking three times per week and a general increase in overall daily physical activity. The second 6 months involved high-intensity exercise in which the subjects progressed to 45 minutes of endurance exercise at 85% of their heart rate reserve. At the conclusion of the 12 months of training, the $\dot{V}O_2$max of the exercising group increased by 30%. The low-intensity training elicited a 12% increase in $\dot{V}O_2$max (25.4 to 28.2 mL/kg/min) while the high-intensity training elicited an additional 18% increase (32.9 mL/kg/min). The authors attributed the increase in $\dot{V}O_2$max to a 14% increase in maximal arteriovenous oxygen difference and a small but significant increase in stroke volume. This study clearly indicated that older persons are able to obtain a training response via peripheral adaptations if the training stimulus is substantial.

There is also strong evidence that the rate of decline in $\dot{V}O_2$max with age can be influenced by long-term exercise training (Fig 1–6). Pollack et al[48] conducted the first longitudinal study on master athletes to investigate the effects of training over time on $\dot{V}O_2$max. Twenty-four master athletes be-

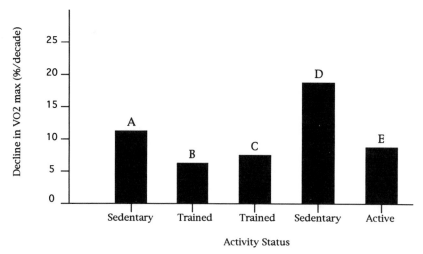

FIG 1–6.
The effects of endurance training on the decline of $\dot{V}O_2$max. The results of four studies. (From Cunningham DA, Paterson DH: Discussion: Exercise, fitness, and aging, in Bouchard C, Shephard RJ, Stevens T et al (eds): *Exercise Fitness and Health: A Consensus of Current Knowledge.* Champaign, Ill, Human Kinetics, 1990, p 703. Used by permission.)

tween the ages of 50 and 82 years were initially tested between 1971 and 1974 and retested 10 years later. During the 10-year period 13 athletes stopped competing but remained physically active. The athletes who maintained their training intensity over the 10-year period suffered only a 2% reduction in $\dot{V}O_2$max. In comparison, the athletes who had reduced their training intensity suffered a 13% reduction in $\dot{V}O_2$max. Over the 10-year period the subjects' body weight did not significantly change.

In a similar study, Rogers et al[54] remeasured $\dot{V}O_2$max after 8 years in 15 well-trained master athletes and 14 sedentary controls. Over the 8-year period the master athletes maintained their training frequency but the duration, intensity, and number of miles per week declined. At the beginning of the study the $\dot{V}O_2$max of the master athletes was 59% higher than that of the control group when expressed in mL/kg/min. After 8 years the authors reported a significant difference in the rate of decline in $\dot{V}O_2$max between the two groups. In the untrained group $\dot{V}O_2$max declined 9.7% from 33.9 to 30.6 mL/kg/min, which is equivalent to 12% per decade. In contrast, the $\dot{V}O_2$max of the master athletes declined 4.1% from 54.0 to 51.8 mL/kg/min, which is equivalent to 5% decline per decade. These results are consistent with the findings of cross-sectional and longitudinal studies, which noted a 9% per decade decline in $\dot{V}O_2$max in sedentary persons.[32] In addition these results verified the suspicions of Heath et al[32] that the age-related deterioration in $\dot{V}O_2$max can be reduced to 5% per decade if training and body weight are maintained.

Thus, the data in these studies indicate that older people are able to increase their $\dot{V}O_2$max between 10% and 20% through regular endurance exercise. In addition, the rate of decline in $\dot{V}O_2$max can be lowered from approximately 9% per decade to 5% per decade if a high level of training is maintained. The physiologic mechanisms responsible for these adaptations are an increase in maximum arteriovenous oxygen difference and an enhanced stroke volume.[29, 56] Figure 1–7 shows that persons who continue to exercise can maintain a high level of $\dot{V}O_2$max.

Older persons with hypertension can both increase their functional capacity and safely lower their blood pressure (BP) through regular endurance exercise training.[10, 21, 31] In a study conducted by Hagberg et al,[31] 33 hypertensive patients (average BP greater than 150/80 mm Hg) between the ages of 60 and 69 years participated in a 9-month training study. Prior to beginning the study all subjects were screened for coronary artery disease and randomly assigned into three groups: the control group, the low-intensity exercise group, or the high-intensity exercise group. Subjects in the low-intensity exercise group walked for 60 minutes at 50% of their $\dot{V}O_2$max three times a week. The high-intensity exercise group slowly progressed from walking at low intensity to fast walking, jogging, cycle ergometry, and treadmill walking at 70% to 85% of their $\dot{V}O_2$max for 45 to 60 minutes three times a week. The authors reported a greater decrease in systolic blood pressure in the low-intensity exercise group (20 mm Hg) compared with the high-intensity exercise group (9 mm Hg). Both training groups experienced a 10- to

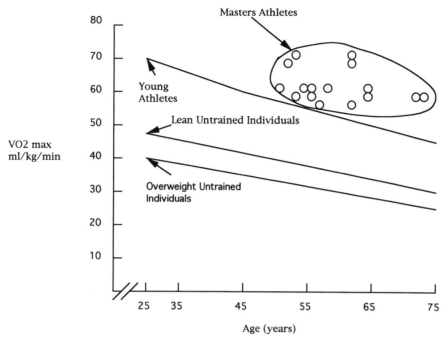

FIG 1–7.
Decline in $\dot{V}_{O_2}$max with age. Note the difference in $\dot{V}_{O_2}$max between master athletes and untrained people. (From Heath GW, Hagberg JM, Ehsani AA, et al (eds): A physio-logical comparison of young and older endurance athletes. *J Appl Physiol* 1981; 51:634–640. Used by permission.)

12-mm Hg decrease in diastolic blood pressure. In a similar study involving 70- to 79-year-old men and women Cononie et al[10] showed that healthy subjects with normal BP to moderate hypertension (between 140/90 and 180/100 mm Hg) could lower their mean, systolic, and diastolic BP by 8, 9, and 8 mm Hg, respectively with endurance exercise. The training protocol slowly progressed from 20 to 30 minutes of walking at 50% $\dot{V}_{O_2}$max three times a week to 35 to 45 minutes of exercise at 75% to 85% $\dot{V}_{O_2}$max for the last 2 months of the 6-month training program. These studies provide evidence that older persons with hypertension can lower their blood pressure with regular endurance exercise training. The underlying mechanisms by which exercise reduces resting blood pressure remains unclear.[49]

Although improving functional capacity is the basic physiologic goal of endurance training, the average older person may not wish to train intensively at the levels described by Rogers et al[54] and Pollock et al.[48] in order to acquire the capacity for peak performance. Instead, the goal may be to increase aerobic capacity, thus augmenting tolerance for daily activities with less fatigue, dyspnea, and perceived exertion. A moderate level of physical activity has been shown to elicit these results.[5, 29, 30, 56]

Aerobic capacity can be developed and maintained if an exercise prescription adheres to the fol-lowing guidelines, recommended by the American College of Sports Medicine[3]:

- Frequency of training: 3 to 5 days per week
- Intensity of training: 60% to 90% of maximum heart rate (HRmax) or 50% to 85% of maximum oxygen uptake ($\dot{V}_{O_2}$max) or HRmax reserve
- Duration of training: 20 to 60 minutes of continuous aerobic activity
- Mode of activity: activities involving large muscle groups that can be maintained continuously and are rhythmic and aerobic in nature, such as walking, hiking, running or jogging, and swimming.

An exercise prescription for older persons should emphasize low to moderate training intensity over a longer period. Low to moderate intensity exercise reduces cardiovascular risk and orthopedic injury and improves compliance[3, 20] (Table 1–2). Depending on the individual's initial level of fitness, exercise intensity as low as 50% of HRmax can provide important cardiovascular benefits.[3]

Exercise intensity is usually prescribed and monitored by heart rate. There are a number of acceptable ways in which to determine the appropriate intensity represented by a target heart rate. For example, target heart rate is frequently determined

TABLE 1–2.

Classification of Intensity of Exercise Based on 20 to 60 Minutes of Endurance Training*

Relative Intensity (%)		
HRmax	$\dot{V}O_2$max or HRmax Reserve	Classification of Intensity
<35	<30	Very light
35–59	30–49	Light
60–79	50–74	Moderate (somewhat hard)
80–89	75–84	Heavy
≥90	≥85	Very heavy

*From Pollock ML, Wilmore JH: *Exercise in Health and Disease: Evaluation and Prescription for Prevention and Rehabilitation*, ed 2. Philadelphia, WB Saunders, 1990. Used by permission.

from a fixed percentage of maximal heart rate. Using this method a healthy 60-year-old person with a maximal heart rate of 160 beats/min would be prescribed a target heart of 112 to 136 beats/min, corresponding to 70% to 85% of HRmax. Another approach to determine target heart rate is the Karvonen formula, which takes resting heart rate into account.[2, 20, 58] Using the Karvonen formula the target heart rate range for the same person would be determined as shown in Table 1–3.

The Karvonen method is advantageous when working with cardiac patients whose resting and exercise heart rates may be affected by medications such as beta-blockers.[20, 58] The target heart rates derived via these two methods are applicable to most activities in which a steady state is achieved. The values obtained are only guidelines to follow and are subject to change depending on variables such as improved functional capacity, cessation of training, and injury.[3]

Target heart rate can be easily monitored at rest and during exercise at either the carotid or radial arteries. Obtaining heart rate by palpating the carotid artery has caused some concern that too much pres-

TABLE 1–3.

Determination of Target Heart Rate for Healthy 60-Year-Old Person Using Karvonen Formula

	Target Heart Rate Range (Beats/min)	
	Lower Limit	Upper Limit
HRmax	160	160
HRrest	− 65	− 65
HRreserve	95	95
Training intensity	× 0.60	× 0.80
(60%–80% HR range)	57	76
HRrest	+ 65	+ 65
Target heart rate	112	141

sure may be exerted while trying to locate and check heart rate, evoking a carotid sinus reflex. Considering that patients with coronary artery disease are particularly sensitive to carotid sinus reflex, it is recommended they be cautious when palpating this site.[20] Some older persons may have difficulty palpating either site due to a loss of sensitivity at their finger-tips and may require assistance.[43]

CORONARY ARTERY DISEASE AND EXERCISE

The prevalence of disease, particularly coronary artery disease (CAD), increases with advancing age. Many older people may at some time experience myocardial infarctions, undergo cardiac surgical procedures, or suffer from stable angina pectoris, chronic arrhythmias, or other cardiovascular disorders. The importance of exercise to this special population cannot be ignored.

A number of randomized and controlled studies have confirmed that a medically prescribed and supervised exercise training program can improve the physical work capacity and $\dot{V}O_2$max of older persons who have suffered a cardiac event or who suffer from CAD.[11, 13, 44, 47] For example, in persons who have experienced either a myocardial infarction or coronary artery bypass graft (CABG) there is evidence that training can improve $\dot{V}O_2$max by as much as 11% to 56% and 14% to 66%, respectively.[27, 46] In general, a supervised program of physical exercise can be expected to increase the $\dot{V}O_2$max in cardiac patients an average of 10% to 20%, with an even more dramatic increase occurring in sedentary older patients with a poor initial level of fitness.[42, 63] The increase in $\dot{V}O_2$max observed in patients with CAD was originally attributed to peripheral adaptations by working muscles involving an enhanced arteriovenous oxygen difference resulting from an increase in blood volume, capillary density, and oxygen extraction, along with a decrease in systemic vascular resistance.[18, 63, 65] The improved ability of the musculature to extract oxygen, along with an increase in vagal tone, lessened catecholamine release, and a number of other factors can decrease the rate-pressure product and other determinants of myocardial oxygen demand by as much as 18%. By reducing the myocardial oxygen demand angina pectoris and ECG changes will occur at a greater work intensity and duration.[63]

Exercise-related cardiac adaptations were originally considered to be highly unlikely in cardiac patients.[65] However, studies conducted by Ehsani et al[18, 19] have suggested that in addition to peripheral adaptations, intense long-term exercise training of progressively increasing intensity, frequency, and duration can elicit central myocardial adaptations. These adaptations produce a reduction in myocardial ischemia and an improvement in both LV function and LV contractile function, thus improving both functional capacity and the probability of surviving an ischemic event.[7, 18, 19]

Considering the goal of exercise in cardiac patients is to both improve and maintain functional capacity, Rogers et al[55] investigated whether the beneficial effects of high intensity training on $\dot{V}O_2$max and myocardial ischemia reported by Ehsani et al[18, 19] could be maintained if cardiac patients continued to train. The study involved nine men (average age 57 years) with documented CAD who had completed a 12-month cardiac rehabilitation program and continued to participate in the program for an additional 6 years. The exercise training regimen involved a 10-minute warm-up consisting of walking and stretching followed by jogging and/or cycling. The frequency, intensity, and duration of the exercise were progressively increased to the point where the patients were training for 50 to 60 minutes per day, 4 to 6 days a week at 70% to 90% of their $\dot{V}O_2$max. At the conclusion of the initial 12 months of training the patients were jogging an average of 18 miles a week at an intensity of 81% of their maximal heart rate. The nine patients continued to train at or slightly below this level for the next 6 years. The mean $\dot{V}O_2$max of the nine patients increased from 1.93 L/min to 2.64 L/min after 12 months of training. Following 6 additional years of regular supervised physical activity the mean $\dot{V}O_2$max of the patients was 2.72 L/min, which was not significantly different from the values obtained after the first 12 months of training. Both heart rate during exercise and maximal oxygen pulse, defined as maximal oxygen uptake divided by heart rate measured at the same time as $\dot{V}O_2$max, increased substantially after the first 12 months and except for a small decline in heart rate they remained unchanged after the additional 6 years of training.

The findings of Rogers et al[55] show that vigorous exercise training performed by selected motivated patients with coronary artery disease can produce and maintain favorable increases in functional capacity ($\dot{V}O_2$max). The authors concluded that the large increase in $\dot{V}O_2$max observed after 1 year of training and maintained for an additional 6 years must be a result of both central and peripheral adaptations.[55]

Cardiac patients receiving medication are also able to improve their functional capacity through aerobic activity. For example, the effects of long-term beta blockade on the exercise conditioning response in coronary patients is well documented (although controversial).[6, 70] Stuart and co-workers[61] reported a substantial increase in $\dot{V}O_2$max (32%) after a 12- to 16-week training program in patients receiving the beta blocker propranolol. The authors attributed this increase to an increase in both stroke volume and peripheral oxygen extraction. Cardiac patients receiving other cardiac medication such as calcium-channel blockers and nitrates are also capable of increasing their functional capacity.[71]

The physiological benefits of exercise for people who have sustained a cardiac event are sound and well documented.[23, 24, 60] These benefits are gained over time as cardiac patients continue to actively participate in an exercise program. In addition, exercise can also yield important gains in self-confidence and self-concept, as well as an enhanced sense of well-being.[15] For many patients these gains can be just as important as the physiologic ones.

CLINICAL HIGHLIGHTS

The clinical effects of aging on the cardiovascular system include:

- Increase in LV wall thickness but no change in cavity size
- Increase in arterial thickness and stiffness
- Increase in systolic blood pressure
- No significant change in resting heart rate
- Decrease in maximal heart rate by approximately 1 beat/min/year
- Reduction in preload and an increase in afterload
- Reduction in resting and maximal stroke volume
- Reduction in resting and maximal cardiac output.

Benefits of endurance exercise training include:

- Maximal oxygen uptake can be enhanced by 10% to 20%
- Rate of decline of $\dot{V}O_2$max can be lowered from approximately 9% per decade to 5% per decade

- Arteriovenous oxygen difference can be enhanced
- Resting blood pressure can be reduced by 8 to 10mm Hg

CONCLUSION

The effects of age on the cardiovascular system cannot be prevented. Exercise however, can help to reduce its severity by slowing the rate of decline in $\dot{V}_{O_2}$max. This enables older people to remain active and independent. Other beneficial effects of exercise include improved quality of life and reduced morbidity and mortality, reduction in platelet aggregation and possible increase in fibrinolysis, weight control, enhanced joint mobility, stability, flexibility, and greater neuromuscular coordination.[5, 60] Endurance training can also have a favorable impact, directly or indirectly, on major CAD risk factors such as hypertension, smoking, and high cholesterol levels.[63]

Hippocrates said, "Speaking generally, all parts of the body which have a function, if used in moderation and exercised in labours to which each is accustomed, become thereby healthy and well developed, and age slowly; but if unused and left idle, they become liable to disease, defective in growth, and age quickly."[66] This statement is certainly true of the cardiovascular system.

Acknowledgment

Special thanks to Sarah Hill for her insightful comments and help in preparing this chapter.

REFERENCES

1. Aitken RCB, Hunter JAA, MacKenzie L, et al: Rehabilitation, in Hughes SPF, Benson MKD, Colton CL (eds): *Orthopaedics: The Principles and Practice of Musculoskeletal Surgery.* New York, Churchill Livingston, 1987.
2. American College of Sports Medicine: *Guidelines for Exercise Testing and Prescription,* ed 4. Philadelphia, Lea & Febiger, 1991.
3. American College of Sports Medicine: Position stand on the recommended quantity and quality of exercise for developing and maintaining cardiorespiratory and muscular fitness in adults. *Med Sci Sports Exerc* 1990; 22:265–274.
4. Berne RM, Levy MN: *Cardiovascular Physiology,* ed 5. St Louis, Mosby–Year Book, 1986.
5. Blair SN, Kohl HW, Paffenbarger RS, et al: Physical fitness and all-cause mortality: A prospective study of healthy men and women. *JAMA* 1988; 262:2395–2401.
6. Blood SM, Ades PA: Effects of beta adrenergic blockade on exercise conditioning in coronary patients: A review. *J Cardiopulmonary Rehabil* 1988; 8:141–144.
7. Blumenthal JA, Califf R, Williams RS, et al: Continuing medical education cardiac rehabilitation: A new frontier for behavioral medicine. *J Cardiopulmonary Rehabil* 1983; 3:637–656.
8. Brandfonbrener M, Landowne M, Shock MW: Changes in cardiac output with age. *Circulation* 1955; 12:557–566.
9. Buskirk ER, Hodgson JL: Age and aerobic power: The rate of change in men and women. *Fed Proc* 1987; 46:1824–1829.
10. Cononie, CC, Graves, JE, Pollock, Ml, et al: Effect of exercise training on blood pressure in 70- to 79-yr-old men and women. *Med Sci Sports Exerc* 1991; 23:505–511.
11. Costill DL, Branam GE, Moore JC, et al: Effects of physical training in men with coronary heart disease. *Arch Phys Med Rehabil* 1974; 59:276–280.
12. Davies HEF: Respiratory changes in heart, sinus arrhythmia in the elderly. *Gerontol Clin* 1975; 17:96–100.
13. DeBusk RF, Houston N, Haskell WL, et al: Exercise training soon after myocardial infarction. *Am J Cardiol* 1979; 44:1223–1229.
14. Dehn M, Bruce RA: Longitudinal variations in maximal oxygen intake with age and activity. *J Appl Physiol* 1972; 33:805–907.
15. DeSouza CA: Patient evaluations of the George Washington University cardiac rehabilitation clinic (unpublished data). George Washington University, 1991.
16. DeVries HA: Physiological effects of an exercise training regimen upon men aged 52 to 88. *J Gerontol* 1970; 25:325–336.
17. Dill DB, Robinson S, Ross JC: A longitudinal study of 16 champion runners. *J Sports Med Phys Fitness* 1967; 7:4–27.
18. Ehsani AA, Biello DR, Schultz J, et al: Improvement of left ventricular contractile function by exercise training in patients with coronary artery disease. *Circulation* 1986; 74:350–358.
19. Ehsani AA, Martin WH, Heath GW, et al: Cardiac effects of prolonged and intense exercise training in patients with coronary heart disease. *Am J Cardiol* 1982; 50:246–253.
20. Fardy PS, Yanowitz FG, Wilson PK: *Cardiac Rehabilitation, Adult Fitness and Exercise Testing,* ed 2. Philadelphia, Lea & Febiger, 1988.
21. Fleg JL: Alterations in cardiovascular structure and function with advancing age. *Am J Cardiol* 1986; 57:33C–44C.
22. Fletcher GF: Exercise in the management of blood pressure, in Fletcher, GF (ed): *Exercise in the Practice of Medicine,* ed 2. New York, Futura Publishing, 1988.
23. Froelicher VF: *Exercise Testing and Training.* St Louis, Mosby-Year Book, 1983.
24. Froelicher VF: Exercise, fitness, and coronary heart disease, in Bouchard C, Shephard RJ, Stephens T, et al (eds): *Exercise Fitness and Health: A Consensus of Current Knowledge.* Champaign, Ill, Human Kinetics Books, 1990.

25. Froelicher VF, Sullivan M, Myers J, et al: Can patients with coronary artery disease receiving beta blockers obtain a training effect? *Am J Cardiol* 1985; 55:155D–161D.
26. Gerstenblith G, Frederiksen J, Yin FCP, et al: Echocardiographic assessment of a normal adult population. *Circulation* 1977; 56:237–238.
27. Greenland P, Chu JS: Efficacy of cardiac rehabilitation services with emphasis on patients after myocardial infarction. *Intern Med* 1988; 1098:671–673.
28. Haber P, Honiger B, Klicpera M, et al: Effects in elderly people of 67–76 years of age of three month endurance training on a bicycle ergometer. *Eur Heart J* 1984; 4:37–39.
29. Hagberg JM: Effect of training on the decline of Vo₂max with aging, *Fed Proc* 1987; 46:1830–1833.
30. Hagberg JM, Graves JE, Limacher M, et al: Cardiovascular responses of 70- to 79-yr-old men and women to exercise training. *J Appl Physiol* 66:1989; 66:2589–2594.
31. Hagberg JM, Montain SJ, Martin WH, et al: Effect of exercise training in 60- to 69-year-old persons with essential hypertension. *Am J Cardiol* 1989; 64:348–353.
32. Heath GW, Hagberg JM, Ehsani AA, et al: A physiological comparison of young and older endurance athletes. *J Appl Physiol* 1981; 51:634–640.
33. Hossack KF, Bruce RA: Maximal cardiac function in sedentary normal men and women: Comparison of age related changes. *J Appl Physiol* 1982; 53:799–804.
34. Hutchins GM: Structure of the aging heart, in Weisfeldt ML (ed): *The Aging Heart: Its Function and Response to Stress.* New York, Raven Press, 1980.
35. Kannel WB, Gordon T, Offutt D: Left ventricular hypertrophy by electrocardiogram. Prevalence, incidence, and mortality in the Framingham study. *Ann Intern Med* 1969; 71:89–105.
36. Kenney RA: *Physiology of Aging, a Synopsis*, ed 2. St Louis, Mosby-Year Book, 1989.
37. Kostis JB, Morerya AB, Amendo MT, et al: The effect of age on heart rate in subjects free of heart disease. *Circulation* 1986; 65:141–145.
38. Lakatta EG: Heart and circulation, in Schneider EL, Rowe JW (eds): *Handbook of the Biology of Aging*, ed 3, New York, Academic Press, 1990.
39. Lakatta EG, Gerstenblith G, Angell CS: Prolonged contraction duration in aged myocardium. *J Clin Invest* 1975; 55:61–68.
40. Lakatta EG, Yin FCP: Myocardial aging: Functional alterations and related cellular mechanisms. *Am J Physiol* 1982; 242:H927–H941.
41. Lansing AI, Alex M, Rosenthal TB: Calcium and elastin in human arteriosclerosis. *J Gerontol* 1950; 5:112–119.
42. Leon AS, Certo C, Comoss P, et al: Position paper of the American Association of Cardiovascular and Pulmonary Rehabilitation: Scientific evidence of the value of cardiac rehabilitation services with emphasis on patients following myocardial infarction—section 1: Exercise conditioning component. *J Cardiopulmonary Rehabil* 1990; 10:79–87.
43. Meisami E: Aging of the nervous system: Sensory changes, in Timiras, PS (ed): *Physiological Basis of Geriatrics.* New York, Macmillan, 1988.
44. Miller NH, Haskell WL, Berra K, et al: Home versus group exercise training for increasing functional capacity after myocardial infarction. *Circulation* 1984; 70:645–649.
45. Niinimaa V, Shephard RJ: Training and oxygen conductance in the elderly. I. The respiratory system. II. The cardiovascular system. *J Gerontol* 1978; 33:354–367.
46. Oberman A: Does cardiac rehabilitation increase long-term survival after myocardial infarction? *Circulation* 1989; 80:416–418.
47. Patterson DH, Shephard RJ, Cunningham D, et al: Effects of physical training on cardiovascular function following myocardial infarction. *J Appl Physiol* 1979; 47:482–489.
48. Pollock ML, Foster C, Knapp D, et al: Effect of age and training on aerobic capacity and body composition of master athletes. *J Appl Physiol* 1987; 62:725–731.
49. Pollock ML, Wilmore JH: *Exercise in Health and Disease: Evaluation and Prescription for Prevention and Rehabilitation*, ed 2. Philadelphia, WB Saunders.
50. Port S, Cobb FR, Coleman RE, et al: Effect of aging on the response of the left ventricular ejection fraction to exercise. *N Engl J Med* 1980; 303:1137–1147.
51. Raven PB, Mitchell JH: Effect of aging on the cardiovascular response to dynamic and static exercise, in Weisfeldt ML (ed): *The Aging Heart: Its Function and Response to Stress.* New York, 1980, Raven Press.
52. Robinson S, Dill DB, Tzankoff SP, et al: Training and physiological aging in man. *Fed Proc* 1976; 32:1623–1634.
53. Rodeheffer RJ, Gerstenblith G, Becker LL, et al: Exercise cardiac output is maintained in advancing age in health human subjects: Cardiac dilation and increased stroke volume compensate for a diminished heart rate. *Circulation* 1984; 69:203–213.
54. Rogers MA, Hagberg JM, Martin WH, et al: Decline in Vo₂max with aging in master athletes and sedentary men. *J Appl Physiol* 1990; 68:2195–2199.
55. Rogers MA, Yamamoto C, Hagberg JM et al: The effect of 7 years of intense exercise training on patients with coronary artery disease. *J Am Coll Cardiol* 1987; 10:321–326.
56. Seals DR, Hagberg JM, Hurley BF, et al: Endurance training in older men and women. I. Cardiovascular response to exercise. *J Appl Physiol* 1984; 57:1024–1029.
57. Sell S, Scully RE: Aging changes in the aorta and mitral valves. Histologic and histochemical studies with observations on the pathogenesis of calcific aortic stenosis and calcification of the mitral annulus. *Am J Pathol* 1965; 46:345–365.
58. Sharkey BJ: *Physiology of Fitness*, ed 3. Champaign, Ill, Human Kinetics Publishers, 1990.
59. Shephard RJ: *Physical Activity and Aging*, ed 2. Rockville, Maryland, 1987, Aspen Publications.
60. Shephard RJ: Exercise regimens after myocardial Infarction: Rationale and results, in Wenger NK (ed): *Exercise and the Heart*, ed 2. Philadelphia, 1985, FA Davis, pp 145–146.
61. Stuart RJ, Foyal SN, Lundstrom R, et al: Does exercise training alter maximal oxygen uptake in coronary artery disease during long-term beta-adrenergic blockade? *J Cardiopulmonary Rehabil* 1985; 5:410–414.

62. Sjorgen AL: Left ventricular wall thickness in patients with circulatory overload of the left ventricle. *Ann Clin Res* 1972; 4:310–318.

63. Squires RW, Gau GT, Miller TD, et al: Cardiovascular rehabilitation: Status, 1990, *Mayo Clin Proc* 1990; 65:731–755.

64. Thomas SG, Cunningham DA, Rechnitzer PA et al: Determinants of the training response in elderly men. *Med Sci Sports Exercise* 1985; 17:667–672.

65. Thompson PD: The benefits and risks of exercise training in patients with chronic coronary artery disease. *JAMA* 1988; 259:1537–1540.

66. Thompson PD, Dorsey DL: The heart of the master athlete, in Sutton, Brock (eds): *Sports Medicine for the Mature Athlete.* Champaign, Ill, Benchmark Press, 1987.

67. Van Camp SP, Boyer JL: Cardiovascular aspects of aging (part 1). *Phys Sports Med* 1989; 17:121–130.

68. Walsh RA: Cardiovascular effects of the aging process, *Am J Med* (Suppl) 1987; 82:34–40.

69. Weisfeldt ML, Gerstenblith ML, Lakatta EG: Alterations in circulatory function, in Andres R, Bierman EL, Hazzard WR (eds): *Principles of Geriatric Medicine.* New York, McGraw Hill, 1985.

70. Weisfeldt ML: Left ventricular function, in Weisfeldt ML (ed): *The Aging Heart: Its Function and Response to Stress.* New York, Raven Press, 1980, pp 297–316.

71. Wenger NK: Cardiovascular drugs: Effects on Exercise Testing and Exercise Training of the Coronary Patient, in Wenger NK (ed): *Exercise and the Heart,* ed 2. Philadelphia, FA Davis, 1985, pp 133–143.

72. Yin CP: The aging vasculature and its effect on the heart, in Weisfeldt ML (ed): *The Aging Heart: Its Function and Response to Stress,* New York, Raven Press, 1980, pp 137–215.

Chapter 2

Physiological and Psychological Benefits of Exercise

Irving E. Weston, M.D.

An octogenarian of my acquaintance, a patient of an associate of mine, was asked the question, "If you were to pick out a 20-year period in your life that was the most enjoyable and satisfying, which 20 years would you pick?" Having grown up, lived, and matured in a society that typically assigns people to certain "pigeonholes" or roles of expected conduct, I found his answer quite startling. Startling, because it was not a usual or typical answer; startling, in that it gave me hope—hope that this sexagenarian would be able to give a similar answer 20 years hence.

This unique person's answer was, without hesitation, "the last 20 years." He did not suggest 20 years in his relative youth, nor the 20 years of his productive zenith. He felt his present state of being was even greater than the excitement and energy of his youth. He had "quality of life."

Implicit in his answer are many things that we need to examine. Researchers might call them variables. The subtle gestalt of this true story is that this man is not suffering pain and he is, therefore, comfortable. His nutrition must be satisfactory, for he is not hungry. His self-image and sense of independence must be at a high level, for he is satisfied with himself and his life-style. What is it in this person's life-style that makes it so comfortable? Is there some magical thing operating for him?

Most of us don't believe in magic. This person's condition, whether talking of the physical or of the mental, is the sum total of life's forces—his loves and experiences. A natural thing happened to him along the way—aging. It happens to everyone.

Whether it was luck, intuition, or intellect, this person instituted an exercise program early on in life and it affected his life in a positive manner. He did other things requiring a decision, like not smoking, that helped his state of health.

But what of the people the same age as the person in our example who are debilitated by the degenerative changes of aging? Or debilitated by injury or disease? They may have had the potential he did but elected a different pathway. Some are in nursing homes. Some require continuous surveillance at home owing to ambulatory deficit from weakness and debility. As a result of their infirmity, depression and despondency manifest themselves. Self-esteem is at low ebb. Coping mechanisms are ineffectual. Cognitive function deteriorates. Physically they feel helpless. The quality of life is lost.

These people exist in a state of dependency. Mental acceptance of that fact, depending on cognitive awareness, is difficult to integrate. Add to it the economic burden each aging person and his or her family must bear. As a person lives longer with disabilities requiring assistance and dependency, the costs go up exponentially.

An appropriate question to ask at this juncture is: is there some way to reduce the economic burden to society for disabilities of the aging population? A number of illnesses related to the aging process are quite costly and consume energies that might be directed to different areas. An example of this is the osteoporosis associated with aging, which results in significant costs for care of hip fractures alone. Attention has been focused upon the cost of medical care on the national scene because of its magnitude, and because of the projected consumption with an aging population. The modalities of diagnosis and the instruments of treatment are extremely costly and this writer would argue that they are necessary. Given the constraints of the budget, there is no alternative but to accept rationed health care.

As a practicing physician, I see the governmental and insurance mandates that come down and they strike heavily at the aging population. Are there things at this stage in life that can be done to reduce the consumption of health care dollars? One study[27] has shown that death is usually preceded by eight to ten years of disability and about one year of total dependency. If one could through some dynamic action reduce the effects of disability or partial dependency by three or four years, there would be a significant economic saving and the cost to society would be limited. Are there habits that can be developed to increase independence and shorten the disability period? Are there protocols of living or axioms of conduct that can be tapped into for the benefit of the aging population or society in general? Exercise is that modality.

In this book and in this chapter, we explore the possibilities of enhancing the well-being of an aging population. And when there is disease, as there will inevitably be disease with disability, what significant interventions can be brought to bear to improve the quality of life? Can we reduce the burden of disease on the individual?

EXERCISE AND WELL-BEING

The 83-year-old man previously mentioned is, to be sure, an exception. He is exceptional in that he has exercised most of his life at an aerobic and conditioning level. He has no major illness or major skeletal abnormalities. He is not overweight and is a nonsmoker. His diet through life has reflected societal trends, including a recent awareness of the need for a low-fat, high-fiber diet. He would seem to have a healthful, comfortable existence. Why should he be this way? As we analyze the subtleties of this person's life, what is it that allows him to enjoy his present status? The one variable that stands out is exercise. Could this act of commission, i.e., exercise, possibly have such a positive effect upon the trajectory of this person's life? Can exercise modify the aging process?

Bortz[6] has studied the biologic changes occurring during the aging process and feels that a part of that change is related to physical inactivity. Support for his premise can be inferred by observing positive changes in elders participating in an appropriate physical exercise program. Does exercise alter the psychological milieu of an individual? Anecdotally, there would appear to be a body of thought stating that this could be true. As one can well imagine, it is difficult to quantify the physical effects of exercise on the body and even more tenuous to quantify those effects on the mind.

The physiology of the body permits the construction of modules of testing, before and after exercise, and we can evaluate some of the physical changes that occur. As the accumulating mass of literature would indicate, some progress has been made in understanding the effects of exercise upon the body. Most, but by no means all, of the data have been collected on younger subjects. It has been established that the data would indicate a positive effect of exercise on the body.

Here in the United States we have become preoccupied with exercise. For the American people, it probably started in Munich in 1972, when Frank Shorter won the Olympic marathon. After his impressive win, there was a crescendo of interest in sports in general, but in endurance sports in particular. There has been some spillover of interest in exercise into all segments of life, the elderly population included. The full effect has not yet been realized. This is extremely gratifying and ultimately will be of great benefit to the participating individual and to society. If a convincing argument can be presented to a receptive audience, in this case an elderly population, there is great potential to change the epidemiology and demography of disabilities of the elderly.

As younger and older groups exercise, are there some parallels between the healthy and younger individual and the elderly or elderly debilitated person that can be utilized to attenuate the health and well-being of that segment of society and its quality of life?

Up to this point, this discussion has included generalities about exercise and the body. In the case of the physiologic effects on the body, it is important to give substance to and document some of the positive changes, particularly in hopes of motivating people to change their course in life. Of extreme importance are the psychological benefits of exercise, and in the latter part of this chapter that will be the focus. It is possible that the quality of life may depend more on this facet of existence than the physical aspect.

PHYSIOLOGIC BENEFITS OF EXERCISE

Twenty-three centuries ago, Hippocrates is reported to have said, "All parts of the body which have a function, if used in moderation and exercised in labours to which each is accustomed, become thereby healthy and well developed and age slowly; but if unused and left idle, they become liable to disease, defective in growth, and age quickly." It is a fair statement to say that he was a good observer.

Physical exercise creates a cascade of physiologic modification. When exercise is carried out in a regular fashion and characterized by intensity, duration, and frequency, a training effect occurs. The training effect requires the prolonged use of large muscle groups against resistance, utilizing large amounts of oxygen, to the stress of which the body adapts. A state of fitness can be attained with three to five sessions a week, each session involving dynamic (isotonic, shortening of muscle fiber) exercise work at 50% to 80% of $\dot{V}O_2$max (maximum oxygen uptake, 60% to 90% of maximal heart rate) continuously for 15 to 60 minutes.[2] That quantity of exercise is what this writer believes to be an "aerobic equivalent."

Cardiovascular Changes

While exercising at the level of an aerobic equivalent, physiologic changes start to occur in the body. Without a doubt, the most significant beneficial effects of exercise are those acting upon the cardiovascular system. The efficiency of this system is increased in a number of ways. The most fundamental of these is maximum oxygen uptake or $\dot{V}O_2$max.[19] As stated by Simon,[33] "$\dot{V}O_2$max is the best overall measure of the training effect and physical fitness." There is a direct relationship between oxygen consumption and muscular work. Therefore, maximum oxygen uptake reflects maximum work capacity.

What the $\dot{V}O_2$max represents circumscribes the entire process of oxygen transport from the atmosphere through the lungs to the vascular system, down to the enzymatic reactions that produced the adenosine triphosphate (ATP) that provides the energy for muscle contraction.[12] In normal individuals the $\dot{V}O_2$max declines about 1% per year.[23] Larsen

and Bruce suggest that oxygen consumption can increase to from 10 to 20 times the original amount with the addition of an exercise program in a person's life. They state that half the increase in oxygen consumption can be attributed to the increase in capacity for aerobic metabolism at the tissue level and the remaining half is attributable to changes in the cardiovascular system. During exercise, cardiac output can increase as much as four times[5] and increases the heart rate (depending upon age) an equal amount, with a corresponding increase in oxygen uptake and again an increase in work capacity.

Heart rate and stroke volume (i.e., amount of blood ejected with each heartbeat) are two factors affecting cardiac output. Herein lies the difference between a fit and a less fit individual. The conditioned heart, having increased myocardial contractility and increased intraventricular volume,[12] can pump greater volumes of blood. Although age has its sanctions on cardiac output with decrease in heart rate, it is possible by increasing stroke volume through exercise to delay the decay curve of cardiac output of aging.

After the age of 20 years, $\dot{V}O_2$max declines slowly. By the age of 60, a person has two thirds of his $\dot{V}O_2$max (i.e., work capacity) at 20 years old. This loss in $\dot{V}O_2$max can be substantially attenuated by aerobic exercise through life. Remember our octogenarian example? It has been shown that three weeks of bedrest can cause a 20% to 25% decline in $\dot{V}O_2$max.[33] As an example, this is what happens to the disabled elderly as they recover from diseases or injuries that require bedrest.

Aerobic exercise has a significant effect upon arterial resistance to blood flow and produces a lowering of the blood pressure.[21] The decrease in arterial resistance results from dilatation of capillary beds in the working musculature. Blood flow can increase tenfold with exercise. As a result, for any given work load, the peripheral vascular resistance is less and the needs of the working muscles are met by extraction of more oxygen by the increase of flow of blood. While all of these changes are occurring in the blood delivery system, if oxygen and appropriate substrates are available, the training or conditioning effect upon muscle occurs.

Musculoskeletal Changes

A point to be emphasized at this juncture is that increasing the functional ability of an organ system, for example the musculoskeletal system, enables the person with a disability to operate at a more efficient submaximal level so that the activities of daily living can be achieved more efficiently and with greater ease. This becomes extremely important in cases of older people who have sustained injuries that require immobilization. This author has observed empirically that the person who is physically conditioned prior to injury or who is able to maintain a reasonable level of aerobic conditioning through the recovery process will invariably return to a higher functional level than those who were less conditioned at the time of the injury.

The genetic complement with which a person arrives in the world is the same genetic complement with which that person exits this life. The chemical reactions, the enzymatic reactions, and the physiologic adaptations that occur early in life are still in place as one ages. The aging process does decrease the virulence of those reactions, but an adaptation response to exercise can attenuate these effects of aging, even in an elderly individual.

An example of this is a recent study in which DeVries[13] subjected a group of men aged 55 to 88 years to an aerobic training program. The exercise lasted for 1 hour and took place three times a week. He was able to show that these aging participants experienced an improvement in oxygen transport capacity, work capacity, decreased body fat, and decrease in the blood pressure. Halloszy and fellow researchers[17] have shown that the training effect can increase muscle mitochondria and oxidative capacity more than twofold. This training effect, which is obtained by isotonic exercise, enhances muscle endurance.

For the aging person with an intact musculoskeletal system this is well and good; but what of the disabled sedentary elderly people who are unable to do aerobic isotonic exercise? Would isometric exercise that builds muscle strength be of benefit to them? Isometric exercise involves slow repetitions of muscle contractions against resistance. This causes the muscle fiber to hypertrophy and therefore become stronger. Curetan and others[12] documented this phenomenon in both men and women. This reaction is certainly much less marked in the aging population, but one can see that it could be put to good use by devising an exercise regimen that would enhance lower extremity muscle strength and strengthen the arm musculature. This might allow someone not able to ambulate the ability to utilize a walker. Elderly people performing these exercises in a prescribed exercise program, as stated by Mead and Hartwig,[23] can improve joint flexibility, muscle tone, and cardiorespiratory endurance. Motivation for exercise can be enhanced by varying the activities.

Preserving Bone Mass

Another great concern in the aging population, especially in menopausal women, is loss of bone mass. Many studies have been conducted to evaluate and quantify variables involved in this very complex problem.

It has been shown in controlled studies that bone mass increases in athletes who are vigorously exercising, as compared with a similar group who were not engaged in any extra physical activity.[8, 21, 26] It has also been demonstrated that osteoporosis develops after inactivity or prolonged immobilization.[1] Given these two observations, it would seem reasonable that exercise can be beneficial to the skeleton. Indeed, Smith[34] has demonstrated that a very modest exercise program for elderly patients in nursing homes can reduce bone loss. The significance of that is that a bone with more mass will be more resistant to fracture. Reducing fracture morbidity at this stage of life is extremely important and beneficial. A fracture might be life-threatening to the elderly person, not to mention the economic sanctions which the fracture engenders.

Coronary Heart Disease

Of all the benefits that exercise can bestow upon the body, probably one of the most important is its effect on the epidemiology of coronary heart disease. Coronary heart disease is the largest single cause of death in the Western world.[9] A number of risk factors predispose people to this disease; some of them like age, gender, heredity, and race cannot be altered. However, a number of risk factors can be altered, such as elevated blood lipid levels, hypertension, cigarette smoking, physical activity, diabetes, diet, behavioral patterns, and stress levels. Some of them can be attenuated by exercise, such as blood lipids, hypertension, obesity, diabetes mellitus, diet, behavioral patterns, and stress level.

Cooper and co-workers[9] analyzed a number of variables of 3,000 men and found an inverse relationship between physical fitness and body weight, percentage of body fat, systolic blood pressure, and serum levels of cholesterol, triglycerides, and glucose. In another study of 2,854 women, a nearly identical inverse relationship between physical fitness and coronary artery disease (CAD) risk factors was found.[16]

In yet another study, Paffenbarger[28, 29] did a retrospective analysis of 16,936 male Harvard alumni and was able to demonstrate that sedentary men were at a 64% higher risk of myocardial infarction than were classmates who expended 2,000 kcal/wk on exercises. Two thousand kilocalories is the amount of energy expended in running 20 miles, which translates to three or four hours of exercise per week.

In 1988, Ekelund et al[14] reported a prospective study of 4,276 American men that revealed an inverse relationship between physical fitness and the risk of death from CAD, which was independent of other coronary risk factors. They concluded that the least fit men were three times more likely to die of cardiovascular disease than those who were most fit.

Blair, Kohl, and Paffenbarger[4] evaluated 10,224 men and 3,120 women and showed that fitness provided similar protection to women. In their study, they concluded that the least fit individuals were eight times more likely to die from cardiovascular disease than those who were most fit. They further concluded that increasing levels of fitness conferred additional protection, and that even modest improvements in fitness and exercise produced significant beneficial responses in both men and women.

Between the years of 1980 and 1987, the Centers for Disease Control (CDC) reviewed studies of exercise and coronary artery disease. They found 43 studies that were methodologically sound.[30] With all data analyzed together, they were able to show that sedentary living increases coronary risk by 1.9 times. So, one has an increased risk of approximately two times just as a result of physical inactivity. The risk associated with inactivity, when compared with other mortality conditioning risk factors such as hypertension, hypercholesterolemia, and cigarette smoking, comes out 2.1 times, 2.4 times and 2.5 times, respectively. Since the sedentary living variable is two to three times more prevalent than the other risk factors, it makes a strong statement for physical exercise as the variant most needed to change the epidemiology of CAD in the United States.[18]

The U.S. Preventive Service Task Force[19] has made the judgment that exercise is cost effective for the prevention of cardiovascular disease and has recommended that physicians prescribe exercise for their patients. We have, of course, been doing this for years, but there is a need for a more global educational process. There is a high percentage of the populace who in the pursuit of making a living, raising a family, and living a certain life-style, are not influenced by some of these statistics. The CDC[8] reported in 1989 that only 8% of the adults in the United States exercise at the recommended level. As an enthusiastic exerciser (runner) for the last 17 years, reaping the benefits of that life-style, and being a physician in primary care tending to the needs of the sedentary and overweight, I am finding it difficult to inspire the "fast food society" appropriately.

Cancer Mortality

Another important observation regarding the benefits of exercise was observed by Blair, Kohl, and Paffenbarger.[4] They noted that if cancer from all sites in both men and women is considered, there is a lower mortality from cancer in physically fit than in sedentary persons. This is good news for the exercising and physically fit person, of course. That bit of information might be motivational for those who would not be otherwise motivated.

HAZARDS OF EXERCISE

With all the positive things that we have seen relative to exercise, it is appropriate to bring to consciousness some hazards of exercise. Most of the hazards come from extremes of intensity and duration. Probably the most important and most serious hazards are those related to cardiovascular risks. Sudden death and nonfatal myocardial infarction head the list. People with suspected CAD should be evaluated, preferably on a treadmill, before an exercise prescription is given. This is especially true in an elderly person who may well benefit from the exercise, but may have latent cardiac disease. There are other organ systems that can be injured by excessive exercise, but as Hippocrates said, "If used in moderation and exercised in labor to which he is accustomed," and with a little common sense, one can avoid most of these problems. It is this writer's opinion that the elderly should be completely evaluated by a physician and a physical therapist before an exercise prescription is written.

PSYCHOLOGICAL BENEFITS
OF EXERCISE

In the preceding pages, we have presented a perspective on the physical benefits of exercise. No matter at what age one starts to exercise, if exercise is conducted within certain parameters, positive changes can occur. The participant becomes stronger, recovers from disease more easily, and is able to attenuate his or her disabilities more effectively. With all of these physical things happening, what happens to the psychology of this person? Anecdotally, people who exercise report a wide range of subjective positive psychological improvements. In Sime's[32] investigations participants reported feelings like elation, relaxation, increased activation, and a sense of accomplishment as positive experiences with regular exercise. Morgan,[24] who has conducted a large amount of research in this area, reports that people often testify to "an improved sense of well being."

Testimonials, whereas they may support a bias commonly held by society, do not go far in establishing a scientific basis for exercise and psychological benefits. There has been some activity by researchers to substantiate these claims. Morgan and Goldston[25] in 1987 reported research evidence of improvements in anxiety and depression with exercise. Martinsen and co-workers[22] demonstrated that clinically diagnosed anxiety disorders can benefit from exercise programs. It is all well and good that exercise impacts these clinical situations, but what of the "internal workings" of the mind of a partially disabled elderly person? Is that person's mind changed by the addition of exercise to his or her life?

Although the research was criticized as simplistic, Sonstroem[35] in 1984 felt that participating in long-term exercise programs improved self-esteem. Sonstroem and Morgan[36] have proposed a new model of exercise and self-esteem as areas for future study. Early data seem to confirm previous observations.

Self-esteem is described as the degree to which people feel positive about themselves.[15] It is the evaluative component of self-concept. Rogers[31] defines self-concept as "an organized configuration of perceptions of the self which are admissible to awareness." Whatever the definitions are, or whatever the hierarchial relationship of these constructs of self are, self-esteem is the energy source and

mechanism that is going to allow us to enjoy a better quality of life. Not strangely, it is what one believes or feels about oneself that is the driving force for change and improvement. This will generate motivation and sponsor responsibility. A "personal judgment of worthiness"[10] (i.e., self-esteem) is that essential personality quality that will go far in setting the stage for a better existence. Self-esteem may allow one to feel good about oneself, but prompts no action. Before there is action, one more level of self-awareness, called perceived self-efficacy, needs to be put into perspective. Bandura[3] states that perceived self-efficacy refers to the level and strength of a belief that one can successfully perform a given activity. Therein lies the ingredient that is often lacking in the aging person's mind that limits his or her response to illness and aging. Are there strategems for changing this?

Having given some scientific background to exercise and psychological state, and having stratified self-esteem, it is not too hard to see that using exercise to enhance the quality of life or attenuate the social condition of the aging person might be a realistic goal. By merely instituting an exercise program in a physical therapeutic setting, we can develop physical strength that leads to self-esteem; that leads to self-efficacy; that activates; that leads to creativity; that leads to self-care; that leads to responsibility; that leads to increased vitality; to decreased anxiety; to decreased depression; to better coping mechanisms; to a sense of accomplishment; to improved socialization; and to a sense of community. These give elderly people a sense of control of their destiny. By realizing these things the quality of life is maintained.

If we could by aiding the exercising elderly extend their independent and responsible life by 3 to 5 years, there would be enormous savings of tight health care budget dollars. But the savings in human misery would make it even more worthwhile.

REFERENCES

1. Abrahamson AS: Bone disturbances and injuries of the spinal cord, cauda equina (paraplegia): Their prevention by ambulation. *Am J Bone Joint Surg* 1948; 30:982–987.
2. American College of Sports Medicine: *Guidelines for Graded Exercise Prescription*, ed 3. Philadelphia, Lea and Febiger, 1986.
3. Bandura A: Self-efficacy: Toward a unifying theory of behavioral change. *Psychol Rev* 84:191–215, 1977.
4. Blair SN, Kohl HW III, Paffenbarger RS Jr.: Physical

fitness and all–cause mortality: A post-prospective study of healthy men and women. *JAMA* 1989; 262:2395.

5. Blomquist CG: Exercise physiology: Clinical aspects, in Wenger NK (ed): *Exercise and the Heart.* Philadelphia, FA Davis, 1978 p 1.
6. Bortz WM: Disease and aging. *JAMA* 1982; 248:1203–1207.
7. Bruer V, Meyer BM, Keele MS, et al: The role of exercise in prevention of involutional bone loss. *Med Sci Sports Exerc* 1983; 15:445–449.
8. Centers for Disease Control: Progress toward achieving the 1990 national objective of physical fitness and exercise. *JAMA* 1989; 262:746.
9. Cooper KH, Pollock ML, Martin RP: Physical fitness levels versus selected coronary risk factors: A cross-sectional study, *JAMA* 1976; 236:166.
10. Coopersmith S: *The Antecedents of Self-Esteem.* San Francisco, Freeman, 1967.
11. Costill DH: *Inside Running: Basics of Sports Physiology,* Indianapolis, Bench Mark Press, 1986.
12. Cureton KJ, Collins MA, Hill DW, et al: Muscle hypertrophy in men and women. *Med Sci Sports Exerc* 1988; 20:338.
13. DeVries HA: Physiologic effects of an exercise regimen upon men ages 52–88. *J Gerontol* 1970; 25:325–336.
14. Ekelund LG, Haskell WL, Johnson JL: Physical fitness as a predictor of cardiovascular mortality in asymptomatic North American men: The Lipid Research Clinic Mortality Follow-up Study. *N Engl J Med* 1988; 319:1379.
15. Gergen KJ: *The Concept of Self.* New York, Holt, 1971.
16. Gibbons LW, Blair SH, Cooper KH: Association between coronary artery disease risk factors and physical fitness in healthy adult women. *Circulation* 1983; 67:977.
17. Halloszy JQ, Rennie MJ, Hickson RC: Physiologic consequences of biochemical adaption to endurance exercise. *Ann NY Acad Sci* 1977; 301:440.
18. Harris SS Caspersen CJ, DeFriese GH: Physical activity counseling for healthy adults as a primary prevention intervention in a clinical setting: Report of the U.S. Preventive Services Task Force. *JAMA* 1989; 261:3590.

19. Kasch FW, Boyer JL, vanCamp SP: The effect of physical activity and inactivity on aerobic power in older men. *Physician Sports Med* 1990; 18:73.
20. Lane NE, Bloch DA, Wood PD: Long distance running, bone density and osteoarthritis. *JAMA* 1986; 225:1147–1151.
21. Larsen EB, Bruce RA: Health benefits of exercise in an aging society. *Arch Intern Med* 1987; 147:353.
22. Martinsen EW, Hoffart A, Solberg O: Aerobic and nonaerobic forms of exercise in the treatment of anxiety disorders. *Stress Med* 1989; 5:115–120.
23. Mead VF, Hartwig R: Fitness evaluation and exercise prescriptions. *Gen Fam Pract* 1982; 13:1039–1050.
24. Morgan WP: Affective beneficiaries of vigorous physical activity. *Med Sci Sports Exerc* 1985; 17:94–100.
25. Morgan WP, Goldston SE: *Exercise and Mental Health.* Washington, DC, Hemisphere, 1987.
26. Nielsson BE, Wesland NE: Bone density in athletes. *Clin Orthop* 1971; 77:179–182.
27. *Ottawa: Health and Welfare,* Canadian Health Survey, Ontario Canada, 1982.
28. Paffenbarger RS Jr, Wing AL, Hyde RT: Physical activity as a heart attack risk in college alumni. *Am J Epidemiol* 1978; 108:161.
29. Paffenbarger RS Jr, Wing AL, Hyde RT: A natural history of athleticism and cardiovascular health. *JAMA* 1984; 252:491.
30. Protective effect of physical activity on coronary artery disease. *MMWR* 1987; 36:426.
31. Rogers CP: The significance of the self—regarding attitudes and perceptions, in Reymert ML (ed): *Feeling and Emotion: The Moosehart Symposium.* New York, McGraw-Hill, 1950.
32. Sime WE: Psychological benefits of exercise, *Advances* 1984; 1:15–29.
33. Simon HB: *Exercise, Health, and Sports Medicine,* New York Scientific American, 1990.
34. Smith EL: Exercise for prevention of osteoporosis: A review. *Physicians' Sports Med* 10:72–83, 1982.
35. Sonstroem RJ: Exercise and self-esteem, in Terjung RL (ed): *Exercise and Sports Science Review,* ed 12. Lexington, Mass, Collamore Press, 1984, pp. 123–155.
36. Sonstroem RJ, Morgan WP: Exercise and self-esteem: Rationale and model. *Med Sci Sports Exerc* 1989; 21:329–337.

Chapter 3

Neuromuscular Considerations

Darrell Menard, M.D.

Epidemiologists estimate that more than 30 million North Americans are over the age of 65 years[18] and that this group is growing so rapidly that by the year 2030 it could constitute as much as 20% of the North American population. This enormous segment of humanity is no longer content to sit back and age gracefully and has begun to challenge the validity of the limited expectations that society has of our older citizens. Until very recently, people anticipated that their "golden years" would involve retirement from their job, a life of leisure, and relative unproductiveness. Today, however, increasing numbers of older adults view these years as a period of change rather then the end of useful life. It is not uncommon to see older persons returning to school to further their education, starting up new businesses, or embarking on a long-dreamed-of adventure. With the advent of the masters athletic movement in the mid-1970s, many aging persons began to look to sports for fun, fitness, and new challenges. Since this time, the sporting participation of aging athletes has grown from a handful of diehards to that of a full-fledged revolution. Masters competitors are not only involved in increasing numbers but they are active in virtually every form of sport and in some cases are winning medals in international competitions. As a result of years of effort by masters athletes, sports organizers, promotions people, coaches, scientists, and the media, the aging athlete is now recognized as a legitimate entity in the world of sports.

One cannot overstate the role that the media have played in the promotion of the masters athletic movement. Over the last 15 years, successful aging athletes have commanded considerable media attention. It appears that the general public is genuinely interested in the life-styles and accomplishments of many senior competitors. This is perhaps because these individuals serve as powerful reminders of what can be achieved if one accepts no artificial limits and simply goes out and gives one's best effort. Some people may feel younger and more worthwhile when they see senior competitors outperforming opponents many years their junior. It is also possible that people simply like a scenario in which the underdog rises to the occasion and succeeds.

Regardless of the rationale, the media have played a very important role in promoting fitness and sporting involvement in our seniors' population. The media have also been instrumental in identifying a number of aging athletic role models who have served to convince many persons that they are by no means "over the hill." Consider for example, Nolan Ryan, who at the age of 45 years remains one of the finest pitchers in the major leagues. Since his rookie year in 1968, he has played 24 seasons and his consistent performances continue to astonish fans and discourage his opponents. During his career to date, he has struck out more than 5,000 batters, won more than 300 games, and pitched 7 no-hitters. What is especially impressive is that his last two no-hit games were thrown when he was in his 40s. While he admits that his fast ball has slowed somewhat in the last ten years, what he has lost in speed he has more than compensated for in terms of improved mechanics and control. He attributes his competitive longevity to his dedication to a rigorous, year-round conditioning program. No one is certain exactly how much longer he will be able to frustrate major league batters but if his 1991 season was any indication, his career is far from being over.

With the growth of the masters athletic movement, there has been increasing scientific interest in the field of aging and human performance. Sports medicine journals, athletic magazines, and reference texts often include topics of direct relevance to the aging competitor. Unfortunately, issues such as longevity and the cardiovascular benefits of exercise have commanded the greatest attention while important issues such as the effect of aging on body structure and function, injury patterns, recovery rates, and performance potential have received relatively little academic investigation. This chapter is aimed at addressing a number of these important issues so that the reader will have a more complete understanding of one of the most important participants in today's sporting world—the aging active adult.

AGING

The concept of aging and why it occurs has been a topic of great interest for centuries and is currently getting considerable attention from scientists in many fields. Advances in molecular biology, immunology, biochemistry, genetics, and nuclear medicine are providing technologies that may one day answer many of the questions pertaining to the aging process. One of the most important discoveries has been the recognition that many of the changes that were once attributed to the aging process are actually the result of other factors such as disease, disuse, and environmental influences (e.g., noise and air pollution). As further research is done, it will almost certainly be demonstrated that many of the structural and physiologic changes currently attributed to the aging process are actually the result of other influences.

Before one can fully appreciate the changes associated with the aging process, one must first understand the concept of aging. Aging is not a sudden transformation that occurs when we reach our 40th birthday. Instead, it is a continuous and unavoidable process that starts at conception and continues uninterrupted until we die. It cannot be foregone or reversed. The best one can hope for is to reduce the rate at which the process occurs by maintaining a healthy life-style.

There are nearly as many definitions of aging as there are authors who are interested in the subject. Strehler[35] offers one of the simplest and yet most comprehensive descriptions of the aging process. He states that the aging process has four basic properties; aging is: (1) universal; (2) decremental; (3) progressive; and (4) intrinsic. In other words, everyone ages, structural and functional losses occur relentlessly with the passage of time, and the aging phenomenon is not a pathological process but rather an innate part of our genetic makeup. Any change in an older person that fails to satisfy these criteria should not be attributed to the aging process. The net result of aging is a gradual erosion of one's organs' built-in functional reserves to the point where one is increasingly less able to compensate for environmental stresses, metabolic disturbances, disease processes, and anything else that can disrupt homeostasis. Several investigators have shown that for most body systems this erosion begins after the third decade of life and follows a linear rate of decline.[30, 33] These decrements remain largely obscure until the person is placed in a situation where physiologic demands exceed their ability to respond. As one ages, progressively smaller and smaller physiologic stresses are necessary to overwhelm the ability to respond.

AGING THEORIES

Aging is an extremely complex process involving changes at the molecular and cellular level in virtually every body system. The exact mechanism by which it occurs has been an academic obsession for many of the world's finest scholars. While numerous theories attempt to elaborate on the mechanism by which the aging process occurs, none of them adequately explains what has been observed. The following is a brief listing of some of the most popular aging theories:

1. The free radical theory—states that tissues age as a result of the cellular damage inflicted by free radicals
2. The aging program theory—contends that the aging process is actually programmed into our genetic makeup
3. The neuroendocrine theory—states that the deteriorating neuroendocrine function associated with aging will have an impact on all tissues
4. The altered protein theory—proposes that with aging, protein formation is altered and these defective proteins become incorporated

into numerous body structures where they have widespread manifestations

5. The waste product accumulation theory—states that as we age, ineffective biologic waste materials accumulate to the extent that they interfere with normal cellular function
6. The cross-linkage theory—contends that increasingly stable intramolecular and intermolecular cross-linkages will significantly inhibit normal cellular and tissue function

These theories represent some of the more popular attempts at explaining how and why we all must grow old. They all contain an element of truth but fall short of explaining all of the changes noted to occur with aging.

INACTIVITY

An inactive life-style is a far greater threat to one's continued health than the aging process. This is of particular concern because inactivity is almost endemic to our industrialized world. In fact, in our highly automated society, inactivity seems to have become a cultural goal. Why climb a set of stairs when an elevator is available? Why shovel snow when you can buy a snow blower? Why walk to the corner store when you could take the car? The enormous number of labor-saving devices we now have were originally intended to improve efficiency and free people to pursue more pleasurable interests. While these devices have succeeded in eliminating much of the mundane labor that once dominated people's working lives, most people elect to use their free time to pursue largely sedentary interests and assume the associated health risks. Results from the Framingham study indicate that physical inactivity may be an independent health risk that increases as we age.[33] Inactivity and its associated health problems are so endemic to our culture that people have begun to recognize a constellation of illnesses known as hypokinetic diseases. These include conditions such as obesity, depression, musculoskeletal inflexibility, osteoporosis, chronic fatigue syndromes, hyperlipidemias, and atherosclerosis.

It is also of great concern that much of our society accepts a sedentary life-style as a natural consequence of aging and that older adults who dare to remain physically active are often considered eccentric, juvenile, and even abnormal. This misconception is so firmly entrenched in people's minds that active seniors are frequently thought to be endangering their lives whenever they exercise. The tragedy of this attitude is that it discourages many older persons from trying something that is not only fun but also good for their health. Remaining active may be viewed as an option for the young, but it is imperative for the continuance of an aging person's health. Inactivity will permit structural and physiologic losses at a rate that will prematurely threaten the person's ability to remain independent.

Many of the changes attributed to the aging process are actually the product of sedentary living. Inactivity is estimated to account for more than 50% of the physiologic and structural decrements that occur in the sedentary adult.[22, 30] This relationship was not fully appreciated until recently. Consequently, much of the research into aging done prior to this period is biased by this "disuse factor." While investigating the effect of exercise and inactivity on the aerobic power of older men, Kasch and co-workers helped to demonstrate the relative roles of inactivity and aging in the deterioration of physiologic function.[18] In this study, 15 men maintained an aerobic program for 23 years while a control group remained relatively sedentary over the same period. Despite the small number of subjects, the results strongly suggested that disuse makes a major contribution to the physical changes noted in most aging people. The maximum oxygen uptake results were especially impressive in that they indicated only 34% of the loss seen in the nonexercisers could be attributed to aging, with the remaining 66% resulting from disuse. This suggests that the decremental influence of inactivity may be even greater than is currently believed. Cooper has conducted extensive physiologic assessments on many international-caliber athletes and based on his findings, he concludes that "Most of the decline that comes with age isn't inevitable at all. It's caused by disuse."[14]

To explain why these disuse changes occur, one must consider one of the basic rules governing the efficient operation of the human body—the "use it or lose it" principle. This principle basically states, "if a particular component of the body is not being utilized, why keep it around?" It is far more economical to mobilize the valuable structural elements from these underutilized areas and incorporate them into areas of the body where they are needed. It is very inefficient to maintain and nurture tissues that are not performing any useful function. To illustrate this, one has only to examine an injured limb after several weeks of immobilization. Invariably the immobilized body parts emerge from the cast with marked atrophy and possibly a reduced range of motion. While these losses are usually temporary, they often require extensive physiotherapy to ensure that the individual is not left with a residual deficiency. Even though the atrophy associated with long-term underuse is not nearly as dramatic as that seen secondary to immobilization, the long-term sequelae are often far more damaging.

STRUCTURAL AND PHYSIOLOGIC CHANGES

The aging process is undeniably associated with a number of well-documented structural and functional changes. These changes probably originate at the cellular level and adversely affect the quantity of cells, their qualitative performance, and the regulatory controls exerted over their operation. The net result is a reduction in the functional reserves of the aging organ systems, rendering them less able to cope with the mechanical and metabolic stresses they encounter. Since the effective operation of the human body depends on the integrated efforts of many organ systems, it would be naive to consider that the age-related changes in the various organ systems occur in isolation of each other. Consider, for example, the potential implications of alterations in the functioning of the central and peripheral nervous systems. With the extensive communication network that these two systems provide, anything influencing their operation would have a considerable impact on the body. It is also critical to recognize that all of the age-associated changes occur so gradually that affected persons are usually unaware that they are taking place until one of their body systems fails completely, or at least fails to respond as expected. The classic example of this is the 75-year-old woman who has no idea she is dangerously osteoporotic until she falls and fractures her hip. The following sections will discuss the specific age-associated changes that have been noted in many of the important tissues in the body.

CONNECTIVE TISSUE CHANGES

Connective tissues form the basic framework of most of the body's structures and so make a signifi-

cant contribution to their mechanical properties. In fact, the mechanical properties of numerous tissues are largely dictated by their specific combination of connective tissues. Using the same basic ingredients in unique combinations, the connective tissues are relied upon to satisfy the radically different physical requirements of structures as functionally diverse as the cornea and the lateral collateral ligament. Fascia, tendons, and ligaments were once believed to be inert structures that were synthesized and then resided passively in the body fulfilling their structural and support roles. Today, however, these tissues are recognized to be highly dynamic in nature, constantly undergoing modifications in order to adapt to the multitude of stresses they experience. Physical activity promotes connective tissue hypertrophy while inactivity promotes atrophic changes, yet another example of the "use it or lose it" principle which is so innate to our physical being.

The properties of compliance and tensile strength of connective tissues are determined by their distinctive mixture of proteins such as collagen, proteoglycans, connectin, and elastin. Collagen is a major constituent of basement membranes, intervertebral discs, blood vessels, teeth, bones, ligaments, skin, and tendons. It is also present in nearly all organs. It is by far the most abundant connective tissue element and accounts for approximately 30% of our total body protein. Five principal types of collagen are recognized, each differing in amino acid composition and sequencing, the extent to which the amino acids are cross-linkage bonded, and the type of cross-linkage bonding it possesses.[36, 39] This diversity of design provides each collagen type with unique properties of compliance and tensile strength based on the amount of cross-linkage bonding it possesses. The greater the amount of rigidity required by a specific tissue, the more extensive its collagen cross-linkage must be. Thus the collagen found in teeth is far more heavily cross-linked than that found in basement membranes. These cross-linkages occur both intermolecularly and intramolecularly and appear to be the site at which the most important age-related alteration to collagen occurs.

As collagen ages, its molecular stability increases and the tissue in which it lies is rendered less compliant. This enhanced stability was initially thought to result from an increase in the number of cross-linkage bonds within the collagen molecule. However, it is now known that shortly after being synthesized, collagen fibers possess all the cross-linkages they will ever have. Instead it is conjectured that during the maturation process, previously reducible cross-linkage bonds undergo molecular stabilization, rendering the collagen fiber progressively less compliant.[3, 39] Factors such as physical activity and hormonal variations influence the rate at which collagen fibers lose their compliance. Exercise promotes collagen turnover and this serves to inhibit the process of maturational stabilization. Thus it would seem that regular utilization is essential to maintaining the youthfulness of collagen containing tissues. Thyroxin, corticosteroids, and insulin have all been implicated in the aging of collagen. Hamlin and associates noted that the collagen isolated from the tissues of a 40-year-old diabetic resembled that extracted from the bodies of nondiabetics over 100 years old.[17] Since endocrine changes accompany the normal aging process, it is reasonable to postulate that these changes may affect the integrity of the collagen fibers in the senior athlete.

Elastin is a connective tissue element found in the elastic fibers of skin, vasculature, and ligaments. Its mechanical properties permit it to return to its original form after being subjected to traction forces sufficient to stretch it to several times its original length. Elastin molecules contain cross-linkage bonds and as they age they undergo the same maturational stabilization that occurs in collagen. An increase in polar amino acid composition occurs in aging elastin.[26] Ultrastructurally, aging elastic tissues appear to lose their regularity and their lamellae become ragged and slender. Collectively these changes render aging elastic fibers increasingly brittle and more easily subject to fracture.[39] This is of considerable importance to aging athletes, who depend on their vasculature and ligamentous tissues during all sporting activities. It should also be noted that aging connective tissues contain less water and so have reduced shock-absorbing capacity and tissue compliance.

Considered in their totality, the connective tissue alterations associated with the aging process are important because they substantially alter the mechanical properties of many tissues and render the aging competitor increasingly vulnerable to injury. This becomes a major issue when one considers the potential for the loss of valuable training time and competitive opportunities.

TENDON AND LIGAMENT CHANGES

Tendons are defined as bands of connective tissue anchoring muscles to bones. A ligament, on the other hand, is a band of connective tissue attaching one bone to another. Both consist primarily of collagen and will experience all of the age-related changes described for other collagen-containing tissues. The bottom line is that aging tendons and ligaments are progressively less compliant and increasingly susceptible to injury. Injured aging ligaments and tendons are relatively unforgiving structures. Severely traumatized ligaments never resume their original length; their stress-strain characteristics are permanently disrupted, and on microscopic examination they show evidence of collagen fiber failure.[6] Aging also appears to be associated with a reduction in the glycosaminoglycans concentration found in tendons.[38]

Inactivity permits a number of deleterious changes to occur in ligamentous and tendinous structures. These changes reduce these tissues' ability to withstand and recover from the mechanical stresses applied to them during physical exercise and include:

1. Reduced tissue water content
2. Reduced collagen fiber thickness, rendering them less able to withstand mechanical strain without injury
3. Diminished rate of collagen fiber turnover, permitting more extensive cross-linkage stabilization and enhancing tissue rigidity
4. Reduced capillary density
5. Decreased glycosaminoglycans concentration
6. Reduced cellular elements
7. Bony resorption at the site of ligament or tendon insertion, rendering these regions more prone to avulsion fractures

All of these changes have been shown to regress when tendons and ligaments are exposed to the repetitive stresses and strains that accompany a regular physical exercise program. In fact, the aging exerciser will develop thicker, stronger, and more supple tendons and ligaments that are better able to tolerate the wear-and-tear effects associated with sports requiring a high volume of repetitive movement, such as swimming and cycling.

CARTILAGINOUS CHANGES

Articular cartilage plays a considerable role in facilitating efficient joint movement. It consists of collagen fibers embedded in a matrix of ground substance that is rich in mucoproteins and chondroitin sulfates. This combination provides it with gel-like physical properties. By reason of these properties, articular cartilage is ideally suited for shock absorption while permitting joints to function as lubricated bearings during movement. Articular cartilage lacks a direct blood supply. Instead, it depends entirely upon imbibition and diffusion processes to meet its nutritional needs. Both of these processes are enhanced by the mechanical loading and unloading of the joint surface. Articular cartilage responds to mechanical stimulation by thickening. Hall's research supports the contention that articular cartilage remains healthy if regularly exposed to compressive and decompressive forces.[16] His work also illustrates that in the absence of such stimulation, cartilage will undergo atrophic changes, leaving it more vulnerable to injury. As with all other tissues, there is a limit to how much mechanical stressing articular cartilage can tolerate before it begins to structurally break down. Overuse will damage chondrocytes, fracture collagen fibers, and reduce the volume of proteoglycans on the cartilaginous surface. This damage will be even more extensive if some degree of joint malalignment exists, whether it be the result of a congenital problem or of previous joint injury. For instance, a torn anterior cruciate ligament will profoundly alter the mechanics within the knee joint such that excessive movement will be permitted between the femoral and tibial contact surfaces. This instability causes excessive wear and tear on the underlying articular cartilage, facilitating the development of early degenerative changes.[13a]

Articular cartilage undergoes a number of age-related alterations, the most important of which is a loss of tissue compliance secondary to the cross-linkage stabilization of collagen molecules. This process renders cartilage increasingly brittle and less able to cope with repetitive mechanical stresses. Aging cartilage also contains less water and has elevated concentrations of chondroitin sulfate and keratosulfate. As a consequence of these changes, aging articular cartilage is increasingly noncompliant, less able to perform its function of shock absorption, and so progressively more susceptible to the structural failure that can accompany overuse injuries.

SKELETAL MUSCLE CHANGES

Skeletal muscle is an essential element in all athletic activities. This is a fact that holds true regardless of the type of sporting activity or the age of the participants. One of the unfortunate realities facing the masters competitor is that aging is accompanied by a loss of muscle tissue. At the cellular level, the total number of muscle fibers diminishes and those fibers that remain undergo atrophic changes.[11] Despite these losses, the contractile proteins appear to remain unaltered.[40] Investigations by Larsson reveal that as an individual ages, the type I (slow-twitch) fiber population remains fairly stable while the type II (fast-twitch) fiber population experiences selective atrophy.[21a] The net result is a relative increase in the aging body's type I fiber population. While these changes have been noted to occur in aging muscle, it is unlikely that they represent a truly age-related phenomenon. They are more likely a consequence of the differential use made of each fiber type as we age. Type II fibers are primarily employed in explosive activities such as sprinting, throwing, or jumping and are generally called into action less frequently as we age. On the other hand, type I fibers are principally utilized in the postural and low-intensity activities that dominate the life-styles of most elderly people. Regardless of the mechanism, the fact remains that as we age there is less muscle available to call upon and the muscle tissue that is available contains a relatively greater volume of type I fibers. Regular use of the fast-twitch fiber population will help minimize the amount of this relative loss that occurs with advancing age.[25, 40]

Aging muscle appears to remain biochemically stable. In terms of their activity per unit of muscle weight, the levels of both the aerobic and anaerobic muscle enzymes remain consistent with those found in younger persons.[40] Thus even though older athletes have less muscle tissue available, what muscle they do have retains its normal enzyme levels and is capable of considerable improvements in terms of strength and endurance when exposed to the appropriate training stimuli. Capillary-fiber ratio refers to the number of capillaries making contact with a given muscle fiber and is important because it determines the maximum distance over which oxygen, energy substrates, and nutrients must diffuse in order to reach each muscle fiber. The larger this ratio, the greater the volume of oxygen that can be delivered to working tissues and the greater the potential aerobic work capacity. Plyley demonstrated that older, sedentary men had a very small decrease in capillary-fiber ratio compared with younger sedentary men.[27] Unfortunately, his research did not compare older and younger athletes. He did, however, comment that aging persons can respond to the stimulus of regular physical activity by increasing their tissue capillary density.[27]

The motor unit is one of the basic elements of neuromuscular organization and consists of a motor nerve and the muscle fibers it innervates. Aging is associated with a reduction in the number of muscle fibers in each motor unit and possibly a reduction in the total number of motor units.[7] As a direct consequence of this change, a smaller amount of contractile tissue can be mobilized when a given motor unit is recruited into action. Despite this, strength appears to decrease very slowly until approximately the age of 50 years when the dropoff occurs more rapidly. For someone who has remained active, the anticipated loss of maximal voluntary strength at 60 years of age normally should not exceed 10% to 20% of an individual's maximal strength.[11, 40] The losses experienced by the sedentary individual would be far greater. With training, older adults can acquire significant gains in strength and possibly experience muscular hypertrophy.

Aging muscle is unable to contract as rapidly as younger muscle tissue, a phenomenon that may be explained by delays in nerve impulse transmission at the motor end-plate. This decrement has important implications for athletic performance, especially in those athletic activities requiring power. Power is defined as the ability to do work over time. In events requiring explosive movements, such as shot-putting, the competitor who can impart the greatest amount of force to the implement over the maximum velocity of muscle contraction will likely enjoy the greatest success. Damon has demonstrated that the maximum velocity of muscle contraction possible against any given mass decreases with age and that this decrement occurs whether the contractions are isometric, concentric, or eccentric in nature.[9] In other words, aging shot-putters are unable to accelerate the shot as rapidly as they were once capable of, so their performance potential diminishes. This helps to explain why aging competitors generally perform poorly in power events in comparison with their younger opponents.

The following is a brief listing of some of the other structural changes observed in aging muscle tissue:

1. Z-band streaming and nemalin-like structures appear in type I fibers.
2. Type II fibers exhibit fragmentation and loss of Z materials.
3. The collagen fiber content increases in aging

muscle, rendering it less compliant and so more susceptible to injury.
4. Lipofuscin granules appear and are of uncertain significance.

The collective effect of the observed age-related changes in muscle tissue is a loss of endurance, strength, mass, contraction speed, and compliance. These losses facilitate a significant deterioration in athletic performance. One thing that does not appear to be lost in aging muscle tissue is the ability to respond to the stimulus of training. Regardless of age, older adults can achieve improvements in muscle structure and function if they undertake the appropriate training.[7] It is difficult to be certain how many of the changes noted to occur in aging muscle are truly age-related and not the product of an inactive life-style. This is a reasonable concern when one considers that many of the structural alterations noted in aging muscle have also been observed in the musculature of younger people who have been immobilized for whatever reason. Perhaps with further research, we will come to discover that muscle tissue experiences less truly age-related change than was once suspected.

OSSEOUS CHANGES

Osseous tissues consist of a mixture of inorganic and organic elements arranged in a matrix that permits them to be relatively light in weight while remaining resilient enough to withstand a lifetime of mechanical stresses. Bones are highly dynamic structures that undergo adaptive changes in direct response to the physical demands made of them. When they are regularly stressed, they respond by becoming mechanically stronger; if they are underutilized, the opposite will occur. This hypertrophic response to exercise is highly specific and will only occur in the areas of the skeleton that are experiencing the extramechanical forces. A classic example of this is the unilateral bony enlargement that is seen in the dominant arms of tennis players. This alteration is undoubtedly aimed at better preparing the dominant arm to cope with the stresses to which it is being exposed. Bassett and Becker have hypothesized that the mechanism for the localized control of bony growth is electrical in nature.[2] In their model, bone tissue functions as a piezoelectric crystal that converts the energy of mechanical deformation into electrical energy. During mechanical stressing, the segment of bone experiencing compressive forces produces a negative electric charge while the extending segment becomes positive. It is through these charges that control over the level of cellular activity in bone is exerted. Conditions that compromise a bone's architectural integrity or its adaptive response will lower its resilience to mechanical stress and leave it vulnerable to structural breakdown through either overuse or direct trauma.

Undeniably, the greatest threat to the skeletal integrity of the aging adult comes from osteoporosis. In this ideopathic condition, the rate of bone resorption exceeds that of bone formation and the resultant imbalance leads to a progressive reduction of bone mass. This is of particular concern because a bone's strength varies directly with its volume of bone mass. Over 25 million North Americans are affected by osteoporosis and most of them are unaware of it. Researchers now recognize the existence of two types of osteoporosis: Type 1 osteoporosis affects women exclusively and is associated with the loss of estrogen production that occurs in and around the menopausal years. As a result of this process, bone mass is lost at a rate of approximately 0.6% per year.[34] Type 2 osteoporosis affects both sexes and is probably the direct result of an age-related decline in osteoblast activity. This form of osteoporosis accounts for a loss of bone mass at a rate of approximately 0.3% per year.[34]

Women experience a far greater rate of bone mass depletion than men. In addition, men often do not experience osteoporotic losses until the age of 50 and usually suffer no sequelae until they are in their 80s, while in women bone mass frequently begins to be depleted in their early 30s. This combination of an earlier onset and a higher rate of loss means that many women reach their 70s having lost more than 30% of their total bone mass.[5, 31, 37] In this state of skeletal compromise, these women are at considerable risk of developing a fracture if they fall or expose their bones to excessive muscle traction forces. Sedentary living is also a major risk factor in promoting an accelerated loss of bone mass. In persons who have been immobilized for various reasons, dramatic bone mass depletion may occur in the affected limbs over relatively short periods of time. Clearly, age-related bone loss is a serious threat to every aging person but especially so for the aging woman.

As far as osteoporosis and aging athletes are concerned, the health care professional should be aware of a number of critical points. First, age-related depletion of bone mass is a universal phenomenon and one must therefore assume that to some extent every aging competitor is osteoporotic. Second, one should not assume that because two persons are the same age that they will have encountered the same volume of bone mass losses. Not only will individual rates of bone mass loss vary, but diet and life-style will have a major impact on the volume of bone mass retained. Third, virtually all female masters athletes will have greater cumulative bone mass losses than similarly aged male athletes. Fourth, osteoporosis is an insidious process that provides no obvious signs or symptoms that it is occurring. The first indication of a problem is usually when the competitor develops a fracture following relatively minor trauma. Fifth, the persons at greatest risk of skeletal failure are those who have lived largely inactive lives and begin a rigorous physical exercise program when they are over 50 years of age. It is very important that these persons start out slowly and progress gradually in order to provide their osseous tissues sufficient time to adapt to the new stresses they are experiencing. Taking this conservative approach to training will greatly reduce the incidence of stress fractures this group of sporting enthusiasts experiences. Sixth, bony tissue appears to respond positively when exposed to mechanical stressing, regardless of the individual's age. The osseous tissues of people in their 80s have been shown to respond to both gravitational forces and muscular traction.[28] Some of the changes observed in the bones of these individuals included increases in cortical thickness, strength, DNA content, calcium concentration, hydroxyproline content, and nitrogen concentration. To date, the scientific evidence suggests that regular physical activity will not only slow down the rate of bony demineralization seen in osteoporosis but to some extent may even reverse it.

SKIN CHANGES

While it is frequently taken for granted, skin is actually a vital component of our body's defense system. It functions as a protective barrier against trauma, an energy storage site, a boundary against infection, a barrier against environmental insults such as wind, rain, and ultraviolet light, and as an integral part of our thermoregulatory system. Considering the diversity of these responsibilities, any age-related change in skin has the potential for far-reaching implications. Cutaneous tissues age as a result of a combination of intrinsic structural and functional changes and extrinsic factors such as wind, ultraviolet light, and thermal stresses. While these extrinsic influences are not innate to the aging process, they have been included here because the very nature of most athletic activities provides the aging active adult with considerable exposure to them.

Wrinkling is a superficial feature readily identified as a sign of aging skin, but below the skin's surface is where most of the age-related changes occur. Many of these changes are of direct relevance to the older active adult. During the aging process the epidermal, dermal, and subcutaneous layers of the skin all become progressively thinner.[13] This loss of tissue substantially compromises the skin's insulatory quality, leaving the person at greater risk of cold-induced injuries. It also reduces the trauma cushion that skin affords the underlying tissues and so a blow of insufficient magnitude to cause a muscle contusion in a younger person might cause one in an older individual. Aging skin contains less elastin and its collagen fibers are increasingly maturationally stabilized. These changes alter aging skin's viscoelastic properties, such that it will be less pliable when subjected to deforming forces. Thus, aging skin is increasingly fragile and more susceptible to damage secondary to even minor trauma. Collisions, abrasions, sheering forces, and wear and tear are hazards common to most sports and when exposed to these various forms of mechanical trauma, aging skin will be damaged at intensities that would leave younger skin unaffected. This should be kept in mind even when attempting to remove adhesive tape from an aging person's skin, as the tape's adhesive properties may exceed the skin's mechanical strength and a tearing injury could develop if one is not careful.

The capillary density in the peripheral tissues diminishes with age and the vasculature that does remain has thinner and more fragile walls. These alterations leave the aging active adult more prone to bruising following trauma. The number of immunocompetent cells present in aging skin is also reduced. T-cell function is diminished and Langerhans' cells die off, making the older individual at increased risk of developing skin infections and neoplasms. Finger and toenails are extensions of the skin and are also affected by the aging process. Aging nails are thinner and so more vulnerable to damage in the athletic environment, where nail-related injuries such as subungual hematomas and fractures

are a common occurance. Since aging nails also grow more slowly, recovery from a nail injury is often delayed.

CARDIOVASCULAR CHANGES

While the aging cardiovascular system has been the subject of considerable investigation, it is often difficult to determine if the changes experimentally observed are truly the result of aging or the result of other factors such as disease processes, environmental factors, inactivity, or a combination thereof. If disease processes are excluded, the aging myocardium appears to undergo only minor structural alterations. Myocardial weight seems to remain relatively constant, even in studies in which subjects 100 years of age have been included. The amount of interstitial elastin, collagen, and reticulin fibers increases, producing a condition referred to as fibrosis. While these increases are generally minor, they do reduce the myocardium's compliance, a change that may be functionally insignificant at rest but at maximum cardiovascular workloads could limit ventricular filling and so lower cardiac output. Lipofuscin and amyloid are proteins that accumulate in aging myocardial tissue, the significance of which is uncertain. The aging process also influences the cardiac electrical conduction system. Not only is there a gradual loss of the specialized conducting tissues, but the tissues that remain are infiltrated with fat, collagen, reticulin, and elastin. By the age of 75, up to 90% of the sinoatrial node's pacemaker cells may be absent.[19] While the functional importance of these changes is unknown, they may contribute to an age-related decline in maximal heart rate. Whether the contractile properties of the heart dwindle with age remains a controversial issue.[3, 7, 19] A number of other myocardial structural and biochemical changes have been observed:

1. Reduced levels of adenylcyclase, norepinephrine, and acetylcholine in cardiac tissues
2. Increased ventricular septal thickness
3. Dilation of the left atrium
4. Reduced left ventricular volume
5. Increased circumference of all heart valves
6. A thicker and less compliant myocardium
7. Collagen, lipid, and calcium deposition on valvular structures

Maximum oxygen uptake ($\dot{V}O_2$max) is considered the single most reliable measure of aerobic fitness. After the age of 35 an inevitable decline in $\dot{V}O_2$ max occurs such that at 60 years of age it is often only 80% of an individual's capacity at the age of 20.[1, 15] In inactive adults $\dot{V}O_2$max may decline at a rate in excess of 1% per year, while elite masters athletes may experience rates of decline as low as 0.1% per year.[33] The more aerobically active an individual is, the more slowly $\dot{V}O_2$max will decrease. Several investigators attribute this decline in $\dot{V}O_2$max to an age-associated reduction in maximum attainable heart rate.[22, 30, 33]

Maximum attainable heart rate (MAHR) shows a linear rate of decline with age.[3] As a general rule, an individual's MAHR can be roughly approximated by the formula:

$$220 - \text{age (in years)} = \text{MAHR}$$

It should be noted that, in addition to maximal attainable heart rate, a number of other physiologic variables such as pulmonary function, cardiovascular function, aerobic fitness level, and muscle function influence an individual's $\dot{V}O_2$max. Since the aging process is associated with changes in all of these areas, it is reasonable to hypothesize that the age-related decline in $\dot{V}O_2$max is multifactorial in origin.

The volume of blood that the heart can pump in a fixed period of time is referred to as the cardiac output *(CO)*. It may be calculated as a product of the heart rate *(HR)* and the stroke volume *(SV)*.

$$CO = HR \times SV$$

At high aerobic workloads, both stroke volume and heart rate have been shown to decline with age and therefore cardiac output will also diminish. The performance implications of this functional loss are enormous in aerobically demanding sports such as endurance cycling, long-distance swimming, cross-country skiing, and marathon running. When cardiac output decreases, the ability to deliver oxygen-rich blood to the working tissues also decreases and hence the ability to perform maximum aerobic workloads will suffer.

As people age, it takes longer for their heart rates to return to normal following maximal and submaximal exercise. This is an important point to keep in mind when one is involved in the physical conditioning of masters athletes. Many training programs employ interval training sessions, in which the athlete is subjected to a workload sufficient to el-

evate heart rate to a desired target range. The individual is then expected to work at that level of intensity for a fixed period of time before he or she is allowed to recover. During the recovery phase, the athlete's heart rate is permitted to fall to a predetermined recovery level, at which time the athlete is expected to repeat the interval. This cycle of events continues until the desired training effect is achieved. Failing to provide a recovery phase of sufficient duration to allow the heart rate to return to the desired resting level will greatly limit the athlete's ability to endure the complete workout and so compromise the objectives of the training session. With this in mind, it is important for coaches to remember that masters athletes will require somewhat longer recovery periods between intervals than would be considered necessary for younger athletes at a similar fitness level. Adjusting the training programs of aging athletes to reflect this difference will ensure that they benefit more from their training, reduce their incidence of overtraining, and decrease their rate of injury.

On the whole, the observed age-related alterations in the cardiovascular system result in a lower $\dot{V}O_2$max, a reduced maximum attainable heart rate, a decreased myocardial compliance, and a diminished cardiac output. Consequently, the aging heart must work harder to meet the metabolic demands of the body at any given workload. This loss of efficiency is a major factor in the progressive decline in aerobic performance noted with increasing age. A review of the age-class world records for any aerobically demanding activity indicates how real this loss actually is.

The vascular system is one area in which the aging process generates a number of important modifications. In any consideration of this system one must, however, be particularly careful to differentiate the changes caused by aging from those resulting from pathological processes such as atherosclerosis. While atherosclerosis is a disease process, it merits discussion because it affects virtually every aging adult in our industrialized world. This insidious disease narrows the lumens of blood vessels and reduces vessel wall distensibility. Consequently, atherosclerotic vessels are less able to deliver blood to the tissues they serve. The extent to which this disease can exist in persons who are apparently asymptomatic is frequently remarkable. Aging vasculature experiences enhanced collagen deposition, independent of any disease process. This collagen undergoes all of the age-related changes witnessed in the collagen of other tissues. The elastin fibers located in the vascular walls encounter calcium deposition, a condition referred to as elastocalcinosis. These collagen and elastic fiber changes result in narrowing of vessel lumens and elevate vessel wall resistance. Thus, greater kinetic energy will be needed to maintain adequate circulation so cardiac workload will be noticeably increased without a demonstrable increase in cardiac output.

Studies employing injection techniques have shown that with aging there is a reduction in the microvascular supply to the peripheral tissues, major organs, and muscle tissues. This reduction in available blood supply creates several problems. First, it decreases the volume of oxygen- and substrate-laden blood that can be delivered to the working tissues. Both of these items are essential if an intense level of work is to be maintained for any prolonged period of time. Second, it limits the functional reserves of the body's major organs, making it increasingly difficult for a person to maintain homeostasis when physically stressed. Finally, it reduces the volume of blood that can be delivered to an injury site and so may delay the rate of injury recovery.

RESPIRATORY CHANGES

An efficient respiratory system is a requisite for success in maintaining an active life-style. Unfortunately, over time, this vital system falls prey to a number of deleterious influences such as tobacco smoke, previous pulmonary illnesses, a sedentary life-style, environmental pollutants, and the aging process itself. It is uncertain to what extent these factors individually contribute to the respiratory changes that accompany aging. Studies that have attempted to control for these variables concluded that there is a progressive deterioration in respiratory structure and function that may be directly attributed to the aging process.[21]

The aging respiratory system undergoes a number of architectural modifications. For example, in the aging thorax the costovertebral joints stiffen, the costochondral cartilages become less elastic and the intercostal musculature becomes less compliant. Collectively, these changes produce a generalized increase in the rigidity of the chest wall so that greater physical effort is needed to overcome chest wall resistance during inspiration. The collagen and elastin fiber content of the pulmonary parenchyma undergo progressive degradation, the rate of which is consid-

erably enhanced in lungs repeatedly subjected to the insult of cigarette smoke and air pollutants. This deterioration of the pulmonary support structures compromises the structural integrity of the aging lung and reduces its capacity for elastic recoil. The normal lung depends on elastic recoil to assist with expiration, and since recoil is a passive phenomenon it serves to reduce the work associated with breathing. As greater amounts of elastic recoil are lost, the active work involved in breathing increases. DeVries estimates that these age-related modifications could account for as much as a 20% increase in respiratory effort.[11]

As respiratory musculature ages, its connective tissue content gradually increases and its strength decreases. These noncompliant and weaker muscles are less able to generate the inspiratory pressures necessary to ventilate the lung's lower lobes, where perfusion is the greatest. The net result is the development of ventilation-perfusion mismatches. In these mismatches, regions of the lungs fail to have concurrent delivery of oxygen and blood to their alveoli, which means that respiratory gas exchange is less efficient and less oxygen is available to deliver to the working tissues. The number of small vessels present in the lung parenchyma is also diminished with aging. Collagen deposition may also occur at the level of the alveolar-capillary basement membrane, increasing the diffusion barrier over which oxygen and carbon dioxide must be exchanged. These structural changes manifest themselves in a number of decrements in respiratory function:

1. Reduced air flow during inspiration
2. Decreased total lung capacity
3. Increased residual lung volume
4. Decrease in vital capacity by as much as 25 mL/yr after the age of 20 years[30]
5. Reduced forced expiratory volume in 1 second (FEV_1);
6. Diminished tidal volume
7. Reduced inspiratory capacity

Considered individually, the practical importance of many of the changes that occur in the aging respiratory system is uncertain. Collectively, however, they leave the respiratory system less efficient and progressively less able to deliver oxygen to the working body tissues. This is one of the principle reasons that with advancing age there is a deterioration of performance in events that demand maximal aerobic efforts. Comparing the marathon world records at ages 40 years (2 hours, 11 minutes, 4 seconds) and

80 years (4 hours, 23 minutes, 55 seconds) serves to demonstrate how truly meaningful these changes are in terms of performance. The rate at which many of these respiratory alterations occur is substantially increased in the inactive person. It should also be noted that the rate at which these changes occur can be substantially reduced via the stimulus of regular aerobic exercise, with the most important contribution coming from the strengthening of the respiratory musculature.

NERVOUS SYSTEM CHANGES

The nervous system forms an incredibly complex communication network and any process affecting its operation will have far-reaching effects on the overall operation of the body. During the aging process, a number of functional and structural changes are imposed upon the nervous system: (1) the brain's ventricles enlarge; (2) in the central and peripheral nervous systems, as many as 100,000 neurons perish on a daily basis[4] (over the course of a lifetime, this can amount to a considerable loss); (3) between the ages of 45 and 85 years, brain weight can diminish as much as 20%. This loss appears to result primarily from a decrease in extracellular fluid levels;[4] and (4) cerebrospinal fluid production and turnover also are reduced. It is uncertain if any of these modifications have a deleterious influence on the effective performance of the human nervous system.

Reaction time is a highly valued athletic ability and in numerous sports it is, in fact, an essential ingredient for success. Consider for example, the need to be able to react in sports such as table tennis, volleyball, boxing, and sprinting. Unfortunately for the aging active adult, reaction time has unequivocally been shown to slow with advancing age. This slowing is not the end result of any single alteration but rather is the culmination of changes manifested in several areas of the aging neuromuscular system.[11] These changes include the following: (1) a reduction in the conduction rate of sensory nerves, (2) a decrease in the rate of perceptual processing, (3) a slowing in the rate at which nerve impulses are propagated; (4) an increase in the time it takes to centrally process sensory stimuli, and (5) a reduction in the speed at which muscular contraction occurs.

While every component of the reflex loop is adversely affected by the aging phenomenon, it is the increase in the time required for central processing that has the greatest detrimental effect on an individual's reaction time. At all ages, the time required for central processing increases significantly when the number of reaction choices that an individual is required to make increases. Thus the quarterback who has only one designated receiver requires less time to think and react than the one who has five potential play options. In these rapid-reaction situations involving multiple possible responses, older athletes' reaction times will slow more than those of their younger colleagues. Thus, as we age, it would appear that our ability to make split-second decisions and react quickly is impaired. This certainly hinders the aging competitor's ability to perform in the "read and react" situations that are such a fundamental part of sports such as volleyball, soccer, tennis, hockey, and football. Inactivity also appears to contribute to the slowing of reaction times, to the extent that young sedentary individuals have been shown to possess reaction times inferior to those seen in many masters athletes.[32]

The special senses are also forced to pay the price exacted by the passage of time. With age, the crystalline lens of the eye becomes increasingly brittle, a change that reduces the eye's power of accommodation. An age-related loss of visual acuity also occurs. These losses are of functional importance because in many sporting events athletes depend very heavily on visual cues to influence their actions and reactions. The aging auditory system is the victum of both the aging process (presbycusis) and the cumulative effect of years of insults from the many sources of noise pollution that abound in our world. Together these influences leave virtually every aging person with some degree of hearing decrement. It is fortunate that the medical technology available today can correct for most of the auditory and visual deficiencies encountered by aging active adults and so facilitate their sporting enjoyment.

FLEXIBILITY CHANGES

Flexibility may be thought of as the range of motion possible for a given joint, and it varies considerably for the various joints found in the human body. An athlete's specific flexibility requirements are dictated by the particular exercise activity in which he or she participates. For example, superior shoulder range of motion may be essential to a successful golfer but of little value to a walker. A number of factors determine the amount of movement possible about any joint:

1. Bony structures—the ball and socket design of the glenohumeral joint is an example of an anatomical arrangement that greatly facilitates the range of motion that can be achieved at the shoulder joint.
2. Fascia and muscle—joint movement will be hindered if these tissues are noncompliant.
3. Tendons, ligaments, and joint capsules—joint movement will also be restricted if these tissues are noncompliant.

For an active adult, the consequences of reduced flexibility are numerous and potentially costly, particularly if the person is involved in an activity that depends heavily on the flexibility of a specific joint or set of joints. Consider, for example, a badminton player who has a limited range of motion in the wrist of his or her dominant arm. Since much of the power in a badminton swing is derived from a snapping action of the wrist, a lack of flexibility in this joint would represent a considerable competitive handicap. Athletes whose lack of flexibility prevents them from assuming certain positions are often less effective. A good example of this is a golfer whose swing is compromised by capsular tightness at the glenohumeral joint. Inflexible tissues provide greater resistance to work and consequently greater volumes of energy must be expended in order to accomplish a given task. It should also be noted that as flexibility decreases, the injury rate will increase.

Controversy exists over whether flexibility is affected by the aging process or whether the losses observed in older adults are a result of inactivity alone. It seems reasonable to assume that if muscle tissue, tendons, ligaments, fascia, and joint capsules become less compliant with age, then the range of motion about the joints they move and support must also diminish. While there is undoubtedly an innate component to the loss of flexibility noted with aging, it appears that for the average person, disuse is by far the dominant factor. Generally speaking, the more inactive a person is the more rapidly his or her flexibility will deteriorate. While age-induced flexibility losses are permanent, inactivity-induced losses are not. In studies where older sedentary people were given a range of motion exercises, significant improvements in flexibility were noted in a relatively short period of time.[7] The greatest gains were

achieved by the individuals who had previously been the most sedentary.

AGING AND INJURIES

The aging process is clearly associated with a number of physiological and structural modifications that leave the excercising older adult increasingly suseptible to injury. Loss of joint range of motion, altered tissue compliance, brittle tendons and ligaments, reduced tissue capillary density, and loss of bone mass all contribute to this enhanced suseptibility. With this in mind, it is only reasonable to expect that the injury pattern experienced by older active adults will differ considerably from that of their younger colleagues.

Older active adults are potentially the victims of two separate sets of injuries: those resulting from the training and competitive program to which they are currently committed and those that occurred in their youth and have come back to haunt them. Either of these sets of injuries has the potential to force a premature retirement from the sporting arena. Regardless of the quality of medical treatment they received, young athletes who experience major joint injuries such as anterior cruciate ligament disruptions, meniscal tears, or shoulder dislocations will have the structural integrity of the affected joint forever compromised. These damaged structures frequently remain quiescent until the individual reaches middle age and initiates a comeback into the world of exercise and fitness. At this time, the person may notice that his or her knee can no longer tolerate the repetitive trauma inherant in an activity such as running. This potentially frustrating situation is seen all too often in aging persons and serves to clearly demonstrate that significant injuries incurred in youth will frequently dictate what athletic activities a person can participate in during their later years.

From clinical experience, it appears that younger athletes incur a much higher incidence of traumatic musculoskeletal injury than do their older colleagues. Athletes' injuries are largely dictated by the sports in which they compete and so it is not surprising to find that younger athletes tend to indulge themselves in sports with a greater potential for violence and body contact. In addition, their relative lack of competitive experience and their tendency to perform with more reckless intensity leave them at greater risk of developing trauma-related injuries. While masters athletes do experience traumatically induced injuries such as internal joint derrangements, these injuries tend to be relatively uncommon, and when they do occur the individual may not present with a classic history. For these two reasons, health care professionals often fail to consider the diagnosis of a significant joint injury in an injured older athlete and mistakenly attribute their complaints to a degenerative process. This is especially true for injuries such as meniscus tears, which can masquerade as overuse phenomena and go undiagnosed for years. These situations can lead to costly delays in obtaining definitive treatment and cause major training schedule disruptions, neither of which is desireable for a serious athlete of any age.

While traumatic injuries are the enemy of the young recreational athlete, the greatest threat to the older active adult comes from excessive "wear and tear" or overuse injuries. Everyone who works with aging active adults should be ever mindful of the threat posed by the "itises." Included in this group are conditions such as tendonitis, fasciitis, bursitis, capsulitis, and arthritis. DeHaven and Littner's research indicates that as we age, the incidence of these inflammatory conditions increases to the extent that at the age of 70 years they represent the top five athletically associated ailments.[10] The incidence of these overuse injuries is greatly facilitated by postural malalignments, which tend to biomechanically overload various components of the musculoskeletal system. For instance, someone who pronates excessively will commonly have tracking problems at the patellofemoral joint. With repetitive use of the knee joint, this individual is at considerable risk of developing patellofemoral syndrome and possibly degenerative changes in the associated articular cartilage—a condition referred to as chondromalacia patellae. It should be noted that most of these injuries start out as minor nagging problems, the point at which they should be identified and treated effectively. Instead, they are commonly ignored or inadequately treated and what were once minor conditions evolve into major problems that require extensive treatment and result in lost training time.

In the management of exercise-induced injuries, the most effective strategy is to prevent them from occurring in the first place. This is especially true for aging active adults because their injury recovery rate is slower. During the aging process anatomic changes occur such that both tissue blood supply and tissue compliance are reduced. With these alter-

ations in mind, in order to reduce the incidence of injuries, it is particularly important that older active adults perform an adequate warm-up prior to every training session and competition. A properly performed warm-up enhances the viscoelastic properties of tissues, increases tissue blood flow, elevates the temperature of the working tissues, and generally "primes" the body for exercise. In general terms, the more compliant tendons and muscles are, the more difficult they are to injure. Warm-ups are often viewed as a waste of precious training time, especially for people who constantly suffer from the constraints of a busy schedule; however, the exercising adult who adheres to an effective warm-up discipline will find the time invested will be more than reimbursed in terms of time saved through injury prevention.

HEALING AND AGING

Classically, the body's response to injury is described as occurring in three phases: (1) the inflammatory phase, (2) the proliferative phase, and (3) the remodeling phase. All three phases are essential to permit proper tissue repair and all three are detrimentally affected by the aging process. Aging dampens the inflammatory response. The cellular migration, proliferation, and maturation that take place during the proliferative phase are also delayed. During the remodeling phase, collagen is laid down more slowly, in smaller volumes, and with altered binding patterns.[12] As a result of these age-associated alterations, when an older person is injured the events associated with the healing process begin later, proceed less rapidly, and do not achieve the same intensity. Some researchers have suggested that the age-related delays in the healing process are the result of an increase in the time it takes to prime the system for the regenerative process.[12] While the etiology of this delay is of academic interest, the bottom line is that once injured, the older athlete's body still effects a quality repair; it simply takes longer to do so. Many former world-class athletes such as Frank Shorter, Al Oerter, and Jack Nicklaus who continue to compete into their forties and fifties, have observed that the injuries they sustain take considerably longer to heal than they did when they were in their 20s.

Just as the rate at which one ages is highly variable, so too there are wide variations in the rate at which individuals recover from injury. To further complicate matters, healing rates are also influenced by tissue changes resulting from disuse, disease processes, environmental insults, and the presence of other body stressors. Anything that reduces tissue capillary density reduces the rate at which oxygen and repair substrates can be delivered to an injury site. It is important to note that the healing delays associated with the aging process do not appear to affect bony tissues. Once skeletal maturity is achieved in late adolescence, there appears to be no age-related decline in the rate of fracture healing.[24]

TREATMENT CONCERNS

It is important for health care professionals to recognize that dedicated older exercise enthusiasts will react to being injured in a manner similiar to most serious competitors and so will be very reluctant to simply discontinue their exercise schedule in order to allow an annoying injury sufficient time to heal. Their sporting life is a highly valued contributor to their positive self-perception, which is seriously threatened when an injury limits their ability to participate. Health care professionals must recognize the existence of this "athletic mind-set" before they will be able to effectively manage the medical treatment and rehabilitation of these individuals. To inform an injured athlete, "The solution to your problem is obvious: if it hurts you to do the front crawl then stop swimming," is not only inappropriate but also insensitive. This approach does little to dissuade many athletes from continuing to participate in their sport. In fact, some people are challenged by such an approach and attack their sport with even greater enthusiasm in an effort to prove the medical community incorrect.

A more effective approach requires that health care professionals take the time to carefully explain the injury and the most likely mechanism by which it occurred. They should also indicate in no uncertain terms that continuing an unrestricted exercise program will not only exacerbate the injury, but may also permanently hamper the person's ability to compete in the future. The primary objective is to convince persons that they are better off accepting short-term losses in order to prevent long-term problems. The magnitude of these short-term losses

can be minimized by having the individual continue to participate in physical activities that stress the various components of fitness necessary for success in their chosen sport, while still permitting the injury site to recover. The more sport-specific these alternate activities are, the greater their potential training value. An excellent example of this is water-running for a distance runner with a tibial stress fracture. Many highly motivated athletes finish these alternate training programs in better condition than they were before they were injured. For some sports, technique modifications offer a way for the athlete to heal while continuing to play. For instance, a baseball player who is afflicted by supraspinatous tendonitis in the dominant arm may find switching from overhead to sidearm throwing is all that is required to permit continued participation with minimal discomfort. In these instances, the specific problem is not directly addressed but what the athlete desires is accomplished—continued participation without further aggravation of their injury. Bracing can also be used to support body parts when the normal musculoskeletal structures have somehow been compromised. While there are injuries and anatomical malalignments that are obviously incompatible with certain sports, the recommendation to change to a new sport should generally be considered as a last resort in the management of injured exercise enthusiasts of all ages.

Injuries of relatively little significance to a sedentary person may cause considerable problems for an active adult, whether that individual is 23 or 63 years of age. An injury that could ordinarily be satisfactorily managed using a conservative approach may demand definitive correction in aging active adults because it prevents them from exercising at a desired level. A classic example of this would be a medial meniscus tear. This injury is generally well tolerated in the average 55-year-old but poorly tolerated in a person of the same age who plays competitively in a tennis league. Left untreated, injured aging competitors often experience the depressive symptoms so commonly seen in younger competitors who are sidelined by an injury. This reaction should not be mistaken for a sign of immaturity but rather is simply a reflection of how seriously these patients take their sporting involvement. Failure to recognize this fact could seriously compromise the health care professional's ability to treat these patients.

When managing any injured older active adult, one must remember that inactivity clearly accelerates the rate at which many age-related changes occur and as such represents a considerable threat to the structural integrity of the aging person. Immobilization is frequently required in the effective treatment of injuries such as fractures and severe ligamentous sprains. Not only is immobilization a frustrating experience, but it threatens the aging exercise enthusiast with all of the deleterious changes associated with disuse. Knortz also suggests that immobilized geriatric patients are doubly disadvantaged in terms of specific muscle fiber alterations that take place.[20] They not only undergo slow-twitch fiber atrophy in response to their immobility but they also continue to experience the selective fast-twitch fiber atrophy that accompanies the aging process. These phenomena suggest a number of management strategies for any aging athlete whose treatment requires them to be immobilized:

1. Immobilization should only be resorted to only when absolutely necessary
2. Immobilization should continue for as brief a period as possible
3. If the injury permits, a weight-bearing cast should be used so as to allow some gravitational loading of the immobilized limb.
4. Once immobilization is no longer necessary, immediate and aggressive physiotherapy should begin in an effort to restore full joint range of motion, reestablish muscle strength, and limit bone mass loss.

The rehabilitation of injured athletically active adults is perhaps the most important aspect of their medical management. It often determines how quickly they can resume training and when they can safely return to competitive or recreational exercise. An effective athletic rehabilitation program strives to restore the athlete to normal function in the shortest possible period of time. Any intervention that enhances recovery time is critically important to older active adults because the longer their exercise regimen is disrupted, the harder they must work to restore their previous level of activity. Once an injury has occurred, rehabilitative efforts should ideally be initiated as soon as possible and should employ a full range of appropriate treatment modalities. Since aging individuals heal more slowly, their rehabilitation program must be adjusted accordingly. As a general rule the rehabilitation time required for a 60-year-old exercise enthusiast, is twice that needed for the average 20-year-old. A person 75 years or older

will likely require three times this standard.[8] These recovery estimates hold true for nearly all injuries and can frustrate both the therapist and the patient, especially if neither is aware that they exist in the first place. It is also very important to remember that a successful rehabilitation program is not so much dependent on a person's age as it is on his or her personal motivation.

SUMMARY

In this chapter we have considered the process of aging and how it impacts on the athletic performance of older active adults. This is becoming an increasingly important topic as more and more older individuals make fitness and competitive sports a regular part of their lives. Reviewing the results from athletic events around the world shows that not only are older athletes participating in increasing numbers, but that an exceptional few are attaining performances that rate them as world-class competitors. Many of these individuals are very serious about their sports involvement and expect that their medical problems will be accorded the same level of concern from the health care profession. Aging is an entirely normal phenomenon that is intrinsic to our nature, universal in its incidence, progressive, and deleterious. The exact mechanism by which we age is yet to be established; however, as individuals age, a number of well-defined functional and structural changes occur in virtually every organ system. These changes not only significantly hinder physical performance but they also influence the incidence of injuries, the rate of wound healing, and treatment considerations. Much of the research in the field of aging has been biased by investigations that failed to control for important variables such as inactivity, disease processes, life-style habits, environmental influences, and medications. Thus, many of the structural and physiological alterations that have been attributed to the aging process may in fact be the result of other factors.

Inactivity is clearly the greatest threat to the general health of our aging population. It is estimated that as much as 50 percent of the physical decrements seen in the average aging individual occur as the direct result of disuse.[30] This lends scientific support to the old saying, "You don't stop playing because you grow old, you grow old because you stop playing." In extolling the virtues of exercise, Shephard, a world-renowned exercise physiologist with a special interest in the effects of aging on human performance, states, "Physical activity has more potential for promoting healthy aging than anything else that science or medicine has to offer today."[29] Our body was designed to be used on a regular basis; when it is deprived of this stimulus a wide variety of atrophic changes will take place. Fortunately, these inactivity-related losses are by no means permanent and people who begin to exercise later in life can make substantial improvements in both their structure and function. Considered in this light, regular exercise is truly a "fountain of youth" from which we all can derive great benefit.

REFERENCES

1. Astrand PO: Exercise physiology of the mature athlete, in Sutton JR, Brock RM (eds): *Sports Medicine for the Mature Athlete.* Indianapolis, Benchmark Press, 1986, pp 3–16.
2. Bassett CA, Becker RO: Generation of electric potentials by bone in response to mechanical stress. *Science* 1962; 137:1063–1064.
3. Berman R, Haxby JV, Pomerantz RS: Physiology of aging: Part 1. Normal changes. *Patient Care* 1988; 22:20–36.
4. Berman R, Haxby JV, Pomerantz RS: Physiology of aging. Part 2: Clinical implications. *Patient Care* 1988; 22:39–66.
5. Beyer RE, Huang JC, Wilshire EB: The effect of endurance exercise on bone dimensions, collagen and calcium in the aging male rat. *Exp Gerontol* 1985; 20:315–323.
6. Booth FW, Gould EW: Effects of training and desire on connective Tissue. *Exerc Sports Sci Rev* 1975; 3:83–112.
7. Brooks GA, Fahey TD: *Exercise Physiology, Human Bioenergetics and Its Applications.* New York, MacMillan, 1985.
8. Brown M: Special considerations during rehabilitation of the aged athlete. *Clin Sports Med* 1989; 8:893–901.
9. Damon EL: *An Experimental Investigation of the Relationship of Age to Various Parameters of Muscle Strength* (doctoral dissertation) University of Southern California, Los Angeles, 1971.
10. DeHaven KE, Littner DM: Athletic injuries: Comparison by age, sport and gender. *Am J Sports Med* 1986; 14:218–224.
11. deVries HA: *Physiology of Exercise for Physical Education and Athletics,* ed 4. Dubuque, Iowa, William C Brown Publishers, 1986.
12. Eaglestein WH: Wound healing and aging. *Clin Geriatr Med* 1989; 5:183–188.
13. Fenske NA, Lober CW: Skin changes of aging: Pathological implications. *Geriatrics* 1990; 45:27–35.
13a. Fetto JF, Marshall JL: The natural history and diagnosis of anterior cruciate ligament insufficiency. *Clin Orthop* 1986; 147:29–38.
14. Fixx JF: The test of time. *Runner,* May 1984; pp 58–62.
15. Goldman R: Speculations on vascular changes with age. *J Am Geriatr Soc* 1970; 18:765–779.
16. Hall MD: Cartilage changes after experimental relief of contact in the knee joint of the mature rat. *Clin Orthop* 1969; 64:64–76.
17. Hamlin CR, Kohn RR, Luschin JH: Apparent accelerated aging of human collagen fibers. *Diabetes* 1975; 24:902.
18. Kasch FW, Boyer JL, Van Camp SP, et al: The effect of physical activity and inactivity on aerobic power in older men (a longitudinal study). *Physician Sportsmed* 1990; 18:73–83.
19. Kitzman DW, Edward WD: Age-related changes in the anatomy of the normal human heart. *J Gerontol* 1990; 45:M33–M39.
20. Knortz KA: Muscle physiology applied to geriatric rehabilitation. *Top Geriatr Rehabil* 1987; 2:1–12.
21. Knudson RJ, Clark DF, Kennedy TC, et al: Effect of aging alone on mechanical properties of the normal adult human lung. *J Appl Physiol* 1977; 43:1054–1062.
21a. Larsson L, Sjodin B, Karlsson J: Histochemical and biochemical changes in human skeletal muscle with age in sedentary males, age 22–65 years. *Acta Physiol Scand* 1978; 103:31–39.
22. McArdle WD, Katch FI, Katch VL: Exercise Physiology—Energy, Nutrition and Human Performance, ed 2. Philadelphia, Lea & Febiger, 1986.
23. Menard DC: The aging athlete. *Top Geriatr Rehabil* 1991; 6:1–16.
24. McRae R: *Practical Fracture Treatment.* New York, Churchill Livingstone, 1981.
25. Molander B, Backman L: Age differences in heart rate patterns during concentration in a precision sport: Implications for attentional functioning. *J Gerontol* 1989; 44:P80–P87.
26. Nejjar I, et al: Age-related changes in the elastic tissue of the human thoracic aorta. *Atherosclerosis* 1990; 80:199–208.
27. Plyley MJ: Fine-tuning muscle capillary supply for maximum exercise performance. *Cardiology* 1990; 6:25–34.
28. Sager K: Senior fitness—for the Health of It. *Physician Sportsmed* 1983; 11:31–36.
29. Shephard JG, Pacelli LC: Why your patients shouldn't take aging sitting down. *Physician Sportsmed* 1990; 18:83–91.
30. Siegel AJ, Warhol MJ, Lang E: Muscle injury and repair in ultra long distance runners, in Sutton JR, Brock RM (eds): *Sports Medicine for the Mature Athlete.* Indianapolis, Benchmark Press, 1986, pp 35–43.
31. Smith EL: Exercise for the prevention of osteoporosis: A review. *Physician Sportsmed* 1982; 10:72–79.
32. Spirduso WW, Clifford P: Replication of age and physical activity effects on reaction and movement time. *J Gerontol* 1978; 33:26.
33. Stauss RH: *Sports Medicine.* Philadelphia, WB Saunders, 1984.

34. Stillman RJ, Lohman TG, Slaughter MH, et al: Physical activity and bone mineral content in women aged 30 to 85 years. *Med Sci Sports Exerc* 1986; 18:576–580.
35. Strehler BL: *Time, Cells and Aging*. New York, Academic Press, 1962.
36. Torp S, Baer E, Friedman B: Effects of age and of mechanical deformation on the ultrastructure of tendon. *Proc Colston Annu Conf Structure Fibrous Biopolymers* 1975; 26:223–250.
37. Twomey L, Taylor J: Age Changes in lumbar intervertebral discs. *Acta Orthop Scand* 1985; 56:496–499.
38. Vailas AC, Perrini VA, Pedrini-Mille A, et al: Patellar tendon matrix changes associated with aging and voluntary exercise. *J Appl Physiol* 1985; 58:1572–1576.
39. Viidik A: Connective tissues—possible implications of the temporal changes of the aging process. *Mech Aging Devel* 1979; 9:267–285.
40. Wiswell RA, Jaque SV, Hamilton-Wessler M: Exercise and muscle strength, in Morley JE, Glick Z, Rubenstein LZ (eds): *Geriatric Nutrition*. New York, Raven Press, 1990, pp 447–456.

Chapter 4

Motivation

Carol Schunk, P.T., Psy.D.

The rehabilitation program for an older person with an orthopedic problem is influenced by the patient's motivation and compliance. Success or failure of the therapeutic intervention often depends upon behaviors such as follow-through with an exercise regimen or cooperation with precautions following surgery. It is essential that the geriatric clinical practitioner be aware of the patient's behavioral pattern as it influences the treatment outcome. Recognition of motivation and compliance as issues in therapy is the initial step. However, for the patient to benefit from a rehabilitation program, the clinician must also understand their role in promoting and improving behavioral patterns that may negatively influence outcome. Behaviors such as motivation and cooperation are often not considered until the patient is being discharged from therapy. At this point motivation and cooperation are cited as a reason or excuse for failure to reach therapeutic goals. Patients are discharged from therapy because they "weren't motivated" or "failed to comply with the therapy regimen." Intervention techniques to modify this behavior are missing from the therapy program. Clinicians underestimate their ability and responsibility to influence motivation and cooperation, factors that enhance the implementation of the treatment plan.

In the health care profession, dealing with motivation and compliance of elderly patients can be complex. Several issues unique to the elderly patient exist that do not exert an influence in the younger population. These include reimbursement policies, chronic medical problems, and a compromised support system. The third-party payers primarily involved with medical care for the elderly often dictate treatment parameters and are not especially lenient with the unmotivated and uncooperative patient. It would be unusual to treat a person over 75 years of age who does not have a secondary medical condition. This might be arthritis or dementia, but will definitely influence program planning for the older patient with an orthopedic condition. Even with full recovery from an orthopedic condition, some elderly people still have a bleak future owing to financial problems or living arrangements. Additionally, the older person's support system, which can be a source of motivation, may be nonexistent or very limited. Given these factors unique to the geriatric population and related to behavior, it is impossible for the health care practitioner to ignore motivation and compliance as treatment issues. It also becomes evident that geriatrics is indeed a specialty area, even when it comes to issues of motivation and compliance.

Persons with uncomplicated orthopedic conditions generally recover. By contrast, recovery from a neurologic condition can be limited by the process or severity of the disability or disease. In elderly orthopedic patients joint replacements are common. In many cases the patient's functional status after surgery exceeds the preoperative level. A younger person who experiences an orthopedic injury is often self-motivated to resume activity. The activity that drives the recovery is the same activity which caused the injury and is often distinct from what might be considered the activities of daily living. With an older person, return to activity is also a force, but the activity may be a basic function like walking, not, for example, competitive downhill skiing. While motivation and compliance are issues in all therapeutic interactions, the elderly patient with an orthopedic problem presents a unique picture that forces the geriatric clinical practitioner to consider these issues and integrate techniques into the treatment program.

COMPLIANCE

The assumption among health professionals is that the patient listens and follows through with instructions as delivered. In reality, estimates of noncompliance range from 20% to 80%.[2] Accurate prediction of compliance is not a talent of physicians, who have been shown to be unable to identify potential noncompliance even among familiar patients.[3] Therefore, health professionals must be consciously aware of the possibility that the patient will not cooperate with treatment guidelines. Once the practitioner views motivation and compliance as part of the treatment, then the program can be modified to accommodate persons whom the therapist may suspect of being potentially uncooperative. Consideration of compliance is essential as the therapist assesses progress toward treatment goals. When progress is not evident the clinician may consider altering a treatment. For example, a therapist may change an exercise program thinking that the lack of progress was a result of the inappropriateness of the prescribed program and the solution is to prescribe different exercises. However, if the lack of progress is a result of noncompliance—the patient never did the exercises—changing the treatment program is inappropriate. Likewise, a physician may substitute a new medication for the initial prescription, which did not produce the desired effect. Upon investigation it becomes evident that the patient did not take the medication as prescribed, accounting for the lack of change. The program is put in jeopardy if noncompliance is not considered as a treatment factor. Once the practitioner is aware that noncompliance may be an issue, assessment of the behavior should follow.

ASSESSMENT OF NONCOMPLIANCE

Although numerous methods of assessing compliance have been researched, most are too cumbersome, costly, or inappropriate for the geriatric clinical practitioner. To be effective and to be used in the clinic, a method must be unintrusive and easy.

While lacking in the sophistication and validity of other techniques, observation and self-report may be the best method currently available that fits the scope of clinical practice. Observation requires the practitioner's experience and visual skill in watching the individual move or asking the patient to repeat an exercise that he or she claims to have been performing all week. A person who has been doing exercises as reported will be able to repeat the regimen upon request. Perhaps the patient's interpretation of the activity will vary from the original; however, a compliant patient will be able to demonstrate as requested. If noncompliance is a factor, requests such as "Show me your exercises" or "I will watch you use the walker" will reveal the lack of follow-through as noted by the inability to perform the activity. If observation reveals the possibility of uncooperative behavior, additional questioning is necessary to identify the reason for failure to follow-through.

Self-report basically involves asking the patient if he or she complied with the prescribed treatment. While not free of bias owing to the desire to report positive behavior, self-report remains an easy, inexpensive, noninvasive method to investigate behavior.[2, 3] The key to maximizing the potential for reporting of truthful behavior is approaching the patient in a nonthreatening, nonjudgmental manner.[4, 5] Essentially, the practitioner is giving the patient permission to report noncompliance without fear of retaliation. An example with an exercise program is to avoid accusatory questioning such as "Did you do your exercises?" Acknowledging the possibility of noncompliance first will draw a more accurate response: "Some people find it difficult to remember to do the exercises; was this a problem for you?" Not only will the practitioner determine if the

TABLE 4–1.

Noncompliance Statements and Responses

Reason	Adjustment
1. I forgot the exercise.	1. What if we have your wife remind you; I'll teach her with you.
2. The weights were too heavy.	2. Perhaps you should do the exercises without weights for a week.
3. My leg got tired.	3. With these exercises, don't be alarmed if your leg gets a bit sore the next day.
4. I was afraid to get down on the floor	4. You don't need to get on the floor if that is a concern; I'll teach you to do the exercises in bed or sitting on a chair.
5. I didn't remember them.	5. We will review the program; I'll write down each one.

program was followed but, as with observation, additional questioning can assess the reason behind the uncooperative behavior.

Table 4–1 gives examples of statements that a patient might give with additional probing by the practitioner after noncompliance has been observed or self-reported. Also prepared are possible statements from the therapist geared to adjustment of the treatment regimen to encourage cooperation.

There are basically three factors involved in improving patient compliance. First is awareness of the behavior as a treatment issue. This includes recognition that compliance can influence treatment outcome. Assessment by observation and self-report is the second factor, with the third being modification of the treatment approach in response to noncompliance.

FACTORS INFLUENCING COMPLIANT BEHAVIOR IN ELDERLY PERSONS

To better help practitioners identify noncompliant behavior it is important to review factors which influence behavior. Several complex health problems put the elderly people at greater risk for noncompliance. Stillwell[11] divides these problems into four groups: communication impairment, prescription complexity, chronic illness, and cognitive dysfunction. Of these four factors communication impairment, prescription complexity, and cognitive dysfunction are issues most pertinent to rehabilitation. If geriatric clinical practitioners are aware of factors that can influence cooperative behavior, they can identify people who have a higher potential for noncompliant behavior.

Communication deficits such as hearing or vision loss should always be considered when an elderly person appears unable to follow directions or perform an exercise as demonstrated. Hearing loss is present in approximately 40% of people over 65 and is often not as obvious to the clinician as a visual deficit.[13] The patient may be characterized as being unmotivated or uncooperative while the actual problem is being unable to hear or see the instructions as given. Speech and language disorders such as receptive aphasia will definitely interfere with the instructional aspect of treatment. The combination of a communication disorder and orthopedic problem would be unusual with a younger person but not so, given the multiple health problems more common

with an older individual. Therefore an assessment of the person's ability to hear, see, and understand should be made prior to initiation of a treatment plan. Depending upon the findings, programs can be modified; for example, oversized figures can be used on home exercise instructions to compensate for visual loss.

Normal aging does not interfere with the ability to learn new material; however, the complication of a cognitive disorder may impair the ability to learn and remember new material. Approximately 15% of the population over age 65 years is affected with some type of cognitive disorder, with the rate increasing to 20% for those over 80 years.[11] There are several cognitive disorders with which therapists should be familiar, as they increase the likelihood of noncompliance. In addition, adjustments may be made in the treatment approach and in goal setting to accommodate a cognitive disorder. Delirium and dementia are the most common mental disorders that could affect the patient's motivation and cooperation with the treatment program. Depression is not characterized as a mental disorder but also can influence behavior.

The primary symptom of dementia is impairment in short- and long-term memory. For a true diagnosis of dementia, the memory loss or other symptoms of decline in judgment and abstract thinking must be severe enough to interfere with work, social activities, or relationships with others.[1] The obvious influence on therapy for the orthopedic patient with dementia is the follow-through and retention of instructions. Maintaining a regimen of partial weight-bearing is going to be a problem for the patient who does not remember the stated precaution from one minute to the next. Within 2 weeks a cognitively intact person with a post surgical orthopedic condition may be an independent ambulator, capable of partial weight-bearing with a walker. A person with a similar orthopedic condition complicated by a cognitive deficit may not be independent until full weight-bearing status is allowed 6 weeks postoperatively. In this case the cognitive disorder has influenced the patient's compliance to maintain partial weight-bearing status and therefore required modification of the treatment and goals. In order to get the patient ambulatory as quickly as possible, the orthopedist and therapist can work together in determining an appropriate gait treatment program with consideration of the patient's physical and cognitive status.

While dementia was once considered to be permanent, there is now evidence that 10% to 30% of those with dementia characteristics actually have reversible dementia. In these cases correction of the condition causing the symptoms will restore intellectual function. Drug complications are the most common cause of reversible dementia.

Especially pertinent to operative orthopedic cases is postsurgical confusion, which may mimic dementia. The affected person will demonstrate dementia-like symptoms while having no previous history of such behaviors. With time symptoms will decrease, distinguishing the condition from true dementia, which is not reversible. Awareness of the therapist can serve to minimize concern by the family and to modify the program until the symptoms clear.

While depression is not technically a cognitive disorder, the symptoms present with a behavior pattern that involves mental function and therefore compliance and motivation. The primary diagnostic symptoms of clinical depression are depressed mood or loss of interest in pleasure in almost all activities for a period of at least 2 weeks. [1] Several additional symptoms may be displayed; those that can have a direct impact on the individual's level of participation and follow-through with treatment are fatigue or loss of energy and diminished ability to concentrate and think. If depression is suspected, the practitioner may have to plan a treatment regimen that is structured to accommodate for the individual's loss of interest without compromising the person's personal goals. Additionally, referral to a psychologist or social worker may be appropriate.

PRACTITIONER COMPLIANCE

A new concept in the compliance literature is physician compliance of accepted and recommended medical practice.[7] While patient compliance was a little-known concept prior to 1970, compliance of the health care practitioner to known medical regimens was rarely mentioned. Of interest is not only the fact that physicians do not comply with acceptable practice but that they perceive that they perform more services than they actually do.[7] Pommerenke identifies several strategies for physicians to improve their own compliance, such as implementation of reminder systems, office organization and logistics, chart review, and reimbursement and cost considerations.[7] If therapists are guilty of forgetting some applicable activity such as a discussion of home safety,

then a method such as inclusion in the assessment form should be initiated. For example, Schreiner et al[8] studied the effectiveness of a reminder system for preventive medicine procedures. Suggestions based on their findings include computer-based prompting techniques, which could easily be incorporated into rehabilitation assessments. The system was successful while operational; however, compliance declined once the reminders were discontinued.

MOTIVATION

It is difficult to separate motivation from compliance. If a person is motivated or has the incentive to participate in the therapy regimen this will usually include cooperation with instructions or home exercise programs. Too often, the term unmotivated is treated as being synonymous with a lack of progress: the patient never reached the goals set by the health care practitioner, so he or she must be unmotivated! Motivation is not simply a character trait. While someone may be described as having a lack of motivation, motivation can also be viewed in terms of a verb, "to motivate the patient." To think that motivation either happens or it doesn't, you have it or you don't, negates the clinician's responsibility in assessing and facilitating a change in the patient's behavior.

Assessment

Assessment of the patient's motivation should be included in the initial evaluation, along with assessment of strength or flexibility. This eliminates the scenario in which motivation is only considered as the final reason to explain the lack of progress toward treatment goals. Shontz[10] proposed a multiple-concept theory of motivation in rehabilitation to describe a person's state rather than function. Modification of his factors produces six considerations that can be assessed and used as a foundation for predicting motivation. The geriatric clinical practitioner can evaluate a patient based on the presence or absence of characteristics as described in Table 4-2.

If the patient is missing the characteristics as described in a specific category, there is a possibility that lack of motivation will be a factor in recovery. With this information the therapist can monitor the patient's progress closely with alterations in the

TABLE 4–2.

Six Considerations for Predicting Motivation

Reality orientation
    Well aware of physical limitation
    Realistic view of potential ability
Energy level
    High degree of energy
    Display of spontaneous activity
    Ability to direct energy
Cooperativeness
    Agreeable
    Follows requests and demands
Involvement
    Willingly participates in program
    Interacts with others
Social requirements
    Discharge plans agreeable with patient
Personal goals
    Incorporation into therapy program
    Desire for personal achievement

treatment approach as needed. For example, a patient with an unrealistic view of his potential for recovery (reality orientation) may be unmotivated to participate in gait training since his perception is that he will never be able to walk again. The assessment criteria not only provide information on potential motivation problems but identify the reason for the behavior.

    Case Example.—An 85-year-old woman who has fractured her hip in a fall is in a skilled nursing facility for rehabilitation. The discharge plan is to have her return to live with her daughter in another city. Upon assessing factors of motivation, the therapist determines that this discharge plan is not agreeable with the patient, who does not want to leave her friends or live with the daughter, who has numerous small children. The patient feels she will be perfectly capable of living alone in her two-story home. Factors that alert the therapist to a potential problem with motivation are threefold. First, the social requirements, the demands and ramifications of relocating, are not agreeable with the patient. The second concern is the issue of personal goals. The therapist's original intent was to get the patient independent enough to live with her daughter. Without the participation of the patient in establishing goals, the therapist may be unaware that the patient's goal is to be totally independent. Lastly, reality orientation is a factor. This woman does not have a realistic view of her potential abilities and the difficulty of maintaining and functioning in a large, two-story home. In response to a motivation assessment the therapist consults with the patient, identifying her goals and social requirements. The patient's potential for independence is discussed, and the possibility of using an assistive ambulatory device

is introduced. A plan is developed to relocate the patient to a small, one-story apartment in her old neighborhood.

    If the clinician in this case had not assessed the factors contributing to motivation, it is possible that the patient would not have cooperated in therapy so as to avoid being discharged to her daughter's home. Therapy goals would not be achieved in the predicted amount of time and the reason given may have been "lack of patient motivation." With the awareness of the role of motivation and the need to assess contributing factors, the initial treatment plan can be modified to accommodate factors that could contribute to unmotivated behavior.

    In an article focusing on the older patient, Lewis and Wagner[6] identified four motivational types of persons seen in physical therapy. The distinguishing characteristics were:

- Type 1, a high degree of motivation in all areas
- Type 2, a high degree of motivation in one nonphysical activity
- Type 3, a high degree of motivation in physical activity
- Not motivated in any area

    Obviously the first group does not present any concerns for participation in therapeutic activities. For the second group of people who focus on nonphysical activities, the concern is the assessment of personal goals as described earlier. The practitioner will experience a higher degree of cooperation if the therapy activities are tied into the patient's nonphysical interests, such as attending a concert or visiting the grandchildren. For example, while the treatment goal is lower extremity exercise for strength and eventual independent gait, therapy is designed with the patient's goal of being able to walk up the aisle at the granddaughter's wedding.

    Persons in Lewis and Wagner's group 3 may appear to be the practitioner's dream: they are highly motivated in physical activity. In reality, problems can arise with this group. Most of the compliance literature focuses on undercompliance—that is, lack of follow-through or not doing what is prescribed. What is ignored is the issue of overcompliance or doing more than prescribed. In an unpublished paper Schunk[9] studied persons suffering from an orthopedic athletic injury. The focus was compliance to a home exercise program as measured by self report. Results showed overcompliance in 30% of the subjects and undercompliance in 30%. With the increasing numbers of older athletes it is worth considering that overcompliance, fueled by the desire to return to competition or to activity, can be an issue. Potential reinjury or overuse syndrome may occur from overcompliance. As opposed to individuals who are noncompliant, those who might be overcompliant are often easier to recognize by their enthusiasm to resume previous activity and reluctance to stop the activity that caused the orthopedic injury. Practitioners' recognition of patient characteristics and awareness of overcompliance will allow for modification of the treatment program. Discussing the harm in doing more than prescribed and giving the person an alternative activity, such as swimming while recuperating from a running injury, will help to minimize the urge to do more than prescribed.

Group four, those not motivated in any area, are the focus of the majority of the practitioner's hard work in making a treatment program effective. The need to assess motivation as part of the initial evaluation as described, and incorporate appropriate motivating techniques into the treatment program becomes an essential part of therapy with the group that is not motivated toward anything. Lewis and Wagner approach the unmotivated individual from the viewpoint that the therapist must "sell" the exercise to the patient.[6]

Intervention

Once a potential motivation problem has been identified, intervention is appropriate, just as one would intervene when a abnormal gait pattern is observed. Techniques will vary depending upon the cause of the behavior, but several can be suggested.

Goal Setting.—Patient participation in setting goals and in designing the therapy program is a factor in motivation. Goal setting incorporates the ultimate social requirements, personal goals, and reality orientation. All practitioners should routinely consult their patients about their expectations and goals of therapy. With this information the treatment program can be oriented to encourage motivated behavior, as the patient is working toward something he or she has identified as important.

Freedom of Choice.—Depending upon the treatment setting, the patient may have limited autonomy, all decisions being relegated to the nursing staff. Patients can feel that the only authority they have remaining is to refuse treatment. The need to take control is rarely directed at the physician, mak-

ing nursing staff and therapists vulnerable. Unfortunately, this situation is intensified as staff members cope with the frustration of working with an uncooperative patient who reduces the therapist to the role of authoritarian dictator. Providing the patient with some power to choose therapy activities may renew interest in the rehabilitation program. Restoration of freedom of choice can be accomplished without compromising therapy by setting up acceptable alternatives. The alternatives do not include refusing therapy but do offer a choice between activities or choice of timing. The therapist can create a situation in which all responses are within the parameters of therapy goals: "Would you like to walk first or do exercises on the mat?" "These are three exercises to strengthen your knee; choose one to do at home this week." The choice is refocused from the issue of participation in therapy toward activities within therapy that still offer the patient control.

Minimization of Failure.—Individuals are more likely to participate in an activity if there is an opportunity to succeed. Guaranteed success or guaranteed failure decreases motivation, as there is no potential for feedback of the effort. Consideration of this concept is the basis for minimizing the failure of patients in therapeutic activities. For example, stating the goal of "walking with crutches" to an elderly person with a lower extremity amputation may result in frustration and reluctance to return to therapy after the initial sessions. Breaking the task into small activities will ensure success along the road to independent ambulation and help to maintain cooperative behavior. Therefore, focusing on standing and walking one length in the parallel bars will increase the patient's potential for a successful session. With positive reinforcement for the accomplishment and verbalization of the anticipated progress, the following day the patient may absorb some of the therapist's enthusiasm for therapy.

One pitfall of this motivational technique is overexuberance by the therapist about small accomplishments. If a person lived alone golfing three times a week prior to the hip fracture the expectations of recovery are high. While a therapist may get excited about a successful exercise of the quadriceps muscle, expectation that the patient will share the enthusiasm is unrealistic and can be discouraging. While minimization of failure encourages breaking the activity into small, manageable tasks with a potential for success, the patient's end goal of playing golf should always be kept in mind. Relating the importance of quadriceps strength to the golf stance keeps the patient encouraged about therapy and willing to participate in the seemingly unrelated tasks necessary for recovery.

Mental Imagery.—Hesitancy of a patient to participate in therapy may not be related to unwillingness but to fear associated with the original injury. When the orthopedic problem is a result of trauma, some older persons are very anxious about the rehabilitation process, especially if pain and discomfort were major factors of the injury. Mental imagery can assist when uncooperative behavior is related to stress, anxiety, or fear. Allowing the patient to relax and imagine a particular activity such as ambulating on stairs with an assistive device may alleviate the reluctance to participate. The practitioner can "walk" the patient through the activity with words in a nonthreatening environment, describing the sequence. If pain is an issue the utilization of relaxation techniques can build in an association of a peaceful event with the anxiety-provoking activity.

REIMBURSEMENT

While motivation may appear to be a therapeutic issue with the older population reimbursement can be jeopardized because of a patient's uncooperative behavior. Medicare and other third-party payers function under the expectation that patients will make progress toward treatment goals as a result of the therapeutic intervention. If payment is denied owing to lack of motivation or cooperation, the therapist will be in a position to appeal the denial. In one case denial was based on lack of cooperation as documented in the subjective portion of the therapy note, even though the patient made steady progress and reached goals. In this instance the therapist probably incorporated motivational techniques into the therapy sessions, thereby achieving success. When this case was heard by the hearings officer the emphasis of the provider was on the role of the geriatric physical therapist in motivating the older individual. Part of the testimony emphasized the geriatrics therapist's training and attention to the unmotivated patient—therapy is not abandoned because a patient states he or she does not want to do something. As a part of the treatment, techniques to enhance motivation and compliance are implemented. In the case cited the denial was overturned. Third-party payers have questioned whether

therapy is appropriate for people with dementia. Given the focus of therapy on learning and education combined with the memory loss characteristic of dementia, can the person with dementia benefit from therapy? It appears that some activities of long standing, such as walking, can be part of therapy; however, introduction of a new activity or technique, such as walking with a walker, may be very difficult. The combination of the medical problems of a total hip replacement and dementia is another example of a difficult therapy situation. Compliance with total hip precautions to prevent dislocation may be an unreasonable expectation of a person with dementia. In this case, the traditional treatment plan and expectations must be modified, with increased nursing involvement and possibly a delay in discharge anticipated. Experience indicates, however, that those with dementia can benefit from therapy with appropriate modifications to the treatment program.

CONCLUSION

An orthopedic condition in an elderly person is rarely simple to treat. The practitioner who focuses only on the physical aspect of treatment is not providing a complete program to the patient. Additionally, the frustration for the therapist is intensified when failure to reach goals is attributed to motivation and cooperation problems. Behavioral issues must be considered, with assessment and intervention techniques incorporated into the therapeutic regimen. There is no guarantee that compliance and motivational problems can be resolved; however, attention to these concepts in rehabilitation provides maximum opportunities for the patient.

REFERENCES

1. American Psychiatric Association: *Diagnostic and Statistical Manual of Mental Disorder,* ed 3, revised. Washington, DC, American Psychiatric Association, 1987.
2. Cumming KM et al: Construct validity comparisons of three methods for measuring patient compliance. *Health Serv Res* 1984; 19:103–114.
3. DiMatteo MR, DiNicola DD: *Achieving patient compliance. The Psychology of the Medical Practitioner's Role.* Elmsford, NY, 1982, Pergamon Press.
4. Fletcher SW, Pappino EM, Harper SJ: Measurement of medication compliance in a clinical setting. *Arch Intern Med* 1979; 139:635–638.
5. Haynes RB, Sackett DL, Taylor DW: How to detect

and manage low patient compliance in chronic illness. *Geriatrics* 1980; 35:91–97.

6. Lewis CB, Wagner M: Motivation for older patients. *Geritopics,* 1991, vol 14.

7. Pommerenke FA, Weed DL: Physician compliance: Improving skills in preventive medicine. *Am Fam Pract* 1991; 43:560–568.

8. Schreiner DT et al: Improving compliance with preventive medicine procedures in a house staff training program. *South Med J* 1988; 81:1553–1557.

9. Schunk CR: Compliance to an exercise program among injured athletes. Unpublished data, 1988.

10. Shontz FC: *The Psychological Aspects of Physical Illness and Disability.* New York, MacMillan, 1975.

11. Stillwell JE: Common health problems that threaten compliance in the elderly. *Top Geriatr Rehabil* 1988; 3:34–40.

12. Teri L, Hughes JP, Larson EB: Cognitive deterioration in Alzheimer's disease: Behavioral and health factors. *J Gerontol* 1990; 45:58–63.

13. Washburn A: Hearing disorders and the aged. *Top Geriatr Med* 1986; 1:61–70.

Chapter 5

Low Back Injuries: An Orthopedic Perspective

Richard J. Nasca, M.D.

Back pain is a common complaint, occurring in 70% to 80% of our population.[13] Fortunately for most, the symptoms are of short duration and resolve with rest.

Aging is an evolutionary process that begins at birth and terminates with death. The aging spine, however, should not be regarded as an isolated structure outside the framework of the human maturation process. Although degenerative changes in the vertebral discs, ligaments, and bones account for most diseases and disorders of the aging spine, systemic disease can coexist and cause the patient's symptoms.[14] Chemical imbalances in calcium, phosphate, and collagen metabolism may result in progressive and disabling osteoporosis and osteomalacia. These conditions often accelerate existing vertebral deformities and result in the unstable collapse patterns commonly seen in scoliosis and kyphosis.

Cancer and infection usually involve the spine secondarily, causing destruction of osseous structures and resulting in spinal instability and neurologic compression. The clinician and therapist must be alert to systemic, as well as local, conditions that can affect the aging spine. The clinical manifestations of these conditions and the treatment methods of benefit to those with disabling spinal complaints will be discussed in the sections below.

GENERAL CONSIDERATIONS OF THE AGING THORACOLUMBAR SPINE

With aging, the spine and appendicular joints become less flexible and range of motion decreases significantly.[5] Elastin tissue degenerates and collagen cross-linking becomes more rigid, resulting in less-supple ligaments and connective tissue. Support of the vertebral elements is provided by the strong anterior longitudinal ligaments, intervertebral disc–vertebral body complex, facet joint capsules, and the highly elastic ligamentum flavum.

With increasing age, there is a steady loss of water and hydration of the intervertebral disk contents, along with wear and tear on the annulus fibrosus. These changes in the disc result in reduced intervertebral disc height and stability of the vertebral body and disc bond.[23] As we age, we lose vertebral stature, in large part because of loss of height in many, if not most, of our 25 intervertebral discs.

Deformities of the disc produce deformities and instabilities of adjacent segments of the spine. The dowager's hump (thoracic kyphosis) is caused by a narrowing of the anterior portion of the disc and loss of anterior vertebral body height in the thoracic spine. Normal kyphosis ranges from 20 to 30 degrees in the second to fifth decades.[15] In the elderly patient with a noticeable dowager's hump, a kyphotic deformity of 50 to 90 degrees may be seen on a standing lateral radiograph of the spine. With the continual axial loading of upright posture, the kyphotic deformity progresses. Compensatory curves occur in the cervical and lumbar spine to balance the spine in the sagittal plane.

In response to a progressive thoracic deformity, an increase in cervical lordosis as well as lumbar lordosis occurs, provided these segments of the spine are flexible. As thoracic kyphosis increases, vertical height often decreases by several inches. Chest and abdominal circumferences increase simultaneously, causing significant changes in body morphology.[15] These findings are often ascribed to an increase in body weight rather than to alterations in the spine's osteoligamentous structure.

Degenerative kyphoscoliosis of the lower thoracic and lumbar spine results in loss of the physiologic swayback posture of lordosis. The lumbar spine becomes flat and the pelvis becomes rotated and asymmetrical. To compensate for reduced lumbar lordosis, the flat-backed person stands with hips and knees flexed. This posture allows affected persons to stand erect in a balanced stance but at the expense of hip and thigh muscle fatigue, thus causing the individual to tire easily.

Secondary compensatory deformities can result in symptoms that need evaluation and careful consideration before initiation of treatment. Progression of deformity can be documented by the patient's history, measurable loss of vertical height, change in clothing sizes, and review of serial photographs. Mild to moderate postural changes in stature are physiologic and are to be expected with advancing age. These changes are usually asymptomatic and require no treatment.

COMMON ETIOLOGIES OF BACK PAIN IN THE OLDER PATIENT

Back pain in the older patient can result from any of a number of common etiologies (Table 5–1). Degeneration of the intervertebral discs and facet joints of the cervical, thoracic, and lumbar spine is responsible for the majority of clinical syndromes.

Lumbar spinal stenosis usually involves the L3-4 and L4-5 vertebral segments. A small-diameter lumbar spinal canal or nerve root canal can be a significant causative factor in this disorder. Degenerative

TABLE 5–1.

Common Etiologies of Back Pain in Aged Persons

Degenerative disc and facet disease
Spinal stenosis
Degenerative scoliosis
Osteoporosis
Spinal fracture
Combinations

changes in the facet joints and intervertebral discs superimposed on a reduced-diameter spinal canal result in bony compression on the spinal neural contents. Patients most often complain of low back pain and neurogenic claudication. The latter is characterized by radicular pain that is intensified by standing and walking and is often relieved with rest in the side-lying flexed position.[8]

The patient can present with bizarre neurologic complaints and a paucity of objective neurologic findings. Often these patients are referred with a diagnosis of peripheral vascular disease. Indeed, the conditions of spinal stenosis and peripheral vascular disease causing claudication can coexist. A careful clinical examination and collaborative diagnostic studies may be necessary to define the cause of the claudication. Patients with neurogenic claudication are able to ride an exercise bicycle in the semiflexed position without complaints of leg pain, in contrast to those with vascular claudication. Impotence, loss of leg hair, and stocking-level loss of sensation are commonly noted in those with peripheral vascular disease. Loss of bowel and bladder control can occur in patients with long-standing spinal stenosis or those who have been inadequately treated. Urinary retention or frequency can also be symptoms of spinal stenosis of the lumbar spine.

Degenerative scoliosis is characterized by progressive deformity of the thoracolumbar spine. Patients complain of back pain, stiffness, and hip, thigh, and leg pain, which is usually relieved by rest. Degenerative scoliosis is more common in women than men. Osteoporosis and osteomalacia accelerate the spinal deformities and instabilities seen in these patients. Spinal stenosis can be a coexisting condition,[20] resulting in nerve root compression, especially on the concave side of the scoliotic curve. Neural deficits may be noted in the L3, L4, and L5 roots. Malrotation and lateral translation of the midlumbar apical vertebrae result in loss of lumbar lordosis and asymmetrical pelvic girdle rotation. Patients who take steroids are especially prone to a collapsing type of degenerative scoliosis.

Compression fractures are commonly seen in patients with osteoporosis, osteomalacia, and degenerative scoliosis. In most cases these injuries heal, but occasionally a nonunion results in marked deformity and extrinsic spinal cord compression. Multiple compression fractures are found in some patients, especially in those taking steroids. They can occur in a sequential pattern with minimal trauma and can lead to months of pain and disability.

Progressive osteoporosis of the spine causes significant disability in otherwise healthy women. Disability resulting from degenerative scoliosis, spinal stenosis and spinal fractures is accelerated by osteoporosis and osteomalacia. Successful treatment of these demineralization and loss-of-matrix diseases enhances patient comfort and reduces deformity and disability. Consultation with a specialist in metabolic bone disease is helpful. Nutritional deficiencies of vitamin D, calcium, and phosphorus cause osteomalacia. Absorption defects in the small intestine and hepatobiliary disease interfere with normal calcium and phosphate uptake and metabolism. Proximal and distal tubular renal lesions result in loss of urinary calcium and phosphate. Primary hyperparathyroidism owing to parathyroid adenomas and hyperplasia causes increased resorption of calcium from bone, resulting in the formation of fibrous cystic areas and brown tumors.[22] Secondary hyperparathyroidism in association with renal osteodystrophies and renal failure also can produce severe osteomalacia. Fractures occur through areas of fibrous tissue replacement and brown tumors. The etiology of osteoporosis is not well defined. It is postulated that increased osteoclastic activity and decreased osteoblastic response coupled with an imbalance in bone turnover rate cause a negative balance in bone reformation.

Other causes of spine pain in the elderly patient are herniated discs, metastatic cancer, spinal infection, Paget's disease and inflammatory arthritis (Table 5–2). A herniated disc, although most often seen in younger patients, can occur in the later years without a significant injury. The onset of acute radicular pain that follows the anatomic course of a nerve root must be investigated if the symptoms are not relieved by rest, medication, and temporary supports.

Cancers of the lung, breast, and prostate commonly metastasize to the marrow of the vertebral bodies. Destruction of the vertebral body and adjacent pedicle causes nerve root or cord compression, or both. Acute paraplegia can result.

Although spinal infection is rare, acute bacterial infection involving the disc and adjacent vertebral

TABLE 5–2.

Less Common Etiologies of Back Pain in Aged Persons

Herniated disc
Metastatic cancer
Spinal infection
Paget's disease
Inflammatory arthritis

bodies can result in severe back and radicular pain. If the infection spreads within the spinal canal, an epidural abscess can cause spinal cord compression.

Paget's disease is characterized by excessive bone resorption and subsequent formation of abnormal bone. The abnormal bone is highly vascular. The cause of Paget's disease is unknown; the most common sites of involvement, however, are the spine, pelvis, skull, hip, and femur. Sarcomatous degeneration can occur and is heralded by a sudden increase in pain.

The inflammatory arthritides of the spine, such as ankylosing spondylitis, commonly seen in men, cause progressive restriction of spinal as well as costovertebral motion. Spondylarthritis may be episodic and fleeting. Rheumatoid arthritis can lead to significant instability in the upper cervical spine and deformity in the thoracolumbar spine.

EVALUATION OF THE AGING THORACOLUMBAR SPINE

A complete, detailed history and physical examination are critical elements in the evaluation of a patient's complaints (Table 5–3). Adequate, high-quality spinal radiographs are also necessary. Standing and dynamic bending views can be valuable in assessing deformities and instabilities involving the spinal segments. Electromyography (EMG) is helpful in evaluating specific nerve root compression and in excluding polyneuropathies, such as those seen in diabetes and demyelinating and degenerative spinal

TABLE 5–3.

Evaluation of the Aging Thoracolumbar Spine

Complete history and physical
EMG, CT-myelogram, MRI
Bone scan, quantitative CT
Calcium, phosphorus, acid and alkaline phosphatase
Sedimentation rate, rheumatoid screen
Vertebral and iliac biopsies

cord diseases.[9] In fact, electrodiagnostic studies were consistent with clinical and operative findings in 75% to 80% of our patients.

Water-soluble myelographic contrast agents coupled with computed tomography (contrast-enhanced CT) provide the clinician with an extremely powerful diagnostic modality for assessing spinal canal and nerve root pathology.[1] These studies are well tolerated by the patient. Using third-generation CT scanners, resolution of nerve root pathology is excellent to the level of the pedicle that corresponds to the end of the dural sac. Magnetic resonance imaging (MRI) provides a superb diagnostic method for visualizing intrathecal spinal cord tumors and syrinxes. Hydration changes in the intervertebral disc produce a variance in the MRI signal that characterizes a normal or an abnormal disc, especially on T_2-weighted sequences.

Occasionally, several adjacent discs demonstrate abnormal MRI signals. In these situations, because of the need to define the disc(s) causing the patient's symptoms, provocative tests such as discography and nerve root blocks are used.[7] Although discography is a controversial procedure, it is generally agreed that if the disc injection *reproduces* the patient's back and extremity pain, the injected disc is symptomatic. Diagnostic lumbar nerve root blocks are helpful in defining radicular pain.[21] These blocks are done with the patient awake and use image intensification for needle placement. A small quantity of water-soluble contrast medium can be placed within the nerve root sheath to verify needle placement and outline the course of the nerve root. Injection of small amounts of local anesthetic agents in the perineural tissues surrounding the nerve root gives temporary relief of symptoms of radiculitis or radiculopathy.

Bone scans provide an excellent method for screening a patient for metastatic cancer, infection, or an occult fracture of the spine. Unfortunately, the bone scan can not determine the causative agent, but it does localize the lesion reliably. Percutaneous needle biopsies of the vertebral bodies and discs are necessary to determine the causes of abnormalities seen on bone scans.

When evaluating patients with significant progressive osteoporosis and osteomalacia, serum calcium, phosphorus, and alkaline phosphatase determinations are necessary in addition to 24-hour collections of urine for determination of calcium and phosphorus content. Iliac crest biopsies and quantitative CT are of value in determining the cause and extent of disease in affected people, who are often very disabled by pain and deformity.

Although the sedimentation rate is a nonspecific test, it is a valuable indicator of occult infection and progressive inflammatory disease, such as rheumatoid arthritis, lupus erythematosus and other inflammatory arthritides.

NONOPERATIVE MANAGEMENT OF THE AGING THORACOLUMBAR SPINE

For most patients with spine problems, simple, straightforward treatment can be very effective (Table 5–4). Rest and reduction of the activities that cause the symptoms can be the first measures to be taken. In spite of this common-sense approach, many people do not heed their bodies' warnings and continue the activities that cause problems. Educating patients in proper exercises or sending them to special classes enables them to make progress in their rehabilitation during the acute and chronic phases of their disorders.[10] Heat, ice, massage, ultrasound, manipulation, and traction modalities are valuable adjuncts in conservative therapy and will be discussed in detail in the rehabilitation chapter. In many instances, these modalities can be used at home by the patient who is aided by a family member or friend. This reduces the need to travel, which often aggravates back symptoms as a result of prolonged sitting.

Walking may be the best exercise for those with spine complaints because it is safe, convenient, and easy to do. Freestyle swimming in a warm pool is also recommended. Swimming increases endurance and flexibility and provides exercise in an antigravity environment. Most patients tolerate the use of a stationary bicycle for 5 to 10 minutes once or twice a day, even those with symptoms and those recover-

TABLE 5–4.
Nonoperative Management of the Aging Thoracolumbar Spine

Rest, heat, cold, massage
Ultrasound, manipulation, traction
William's and Mackenzie exercises
Anti-inflammatory drugs
Weight reduction
Replacement therapy for osteoporosis
Functional bracing

ing from surgery. William's flexion exercises and MacKenzie extension exercises or similar exercises, may be helpful and will be discussed in detail in the companion chapter. If a patient's symptoms are exacerbated by a particular exercise even though it is being done properly, it should be discontinued. Monitoring for proper performance of exercises is essential and should be done by a physical or occupational therapist.

Anti-inflammatory medication helps reduce pain, but may cause adverse gastrointestinal effects. It may be necessary to try several nonsteroidal anti-inflammatory drugs (NSAIDs) before finding one that is effective and well tolerated by the patient. Muscle relaxants and oral pain medication used for short periods of time are beneficial during acute phases or periods of exacerbation. Long-term reliance on muscle relaxants and oral narcotic analgesics is discouraged.

Weight reduction is mandatory to reduce excessive vertical loading on the spine. In the patient who cannot or will not exercise because of pain, however, it is difficult to lose weight even with reduced caloric intake.

Temporary bracing is helpful in alleviating pain associated with inflamed motion segments. Lumbosacral supports are effective. Custom-fitted, lightweight thermoplastic braces can be used to support unstable and deformed spines, as well as those with recent fractures. For a brace to be effective, however, it must be worn. A properly fabricated and fitted orthosis increases patient compliance.

Osteoporosis and osteomalacia require aggressive medical therapy. Calcium, vitamin D, and estrogen supplements are proven effective replacement therapy. Weight-bearing exercises, such as resisted swimming and progressive exercise, are helpful and usually well tolerated. Lightweight custom brace supports are necessary for patients with compression fractures; however, in older patients with poor posture, comfort may be a problem. Abstinence from alcohol and tobacco is another important, although often overlooked, aspect of treatment.

Epidurally administered steroids are useful in alleviating sciatica in a significant number of patients.[4] If the sciatica is the result of an irritated nerve root, relief can be long-lasting; however, if symptoms are caused by a truly compressed root, relief will usually be of short duration. Epidural steroids are contraindicated in the presence of infection. Repeat injections of steroids within a 4- to 6-week period are safe and necessary in some patients. Care must be taken

to properly place the needle within the confines of the epidural space.

OPERATIVE TREATMENT OF THE AGING THORACOLUMBAR SPINE

It is this author's opinion that replacement of major weight-bearing joints with internal prosthetic components has revolutionized the surgical management of patients with crippling arthritis during the last 25 years. In spite of age, disuse atrophy, and often fragile general health, patients tolerate these surgical procedures well and achieve significant functional improvement. Spine surgery has not met with the same dramatic success that hip and knee surgery have, although recent diagnostic and therapeutic breakthroughs are enabling spine surgeons to do more for patients with debilitating spine injuries and diseases (Table 5–5).

Whereas the joint replacement surgeon relies on high-performance artificial components as a substitute for damaged bone and joint structures, the spinal surgeon must depend on the patient's ability to heal and the ability of bone to regenerate in the fusion area. It is estimated that in 13% to 15% of patients bone does not heal in a satisfactory manner.[19] In some patients, failure of fusion after surgery (pseudoarthrosis) does not cause pain, whereas in others it does. Several investigators are currently designing and testing safer and more efficient types of spinal implants. Synthetic materials such as calcium hydroxyapatite and tricalcium phosphate show promise as bone substitutes and extenders in arthrodesis surgery.[17]

Conditions that often require surgical intervention are described.

Spondylolisthesis

Although there are several types of spondylolisthesis, the isthmic type is most commonly seen in

TABLE 5–5.
Operative Treatment of the Aging Thoracolumbar Spine

Decompression and fusion for spinal stenosis
Instrumentation and fusion for scoliosis
Stabilization of spinal fractures
Excision and stabilization of tumors
Debridement and fusion for chronic infection

the adult. Spondylolisthesis is forward displacement of a vertebra over an adjacent vertebra, usually at the level of L5-S1 or L4-5. Hyperextension forces fracture the pars interarticularis, usually bilaterally. Once these pars, or isthmic, stress fractures occur, stability is lost and the superior vertebra slides forward on the inferior vertebra of the motion segment. This condition is seen in 5% of people with spinal problems.[12] Symptoms include lumbar and extremity pain. The latter may be radicular and follow the L5 root dermatomes. Occasionally there is an associated disc herniation at the level above the spondylolisthesis. Patients usually respond to bed rest and bracing since in most instances the pain is generated by mechanical instability.

If conservative therapy fails and recurrences cause long periods of disability, a spinal fusion is indicated. Although several techniques are used, the most reliable is a posterolateral or lateral fusion. This consists of decortication of the posterior surfaces of the lamina and transverse process, as well as removal of the facet articular cartilage to create a fusion bed to which bone graft is added. Removal of the loose posterior element of L5 is usually not necessary and can result in a lower rate of bony union because of a reduced surface area.[12] Occasionally, decompression of the L5 nerve roots and disc excision are done in conjunction with arthrodesis. Decompression alone is rarely successful for this condition. Results of surgical treatment are good to excellent in 85% to 90% of patients with isthmic spondylolisthesis and complications are uncommon.[12] Recently, intraoperative reduction of significantly displaced spondylolisthesis has been popularized.[2] Neuropraxia resulting from stretching of the L5 nerve roots occurs in approximately one third of the patients treated by reduction and rigid internal fixation.

Degenerative spondylolisthesis occurs most commonly at the L4-5 level in women. This is the result of a combination of an unstable degenerative L4-5 disc and degeneration of the facet joints. Severe lumbar and radicular pain in the lower extremities are common in these patients. The L5 roots are often irritated and may be stretched or compressed. Patients experience a worsening of these symptoms after diskectomy. In most cases, a limited nerve root decompression and spinal fusion of the L4-5 motion segment is successful. Internal fixation adds immediate stability and a good deal of pain relief occurs in the early postoperative period. Reduction of degenerative spondylolisthesis is not necessary.

Lumbar Spinal Stenosis

Spinal stenosis involving the lumbar motion segments most commonly occurs at L3-4 and L4-5 in middle-aged adults.[14] Some patients have a small spinal canal with a reduced anteroposterior diameter and cross-sectional area. Small disc herniations and mild degrees of spinal canal and facet joint arthritis can cause significant compression in patients with these anatomic variants. These patients usually present with spinal stenosis in the early decades and may be helped by decompression and arthrodesis. Diskectomy alone seldom is effective in these patients and may exacerbate their lumbar and radicular symptoms.

Central-mixed spinal stenosis is commonly encountered in middle-aged and older patients. Most of these patients have degeneration of the L3-4 and L4-5 discs as well as facet joint osteoarthritis. Some retain stability in spite of marked degeneration of their motion segments, whereas others have marked instability associated with their stenosis. The former group can be effectively treated with decompression alone. This consists of removal of the laminae and a portion of the facet joint to widen the spinal and nerve root canals. Herniated and sequestered discs require removal. It is best to leave bulging and protruding discs alone. In cases of stenosis in which there is instability, arthrodesis is indicated with or without internal fixation.[16] Postoperative brace support is usually required for 4 to 6 months after surgery. In patients who have had previous laminectomies or fusions and who subsequently develop spinal stenosis, the addition of fusion to the decompression, in our experience, produces a more successful result. Women with osteoporosis and deformed vertebral elements as a result of bone collapse benefit from spinal arthrodesis. Despite their metabolic bone imbalances, these patients appear to have satisfactory bony healing. When freshly frozen allograft bone is placed on a properly decorticated spine, a satisfactory arthrodesis results in 87% of patients. These results compare favorably with those in patients who received autogenous bone.[19] The value of internal fixation in promoting spinal fusions is presently not resolved by a short arthrodesis of one to three motion segments. However, in long multisegment fusions, internal fixation is necessary to maintain corrective forces and support during the healing period.

Degenerative Scoliosis

Scoliosis has long been considered an adolescent problem. Today, in a busy spine center, adults are being treated as often as adolescents. In some patients, moderately severe adolescent idiopathic scoliosis progresses and becomes painful in their third and subsequent decades. Pain is usually noted at the curve apex, is relieved with rest and is aggravated by increased activity in the upright posture. Fatigue, shortness of breath, and reduced work capacity are common. Occasionally, radicular symptoms occur; these may be the result of spinal stenosis and compression of nerve roots on the concave side of the curve.[20] Significant anatomic compression associated with scoliosis and spinal stenosis usually results in objective signs of nerve root compression. Surgical decompression combined with spinal stabilization is necessary in these patients. Decompression alone is usually not successful. Correction and stabilization of the major curves by instrumentation and arthrodesis relieves both mechanical and radicular pain, increases work tolerance, and improves physical appearance. Care must be taken during surgical correction to maintain adequate lumbar lordosis and to avoid creating a "flat back" deformity. Straightening the normal lordotic lumbar spine places the patient in a forward, off-balanced posture. This posture requires compensation with flexed hips and knees and leads to fatigue.

Two-stage or combined single-stage anterior and posterior fusions are commonly done for degenerative scoliosis. The initial procedure consists of disc excision with anterior interbody bone grafting at several spinal levels followed by posterior arthrodesis and instrumentation. Despite the duration of the procedure, the combined operation is well tolerated by most patients. Advantages of the front-and-back approaches are better correction and more successful arthrodeses. Some surgeons use anterior instrumentation in conjunction with anterior arthrodesis in thoracolumbar curves located between T10 and L4. Short degenerative lumbar curves can cause significant disability from one or two motion segment instabilities. These patients obtain significant relief from a solid arthrodesis with or without attempts at curve correction.

Spinal Fractures

Compression fractures are commonly seen in osteoporotic adults. Rest, mild analgesics, and light bracing is all the treatment necessary for most patients. Fortunately, most of these fractures heal with little, if any, resultant disability. However, some patients experience continued severe pain after compression fracture. Whether this is the result of a nonunion of the fracture, instability, or a combination of the two may not be apparent. Prolonged bracing and rest only increase disability. Physical therapy can be helpful with modalities and exercise. Although it is rarely necessary, surgical stabilization can benefit these disabled patients, especially those with multiple fractures that occur in rapid sequence.

Rigid forms of internal fixation using pedicle screws can fail because of osteoporosis of the pedicles and vertebral bodies. Rod and hook systems, interspinous wires, and sublaminal wires in combination with cross-linked longitudinal rods are useful in stabilizing these patients. Posterolateral fusion using local autogenous bone provided by decortication and supplemented with large quantities of fresh frozen allograft bone has been successful in these patients. Bracing is used until the fusion is structurally mature, which may require 6 to 9 months. Calcium, vitamin D, and estrogen supplements are necessary and alcohol, tobacco, and steroids should be avoided.

Spinal Infection

Although rare, bacterial infection can be a complication of urologic, gastrointestinal, or cardiopulmonary surgery. Batson's plexus provides a direct route to the epidural venous system surrounding the dura as well as to the veins to the vertebral body. Urinary and pelvic infections commonly spread along Batson's plexus, causing vertebral osteomyelitis or disc space infections. Patients experience severe back pain and bilateral radicular pain. Slight, unexpected movement of a patient's bed often markedly intensifies pain.

Delay in diagnosing infection is common. In a series of 65 patients studied by Eismont and colleagues, the average time from onset of symptoms to hospitalization was more than 50 days and the delay in arriving at the correct diagnosis was more than 30 days.[6] Fever and leukocyte response may not be significantly elevated; however, a high sedimentation rate, usually greater than 60 mm/hr, is common. Blood cultures are negative in many of these patients. The infection is usually diagnosed by percutaneous needle biopsy performed using image intensification.

The clinician and therapist must be aware of the prevalence of gram-negative bacterial infections in intravenous drug users. Although much less common today, tuberculosis of the spine can occur, especially in debilitated patients and in those receiving steroids and chemotherapy. Fungal infections often occur in these patients.[18]

If the diagnosis is made early and the pathogen is identified, most disc and vertebral body infections can be treated successfully with rest, immobilization, and antibiotics. Patients who have a well-established disc space infection with paravertebral abscess formation, destructive vertebral body osteomyelitis with collapse and instability, or an epidural abscess will require surgical drainage and decompression. The anterior approach to the spine popularized by Hodgson and Stock for eradication of tuberculosis provides us with an effective route of attack on chronic bacterial and fungal infection involving vertebral bodies and disk spaces.[11] A timely diagnosis and prompt surgical decompression, when indicated, should produce a satisfactory outcome. Paraplegia is a rare but disastrous complication of undiagnosed or improperly treated vertebral osteomyelitis. After adequate anterior debridement and drainage, a bone graft is placed between the resected margins of healthy vertebrae to provide a scaffold for interbody fusion. Once fusion occurs the patient usually can resume all activities without restriction. Recurrence of an adequately treated spinal infection is rare.

In patients who develop infection following an elective spinal surgical procedure, prompt debridement of infected tissue and closure of the incision over a suction-irrigation system is usually successful. Appropriate antibiotics are given until the incision heals. Spinal implants are not removed. Bone grafts are debrided, washed, and replaced over the areas to be fused.

COMPLICATIONS OF SURGICAL TREATMENT OF THE AGING THORACOLUMBAR SPINE

Although the medical and anesthetic risks are greater for the older patient, these patients usually do well during spinal surgery, even that of several hours' duration (Table 5–6). Modern anesthetic techniques make time-consuming surgical procedures quite safe. Preoperative autologous blood donation and relative hypotensive anesthesia have been effective measures in combating intraoperative blood loss. In situations where significant blood loss is anticipated, a cell saver is used to harvest lost blood and return it to the patient during surgery.

TABLE 5–6.

Complications of Surgical Treatment of the Aging Thoracolumbar Spine

Greater medical and anesthetic risks
Postoperative hemorrhage; thromboembolism
Osteoporotic bone heals but may not hold
Need for care in placing pedicle screws, hooks, etc.
Bank bone useful in osteoporosis
Broken or loose spinal fixation
Cardiac, pulmonary, and vascular disease

Administration of potent, short-acting narcotics reduces the need to use high concentrations of anesthetic gases. Precise monitoring of cardiopulmonary function is performed constantly during the surgical procedure by a variety of invasive and noninvasive techniques. Intensive care postoperative management benefits patients who require ventilatory support, close monitoring of cardiac status, and one-on-one nursing care.

Excessive postoperative hemorrhage owing to imbalances in the coagulation process is a potentially life-threatening complication that can be successfully treated with the appropriate blood products. Thromboembolism is another complication requiring prompt diagnosis and aggressive therapy. The value of preoperative anticoagulation has not been uniformly established. Overanticoagulation can result in operative site bleeding and wound disruption, which can be complicated by secondary infection that requires return visits to surgery.

Because older bone is usually osteoporotic, it must be handled with great care. Decompressive procedures require rapid but precise removal of bone-compressing neural elements without damaging neural structures or their protective coverings. The various hooks and screws used to anchor spinal implants must be carefully placed. Augmentation with polymethyl methacrylate is not recommended because in liquid form the acrylic is hard to control and in the solid state it has virtually no shear- or tensile-resisting strength. If internal fixation cannot be applied safely and securely, it is best left out.

Allograft-banked bone has enabled surgeons to augment extensive areas of bone loss. It is especially valuable in patients who need multisegmental fusions, but who have inadequate autogenous bone or bone of poor quality, as is often the case in older, osteoporotic patients. The increased vascularity of osteoporotic bone and the paucity of dense lamellar and cortical bone appears to be a good environment for an arthrodesis; however, the mechanical strength of the resultant fusion may be such that external forces can cause further deformity through bending. Judicious postoperative protection with well-designed and mechanically sound spinal orthotics is necessary until the spine and graft reach maximum strength.

Loss of correction, loose or broken spinal implants, and continued mechanical pain complaints are indicative of pseudarthroses. These are difficult to detect even with tomography and CT scans. In most cases, pseudarthroses require repair. Broken or loose spinal fixation needs removal. Intact spinal implants are well tolerated and usually do not require removal unless bursal reactions occur over prominent metallic surfaces in thin patients. Stress shielding has not been a significant problem with rigid spinal implants.

The author has observed that, postoperatively, early mobilization of the patient in a protective orthosis results in less morbidity, maintenance of deformity correction, and a happier patient. Daily walks are encouraged. Personal hygiene care and household activities that are not physically demanding are resumed during the first 4 to 6 weeks after surgery. Subsequently, more home and away-from-home activities are added. Usually by 3 months patients can resume activities that do not require significant lifting, bending, or climbing. Patients can usually be weaned off braces at 6 to 9 months unless there is significant osteoporosis, potential instability, or delay in healing of the fusion.

Significant vascular disease of the aorta and its branches may preclude surgery of the anterior spine since these large diseased vessels must be mobilized and manipulated, thus increasing the risk of atheroma dislodgement. If dislodgement occurs, timely removal of the atheroma and thrombus usually results in restoration of the arterial circulation. Sensory and motor evoked potential monitoring of spinal cord function has added another safety factor to spinal surgery. These noninvasive monitoring techniques are sensitive and effective modalities that alert the operative team to change in spinal cord function during decompression and instrumentation procedures.

SUMMARY

Aging is an evolutionary process. The aging spine must not be regarded as an isolated structure. The clinician and therapist must be alert to systemic as well as local conditions that affect the spine. With increasing age, hydration of the intervertebral disc decreases along with wear and tear on the anulus fibrosus. Deformities and instabilities of the spine may occur and result in pain. Lumbar spinal stenosis results in radicular pain in the lower extremities, intensified by standing and walking and often relieved by rest in the side-lying position. Spinal stenosis and peripheral vascular disease causing claudication in the legs may coexist. Degenerative scoliosis, seen commonly in women, may present with both back and radicular pain as a result of nerve root compression. Compression fractures are commonly seen in patients with osteoporosis and osteomalacia. Primary and secondary hyperparathyroidism can result in severe osteomalacia caused by increased osteoclastic activity and decreased osteoblastic response. Metastatic bone cancer is common in aged people and should not be overlooked as a cause of pain.

A complete history and physical examination is critical in the evaluation of patients with spine and radicular complaints. High-quality radiographs, electrodiagnostic tests, contrast-enhanced CT, and MRI are valuable diagnostic tools. Metabolic evaluation and iliac crest biopsies may be necessary in those with progressive osteoporosis and osteomalacia.

Nonoperative management includes rest, heat, ice, massage, ultrasound, manipulation, traction. Referral to a physical therapist who is knowledgable and skilled in working with these patients is to be encouraged and greatly facilitates their treatment. Walking, swimming, and the use of a stationary bicycle are therapeutic and well-tolerated forms of active exercise. Temporary bracing, epidural steroids, and use of NSAIDs may be beneficial. Calcium, vitamin D, and estrogen replacement has proven effective for patients with osteoporosis and osteomalacia.

Spinal surgery is well tolerated in the older motivated patient. Although the spine is not replaced with a prosthetic implant, a solid spinal fusion allows the patient to carry out most normal activities without pain or repeated disability. Anesthetic and medical complications can be anticipated and minimized by proper preoperative planning, intraoperative monitoring, and skillful postoperative care and surveillance. Functional results and improved quality of life can be gratifying for patients with spine disorders that have been properly diagnosed and treated. The future is bright, with technical advances in medicine, anesthesia, and surgery that should continue to improve the care of these individuals.

REFERENCES

1. Bolender NF, Schonstrom NSR, Spengler DM: Role of computed tomography and myelography in the diagnosis of central spinal stenosis. *J Bone Joint Surg (Am)* 1985; 67:240–246.
2. Bradford DS: Treatment of severe spondylolisthesis. A combined approach for reduction and stabilization. *Spine* 1979; 4:423–429.
3. Cervical Spine Research Society (ed): *The Cervical Spine.* Philadelphia, JB Lippincott, 1983.
4. Cuckler JM, Bernini PA, Wiesel SW, et al: The use of epidural steroids in the treatment of lumbar radicular pain. *J Bone Joint Surg (Am)* 1985; 67:63–66.
5. Einkauf DK, Gohdes ML, Jensen GM, et al: Changes in spinal mobility with increasing age in women. *Phys Ther* 1987; 67:370–375.
6. Eismont FJ, Bohlman HH, Soni PL, et al: Pyogenic and fungal vertebral osteomyelitis with paralysis. *J Bone Joint Surg (Am)* 1983; 65:19–29.
7. Gibson MJ, Buckley J, Mawhinney R, et al: Magnetic resonance imaging and discography in the diagnosis of disc degeneration. *J Bone Joint Surg (Br)* 1986; 68:369–373.
8. Grabias S: The treatment of spinal stenosis. *J Bone Joint Surg (Am)* 1980; 62:308–313.
9. Haldeman S: The electrodiagnostic evaluation of nerve root function. *Spine* 1984; 9:42–48.
10. Hall H, Iceton JA: Back school; an overview with specific reference to the Canadian back education unit. *Clin Orthop* 1983; 179:10–17.
11. Hodgson AR, Stock FE: Anterior spine fusion for the treatment of tuberculosis of the spine. The operative findings and results of treatment in the first one hundred cases. *J Bone Joint Surg (Am)* 1960; 42:295–310.
12. Johnson LR, Nasca RJ, Dunham WK: Surgical management of isthmic spondylolisthesis. *Spine* 1988; 13:93–97.
13. Kelsey JL, White AA III: Epidemiology and impact of low back pain. *Spine* 1980; 5:133–142.
14. Kirkaldy-Willis WH, Wedge JH, Yong-Hing K, et al: Pathology and pathogenesis of lumbar spondylosis and stenosis. *Spine* 1978; 3:319–328.
15. Moe JH: in Bradford DS, et al (eds) *Moe's Textbook of Scoliosis and Other Spinal Deformities,* ed 2. Philadelphia, WB Saunders, 1987.
16. Nasca RJ: Surgical management of lumbar spinal stenosis. *Spine* 1987; 12:809–816.
17. Nasca RJ, Lemons JE, Deinlein DA: Synthetic biomaterials for spinal fusion. *Orthopaedics* 1989; 12:543–548.
18. Nasca RJ, McElvein RB: *Aspergillus fumigatus* osteomyelitis of the thoracic spine treated by excision and interbody fusion. *Spine* 1985; 10:848–850.
19. Nasca RJ, Whelchel JD: Use of cryopreserved bone in spinal surgery. *Spine* 1987; 12:222–227.
20. Simmons EH, Jackson RP: The management of nerve root entrapment syndromes associated with the collapsing scoliosis of idiopathic lumbar and thoracolumbar lumbar curves. *Spine* 1979; 4:533–541.
21. Tajima T, Furukawa K, Kuramochi E: Selective lumbosacral radiculography and block. *Spine* 1980; 5:68–77.
22. Urist MR: *Fundamental and Clinical Bone Physiology.* Philadelphia, JB Lippincott, 1980.
23. White AA III, Panjabi MM: The basic kinematics of the human spine: A review of past and current knowledge. *Spine* 1978; 3:12.

Chapter 6

Low Back Injuries: A Rehabilitation Perspective

Carole B. Lewis, P.T., Ph.D.
Therese McNerney, P.T.

Treating back pain is a critical part of any rehabilitation strategy for an elderly person. The list of possible diagnoses related to low back pain for this segment of the population is long; however, the current treatment techniques and modalities available to rehabilitation therapists for treating these conditions is even longer. It is therefore important for therapists working with older patients to address each component of the rehabilitation strategy and treatment program.

In the current atmosphere of practice without referral, the therapist's evaluation skills and treatments must reflect the most up-to-date knowledge base. In addition, the insurance crisis and the threat of incomplete reimbursement necessitate that the efficacy of treatment approaches be documented.

This chapter will briefly discuss the anatomy and physiology of the thoracic and lumbar spines and the normal changes that occur with age.

ANATOMY

The aging spine reaches its skeletal mass peak by age 40. Progressive bone loss after the age of 40 years has been termed *negative bone balance*, as bone is resorbed at twice the rate at which it is formed.[5] Women are particularly affected by the decreased bone formation as loss of estrogen allows a doubled rate of calcium resorption in bone and a decreased ability to absorb calcium from the intestines.[5]

With each passing decade, both men and women experience a 3% loss in cortical bone and a 6% to 8% loss of both horizontal and transverse trabecular bone.[12] Horizontal trabecular loss in older vertebral bodies leads to gradual increases in vertebral end-plate concavity, resulting in a ballooning of the center of the disc into the adjacent vertebral bodies.[18] Transverse trabecular loss results in a horizontal spreading or "thickening at the waist" of the vertebral bodies. Both horizontal and transverse trabecular loss leads to the decreased stature of older persons. Previously a "thinning" disc was thought to be the cause of decreased height, but alternately it has been noted that there may be an actual decrease in bone density with subsequent vertebral end-plate collapse that leads to this decrease.[18]

The aging disc also undergoes significant change. A 40% increase in disc stiffness has been noted as a result of histologic and biochemical changes.[17] These changes include decreased water-binding capabilities, increase in total number of collagen fibers and a decreased differentiation between the nucleus and the anulus.[18] The changing shape of the disc acts as a shock absorber as vertical forces are redistributed in horizontal directions.

In old age, the sexual differentiations between vertebral shape, posture, and spinal range of motion become less pronounced. As shown in Table 6–1, Twomey and Taylor have shown that all movements

TABLE 6–1.

The Mean and Standard Deviation for the Total Ranges of Sagittal, Horizontal and Coronal Plane Movements in Living Subjects (Population 960 Persons)*

| | Ranges of Movements | | | | | |
| | Sagittal Range (Flexion-Extension) | | Horizontal Range (Rotation to Both Sides) | | Coronal Range (Side Flexion) | |
Age	M	F	M	F	M	F
5–12 yr	58° ± 9°	58° ± 9°	34° ± 6°	34° ± 6°	47° ± 6°	47° ± 6°
13–19 yr	45° ± 10°	57° ± 8°	30° ± 4°	34° ± 4°	38° ± 5°	37° ± 4°
19–35 yr	42° ± 6°	42° ± 7°	33° ± 6°	33° ± 6°	40° ± 5°	40° ± 5°
35–59 yr	38° ± 7°	38° ± 7°	26° ± 6°	27° ± 6°	32° ± 4°	30° ± 3°
60+ yr	30° ± 7°	28° ± 6°	22° ± 5°	20° ± 4°	28° ± 4°	30° ± 5°

*From Twomey LT, Taylor JR: *Physical Therapy of the Low Back.* New York, Churchill Livingstone, 1987. Used by permission.

of the lumbar spine decrease with age.[18] Lumbar lordosis also has been shown to flatten in 32% of females and 20% of males after adolescence.[18]

Muscles can atrophy in both size and type with age.[2] A general increase in type I muscle fibers and a decrease in type II fibers is noted.[8] A general loss of skeletal muscle occurs as larger numbers of motor units are needed to produce a given force. Maximal muscle strength declines. All of these changes reflect a decrease in the older spine's ability to adapt and therefore dictate the type of rehabilitation programs that must be created.

STENOSIS

Lumbar stenosis is a pathologic condition rarely affecting people under the age of 60 years. It is commonly identified in conjunction with radiographic changes of advanced degenerative disc disease and electromyographic (EMG) results showing multilevel involvement.[9] Stenosis is defined as a narrowing of the lumbar spinal cord of such magnitude that pressure is exerted on the nerve roots prior to their exit from the foramina.[20] The nerve root impingement is caused by a combination of narrowed disc space, enlarged facet joints and laminae, and hypertrophy of the ligamentum flavum.[6] The bony encroachment of the lumbar spinal canal with subsequent neurologic pressure is greatest with the lumbar spinal position of extension and with activities such as ambulation. Extension positioning or activities that involve lumbar extension may lead to neural tissue ischemia. Neural ischemia, also referred to as neurogenic clau-

dication, may result in bowel and bladder dysfunction, numbness, and significant weakness of the lower extremities.[21]

Patients with lumbar stenosis will report in their subjective evaluations that activities such as sitting and touching their toes (lumbar flexion) will relieve their symptoms. Prolonged standing or walking (lumbar extension) will bring on back, buttock, or leg pains that start proximally and progress distally. Once irritated, nerve pain may take 30 minutes or longer to subside.[21] In severe cases, a patient may report episodes of falling because of lower extremity weakness or foot drop that results from the progression of the disease process. Objective evaluation findings may include active range-of-motion test results in which lumbar flexion relieves pain and symptoms, while lumbar extension may increase the symptomatology.

Neurologically, the patient may have decreased deep tendon reflexes both at the knee and the ankle.[21] Progressive neurologic symptoms include loss of bowel and bladder control and feelings of numbness in the buttock area.[21] The evaluation should focus on flexibility and strength testing of the hip, low back, and abdominal muscles.

The orthopedic treatment for this progressive pathology that offers a good prognosis is the surgical decompression of the involved segments.[13] The potential relief gained from the surgery, however, must be weighed against the postoperative complications experienced by many elderly persons. For patients who are not candidates for surgery, conservative physical therapy management includes education, strengthening, stretching, and rest. Patients must be educated about their progressive condition.

Exercise and its relationship to lumbar position-

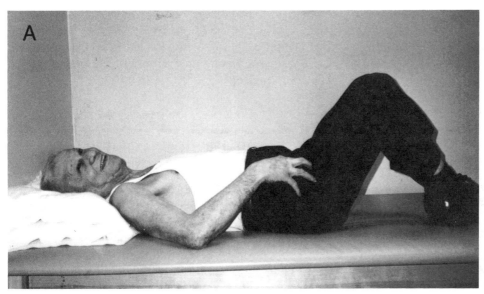

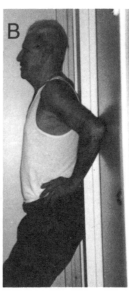

FIG 6–1.
A, active posterior pelvic tilting, supine. Patient places hands on pelvis to assist in feeling posterior movement or flattening of lower back to bed. **B,** standing posterior tilt. Patient places feet 1 foot from the wall and slides back down the wall keeping lower back flat against the wall.

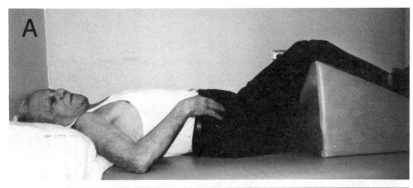

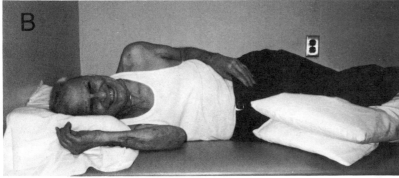

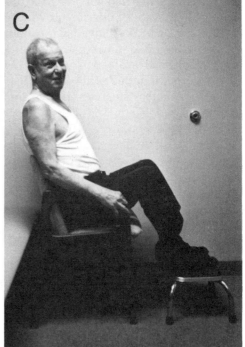

FIG 6–2.
Passive posterior pelvic positioning. **A,** supine. **B,** side-lying. **C,** sitting.

ing cannot be overemphasized. Patients are instructed in a progressive posterior pelvic tilting program that can be translated into both sitting and standing postures. By maintaining some form of posterior pelvic tilt that encourages abdominal and gluteal strengthening, patients are able to symptomatically control their pain and maintain their function through relief of compressive neurologic forces in the spine. Figure 6–1 illustrates active posterior pelvic tilting in both the supine and standing positions.

Patients are also instructed in passive positioning. In bed, patients are instructed to use positions that facilitate lumbar flexion (i.e., side-lying in the fetal position or supine with the legs over pillows.) In sitting, patients are also encouraged to sit with their knees flexed higher than their hips midday for 20 minutes. Figure 6–2 illustrates passive posterior pelvic positioning in supine, side-lying and sitting positions.

Patients are also encouraged to take frequent rests from walking. Stationery bike riding is suggested as an alternative to walking because patients are less likely to irritate neural structures, since they naturally go into a posterior tilt when riding, while maintaining good cardiovascular conditioning.

Clinically, it is imperative that a thorough initial musculoskeletal evaluation be performed to detect and record strength and flexibility changes. The patient with lumbar stenosis may benefit from a wide variety of modalities (moist heat, electrical stimulation, massage, and ultrasound) that encourage relaxation of tight lumbar muscles. Strengthening and flexibility exercises are an essential part of the reha-

bilitation strategy. Functional electric stimulation also has been found to be efficacious in the treatment of foot drop if detected in its early stages.

Evaluation and treatment of lumbar stenosis are summarized in Table 6–2.

VERTEBRAL COMPRESSION FRACTURE

Vertebral compression fractures usually affect the vertebral levels T8-L3.[4] These fractures are related to a loss in trabecular bone owing to decreased bone mineral content.[4] The weakened bone causes the anterior elements of the vertebral bodies to compress into a wedged-shaped configuration. The fractures typically occur during routine activities such as bending to tie a shoe, rising from a chair, or simply getting out of bed. The acute symptomatic fracture will result in subjective complaints of immediate, severe local pain in the back at the level of the fracture. This pain usually subsides within months, but may persist for years. Some vertebral compression fractures, however, do not cause pain. These gradual asymptomatic fractures are only detected on radiographic examination or by the loss of body height

TABLE 6–2.
Summary of Evaluation Findings and Treatment Techniques for Lumbar Stenosis

1. History of weakness in lower extremities: "I am unable to walk as far as I'm used to."
2. "Sitting feels good."
3. "I get leg pain when I stand or walk for any length of time."

Objective evaluation findings
1. Lumbar flexion relieves leg pain and symptoms.
2. Lumbar extension increases pain and symptoms.

Treatment techniques
1. Modify environment
   A. Sit midday with knees flexed higher than hips for 20 minutes.
   B. Use posterior pelvic positioning in activities of daily living (e.g., sleeping in the fetal position).
2. Use modalities (i.e., moist heat, ultrasound, electrical stimulation, massage) to reduce erector spinae muscle guarding.
3. Follow active and passive posterior pelvic tilting program.

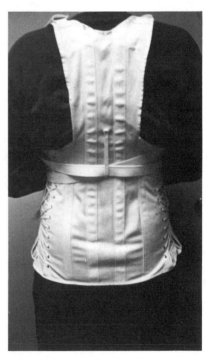

FIG 6–3.
Thoracolumbar corset.

that presents as an increase in thoracic kyphosis known as the dowager's hump.[19]

Complications of multiple vertebral compression fractures and resultant shortening of the spine include respiratory dysfunction arising from chronic alveolar hypertension and retention of bronchial secretions leading to repeated episodes of pneumonia.[7] Abdominal symptoms such as bloating and constipation also may be present due to restrictions in digestive tract space. If the fractures become severe enough, the patient may experience spinal cord damage resulting in bowel and bladder dysfunction and paresthesias.[7]

On objective evaluation, palpation may reveal sharp pain at the specific vertebral level and increased muscle guarding surrounding the fracture site. Flexion activities that put more pressure on the already-weakened anterior vertebral bodies will increase pain. Extension activities that decrease the damaging compression forces will decrease the pain if the patient is able to tolerate the positioning. Because many of these elderly forward-flexed patients have trouble attaining any vertebral extension, several braces have been developed to assist them. Braces can prevent flexion, but the classic extension brace (Cash orthosis, Jewett) is not tolerated well by

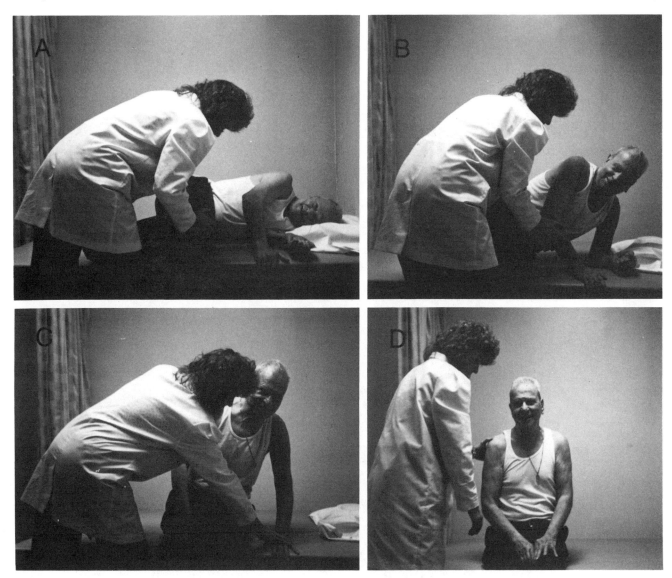

FIG 6–4.
Rolling from supine to sitting while stabilizing in pain-free position. **A,** patient squeezes buttocks and tightens abdomen in pain free position and then log-rolls while tightening abdominals and buttocks muscles. **B** and **C,** patient pushes to sitting position while continuing to tighten muscles. **D,** patient sits up completely and relaxes muscles.

elderly patients because of uncomfortable pressure exerted on the sternum and pubis.

The authors find that the thoracolumbar corset is the only brace tolerated with any level of comfort because the patient can rest into the shoulder harnesses, as shown in Figure 6–3.

The treatment for vertebral compression frac-tures can be separated into two phases: the initial phase and the chronic phase. During the initial phase, lasting from 1 day to between 4 and 6 weeks, the patient is confined to some form of bed rest. The therapist may apply ice packs or moist heat to the symptomatic area for pain relief. The authors have found that functional electrical stimulation can be

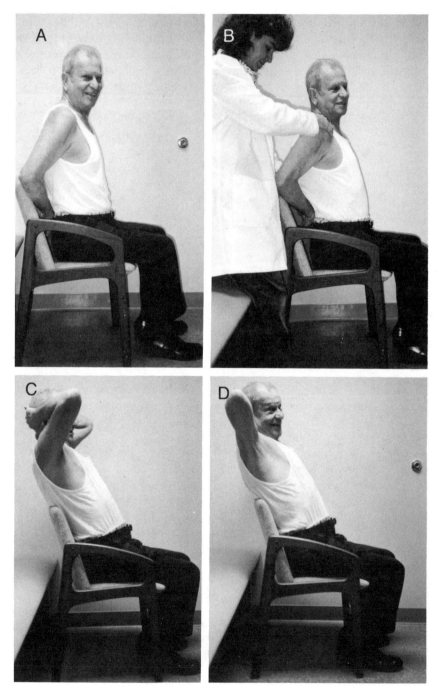

FIG 6–5.
Osteoporosis exercises. **A** and **B,** patient places hands in the small of the back and arch backward. **C** and **D,** patient places hands behind the head and pull shoulder blades to-gether.

very efficacious in the treatment of compression fractures during this phase by increasing strength and providing significant pain relief.

While in bed, patients are instructed in a series of isometric exercises that emphasize extension. These exercises consist of gluteal squeezes, quadriceps sitting, back arches, rhomboid tightenings, neck extensions, and pressing the entire body into the bed. These isometrics should be held to a count of 10 while breathing or counting out loud.

It is imperative that as soon as the patient can get out of bed he or she be instructed to do so for 10 minutes out of every hour.[4] The vertebral fractures linked to bone mass reduction (osteoporosis) need weight-bearing to maintain their bone mineral content. For patients to be compliant with out-of-bed orders, it is important to instruct them in the proper ways of getting out of bed while avoiding flexion and the pain associated with it. Neutral position stabilization of the involved segment using abdominal bracing followed by instruction in "log-rolling" will minimize forward-flexed positioning. Figure 6–4 presents the progression for teaching patients to roll to stabilize the painful area.

Once the patient with a subacute condition is out of bed, he or she should be instructed in exercises to decrease muscle guarding and improve posture to prevent further injury. These exercises can be found in *The Osteoporosis Exercise Book*.[10] Patients should be encouraged to perform these exercises three times a day for 6 to 8 weeks. Several of these exercises are shown in Figure 6–5.

As the patient begins to return to normal activities, he or she must be instructed in the avoidance of flexion activities such as bending from the waist to pick up objects and avoiding poor postures. The strengthening program after the subacute phase may progress to resistive exercises emphasizing extension. The emphasis on extension exercises in relation to vertebral compression fractures comes from the work of Sinaki and Mikkelsen.[14]

In their study, flexion, extension, and flexion-extension exercise programs were undertaken by people with a history of vertebral compression fractures. In their 2-year follow-up study, 89% of the patients following flexion exercise programs had a recurring vertebral compression fracture, as did 67% of those on a flexion-extension program and 56% of the control group. Only 16% of the extension exercise group suffered a recurring fracture. This strongly illustrates the importance of having patients who have had or who are susceptible to compression fractures continue to follow an extension exer-

TABLE 6–3.

Summary of Evaluation Findings and Treatment Techniques for Vertebral Compression Fractures

Subjective evaluation findings
1. Complains of sharp pain along the spine.
2. "Sitting up in a chair for too long makes me feel worse."
Objective evaluation findings
1. Presents with increased muscle guarding at the fracture site.
2. Flexion increases the pain; extension decreases it.
Treatment techniques
Acute phase
1. Horizontal bed rest, out of bed for 10 minutes of every hour.
2. Position of comfort, emphasizing extension in sleeping, standing, and sitting.
3. Isometric extension exercises in bed.
4. Work on proper posture when standing.
Chronic phase
1. Teach patient extension exercises.
2. Teach proper posture.
3. Begin progressive resistive extension exercises (see Fig 6–13).
4. Avoid flexion activities.
5. Use modalities (ice, heat, electricity) as needed.
6. Modify the environment (e.g., soft-soled shoes to decrease vertebral loading).

cise program. As exercise specialists, rehabilitation therapists must instruct patients in the correct form of exercise and encourage compliance. Evaluation and treatment of vertebral compression fractures are summarized in Table 6–3.

MECHANICAL LOW BACK PAIN

The final diagnosis to be discussed in this chapter is mechanical low back pain. Before continuing, it must be noted that the causes of low back pain in the elderly may be nonmechanical and unrelated to musculoskeletal conditions. For example, 85% of spinal metastases present themselves in the thoracolumbar spine.[5] Back pain can also be related to or referred from dysfunctional kidneys, ovarian cysts, prostrate problems, gastrointestinal dysfunctions, and aortic aneurysms.[5]

The key to distinguishing between mechanical and nonmechanical low back pain is a thorough evaluation that demonstrates an increase or decrease in the patient's symptoms with some combination of physical movement. If symptoms cannot be replicated, the patient should be referred back to a physician for management of nonmechanical low back pain.

A clinical example may help in clarifying this point.

Case Example.—An 80-year-old patient arrived in the clinic, sent on an emergency basis by an internist. The prescription read, "Low back pain: please apply heat and ultrasound." The patient complained of severe pain in the L2-3 area. On evaluation, the soft tissue was not tender to palpation, but the patient continued to report extreme pain.

On evaluation of active and passive range of motion of the thoracolumbar spine, no combination of movements replicated the symptoms, no positioning alleviated the pain, and no position intensified the pain. The therapist at this point suspected a nonmusculoskeletal basis for the patient's complaints. The patient was sent home and asked to rest and call the therapist the next day. During a follow-up phone call the next day the patient complained of a rash along the L2 dermatome.

On return to the internist, the patient was diagnosed as having herpes zoster, or shingles. If the therapist had followed the prescription without performing a thorough evaluation, the patient would have received a treatment possibly contraindicated for shingles. It is therefore imperative if a therapist can not replicate the symptoms through the evaluation process to refer the patient back to the physician.

Mechanical low back pain is therefore defined as a condition with reproducible signs and symptoms. These signs may range from decreased flexibility and strength to increased muscle guarding, postural changes, and structural asymmetries. The authors find the use of the flexion-extension-asymmetry principles helpful in determining a baseline from which to begin their evaluation and base their treatments. These principles are summarized in Table 6–4.

A case study may help illustrate the use of the flexion-extension-asymmetry principle in determining a course of treatment.

Case Example.—A 72-year-old woman came to the clinic with a prescription that read, "Low back pain: evaluate and treat." The patient's subjective history was relatively uninvolved because this was her first episode of back pain. She reported that the back pain started approximately 2 weeks earlier after she quickly bent down to pick up the newspaper. Subjectively, she complained of pain with walking, stooping, or rising from a chair. She also complained of pain with turning in bed and while climbing stairs. Posturally, she had decreased lumbar lordosis and pelvic asymmetry both in sitting and standing.

In terms of flexibility, she had tight hamstrings bilaterally and extremely tight external rotators on the

TABLE 6–4.

Flexion-Extension-Asymmetry Principles

Most frequent signs—flexion principle
Increased lumbar lordosis, but may slouch in sitting position.
No lordotic reversal noted in forward bending.
Does not have full range of motion of forward bending.
Extreme range of backward bending—painful at end range.
Sustained forward bending eases pain.
Repeated backward bending increases pain.
Sustained backward bending increases pain.
Repeated forward bending causes pain but does not worsen it.
Tight iliopsoas.
Short erector spinae.
Large gluteal mass.
Tight latissimus dorsi and pectorals.
Weak lower abdominals, increased lordosis.
Most frequent symptoms—flexion principle
Feels better sitting.
Pain occurs with walking and is most severe when standing.
Pain increased by prone lying (may also be worse with supine lying with knees straight).
Pain worse with overhead work.
Most frequent signs—extension principle
Decreased lumbar lordosis.
Lordotic reversal noted in forward bending.
Lumbar extension limited.
Tight hamstrings.
Small gluteal mass.
Weak gluteals.
Sustained forward bending increases pain.
Repeated forward bending increases pain.
Sustained backward bending eases pain.
Most frequent symptoms—extension principle
Pain is worse with prolonged sitting.
Pain is worse with driving.
Pain is worse with stooping and bending.
More comfortable lying.
Feel better walking.
Increased pain upon rising from a seated position.
Most frequent signs—asymmetry principle
Unequal hip height in standing and/or sitting.
Leg length difference.
Unequal strength from right to left in selected muscles of hip and back (most common: hip abduction weakness in one side).
Unequal flexibility from right to left in selected muscles of hip and back (most common: tight piriformis on one side).
Most frequent symptoms—asymmetry principle
Painful to stand on one leg (so may avoid and stand on other).
Relief when legs are crossed in sitting.
Painful when walking on uneven surfaces.
Tender to touch at posterior/superior iliac spines.

low side of the pelvic asymmetry. Her gluteal strength bilaterally was 3/5. On palpation, she had exquisite tenderness over the quadratus lumborum musculature. Her treatment program included moist heat and electrical stimulation to the lumbar paraspinal and gluteal muscles, followed by ultrasound and ischemic compression to the involved trigger points. Stretching of the quadratus lumborum hamstrings and external rotators was then performed. The patient was then instructed in a therapeutic exercise program, which included neutral stabilization strengthening and hamstring stretches. A reevaluation of her pelvic asymmetry revealed that following the stretching and soft tissue work, her pelvis was level and her apparent leg length discrepancy resolved.

Unfortunately, because of the amount of muscle guarding with which she presented her pelvic asymmetry recurred. She was then given the environmental modifications of a shoe lift and a "butt lift" as a temporary means of reducing the asymmetrical forces she was encountering. After 2 weeks of continued use of modalities, exercise, and environmental modifications, she was slowly weaned from the shoe lift and the butt lift; her pelvis remained symmetrical and she remained asymptomatic. She was then instructed in a more progressive exercise program, which included cardiovascular conditioning and pain-free range-of-motion exercises.

It is not the authors' intention to simplify the treatment of thoracolumbar mechanical low back pain into three categories. Rather, therapists are challenged to use this information combined with additional facts gained from the initial evaluation, subsequent treatments and the literature to develop appropriate and comprehensive rehabilitation programs (Table 6–5).

TABLE 6–5.

Summary of Treatment Techniques for Flexion, Extension, and Asymmetry

Flexion treatment techniques
1. Modalities to relax and loosen lumbar musculature.
2. Soft tissue mobilization and stretching of lumbar muscles.
3. Flexion and stabilization exercises.
4. Modify the environment:
    a. Sit frequently if needed for relief of soreness.
    b. Sleep in the fetal position.
Extension treatment techniques
1. Modalities to relax and loosen lumbar musculature.
2. Soft tissue mobilization and stretching of lumbar muscles.
3. Extension and stabilization exercises.
4. Avoid flexion activities.
5. Modify the environment:
    a. Use a lumbar roll when sitting.
    b. Stand and arch frequently.
    c. Sleep prone or supine without pillows.
Asymmetry treatment techniques
1. Modalities to relax and loosen lumbar and hip musculature.
2. Soft tissue mobilization and stretching of lumbar muscles.
3. Stretch asymmetrically shortened muscles.
4. Strengthening asymmetrically weak muscles.
5. Modify the environment:
    a. Use a heel lift or butt lift if the hips are unequal.
    b. If side-lying, place pillows between knees.

EVALUATION

In the conservative management of thoracolumbar pain, a thorough initial evaluation cannot be overemphasized. An example of a geriatric low back evaluation is shown on p. 70. (Fig 6–6).

The low back evaluation could be used on any aged person. What is specific to the geriatric patient will be covered in the next few pages.

The subjective evaluation will, in most instances, indicate not only what is wrong with the patient, but how to treat that patient effectively. Defining loss of functional activities (e.g., shooting pain into right lower extremity after 10 steps) not only makes the clinician aware of important functional deficits but provides good documentation material. Writing skilled notes is just as important as performing skilled care.

The visual analog scale is another documentation tool used to write skilled notes in reference to defining subjective complaints of pain. Figure 6–7 is a visual analog scale with a description of how to use it. An example of an initial scale given to a patient is on the left; on the right is a discharge scale after the therapist has evaluated it.

The patient is asked to mark on the figure (see Fig 6–7, A) where he or she would rate his or her pain on a scale from unbearable pain to no pain. The therapist then measures the line from 0 to 100 mm (see Fig 6–7,B). At discharge or to record progress, the therapist gives the patient a new scale. Again, a number is recorded after the therapist remeasures the new line. A patient should not be shown the previous analog scale when performing the discharge analog scale.

Specific postural changes noted in elderly people have already been briefly discussed in the anatomy section. Forward head position, rounded shoulders, increased thoracic kyphosis, and decreased lumbar lordosis may all be noted. Postural screening tools (such as the Reedco posture score sheet, Fig 6–8) that give quantitative feedback may be helpful in objectively evaluating the older person.

Active range of motion of the thoracolumbar spine has been shown to decrease in all planes in elderly people. Many elderly people will tolerate a standing range of motion evaluation, but the authors' experience is that repetitions of active movement will many times severely exacerbate the problem therapists are trying to treat. The geriatric clinician must become skilled at evaluating motion

Back Pain Evaluation

Date _____

Name _____ Diagnosis _____

Age _____ Blood pressure _____

Present History _____ General health _____
_____ _____
_____
  Bowel/bladder _____
Past history _____ _____
_____
_____ Numbness/tingling _____
  _____
Medications _____ _____
_____
_____ Shooting pain _____

Testing (X-ray, MRI) _____ _____
_____ Visual analog score _____

Posture _____ Flexibility
_____ Hamstrings _____
_____ Iliopsoas _____
  Rectus femoris _____
Active ROM Iliotibial band _____
Flexion _____ Gastrocnemius _____
Extension _____ Soleus _____
Right rotation _____
Left rotation _____
Right sidebending _____ Reflexes
Left sidebending _____ Ankle jerk _____R _____L
  Knee jerk _____R _____L
Passive ROM
Flexion _____ Strength
Extension _____ Abdominal _____
Right rotation _____ Hip flexor _____
Left rotation_____ Hip extensor _____
Right sidebending _____ Hip abduction _____
Left sidebending _____ Hip adduction _____
  Knee extension _____
Palpation/muscle guarding _____ Knee flexion _____
_____ Dorsiflexion _____
_____ Plantarflexion _____

Gait _____ SLR _____R _____L
_____
_____

Balance _____
_____

FIG 6–6.
Low back evaluation form.

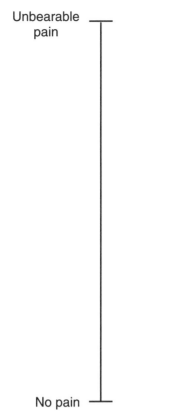

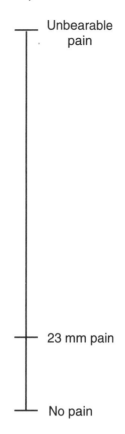

FIG 6–7.
Visual analog scale. **A,** patient is given this scale and asked to mark on the line indicating level of pain at the present time. The therapist then measures the distance from "no pain" to the mark. **B,** therapist's evaluation of pain level. This patient had 23 mm of pain on the visual analog scale, measured from "no pain" or 0 mm to the patient's mark.

with one repetition for all the planes of movement. For many geriatric patients, the standing evaluation in itself is too rigorous and a modified sitting evaluation must be performed. Figure 6–9 illustrates the modified sitting range of motion evaluation.

Standing balance is also included in the evaluation of the geriatric patient. Richard Bohannon's balance scores provide a norm for someone 70 years old (14 seconds).[1] In our clinic, we use this value as a screening mechanism for the relationship between standing balance and lower extremity weakness, as a possible screen for referred low back pain or sacroiliac joint dysfunction. If a patient is unable to stand for 14 seconds, then this cues the therapist to investigate the above-noted possibilities.

Gait is also evaluated. Below is a list of normal gait changes noted in the elderly:

- Fewer automatic movements
- Decreased speed and amplitude of automatic movements

- Increased muscle activity in the gait cycle
- Less accuracy and slower movement, especially in the hip
- Decreased swing-to-stance ratio
- Decreased vertical displacement
- Broader stride width
- Increased toe-floor clearance
- Decreased heel-floor angle
- Slower cadence
- Decreased rotation of the hips and the shoulders
- More abnormalities in posture
- Mild rigidity, particularly in proximal regions[3]

Patients with hip problems will often lurch over the affected hip. Patients with low back problems may lurch away from the painful side. Limping because of pain or weakness, as well as significant decreased trunk rotation owing to pain and muscle guarding may also be noted.

POSTURE SCORE SHEET	Name _____			SCORING DATES				
	GOOD - 10	FAIR - 5	POOR - 0					
HEAD LEFT RIGHT	HEAD ERECT GRAVITY LINE PASSES DIRECTLY THROUGH CENTER	HEAD TWISTED OR TURNED TO ONE SIDE SLIGHTLY	HEAD TWISTED OR TURNED TO ONE SIDE MARKEDLY					
SHOULDERS LEFT RIGHT	SHOULDERS LEVEL (HORIZONTALLY)	ONE SHOULDER SLIGHTLY HIGHER THAN OTHER	ONE SHOULDER MARKEDLY HIGHER THAN OTHER					
SPINE LEFT RIGHT	SPINE STRAIGHT	SPINE SLIGHTLY CURVED LATERALLY	SPINE MARKEDLY CURVED LATERALLY					
HIPS LEFT RIGHT	HIPS LEVEL (HORIZONTALLY)	ONE HIP SLIGHTLY HIGHER	ONE HIP MARKEDLY HIGHER					
ANKLES	FEET POINTED STRAIGHT AHEAD	FEET POINTED OUT	FEET POINTED OUT MARKEDLY ANKLES SAG IN (PRONATION)					
NECK	NECK ERECT, CHIN IN, HEAD IN BALANCE DIRECTLY ABOVE SHOULDERS	NECK SLIGHTLY FORWARD, CHIN SLIGHTLY OUT	NECK MARKEDLY FORWARD, CHIN MARKEDLY OUT					
UPPER BACK	UPPER BACK NORMALLY ROUNDED	UPPER BACK SLIGHTLY MORE ROUNDED	UPPER BACK MARKEDLY ROUNDED					
TRUNK	TRUNK ERECT	TRUNK INCLINED TO REAR SLIGHTLY	TRUNK INCLINED TO REAR MARKEDLY					
ABDOMEN	ABDOMEN FLAT	ABDOMEN PROTRUDING	ABDOMEN PROTRUDING AND SAGGING					
LOWER BACK	LOWER BACK NORMALLY CURVED	LOWER BACK SLIGHTLY HOLLOW	LOWER BACK MARKEDLY HOLLOW					
ALL REPRODUCTION RIGHTS RESERVED © **REEDCO** "The Good Posture People" P.O. BOX 345 • 51 NO. FULTON ST. AUBURN, N.Y. 13021 (315) 252-0020 COPYRIGHT 1974		**TOTAL SCORES**						

FIG 6–8.
Reedco posture score sheet. (Reprinted with permission of Reedco Research.)

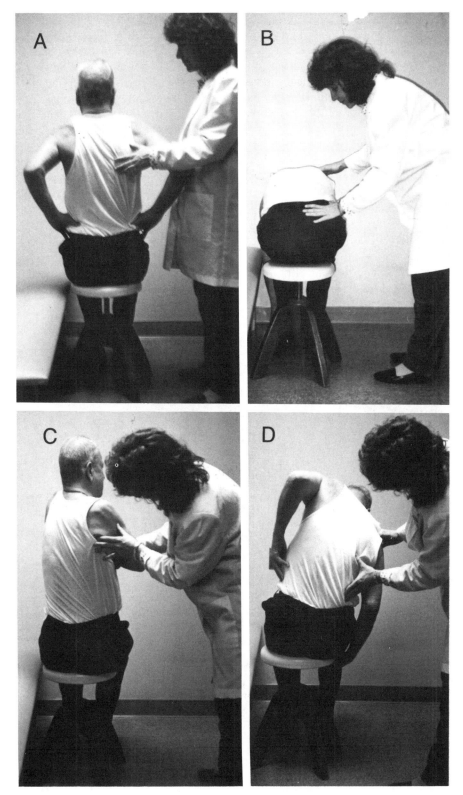

FIG 6–9.
Modified lumbar spine sitting range of motion. Patient is asked to flex (**A**) and extend (**B**), rotate in both directions (**C**), and laterally flex in both directions (**D**). Decrements in motion in all directions are noted by the therapist, as are discrepancies from left to right.

TREATMENT

Unfortunately, in many instances medical attention is not sought until an actual functional activity can no longer be performed (e.g., unable to climb stairs).

As health care providers, we realize that the functional ability to go up and down stairs was not lost in 1 day as many patients will describe. Rather, a slow, gradual decline in strength, flexibility, and endurance occurred, which caused a decreased ability to climb the stairs. Postural changes occur in a similar fashion. In the elderly, gradual muscle weakness and decreases in flexibility are not easily corrected with stretching or strengthening. Environmental modifications may be the best alternative.

Environmental modifications also include positioning. Finding a comfortable sleeping position for

the patient that allows him or her to wake up in less pain is important (See Fig 6–2,A and B).

In addition, posture, for example, reveals specific pelvic asymmetries, such as one iliac crest or posterior superior iliac spine that is higher than another. The supine evaluation may reveal one malleolus lower than another. These asymmetries are typically associated with both flexibility and strength changes most commonly noted in the hip musculature. Travell's work suggests a pelvic lift under the involved lower ischial tuberosity and a heel lift under the involved foot to correct asymmetries that do not respond to stretching and strengthening exercises.[16]

The authors have mentioned modalities as adjuncts to treatment. They may play a critical role in the rehabilitation strategy if used effectively. Application of heat prior to stretching and ice used to decrease inflammation are a regular part of the treatment progression. Gentle oscillation and mobi-

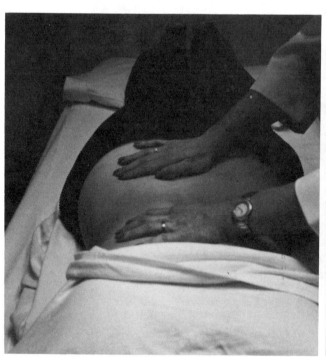
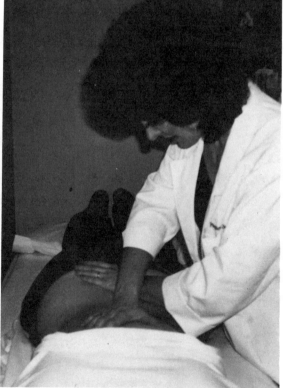

FIG 6–10.
A, rotation oscillation. Therapist places hands on sacrum and upper lumbar spine and gently rocks the sacrum and pelvis side-to-side while stabilizing with upper hand. For more specific joint mobilization, the therapist can block the spinous processes at various levels while rocking with hand on sacrum. **B,** posterior distraction. With hand placement and gentle rocking motion as in **A,** therapist pushes upper hand cephalad and sacral hand caudally, thus providing a gentle distraction in the lumbar spine.

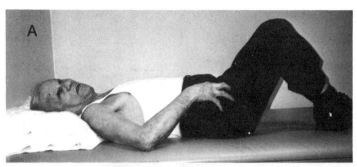

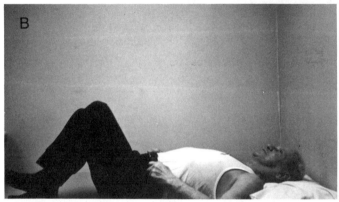

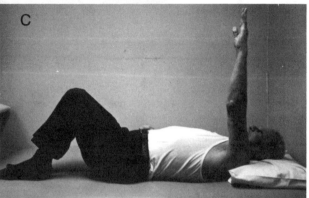

FIG 6–11.
Neutral stabilization progression. The patient is assisted to find the position of comfort. **A,** once this is done, the patient stabilizes this position by tightening abdominal and buttock muscles. **B,** while maintaining this position, the patient adds

his own body resistance by gently lifting legs alternately, one at a time, and **C,** lifting alternating arms. The authors feel this arm on body motion closely approximates functional activity.

lization techniques are tools used in the treatment of hypomobility and muscle guarding. Figure 6–10 illustrates both oscillation and mobilization techniques.

Therapeutic exercise that activates the muscu-

loskeletal system is the only noninvasive means by which the structure and function of the spine can be effectively influenced.[11]

Therapists are challenged to find the pain-free position and exercise program that will allow their

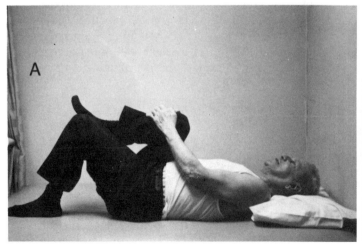

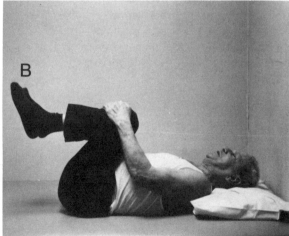

FIG 6–12.
Flexion exercises. **A,** single knee to chest; **B,** double knee to chest.

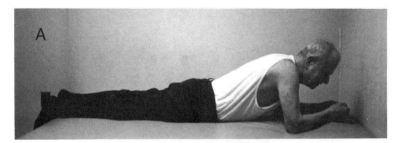

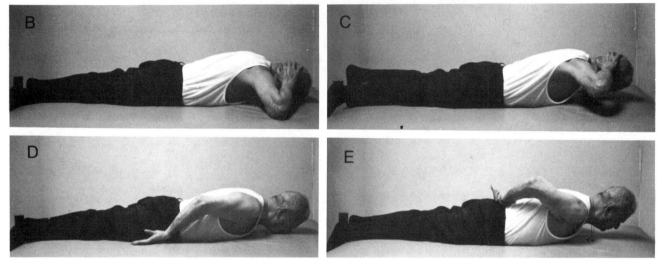

FIG 6–13.
Extension exercises. **A,** prone props; **B** and **C,** upper thoracic extension; **D** and **E,** lumbar extension.

patients to begin their earliest exercise progression. Patients will not comply with painful exercise programs; thus, pain-free stabilization and strengthening programs leading to pain-free active range of motion are needed. Figure 6–11 represents neutral stabilization progression.

Figures 6–12, 6–13, and 6–14 are examples of flexion, extension, and asymmetry exercises. Sinaki and Lutness did an excellent study involving spondylolisthesis patients. Their research indicates that spondylolisthesis patients did substantially bet-

ter with flexion exercises as opposed to extension exercises.[15] McKenzie suggests that centralization of peripheral pain caused by a protruding disc will, however, benefit from extension exercises.[12a]

The type of exercise programs developed can be creative but must be appropriate. Prescribing flexion exercises for a compression fracture is not only inappropriate but borders on malpractice. Therapists must become experts at combining exercise, stretching, modalities, and manual techniques into the individual program that will get patients better.

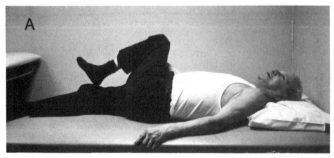

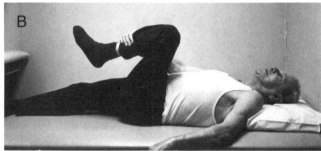

FIG 6–14.
Asymmetry exercises. **A,** piriformis stretch; **B,** sacroiliac stretch.

CONCLUSIONS

Appropriately evaluating and treating low back pain in any aged person is an exciting challenge. When the pain occurs in an older person, the task can become overwhelming. This chapter attempts to consolidate research information on the aging lumbar spine with clinical techniques from various disciplines to provide options in the treatment of these conditions.

REFERENCES

1. Bohannon RW: Decreases in timed balance test scores with aging. *Phys Ther* 1984; 64:1067–1071.
2. Costell R: Age related strength changes (lecture notes). Cybex seminar, San Diego, Calif, August 1989.
3. Findley FR, Coaly KA: Locomotion patterns in elderly women. *Arch Phys Med Rehabil* 1967; 50:140.
4. Frost H: Clinical management of the symptomatic osteoporotic patient. *Orthop Clin North Am* 1981; 12:671–681.
5. Gandy S, Payne R: Back pain in the elderly: Updated diagnosis and management. *Geriatrics* 1986; 41:12.
6. Grabias S, Mankin H: Pain in the lower back. *Bull Rheum Dis* 1980; 30:1040–1044.
7. Kaufmann T: Osteoporosis. *Geritopics* 1984; 7:1–9.
8. Knortz K: Muscle physiology applied to geriatric rehabilitation. *Top Geriatr Rehabil* 1987; 2:1–9.
9. Lee BC, Kazam E: Computed tomography of the spinal cord. *Radiology* 1978; 129:717–719.
10. Lewis C: *Osteoporosis Exercise Booklet.* Rockville, MD, Aspen, 1987.
11. Liemohn W: Exercise and the back. *Rheum Dis Clin North Am* 1990; 16:945–951.
12. MacKinnon JL: Osteoporosis: A review. *Phys Ther* 1988; 68:1553–1540.
12a. McKenzie RA: *The Lumbar Spine: Diagnosis and Therapy.* New Zealand, 1981, pp. 4–8.
13. Mooney V: Surgery and postsurgical management of the patient with low back pain. *Phys Ther* 1979; 59:1000–1006.
14. Sinaki M, Mikkelson B: Postmenopausal spinal osteoporosis: Flexion vs extension exercises. *Arch Phys Med Rehabil* 1984; 65:593–596.
15. Sinaki M, Lutness M: Lumbar spondylolithesis: Retrospective comparison and three-year follow-up of two conservative treatment programs. *Arch Phys Med Rehabil* 1989; 70:594–598.
16. Travell J, Simons D: *Myofascial Pain and Dysfunction.* Baltimore, Md, Williams & Wilkins, 1983, pp. 650–654.
17. Twomey LT, Taylor JR: Sagittal movements of the human lumbar vertebral column: A quantitative study of the role of the posterior vertebral elements. *Arch Phys Med Rehabil* 1983; 64:322.
18. Twomey LT, Taylor JR: *Physical Therapy of the Low Back,* New York, Churchill Livingstone, 1987, pp. 38–79.
19. Wiesel S, Bernini P: *The Aging Lumbar Spine.* Philadelphia, WB Saunders, 1982.
20. Wilson ES, Brill RF: Spinal stenosis: The narrow lumbar canal syndrome. *Clin Orthop* 1977; 122:244–248.
21. Watkins R, Campbell D: The older athlete after lumbar spine surgery. *Clin Sports Medicine* 1991; 10:391–399.

Chapter 7

Cervical Spine Complications: An Orthopedic Perspective

Richard J. Nasca, M.D.

Pain originating in the cervical spine is a common complaint. Most of us have experienced getting out of bed with a stiff neck, which usually improves spontaneously. Often neck and upper extremity radicular pain will occur without any provocation. Such a clinical presentation is most likely related to changes in the health of the cervical intervertebral discs and irritation of their corresponding nerve roots. Fortunately, these symptoms are usually of short duration. Aging of our cervical spine begins during infancy. During the third decade, degenerative changes can be documented by discography and histologic evaluation of the cervical discs.[5, 17] Like the thoracic and lumbar spine, the cervical spine must not be regarded as an isolated structure, but rather as an integral part of the body, susceptible to systemic as well as local diseases and disorders. Although osteoporosis and osteomalacia are not as common in the cervical spine as in other skeletal areas, these conditions may occur alone or in combination with other systemic diseases and inflammatory arthritis.

Cancer and infection may affect the cervical spine, causing destruction of bone resulting in instability and spinal cord compression with paralysis. The therapist and physician must be aware of systemic as well as local pathologic conditions affecting the cervical spine. Common clinical disorders and diseases involving the cervical spine will be discussed here, as well as the diagnostic methods and treatment modalities.

GENERAL CONSIDERATIONS OF THE AGING CERVICAL SPINE

As we age, our cervical spines become less flexible and less resistant to axial, shear, and torsional forces. Elastin and collagen fibers degenerate, resulting in less-supple connective tissue support for the vertebral motion segments. Water content in the nucleus pulposus and in the surrounding annulus fibrosis is progressively reduced with age. As a result of these histologic and chemical changes, fissures occur within the intervertebral disc. These defects often progress into the annulus and result in tears. Once this process of degeneration starts, it progresses. During the fourth and fifth decades multilevel disc degeneration can be observed in the majority of cervical spines.[5, 7] As the disc degenerates, disc height and functional stability are reduced. Loss of vertebral stature is in large part a result of loss in height of most of our intervertebral discs. Increase in shirt collar size may result from the shortening associated with multilevel disc degeneration. As the disc degenerates, the facets also become incongruent. Facet articular cartilage wears out. Depending on the healing response, through production of osteophytes, various degrees of spinal instability may result.[1] If the spine does not self-stabilize, segmental instability may result in pain with motion, irritation, or compression of adjacent nerve roots or the spinal cord. Progressive disc space narrowing may result in a loss of normal cervical lordosis, cervical scoliosis, and kyphosis. Because of its linkage to the thoracic spine, fixed deformities of the former may cause compensatory changes in the cervical spine such as hyperlordosis in response to progressive thoracic kyphosis.

As disc height decreases, osteophytes form around the periphery of the disc at the disc-vertebral margins in an attempt to "heal and stabilize" the pathologic process. Osteophytes also form in and around the Luschka joints and in the vicinity of the neural canals. These osteophytes, along with reduced space and supporting function of the disc, may result in intermittent nerve root irritation and/or compression. Recent work by Weinstein[21, 22] has shown chemical substances such as substance P, prostaglandins, and various peptides can have a direct irritant effect on the dorsal root ganglion of the nerve root at the spinal level in which degeneration of the disc is progressing. Osteophytes also form along the posterior peripheral margins of the vertebral bodies and result in compromise of spinal cord circumference through reduction in the anterior-posterior diameter. Degeneration is most common in the C4–5, C5–6, and C6–7 high-motion segments.

Acute disc herniation results from extrusion of nuclear material through defects in the annulus fibrosus. These extruded discs can cause acute compression of the adjacent nerve root or spinal cord. Rarely, free fragments of disc material can find their way into the epidural space. Cervical cord compression may result from pressure on the delicate anterior spinal artery and its branches to the cervical cord.[1]

COMMON CAUSES OF NECK PAIN IN THE OLDER PATIENT

Cervical degenerative disc disease may result in significant neck and upper extremity radicular pain (Table 7–1). The radicular pain may be associated with muscle weakness, loss of sensation, or decrease in deep tendon reflexes.[17] Because of their high degrees of motion and stress, the C4–5, C5–6, and C6–7 levels are commonly the most symptomatic.[20] If cord compression occurs as a result of cervical spondylosis, appendicular spasticity and loss of bowel and bladder control may occur. These symptoms can be insidious at onset, but should raise the

TABLE 7–1.

Causes of Neck Pain in Aged People

Common Causes
   Degenerative disc and facet joints
   Cervical spondylosis without myelopathy
   Cervical spondylosis with myelopathy
   Spinal fractures
   Soft tissue injuries
Less common causes
   Herniated disc
   Metastatic disease
   Spinal infection
   Inflammatory arthritis
   Congenital anomalies

examiner's suspicion. A careful and complete neurologic evaluation is necessary.

The typical acute cervical disc herniation occurs in patients in the third, fourth, and fifth decades, often after minimal or no trauma. Very severe radicular pain into the shoulder, arm, forearm and hand may divert the examiner's attention away from the neck. At times, range of motion of the neck is maintained with an acute cervical disc herniation. Patients will obtain relief of their radicular pain by positioning the affected upper extremity in abduction, flexion, and external rotation, typically with the palm of the hand resting behind the head. This reduces tension on the cervical-brachial plexus and the affected nerve root.

Cervical spondylosis usually involves the C3–4, C4–5, C5–6, and C6–7 motion segments. A reduced cervical spinal canal diameter may be a significant contributing factor. Degenerative changes in the facet joints and intervertebral discs superimposed on a reduced spinal canal diameter result in bony compression of the cervical spinal cord and adjacent nerve roots.

Patients with cervical spondylosis and cervical myelopathy most often complain of abnormal sensations in the extremities associated with clumsiness and weakness. Walking at night may become difficult owing to lack of proprioception in the lower extremities. Wasting and atrophy of the extremity musculature may be seen. A broad-based, jerky gait may result. Frequent dropping of objects may occur as a result of loss of proprioception and intrinsic muscle strength.[1, 17] Loss of pain, temperature, position, and vibratory sensation is caused by involvement of the spinothalamic tracts and the posterior columns. Bowel and bladder sphincter control are usually preserved. Cervical spondylosis may coexist with lumbar stenosis, making it necessary to evaluate thoroughly the lumbar as well as the cervical spine and its contents.

Pathologic evaluation of cadaver cervical spines removed from those affected with cervical spondylosis and myelopathy demonstrates indentations of the cervical cord owing to osteophytes arising from the affected posterior disc levels.[14] Progressive disc space narrowing coupled with facet joint overriding, degeneration, and thickening of the ligamenta flava result in dorsal compression of the spinal cord around the posterior columns. This combination of ventral and dorsal osteophytosis produces significant compression of the cervical cord and its blood supply.

As the disc degenerates, the corresponding Luschka joints also show signs of osteophyte formation. In an unpublished study, we noted that when Luschka joint osteophytes were seen on plain radiographs of the cadaver cervical spine, degeneration of the disc verified by discography and pathologic examination was confirmed to be present. As the Luschka joint osteophytes progress, ventral compression of the corresponding nerve root occurs. As the facet joint degenerates and forms bony spurs, the corresponding nerve root is compressed dorsally. The combination of Luschka and facet joint osteophyte formation can result in circumferential nerve root compression within the nerve root canal.

Congenital anomalies resulting from defects in vertebral segment formation or failure of segmentation occurs infrequently yet may cause significant problems in the cervical spine. Congenital anomalies of the odontoid process may lead to C1–2 instabilities and spinal cord compression. Klippel-Feil syndrome is characterized by an unusually short neck, low hairline, and severe restriction in range of motion. Usually several vertebrae fail to segment and appear as "fused vertebrae." Flexion and extension motion may occur at only one or two segmented interspaces. Rotation and lateral bending are usually significantly compromised. Congenital elevation of the scapula (Sprengel's deformity) may be associated with Klippel-Feil syndrome.

Congenital hemivertebrae may interpose themselves between normal vertebrae and result in a lateral scoliosis of the cervical spine. Kyphotic and lordotic deformities may occur owing to congenital spinal anomalies. Often these deformities remain asymptomatic until midlife when progressive degenerative changes occur and result in cord and or nerve root compressive syndromes.

Traumatic fractures and dislocation of the cervical spine result in significant morbidity when cord involvement occurs. Spontaneous compression fractures of the cervical spine associated with osteoporosis and osteomalacia are rarely seen, in contrast to those occurring in the thoracic and lumbar spine. Patients with severe rheumatoid arthritis commonly present with a kyphotic, collapsing cervical spine. Loss of bone integrity and density owing to osteoporosis, steroid administration, and the rheumatoid disease process itself make this a difficult problem to manage nonoperatively. Metastatic cancer from the lung, breast, and prostate commonly seed the marrow of the vertebral bodies. Destruction of the vertebral body and posterior elements can result in acute quadriplegia. Although spinal infection is rare, acute bacterial infection can involve the vertebral body and disc. Severe neck and radicular pain may result. Bacterial, tuberculous, and fungal infections involving retropharyngeal and paravertebral structures may invade the cervical spine through direct penetration, as well as by blood-borne routes. Epidural spread with pus under pressure may result in cord compression.

Ankylosing spondylitis of the cervical spine results in reduced neck motion in all directions. Progressive kyphotic deformity of the thoracic spine and a lordotic posture of the cervical spine are commonly seen. Patients with ankylosing spondylitis need to be warned that a sudden improvement in motion after a fall or other trauma is the result of a fracture, which must be quickly stabilized to protect the cord from damage resulting from instability.

EVALUATION OF THE AGING CERVICAL SPINE

A carefully taken, detailed history is necessary in order to properly evaluate cervical spine complaints. Older people may be unaware of or reluctant to report mild to moderate functional deficiencies such as proprioceptive loss and clumsy gait. A thorough examination of the spine and extremities as well as a careful neurologic examination is required. The examiner must search for clonus, exaggerated deep tendon reflexes, and proprioceptive and coordination deficits. Combinations of upper and lower motor neuron involvement are commonly seen in cervical spondylosis. Upper motor neuron involvement results from cord myelopathy, whereas the lower motor neuron deficits are caused by root level compression.

High-quality radiographs of the spine are necessary. Dynamic bending views can be of value in assessing deformities and instabilities. Electromyography (EMG) is of value in detecting specific nerve root compression and in excluding polyneuropathies such as those seen in diabetes and demyelinating spinal cord diseases. Contrast-enhanced computed tomography (CT) allows for critical assessment of the spinal and nerve root canals and their contents. Because of rapid flow and reduced volume and in the interest of keeping contrast medium out of the cerebrospinal fluid, water-soluble myelography of the cervical spine requires more attention to positioning and technique than does lumbar myelography. Image quality may be less than optimal on spot films taken during cervical myelography; however, postmyelography CT will usually allow for better definition of suspected pathologic areas. Magnetic resonance imaging (MRI) provides an excellent method of visualizing the spinal cord and its thecal coverings. Degenerative and herniated discs produce abnormalities on the T_2-weighted signals owing to changes in hydration. The image quality in cervical MRI often makes it possible to readily appreciate pathologic degrees of compression of the neural elements that may not be as well defined on contrast-enhanced CT. As in the lumbar spine, several adjacent discs in the cervical spine may demonstrate abnormal MRI signals. Cervical discography may be helpful in determining the symptomatic level. Cervical nerve root blocks may be of value in defining the root transmitting the radicular pain. Injection of small quantities of local anesthetics around the symptomatic nerve root must be done with care to avoid intrathecal administration, which can lead to a high spinal anesthesia requiring ventilatory support. Radionuclide bone scans are useful in ruling out metastatic cancer, infection, or an occult fracture. Percutaneous needle biopsies of the vertebral bodies and discs using image intensification to aid in proper needle placement may be necessary to obtain tissue for pathologic and microbiologic examination to determine the etiology of the patient's complaints.

A complete blood cell count, sedimentation rate, and chemistry profile, including calcium, phosphorus, and acid and alkaline phosphantase determination can be useful, as discussed in the section on evaluation of the aging thoracolumbar spine. A summary of the factors in cervical spine evaluation appear in Table 7–2.

NONOPERATIVE MANAGEMENT OF THE AGING CERVICAL SPINE

For the majority of patients with cervical spine symptoms, simple, common sense treatment is effective (Table 7–3). Rest and reduction of the stressful activities that are implicated as causative factors are the first measures to be taken. Referral to a physical therapist skilled in assisting patients with spine disorders is indicated, not only to provide therapeutic modalities, but for education, support, and encouragement during the rehabilitative phase. Heat, ice, massage, traction, and gentle manual manipulation are helpful. Contoured cervical pillows are useful aids for sleep. Soft cervical collars are of value for short periods during acute attacks and exacerbations. Home cervical over-the-door traction may be beneficial, but the patient must be carefully instructed in its use. Positioning the head and neck in a slight flexion or neutral rather than extension is usually best, since this position allows more space for the spinal contents. Isometric exercises to increase strength of the cervical musculature are beneficial. Activities that require rotation, lateral neck flexion and hyperextension should be avoided. Free-style swimming can be done with the use of a mask and snorkel to facilitate breathing without head turning.

Nonsteroidal anti-inflammatory drugs (NSAIDs) are effective in reducing inflammation. It may be necessary to try several types of NSAID before finding one that is of value and well tolerated. Adverse gastrointestinal side effects occur in approximately

TABLE 7–2.
Evaluation of the Aging Cervical Spine

Complete history and physical
EMG, MRI, CT with contrast
Bone scan
Sedimentation rate, arthritis screen
Calcium, phosphorus, acid and alkaline phosphatase levels

TABLE 7–3.
Nonoperative Management of the Aging Cervical Spine

Rest, heat, cold, massage
Ultrasound, manipulation, traction
Isometric exercises
Anti-inflammatory drugs
Cervical collar
Epidural steroids

one of three patients. Also, with time an NSAID may no longer be effective for a particular patient, requiring a change to another class of anti-inflammatory drugs. Compliance may also be a factor with three- or four-times daily dosages. Muscle relaxants and oral pain medications are useful during acute phases or periods of exacerbation, but long-term reliance on these medications is discouraged. Epidural instillation of steroids may be of benefit in relieving cervical radiculitis; however, if symptoms are caused by a compressed nerve root, relief will usually be only temporary. Epidurally administered steroids are contraindicated in the presence of infection.

OPERATIVE TREATMENT OF THE AGING CERVICAL SPINE

Reconstructive surgery of the spine has progressed during the last decade. Recent diagnostic and therapeutic developments have enabled surgeons to carry out restorative procedures for patients with debilitating spine injuries and disorders (Table 7–4). Presently there are no effective replacement parts for the spine equivalent to those used for total joint arthroplasty; however, during the past few years, a number of spinal implants have been developed and are useful in stabilizing the traumatic and degenerative spine.[16, 23] As in the lumbar and thoracic spine, the spinal surgeon must depend on the patient's ability to heal and make bone in the fusion area. Allograft bone, calcium hydroxyapatite, and tricalcium phosphate show promise as useful biomaterials in spinal arthrodesis surgery.[12, 13]

The following conditions often require surgical management:

Herniated Disc Causing Nerve Root Compression

A herniated cervical disc causing nerve root compression not responsive to conservative treatment may require surgery.[2, 3] Disc herniation com-

TABLE 7–4.

Operative Treatment of the Aging Cervical Spine

Disc excision with or without fusion for herniated disc
Anterior decompression and fusion for spondylosis
Laminoplasty decompression for spondylosis
Anterior or posterior stabilization of fractures
Excision and stabilization for tumors and infection

monly occurs at the high-motion segments of C4–5, C5–6, and C6–7. As the intradiscal contents leave the annulus, they may migrate around the adjacent nerve root resulting in radiculopathy. If the herniated disc displaces into the epidural space, cord compression may result. Uncommonly, free fragments of disc material may be found in the epidural space. Patients usually present with severe radicular pain involving the upper extremity and shoulder girdle area. Commonly in a C5–6 disc herniation, the patient loses the biceps reflex and biceps muscle strength. Numbness along the dorsal aspect of the thumb and index finger is typical. Disc herniation of C4–5 results in numbness around the shoulder and weakness of the deltoid muscle. Deep tendon reflexes are not altered. Herniations of the C6–7 disc cause depression of the triceps reflex, weakness of the triceps muscle, and numbness of the long and ring fingers. Because of variation in neural anatomy, this classical presentation may not be present. The clinician and therapist should be cognizant that brachial plexus neuropathies of various etiologies, herpes zoster radiculitis, and spinal cord and nerve root tumors may mimic cervical disc herniation in their initial symptoms.

If conservative therapy fails, surgical disc excision is performed using either an anterior or posterior approach.[2, 10, 19] The posterior approach requires a cervical laminectomy and exposure of the compressed nerve root in conjunction with disc excision. The anterior approach has gained popularity in the last three decades. Through this approach, the disc is removed, a search is made for free fragments, and an interbody fusion is done using the patient's own or banked bone. The purpose of the fusion is to restore stability to the involved motion segment and to prevent further collapse and kyphotic deformity of the disc space. Results of surgical treatment are good to excellent in 85% to 90% of patients treated by anterior disc excision and fusion.[2, 6, 10] With either approach, careful documentation of the involved level with intraoperative x-ray is mandatory. It requires 8 to 10 weeks for the anterior cervical bone graft to heal. Patients are protected during this time with a cervical collar. Reduction of cervical range of motion is rarely noted by the patient undergoing a one- or two-level anterior cervical fusion.

Degenerative Cervical Disc Disease (Spondylosis), With and Without Myelopathy

Cervical spondylosis most commonly involves the C4–5, C5–6, and C6–7 motion segments.

Symptoms of nerve root irritation or compression may result from degenerative discs, osteophytes, and/or instabilities. Cervical myelopathy resulting from cord compression may occur with the progression of cervical spondylosis. Anterior cervical decompression and fusion has gained popularity in treating cervical spondylosis with myelopathy.[9] The procedure consists of excision of degenerative discs, as well as anterior and posterior lateral osteophytes. Removal of the collapsed disc contents and adjacent vertebral body allows access into the anterior epidural space. Decompression may be necessary at several levels. Usually a longitudinal strut bone graft is placed to support the resected area, which results in fusion. The Japanese have popularized the procedure of cervical laminoplasty decompression for cervical myelopathy.[11] This procedure consists of cutting the laminae so they can be lifted off the posterior epidural space. The laminae are then repositioned by sutures during healing. Postoperative CT scans confirm enlargement of the cervical epidural space after laminoplasty.[9, 11] Resection of the spinous processes and laminae and partial cervical facetectomy has resulted in cervical kyphotic deformities after posterior decompression. For this reason, long and wide posterior decompressive procedures without fusion or laminoplasty have lost popularity. The indications for multilevel anterior interbody fusion for degenerative disc disease with radiculitis is less clear. In patients whose symptoms are recurrent, disabling, and not responsive to conservative therapy, arthrodesis may be helpful. Cervical discography can be useful in evaluating these patients. Results are 80% to 90% good to excellent in patients undergoing one- or two-level anterior cervical fusions.[2, 6, 19] Patients with disease at multiple levels fare less well and a nonsurgical approach is favored in such cases.

Traumatic Fracture and Dislocations of the Cervical Spine

Although cervical fractures and dislocations most commonly occur in young patients, motor vehicle trauma respects no age group. Compression fractures owing to axial loading may be stable or unstable, depending on the degree of displacement and associated soft tissue injury. Axial cervical burst fractures are usually unstable, result in neurologic damage, and require surgical decompression and stabilization.[16] Dislocation of the cervical facet joints may occur unilaterally or bilaterally in association with forward displacement of the craniad vertebral

body on the caudad. Neurologic injury may vary from none to complete quadriplegia. Closed reduction and immobilization may be all that is required to treat unilateral facet dislocation in contrast to bilateral facet dislocation, which necessitates reduction and stabilization because of the associated soft tissue and disc vertebral body disruption. Injuries to the upper cervical spine may result in C1–2 instabilities owing to rupture of the transverse and alar ligaments that bind the odontoid process to C1. If significant displacement occurs in a symptomatic patient, a posterior C1–2 arthrodesis is indicated. Fractures of the C1 posterior ring and body, the so-called Jefferson fracture, can usually be treated effectively with immobilization, as can pedicle level fractures resulting in traumatic spondylolisthesis of C2. Odontoid fractures occurring through the junction of the odontoid process and the body of C2 may not heal with immobilization and may require a C1–2 fusion to control the resultant instability between the atlas and the axis.

The halo brace has been a useful adjunct in the management of cervical spine injuries and is tolerated quite well by patients. The halo ring can be used as a traction device during acute fracture management as well as for intraoperative and postoperative immobilization. Recently anterior decompression and fusion with plate and screw fixation has been successful in the management of unstable cervical fractures and dislocations.[16] Because of the rigid internal fixation provided by the anterior plate and screws, halo immobilization is not necessary as it is with traditional posterior wire fixation methods, which do not provide such stable fixation. Physical and occupational therapists play a vital role in the postoperative day-to-day management of these patients and in their education regarding activities of daily living.

Surgical Management of the Rheumatoid Cervical Spine

Rheumatoid arthritis causes a cascade of instabilities in the cervical spine owing to destruction of capsule and ligamentous support as well as small-joint destruction. In many respects, a process similar to that occurring in the small joints and soft tissue of the hand resulting in subluxation and dislocations occurs in the cervical spine. The occipital C1–2 area is commonly invaded with destructive rheumatoid pannus which, results in instability especially in flexion, extension, and rotation. Patients complain of suboccipital headaches and upper neck pain, which improves with rest and immobilization. Occasionally bizarre shock-like sensations will occur in the upper and lower extremities with extreme neck flexion (Lhermitte's sign) owing to stimulation of the cervical cord. Occipital-upper cervical fusion with internal fixation is successful in alleviating the patient's symptoms and instability.

Although less commonly seen, instability in the mid and lower cervical spine may occur owing to multisegment rheumatoid disease. Steroid-associated osteoporosis compounds the destructive effects of the rheumatoid process, further reducing the stability and integrity of the cervical spine. Short-term use of soft and semirigid neck supports is helpful in reducing symptoms in these patients. Great care must be taken during elective surgical procedures in placing endotracheal tubes and in positioning the patient with rheumatoid involvement of the cervical spine in order to prevent cord compression.

Ankylosing Spondylitis of the Cervical Spine

Ankylosing spondylitis occurs primarily in men and results in ossification of the major and minor supporting ligaments and capsules of the spine. The end result of this process is markedly reduced spinal mobility and deformity. A severe flexion deformity of the cervical spine may result in a "chin-on-chest" deformity. Rotational deformities may occur in conjunction with flexion deformities. A sudden increase in cervical spine motion following a fall or accident is the result of a fracture through the "fused" spine. These fractures are unstable, may cause cord trauma, and require emergency immobilization in traction.[15]

Osteotomy to improve the position of the neck in ankylosing spondylitis has been popularized by Simmons.[18] A closing laminectomy of the lower cervical spine performed under local anesthesia and sedation has been effective and safe in repositioning the cervical spine in a neutral to extended attitude. This allows the patient to see straight ahead and to eat in a more normal fashion. Hip and shoulder involvement are commonly seen in ankylosing spondylitis and can be effectively treated with hip and shoulder joint arthroplasties.

Metastatic Disease of the Cervical Spine

Implants of malignant tumor reach the cervical spine by way of the veins in the epidural plexus. Since a majority of these tumors are radioresistant and have not responded to systemic chemotherapy, surgical removal and stabilization is an option. Lesions of the vertebral body require vertebrectomy and replacement with an implant, methyl methacrylate and/or a bone graft.[23] Lesions of the laminae, facets, and pedicles require resection and posterior stabilization with fusion using bone grafts, methyl methacrylate, and external fixation. Pain relief following these procedures is immediate and frees the cancer patient from cumbersome immobilization devices, thus allowing increased activity. Intraoperative monitoring of spinal cord function during resection is necessary. Use of an intraoperative blood recovery system to enable autotransfusion is highly recommended since blood loss can be significant from these vascular lesions.

Patients with metastatic spine lesions should be offered the option of surgical resection and stabilization in order to relieve pain, protect neurologic function, and improve their life-style. It has been the author's experience that although methyl methacrylate has no resistance to shear or tensile forces, its use to fill bone defects due to tumor in the cervical spine has met with short-term clinical success and appears safer to use than in the thoracolumbar spine where shear and tensile forces are of greater magnitude.

Complications and Outcomes of Cervical Spine Surgery

As with thoracolumbar surgery, cervical spine reconstructive surgery is well tolerated by the older patient. Utilizing modern anesthetic techniques, procedures requiring several hours to perform can be done safely in the elderly patient. The most common complaint after anterior cervical surgery is a sore throat and difficulty swallowing, both of which resolve within a few days. Temporary hoarseness owing to edema of the larynx also occurs. Paralysis of a vocal cord as a result of injury to the recurrent laryngeal nerve is rare. This results in hoarseness, which usually resolves unless the nerve has been transected. Pain, hematoma, and drainage from the iliac crest donor site can be obviated by using precut cryopreserved or freeze-dried allograft bone.[13] Complete extrusion of a properly placed graft between the vertebral bodies rarely occurs. Partial extrusion may occur on occasion but does not effect the end result. That portion of the graft projecting from the anterior surface of the cervical spine resorbs during bone healing and incorporation. Graham found a higher incidence of neurologic complications in posterior approaches than in anterior procedures in the cervical spine.[8] Complications of surgical treatment are summarized in Table 7–5.

In a study by Flynn, a 0.1% rate of myelopathy was documented in over 45,000 cases performed by 501 surgeons.[4] Surgical injury to the carotid artery, esophagus, and trachea is rare. Failure to heal of a properly placed bone graft in an anterior cervical fusion at one level is uncommon; however, the rate of pseudoarthrosis may increase with additional levels done. Long strut grafts placed over a distance between vertebral bodies may displace or fracture without additional external fixation or external support. Incorporation and healing of the bone graft is usually quite rapid, taking 8 to 12 weeks. Patients who undergo a one- or two-level anterior interbody graft are placed in a soft or semirigid collar after surgery; they are allowed to remove the collar for bathing and are cautioned to avoid excessive neck range of motion, especially hyperextension, until graft healing is confirmed by radiographs. Bilateral multiple-level laminectomy for cervical spondylosis may result in cervical spine instability in the postoperative period. Instability following posterior decompression is characterized by pain, limitation of extension, and development of a cervical kyphotic deformity. The latter is difficult to treat and is best avoided by performing a concomitant fusion at the time of extensive decompression or a cervical laminoplasty.

Herkowitz did a comparative study of anterior cervical fusion, cervical laminectomy, and cervical laminoplasty for the surgical treatment of multilevel spondylitic radiculopathy.[9] He found that the anterior cervical fusion provided the best results followed by cervical laminoplasty; although range of motion was most limited by laminoplasty. Cervical laminectomy provided the least favorable results in the treatment of multilevel cervical spondylosis.

Patients with cervical myelopathy caused by cervical spondylosis may not recover lost neurologic function following decompression. The longer the myelopathy has been present, the less chance of reversing it regardless of the surgical technique employed. Early referral of patients with cervical spondylolytic myelopathy is imperative. The degree of vascular as well as cord compression due to bony cervical stenosis is a major factor in determining the prognosis for improvement.

SUMMARY

Aging of the cervical spine is a gradual process resulting from reduction in disc hydration and nutrition coupled with wear and tear on the annulus fibrosus and articular cartilage of the facet and Luschka joints. Deformities, diseases, and instabilities of the cervical spine may result in significant morbidity. The clinician and therapist must be vigilant to recognize systemic as well as local etiologies for cervical spine complaints.

Acute cervical disc herniation is heralded by severe radicular pain, muscle weakness, sensory loss, and decrease in deep tendon reflexes. If nonoperative treatment is not effective, anterior cervical disc excision and interbody fusion is the preferred surgical approach. Cervical spondylosis without myelopathy or radiculopathy is best treated without surgery. Patients with documented nerve root or cord compression will benefit from anterior decompression and fusion. Laminoplasty is an option; however, functional results may not be as good. Multilevel laminectomy may result in a progressive kyphosis due to removal of the posterior elements and their supporting ligaments and capsules. Management of upper cervical spine instabilities associated with rheumatoid arthritis may be complicated by osteoporosis and long-term steroid use. Sudden increase in neck range of motion in a patient with ankylosing spondylitis after a fall or trauma indicates a fracture and the need for immediate immobilization with traction. Cervical spine fractures and dislocations that are judged to be unstable respond well to internal fixation and fusion. Recent data are supportive of anterior reduction, decompression, and plating for these injuries, which have traditionally been treated with posterior fusion and wiring followed by halo brace immobilization.

Patients with congenital anomalies resulting from failure of segmentation or formation may develop significant degenerative disease and instability at segments adjacent to their abnormalities. Decompression and fusion are often necessary to relieve their radiculopathy and/or myelopathy. Metastatic

TABLE 7–5.

Complications of Surgical Treatment of the Aging Cervical Spine

Greater risks than in younger patients
Injury to spinal cord (0.1%)
Vocal cord paralysis (rare)
Vascular, tracheal, esophageal injury (rare)
Instability, graft dislodgment (2%–3%)
Failure of fusion (5%)

disease in the cervical spine not responsive to radiation or chemotherapy can be palliated with surgical resection and stabilization.

A detailed history and physical assessment are critical in the evaluation of patients with neck complaints. High-quality plain radiographs, contrast-enhanced CT, and MRI are valuable diagnostic tools. Electrodiagnostic tests of the central nervous system complement the imaging studies. A skilled and knowledgeable physical therapist is an invaluable resource in facilitating the nonoperative treatment of these patients.

REFERENCES

1. Bohlman HH, Emery S: The pathophysiology of cervical spondylosis and myelopathy. *Spine* 1988; 13:843–846.
2. Cloward RB: The anterior approach for removal of a ruptured cervical disc. *J Neurosurg* 1953; 10:154–168.
3. Dillion W, Booth R, Cuckler J, et al: Cervical radiculopathy. *Spine* 1986; 11:988–991.
4. Flynn TB: Neurologic complications of anterior cervical fusion. *Spine* 1982; 7:536–539.
5. Friedenberg Z, Miller W: Degenerative disc disease of the cervical spine. *J Bone Joint Surg Am* 1963; 45:1171–1178.
6. Gore D, Sepic S: Anterior cervical fusion for degenerative and protruded discs. *Spine* 1984; 9:667.
7. Gehwheiler J, Nasca R: Luschka joint osteophytes and cervical disc disease, a discographic and pathologic study (unpublished study). Duke University Medical Center, 1969.
8. Graham JT: Complications of cervical spine surgery. *Spine* 1989; 14:1046–1050.
9. Herkowitz HN: A comparison of anterior cervical fusion, cervical laminectomy and cervical laminoplasty for the surgical management of multi-level spondylotic radiculopathy. *Spine* 1988; 13:774–780.
10. Herkowitz HH, Kurz LT, Overholt DP: Surgical management of cervical soft disc herniation. *Spine* 1990; 15:1026–1030.
11. Nakano N, Nakano T, Nakano K: Comparison of the results of laminectomy and open-door laminoplasty for cervical spondylotic myeloradiculopathy and ossification of the posterior longitudinal ligament. *Spine* 1988; 13:792–794.
12. Nasca RJ, Lemons JE, Deinlein DA: Synthetic biomaterials for spinal fusion. *Orthopaedics* 1989; 12:543–548.
13. Nasca RJ, Whelchel JD: Use of cryopreserved bone in spinal surgery. *Spine* 1987; 12:222–227.
14. Ono K, Ota H, Tada K, et al: Cervical myelopathy secondary to multiple spondylotic protrusions. *Spine* 1977; 2:109–125.
15. Raycroft JF, Broom MJ: Complications of fractures of the cervical spine. *Spine* 1988; 13:763–766.
16. Ripa DR, Kowall MG, Meyer PR, et al: Series of ninety-two traumatic cervical spine injuries stabilized with anterior ASIF plate fusion technique. *Spine* (Suppl) 1991; 16:S46–S55.
17. Rothman R, Simeone F: Cervical disc disease, in Rothman R, Simeone F (eds): *Spine.* Philadelphia, WB Saunders, 1991, pp 440–453.
18. Simmons EH: The surgical correction of flexion deformity of the cervical spine in ankylosing spondylitis. *Clin Orthop* 1972; 86:132.
19. Smith GW, Robinson RA: The treatment of certain spine disorders by anterior removal of the intervertebral disc and interbody fusion. *J Bone Joint Surg Am* 1958; 40:607–624.
20. The Cervical Spine Research Society (ed): *The Cervical Spine.* Philadelphia, JB Lippincott, 1983.
21. Weinstein J, Claverie W, Gibson S: The pain of discography. *Spine* 1988; 13:1344–1348.
22. Weinstein J: Mechanisms of spinal pain. The dorsal root ganglion and its role as a mediator of low back pain. *Spine* 1986; 11:999–1001.
23. White AA: Clinical biomechanics of cervical spine implants. *Spine* 1989; 14:1040–1045.

Chapter 8

Cervical Spine Complications: A Rehabilitation Perspective

Carole B. Lewis, P.T., Ph.D.
Therese McNerney, P.T.

One of the most notable postural changes of some older persons is the positioning of the head and the shoulders in relationship to the torso. The visual image of an older person illustrates the changes that may occur gradually as cervical spine height is reduced, posterior neck muscles shorten, and upper back muscles become overstretched.

Morphologic changes in the neck and the shoulder structures may lead to increased pain and limited flexibility, but the literature does not indicate that these complications must occur with age. In fact, most pathologies of the neck and surrounding areas are just as prevalent in younger as older segments of the population.[6]

This chapter will describe the anatomy and physiology involved in the neck area and normal as well as pathologic changes occurring with age in the cervical spine. Evaluation, environmental modifications and rehabilitation programs will be discussed.

ANATOMY

The structures composing the cervical spine are numerous. The main focus of this section will be to describe the age-related changes of the vertebrae, ligaments, intervertebral discs, and muscles.

The first normal age-related change that occurs in the vertebral body, which is composed of trabecu-

lar and cortical bone, is the loss of bone mineral content. With age, a 3% decrease in cortical bone and a 6% to 8% decrease in horizontal and transverse trabecular bone is observed.[11] This decrease in bone density may lead to a gradual collapse in vertebral end-plates and subsequent reduction in cervical height.

Degenerative changes in cartilaginous end-plate morphology begin early in the aging process. These cartilaginous end-plates composed primarily of hyaline cartilage serve to separate the nucleus and the anulus from the vertebral bodies. It has been shown that the calcification process begins as early as the third decade and that by the eighth decade, 93% of the end-plate is calcified.[15]

This calcification does not lead to serious manifestations of symptoms as long as the calcific process remains inside the end-plate. If the calcification process begins to present itself outside the end-plate, degeneration of the nucleus pulposus may occur, leading to symptomatic conditions such as nerve root irritation.

The cervical spine may develop both anterior and posterior osteophytes. Anterior osteophytes are commonly found at all levels of the aging person's cervical spine. Posterior osteophytes are less common but when observed are typically noted at C5-6 and C6-7.[14]

The intervertebral disc also changes with age. The anulus fibrosus becomes less elastic and the nucleus pulposus has a decreased ability to maintain extracellular water.[14] The aging disc is less absorbent and less resilient and therefore less able to redistribute spinal pressures and reduce common postural changes seen with aging.[3]

Muscles can atrophy in size and type with age.[4] Muscles receive less nourishment from the cardiovascular system and therefore are less able to generate vigorous contractions.[8] By age 65, from 20% to 40% of the maximal muscle strength is lost.[7] A general loss of skeletal muscle is noted as larger numbers of motor units are needed to produce a given force. A general increase in type I muscle fibers and a decrease in type II muscle fibers is also noted.[7]

The major role of muscles in the cervical spine is the facilitation of range of motion and support. Cervical range of motion decreases in all directions with age. Lind's study of both males and females between the ages of 12 and 79 demonstrated the linear relationship between age and decreased cervical motion.[10] The decrease in cervical range of motion starts in the third decade and continues until the eighth decade.[10] Significant differences between men and women were not noted. The norms for range of motion are noted in Table 8–1.

All of the factors listed above contribute to the postural changes noted with age. Habitual forward head posturing can lead to thoracic hypomobility known as the dowager's hump. Rounded shoulders typically accompany this forward head position and cause suboccipital and anterior chest tightness with subsequent upper back overstretching. The suboccipital muscular tightness is compensated for by a counterweighing of the forward head position, with the head held in cervical extension. All of these postural changes may be exacerbated by decreased activity.[16]

At this point special note should be made of specific structures that may affect the elderly. The cervical mechanoreceptors located in the facet capsule provide postural, dynamic, inhibitory and nociceptor information.[16] For the receptors to fire, they must receive a stretch. As one ages, the cervical

mechanoreceptors decrease input into the cervical cord owing to hypokinetics (decreased activity level). The older person therefore receives less proprioceptive (position sense) information about the environment.[19] An older person who is restricted by a forward head position or decreased motion in the cervical spine will not receive adequate mechanoreceptor input.[19] Rehabilitation of the cervical spine that seeks to improve posture, stretch tight muscles and increase range of motion will make the elderly patient not only more functional but more aware of the environment.[16]

The normal degenerative process results from an attempt to maintain stability. Poor posture resulting in a forward head position leads to cervical joint trauma. Constant pressure on the facet joint develops into an overstretch of the joint capsule that begins to initiate end-plate damage. Eventually, circumferential followed by radial tears of the disc may occur.[14] Once the cervical spine becomes unstable, the bone begins to protect the joint structure, which results in osteophyte or spur formation. The process of joint ankylosis and resulting hypomobility has begun.

It is the authors' belief that this scenario can be delayed or preempted at any point with appropriate prevention and treatment techniques that include stabilization, strengthening, and range of motion exercises.

CERVICAL PATHOLOGIES IN THE OLDER PERSON

Numerous pathologic conditions can cause neck pain in elderly people. This section will describe the most common.

Cervical Spondylosis

Cervical spondylosis is a degenerative change in the cervical spine that is characterized by radiographic changes indicating the narrowing of the intervertebral foramina and the formation of osteophytes. The degeneration results in subsequent nerve root compression, most commonly observed at the C6 and C7 levels. Fifty percent of people over the age of 50 will complain of neck pain and stiffness secondary to this condition.[17]

The degenerative changes may be a result of the cervical hypermobility commonly found in patients

TABLE 8–1.

Range of Motion Norms, in Degrees

	Age, yr		
	10	30	80
Flexion	35	30	27
Lateral flexion	60	50	30
Rotation	165	150	130
Extension	60	50	35

presenting with a forward head position. Evaluation during the early stages of spondylosis may reveal mechanical shortening of the cervical musculature with subsequent pain and stiffness, without the neurologic component. Nerve root irritation or arm pain, however, occurs in 25% to 40% of the patients complaining of the neck pain.[14]

Evaluation of this problem reveals a limitation in range of motion, pain, stiffness, and radicular symptoms. The progression of the pathology may lead to muscular atrophy and sensory deficits of the involved nerve roots. Posterior osteophyte formation in the spinal canal may result in lower-extremity weakness and positive Babinski signs.[2]

Conservative management can be extremely beneficial for these patients. Anti-inflammatory medication and cervical traction followed by pain-free range of motion exercises are the treatment of choice. Prior to traction or exercise, however, special attention should be placed on addressing the common tightness of the suboccipital muscles. Moist heat, massage, and gentle stretching to this area may enhance the benefits of cervical traction and postural retraining, which should emphasize axial extension.

Evaluation findings and treatment for cervical spondylosis are summarized in Table 8–2.

Vertebral Artery Syndrome

Vertebral artery syndrome often occurs as a result of spondylotic changes in the cervical spine. Osteophyte formation in combination with reduced cervical height and a forward head position may cause encroachment on the vertebral foramina. This

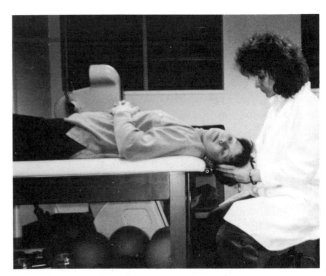

FIG 8–1.
Evaluation for vertebral artery syndrome. Extend and rotate neck; look for nystagmus, nausea, dizziness, or other neurologic signs. Hold the patient's head in this position for 60 seconds or until signs are noted.

encroachment, which may be further irritated by cervical position, results in a decreased flow of blood through the vertebral artery to the brain.

The patient with vertebral artery syndrome will avoid a combination of positions including rotation, extension, and lateralization of the head. This positioning reproduces symptoms of dizziness, blurred vision, and nystagmus.[12]

The objective evaluation for vertebral artery syndrome is illustrated in Figure 8–1. Figure 8–2 is a

TABLE 8–2.
Summary of Evaluation Findings and Treatment for Cervical Spondylosis

Evaluation findings
1. Pain and stiffness in the neck area that may radiate into the upper extremity.
2. Limitation in cervical range of motion secondary to the rate of degeneration.
3. Suboccipital muscle tightness.

Treatment in acute phase
1. Anti-inflammatory medication.
2. Cervical traction following suboccipital relaxation.
3. Pain-free cervical range-of-motion exercises.

Treatment in subacute phase
1. Modalities as needed for pain and muscle relaxation.
2. Cervical range-of-motion and stretching exercises in pain-free range.
3. Progressive resistive exercises, isometrics, progressing to isotonics.

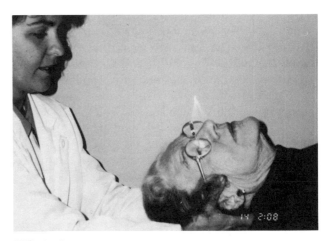

FIG 8–2.
Modification of test for vertebral artery syndrome for older persons. Patient's head is kept in extension while rotating to each side. Examiner keeps the head in extension by using the hand under the neck. Continue examination as in Figure 8–1.

modification of the test for older persons. Application of this test involves asking the patient to rotate, laterally flex, and extend the head, maintaining this position for 30 to 60 seconds.[12] (As noted in Figure 8–2, many elderly patients, because of their forward head posture, are already in cervical extension.) Laterally flexing and rotating the cervical spine is all that is necessary.

Dizziness, nystagmus, nausea, and unilateral pupil dilation are positive indications that vertebral artery syndrome is present. Vertebral artery syndrome can be differentially diagnosed from vestibular dysfunction in that position, rather than movement, of the head, reproduces the symptoms.[12]

The subjective evaluation for this problem may reveal patient complaints of pain in the neck, but more commonly they will complain of dizziness when reaching into cabinets or when looking up while sitting in a wheelchair. On an objective evaluation, the patient will have a positive test result for vertebral artery syndrome.

Treatment for patients suffering from vertebral artery syndrome may include the use of cervical collars to maintain the head in a neutral position. Cervical collars can be detrimental to the older person, however, owing to the decrease in input from the mechanoreceptors. Cervical collars are therefore only recommended in cases where the patient has experienced drop attacks secondary to vertebral artery occlusion. Clinically, the authors have found that effective treatment includes postural instruction in axial extension positioning, suboccipital relaxation techniques, stabilization exercises, and education regarding the cervical position that may reproduce the symptoms. The treatment goals are to maintain a neutral head position with muscular strength and avoid position of discomfort and dizziness. Modifying the patient's activities and environment through a home evaluation may identify the activities that compromise the vertebral artery and place the patient in daily jeopardy of falls or dizziness from vertebral artery occulsion.

The evaluation and treatment of vertebral artery syndrome are summarized in Table 8–3.

Rheumatoid Arthritis

Rheumatoid arthritis is a chronic illness characterized by inflammation of the synovium of the diarthroidal joints. Unlike osteoarthritis, the incidence of rheumatoid arthritis actually declines after age 65.[1] However, of those diagnosed with rheumatoid arthritis, 50% report involvement in the neck.[13] The

TABLE 8–3.

Summary of Evaluation and Treatment of Vertebral Artery Syndrome

Evaluation of findings
1. Positive vertebral artery test.
2. Complaints of dizziness on extension, rotation, and lateral side-bending of the cervical spine.
3. Possible pain and stiffness in the cervical area.

Treatment
1. Modify environment and daily activities to avoid positions of extension, rotation, and lateralization of the head.
2. Teach axial extension
3. Teach stabilization (isometrics)
4. Cervical collar, if patient is unable to maintain cervical spine in a neutral position.

patient diagnosed with rheumatoid arthritis will typically complain of pain in the occipital and middle posterior areas. Prior to evaluation or treatment a radiograph or magnetic resonance imaging (MRI) scan should be obtained to rule out the possibility of atlanto-occipital subluxation. MRI is the more definitive test when dealing with a rheumatoid arthritic older patient.

In the presence of atlanto-occipital subluxation, manipulation is strictly contraindicated. Care must also be taken in the evaluation of passive range of motion of the cervical spine. In the presence of severe rheumatoid arthritis, cervical rotation can rupture the transverse and alar ligaments, resulting in an atlantoaxial dislocation.[12] Pain relief for the patient with rheumatoid arthritis can be accomplished by support of the head. During acute cervical flare-up in a rheumatoid arthritic patient, the use of a cervical collar may be indicated. Environmental modifications such as evaluating the way a person sleeps as well as the number of pillows they sleep with may help alleviate positional stresses and give good support to the head and neck.

Treatment consists of pain relief modalities such as heat, ultrasound, and massage for soft tissue relaxation followed by gentle range-of-motion and progressive resistive exercises for strengthening. It is imperative to use pain tolerance as the guide to the number of resistive exercises prescribed.

The evaluation and treatment of rheumatoid arthritis are summarized in Table 8–4.

Ossification of the Posterior Longitudinal Ligament

Ossification of the posterior longitudinal ligament is commonly known as the Japanese disease because it is primarily seen in people of Japanese de-

TABLE 8–4.

Summary of Evaluation and Treatment of Rheumatoid Arthritis

Evaluation findings
 1. Positive medical test results for rheumatoid arthritis.
 2. Check for subluxation of atlanto-occipital joint.
 3. Assess range of motion and strength within the patient's pain tolerance.

Treatment—acute phase
 1. Use anti-inflammatory agents such as ice, ultrasound (0.5 W/cm²)[5]
 2. Work on gentle active-assistive exercises within the patient's pain tolerance.
 3. Use isometric exercises as tolerated by the patient.

Treatment—subacute phase
 1. Use heat, ultrasound, and massage to reduce muscle guarding and relieve pain.
 2. Work on active-assistive exercises to increase active range of motion in the patient's pain tolerance.
 3. Work on strengthening exercises, starting with isometrics and progressing to resistive exercises if tolerated.

scent; however, it has also been noted in Caucasian cultures as well. The posterior longitudinal ligament becomes hard and fibrous because of increased deposits of calcium. The ligament can actually be observed on a cervical radiograph. This condition is rarely noted in people under the age of 50.[14]

On initial evaluation, the rehabilitation therapist will note restrictions in forward flexion of the cervical spine as well as pain on any increased activity of the neck.

Treatment for this condition is rest and the avoidance of stressful activities. Increasing active range of motion, stretching, and progressive resistive exercises are implemented to increase the ability of the muscles to hold the neck in a nonstressed position. Rehabilitation therapists must be aware of possible radicular symptoms. Neurologic involvement warrants change in the treatment progression. The goal of the rehabilitation therapist is therefore to stretch the posterior aspect of the cervical spine

TABLE 8–5.

Summary of Evaluation and Treatment of Ossification of the Posterior Longitudinal Ligament

Evaluation findings
 1. X-rays indicate calcification of the posterior longitudinal ligament.
 2. Patient presents with restriction of cervical flexion.
 3. Patient may present with cervical pain and possible radicular symptoms.

Treatment
 1. Heat, ultrasound, and massage to relieve muscle guarding.
 2. Stretching of posterior neck muscles.
 3. Progressive resistive exercises.

without increasing neurologic symptoms. Evaluation and treatment are summarized in Table 8–5.

MYOFASCIAL PAIN

The myofascial pain syndrome as defined by Travell is "a pain and/or autonomic phenomena referred from active myofascial trigger points with associated dysfunction."[18] Myofascial trigger points can refer pain that is characterized as aching and dull, often deep, and ranging from uncomfortable to incapacitating. Trigger points not found in normal muscles are described as either active or latent and both have been found to cause dysfunction.[18]

Active trigger points are defined as hyperirritable areas of skeletal muscle tissue that cause pain. Latent trigger points, although not painful, may cause weakness and restriction of movement.

On evaluation, patients presenting with active trigger points will demonstrate a "jump sign." Application of pressure to the affected trigger point will cause the patient to jump or move away from the point of pressure. As activity levels decrease, the older patient will tend to have the associated stiffness and restricted motion of latent trigger points rather than the more acute pain of active trigger points. The older patient presenting with latent trigger points may convert these to active trigger points through muscle overuse and irritation.. The therapist must therefore take a dual approach to the treatment of active and latent trigger points.

The latent and active trigger point evaluation addresses three areas; structural inadequacies, postural stresses, and constriction of muscle.[18] Body asymmetry is a common structural inadequacy. A 0.16-cm leg length discrepancy, which will remain with them throughout life, was found in 80% of schoolchildren between the ages of 5 and 17.[18] Cervical trigger points, specifically the scalenes, may be activated by a tilted shoulder-girdle axis due to a short leg length in standing.

Postural stresses such as misfitting furniture, poor posture, abuse of muscles and poor body mechanics can all activate trigger points. Finally, and most applicable to the elderly woman, is constriction of muscle or constricting pressure on a muscle. Narrow bra straps may activate the trapezius, knee-high pantyhose may activate the gastrocnemius, and tight brassieres may activate the latissimus muscles. For men, tight ties or shirt collars may activate the sternocleidomastoid muscle. These are just a few areas that need to be considered but it opens up the scope of perpetuating factors which can convert latent to active trigger points.

Two common areas of myofascial involvement of the cervical spine are the levator scapulae and scalenes. These are described in more detail below.

Scalenes

The anterior, middle, and posterior scalene muscles act to stabilize the cervical spine against lateral movement and elevate the first and second ribs during inspiration. The scalene muscles are referred to as the great entrappers owing to their positional relationship to the brachial plexus. Tightness in these muscles may occlude nerves and blood vessels to the proximal and distal part of the arm. Physical symptoms include morning edema specifically on the radial and dorsal aspect of the hand.[18]

Neurologic symptoms include numbness and tingling in the hand especially along the ulnar border. These patients may have problems pulling or lifting objects, especially above waist level, and have a tendency to drop things.[18] They may also move their arms restlessly as if trying to relieve certain muscles. Objective evaluation reveals lateral side-bending of the cervical spine restricted by at least 30 degrees to the opposite side and cervical rotation, which is normal.[18]

Three tests help in the differential diagnosis of this condition. The cramp test is performed as the patient fully rotates the head to the affected side and drops the chin into the hollow behind the clavicle. The test is positive if a hard contraction or cramp of the scalene muscles occurs, indicating active trigger points.[18] Elderly patients who are hearing-impaired must be instructed to turn their bodies, not their heads, so as not to elicit the cramp sign.

The finger-flexion test is positive for scalene trigger points if, with extended proximal phalanges, all the medial fingers tips do not press tightly against the metacarpophalangeal joints.[18] Finally, the scalene relief test involves elevation of the arm and clavicle, thereby lifting the clavicle off the underlying scalenes. This is accomplished by having the patient place the forearm of the involved side across the forehead. This arm and clavicular positioning should produce pain relief within several minutes.[18]

Treatment for this condition includes various modalities (hot packs, ultrasound, gentle massage) that facilitate relaxation, followed by stretching and active range-of-motion exercises.

Postural retraining, concentrating on axial extension, and instruction in diaphragmatic breathing are essential. Also important are body mechanic instructions of how to carry objects without extending them too far from the body. For patients who continue to get good relief from treatments but return with symptoms, sleeping and sitting posture should

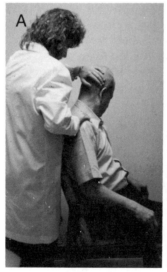 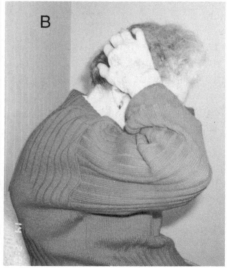

FIG 8–3.

A, levator scapulae stretch. Patient looks down and away from involved side. Therapist applies gentle stretch as shown, holding 20 seconds. **B,** home levator stretch. Patient gently presses down against the back of head, thereby stretching the posterior cervical musculature and the levator. Stretch is held 20 to 30 seconds.

be investigated. Slightly elevating the head of the bed or adjusting the arm levels of their wheelchairs will decompress the clavicular area and may give patients long-term relief of the symptoms.

Levator Scapulae

The levator scapulae muscle primarily acts to rotate the cervical spine to the same side and elevate the scapula. Patients with levator scapulae tightness are the classic "stiff neck" or torticollis patients. These patients have difficulty rotating the head, specifically to the side of involvement. The levator scapulae is the shoulder girdle muscle most likely to have trigger point involvement.[18]

Physical symptoms include decreased rotation

TABLE 8-6.

Summary of Evaluation of Treatment of Myofascial Pain

Evaluation findings: myofascial pain
1. Patient may display a "jump sign."
2. Patient may complain of pain and fatigue.
3. X-rays are negative.
4. Patient will present with range-of-motion limitations and weakness.

Treatment: myofascial pain
1. Heat the involved muscle group for 15–20 minutes (ultrasound at low intensities inactivates trigger points)
2. Application of ischemic compression or acupressure to the activated trigger points.
3. Fluoromethane spray and stretch to the involved muscle.
4. Reheat the affected muscle for 5 minutes to decrease possible soreness and help facilitate pain-free range of motion.
5. Perform pain-free range-of-motion exercise in all directions.

Evaluation findings: activated scalene trigger points
1. Lateral side-bending of the cervical spine is restricted by 30 degrees to the opposite side.
2. Cervical rotation is full.
3. Cramp test, finger flexion test, and scalene relief test are all positive.

Treatment: activated scalene trigger points
1. Stretch scalene muscles.
2. Teach diaphragmatic breathing.
3. Elevate the head of the bed.
4. Instruct patients not to carry heavy objects with arms extended.
5. Instruct hearing-impaired patients to turn the body instead of the head in the acute stages.

Evaluation findings: activated levator scapulae trigger points.
1. Patient presents with a "stiff neck."
2. Unable to rotate the head to the side of involvement.
3. Patient may be walking with a cane that is too long.
4. End range flexion and/or rotation is limited.

Treatment: activated levator scapulae trigger points.
1. Stretch levator scapulae muscles.
2. Adjust cane to proper height.
3. Instruct in home heating and strengthening program.

and end-range flexion of the cervical spine. Cervical extension is unaffected. Decreased scapular rotation may also be present, limiting full-range abduction of the arm on the affected side.[18]

Elderly patients may activate levator scapulae trigger points by overfatiguing muscles, sitting in drafty places, or sleeping with the neck in a tilted position. Common ergonometric problems that irritate patients include armrests that are too high and canes that are too long. Both of these cause the scapula to be elevated and may activate the underlying latent trigger points. Ergonometric modifications include adjusting canes to the appropriate height and finding chairs with armrests that do not elevate the scapulas.

Treatment for these patients includes various modalities (hot packs, ultrasound, gentle massage) to facilitate relaxation. Fluoromethane spray followed by stretching is extremely effective, particularly if the patient follows through with a home stretching program. The stretch specific to the levator scapula is described in Figure 8–3.

Evaluation and treatment of myofascial pain and trigger points is summarized in Table 8–6.

DISC HERNIATION

True disc herniation is relatively uncommon in the elderly because of the decreased water content of the nucleus pulposus.[16] When disc herniation does occur, it is usually but not always triggered by some form of trauma. Symptoms may include sudden and severe neck and arm pain as well as paresthesia along the involved nerve root. Neck movements, especially lateral flexion toward the affected side will typically aggravate the pain. These symptoms will usually resolve themselves in 4 to 6 weeks although the paresthesia may persist longer.[14]

Acute treatment of this condition may include a cervical collar for head support. It may be necessary for the patient to sleep with the collar on if a comfortable sleeping position cannot be found. The authors have found that heat and ultrasound for muscle relaxation followed by manual cervical traction and ice are an effective way to alleviate symptoms. Pain-free range-of-motion exercises and isometrics are started as soon as possible. Evaluation and treatment of disc herniation are summarized in Table 8–7.

TABLE 8–7.

Summary of Evaluation and Treatment of Disc Herniation

Evaluation findings for disc herniation
1. Patient presents with severe neck and arm pain.
2. Symptoms are usually related to some type of trauma.
3. Lateral cervical flexion toward the affected side will increase the symptoms.

Treatment for disc herniations: acute phase
1. Cervical collar.
2. Manual cervical traction.
3. Ice.
4. Pain-free active assistive exercises.

Treatment for disc herniation: subacute phase
1. Hot packs, ultrasound, and massage for muscle relaxation.
2. Pain-free range of motion exercises.
3. Isometrics.

EVALUATION OF CERVICAL PROBLEMS

A systematic evaluation of the cervical spine starts with subjective questioning. Prior to asking specific questions about a particular condition, therapists must ask themselves, Why is the patient here to see me? What is it that he or she expects to achieve from the visit with me, and what is his or her particular functional problem? Mentally answering these questions during the course of the evaluation will facilitate the implementation of the most appropriate plan of cure.

Specific subjective questioning includes: What aggravates or eases the condition? What are the symptoms like in the morning compared with the evening? What type of assistive devices (bifocals, hearing aid, cane) is the patient using?

Figures 8–4,A and 8–4,B provide a cervical spine evaluation form.

Different patient populations need different types of assessments. The authors have developed an evaluation that combines objective clinical information with documentation material. In this era of Medicare guidelines, it is imperative for rehabilitation therapists to note functional limitations.

In the "functional problem" section a well-documented evaluation might include: (1) Patient unable to sleep for more than 2 hours without significant pain of 9/10. (2) Patient unable to drive a car because rotation of the neck is limited to 8 degrees on the right.

The "short-term goal" section might read: (1) Increase pain-free sleeping time to 4 hours. (2) Increase pain-free cervical rotation to the right 16 degrees. "Long-term goals" may read: (1) Pain-free sleeping throughout the night. (2) Pain-free range of motion of 35 degrees of the cervical spine to the right so that the patient may drive a car independently.

The time of day that the patient experiences pain may give an indication of whether the problem is systemic or mechanical in nature. Morning stiffness lasting longer than 1 hour that lessens as the day progresses may indicate a systemic dysfunction such as rheumatoid arthritis.

In contrast, morning stiffness that dissipates within half an hour may indicate osteoarthritis. Pain and fatigue noted at the end of the day may indicate myofascial involvement or degenerative changes.

Sleeping positions are noted initially because morning pain may indicate arthritis, but it may also indicate that the patient is not getting good support throughout the night. Number of pillows and position are discussed and modified. Something as simple as changing a sleeping position may give the patient significant morning pain relief.

Active and passive range of motion, posture, and muscle guarding are all evaluated. Norms for the elderly have been included. Neurologic problems such as abnormal reflexes and myotome involvement are also assessed. "VAS" indicates vertebral artery syndrome; positive testing should indicate if the involvement is right or left sided.

TREATMENT

Treatment suggestions have been presented under the various pathologies. This section will provide the treatment techniques that were not described in detail.

The use of modalities cannot be overlooked when treating the elderly patient. Studies have indicated that the collagenous nature of older tendons makes them more easily stretched with a prior application of heat.[9] Ultrasound has been shown effective in deactivating trigger points and ice is an excellent topical analgesic. All of these treatments in combination with exercise and education may accelerate the recovery of the older patient.

Exercise is obviously an essential part of any rehabilitation program. The first area that is often addressed in elderly people is postural reinstruction. Patients must be able to correct a forward head posi-

Geriatric Cervical Evaluation

Name _____   Date _____ Age _____

Primary Diagnosis   History _____

_____   _____

_____   _____

Functional Problems   _____

1. _____   _____

2. _____   Sleeping Position _____

3. _____   _____

Medications   Muscle Guarding

1. _____   _____

2. _____   _____

3. _____   Pain   0   none

                                                                 10   excruciating
Assistive Devices (glasses, hearing aid, cane)   Score _____

1. _____   Pain Descriptors

2. _____   Sharp _____ Dull _____ Localized _____

3. _____   Diffuse _____ Burning _____

_____

Posture   0   extremely helpful
                10   normal   Blood Pressure _____

Shoulders   Pulse _____
        Forward _____
                                             V.A.S. Right _____ Left _____
        Lateral Tilt_____

Kyphosis _____

Pain Location _____

Related Pain
        When it occurs (am/pm) _____

        Frequency and duration _____

        Aggravating /easing activities _____

FIG 8–4.
Geriatric cervical evaluation form (*front*).

(Continued.)

Range of Motion of the Cervical Spine

Active Flexion _____	Active Extension _____
Passion Flexion _____	Passive Extension _____
Normal _____30_____	Normal _____30_____
Active Right Lateral Flexion _____	Active Left Lateral Flexion _____
Passive Right Lateral Flexion _____	Passive Left Lateral Flexion _____
Normal _____40_____	Normal _____40_____
Active Right Rotation _____	Active Left Rotation _____
Passive Right Rotation _____	Passive Left Rotation _____
Normal _____45_____	Normal _____45_____

Reflexes

      Biceps C5 _____

      Brachioradials _____

      Triceps C7 _____

Myotomes

C1 C2 Neck Flexion _____	C6 Elbow Flexion _____
C3 Lateral Flexion _____	C7 Elbow Extension _____
C4 Shoulder Elevation _____	C7 Wrist Flexion _____
C5 Shoulder Abduction _____	C8 Thumb Extension _____
C6 Elbow Flexion _____	T1 Thumb Abduction _____

Treatment Goals

1. _____

2. _____

3. _____

4. _____

FIG 8-4 (cont.).
Geriatric evaluation form (*back*).

tion that may limit respiratory volume and active range of motion, and may facilitate suboccipital musculature shortening.[16] The patient must learn to maintain a position of axial extension. The authors have found that overemphasizing the forward head position followed by repositioning and visualization is often an effective means of attaining the axial extension position. If the patient is limited in axial extension or in attempting axial extension he or she experience pain, the therapist should check for subsequent suboccipital muscle tightness. The occipital release technique illustrated in Figure 8–5 may be the treatment of choice prior to painful postural reinstruction.

Patients may also benefit from the use of assistive devices such as stretch wraps and a clavicular strap when treating the problem of rounded or protracted shoulders. This technique should be discouraged, however, when the main problem is a forward head position. The authors have found that pulling the shoulders back prior to correcting the forward head position may actually worsen the head position. It is therefore imperative to work on axial extension positioning prior to shoulder retraction activities.

Pectoral doorway stretching illustrated in Figure 8–6 has also be found an effective active way to correct the shoulder protraction problem and stretch the anterior chest musculature. Axial extension head positioning is emphasized as the patient performs the stretch.

Pain-free range-of-motion exercises are started

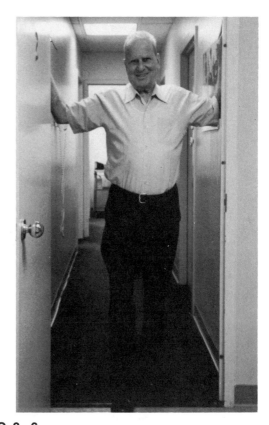

FIG 8–6.
Pectoral door stretch. Patient stands with arms propped in the doorway as shown. Patient leans through the door and holds the stretch 20 to 30 seconds. To stretch various parts of the pectoral muscles, hands are placed at shoulder level to stretch upper pectoral muscles, at head level to stretch middle pectoral muscles and above the head to stretch lower pectoral muscles.

as soon as the patient can tolerate them. Isometric exercises may be started prior to isotonics if the patient cannot tolerate any cervical motion. Therapists must be cautious in the use of isometrics in the elderly, because they have been shown to increase blood pressure. Isometrics may, however, be the only pain-free exercises the patient can perform. Figure 8–7 is an example of how to monitor blood pressure while performing the cervical isometric exercise.

In order for treatment strategy to be effective, ergonometric assessment and modification must be included. Considerations of the patient's environment may lead to some important discoveries in the patient's treatment. For example, the patient may wear bifocals when using a computer or reading a newspaper and extend the head backward placing pressuring on the suboccipital region of the cervical spine. Also, patients who sleep with too many pil-

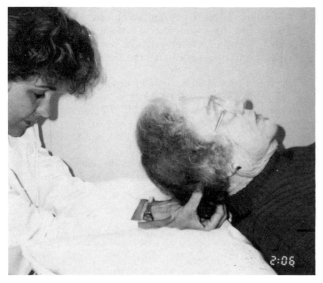

FIG 8–5.
Occipital release. Pressure is applied with fingertips just proximal to the occiput until the suboccipital muscles relax.

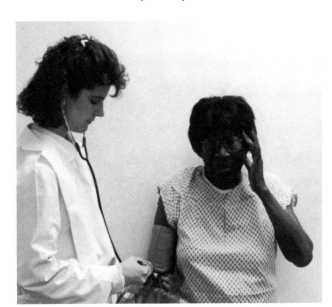

FIG 8–7.
Monitoring blood pressure while doing a cervical isometric. The patient is asked to press head into his or her fingers and hold 10 seconds. The therapist monitors blood pressure and gives patient feedback on breathing and relaxation to decrease pressure, if it rises.

lows may flex the suboccipital spine, contributing to irritation of painful end-range postures. If the therapists are aware of these positions and correct them, then they can be more effective in their treatment program.

SUMMARY

Older patients with neck pain can benefit from the use of modalities, ergonometric assessment and a comprehensive exercise program. The authors have described normal and pathologic changes that cause neck pain and presented various options in evaluation and treatment strategies. Older patients are living longer and the average life expectancy has increased dramatically since the early 1900s. Older patients are not willing to live at age 60 with neck pain that they know may last for the next 20 years. It

should be the job of the rehabilitation professional to provide a thorough evaluation and an appropriate rehabilitation program to keep these patients pain-free and improve their quality of life.

REFERENCES

1. Abrams WB, Berkow R (eds): *Geriatric Merck Manual*, Rathway, NJ, Merck, Sharp & Dohme, 1990.
2. Berkow R (ed): *Merck Manual*, ed 14. Rahway, NJ, Merck, Sharp & Dohme, 1982.
3. Burkart S, Beresford W: The aging invertebral disc. *Phys Ther* 1979; 59:969–970.
4. Costell R: Age related strength changes (lecture notes). Cybex seminar, San Diego, CA, August 1989.
5. Dyson M: Therapeutic applications of ultrasound, in Nyborg W, Zisken M (eds): *Biological Effects of Ultrasound.* New York, Churchill Livingstone, 1985, pp 121–135.
6. Hayashi H, Okada K: Etiologic factors of myelopathy. *Clin Orthop Rel Res* 1987; 214:200–208.
7. Jokl P: The biology of aging muscle, in Nelson CL, Dwyer A (eds): *The Aging Musculoskeletal System.* Lexington, Mass, Collamore Press, 1984, pp 17–33.
8. Knortz K: Muscle physiology applied to geriatric rehabilitation. *Top Geriatr Rehabil* 1987; 2:1–9.
9. LaBella FS: Structure of collagen form human tendon as influenced by age and sex. *J Gerontol* 1965; 20:54–59.
10. Lind B, Sihlbom H: Normal range of motion of the cervical spine. *Arch Phys Ther Rehabil* 1989; 70:692–695.
11. Mac Kinnon JL: Osteoporosis: A review. *Phys Ther* 1988; 68:1533-1541.
12. Maitland GD: *Vertebral Manipulation.* London, Butterworths, 1986.
13. Maricic MJ, Gall EP: Cervical arthritis: Which therapy for your patient? *J Musculoskeletal Med* 1989; 6:66–76.
14. Moskovitz R: Neck pain in the elderly: Common causes and management. *Geriatrics* 1988; 43:65–89.
15. Oda J, Tanaka H: Intervertebral disc changes with aging human cervical vertebrae. *Spine* 1988; 13:1205–1211.
16. Paris S: Cervical symptoms of forward head posture, *Top Geriatr Rehabil* 1990; 5:11–19.
17. Payne R: Neck pain in the elderly: A management review, part I. *Geriatrics* 1987; 42:59–65.
18. Travell J, Simons D: *Myofascial Pain and Dysfunction.* Baltimore, Md, Williams & Wilkins, 1983.
19. Wyke B: Cervical articular contributions to posture and gait: Their relation to senile disequilibrium. *Age Aging* 1979; 8:251.

Chapter 9

Shoulder Disorders: An Orthopedic Perspective

John G. Yost, Jr., M.D.

Daniel W. Schmoll, M.D.

As we age, our connective tissue undergoes degeneration. We develop gray hair and wrinkles, and degenerative changes occur in the tendons and joints of the body. This degenerative change is associated with the three most common shoulder problems found in the geriatric population: impingement, degenerative arthritis of the glenohumeral joint, and degenerative arthritis of the acromioclavicular joint. The anatomy of the shoulder and the effects of aging on the shoulder are discussed extensively in another section of the book and will not be discussed here.

The goal of this chapter is to help the examiner diagnose and treat the most common causes of shoulder pain and weakness in the geriatric population. Simply put, there are only four possible sources of shoulder pain.

1. The subacromial space: most commonly impingement syndrome and rotator cuff tears.

2. The glenohumeral joint: most commonly degenerative arthritis of the glenohumeral joint, or frozen shoulder syndrome. Instabilities and dislocations of the glenohumeral joint rarely occur in this age group.

3. The acromioclavicular joint: often the site of degenerative arthritis with spurs. On rare occasions, acromioclavicular joint separation and osteolysis can be encountered.

4. Elsewhere: the examiner must be aware that pain is referred to the shoulder region from cervical spine pathology, lung pathology, and certain abdominal pathology. By determining the area of origin of the pain, the examiner will have the highest yield of successful diagnoses and happy patients.

NORMAL EXAMINATION

Normal examination of the shoulder includes an assessment of range of motion (Fig 9–1) and power (Fig 9–2), palpation (Fig 9–3), and common maneuvers used to discern the source of pain in the shoulder (Fig 9–4).

THE SUBACROMIAL SPACE

The subacromial space is the most common site of symptoms in older active adults. Here impinge-

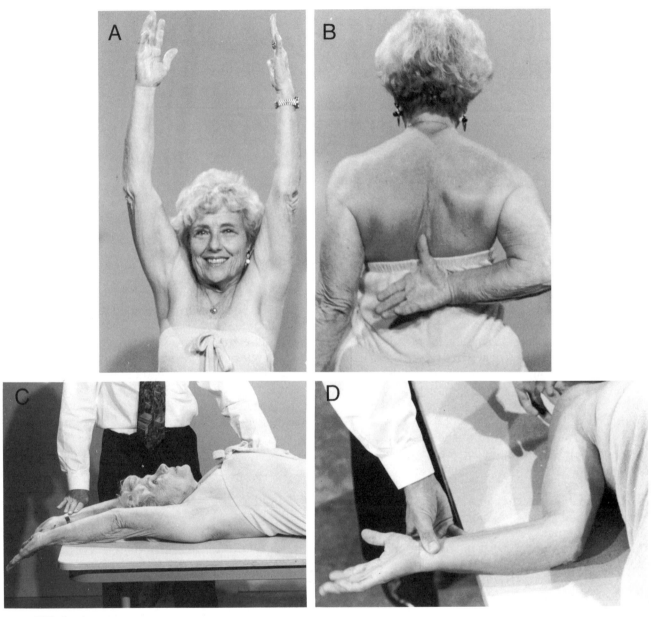

FIG 9–1.
Range of motion of the shoulder. **A,** active elevation. **B,** internal rotation. **C,** passive elevation. **D,** external rotation.

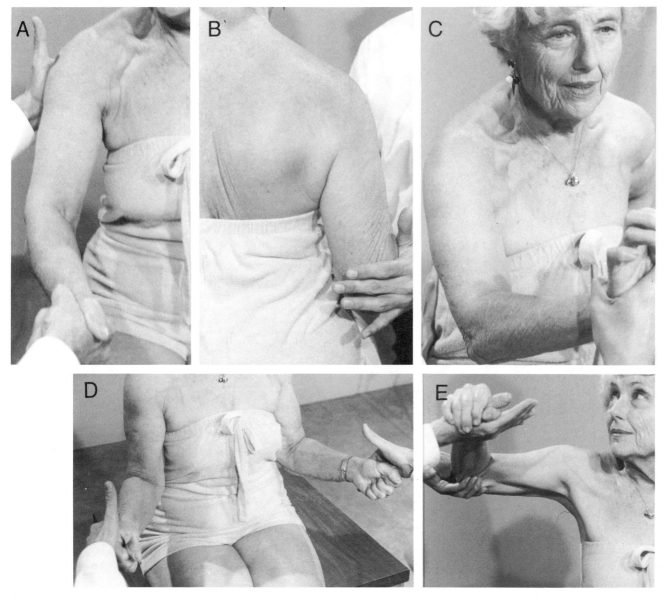

FIG 9–2.
Strength evaluation of the shoulder. **A,** anterior deltoid: axillary nerve, C5 root innervation. **B,** posterior deltoid: axillary nerve, C5 root innervation. **C,** triceps: radial nerve, C7 root innervation. **D,** external rotators: suprascapular nerve, C5 innervation. **E,** subscapularis: nerve to the subscapularis, C4 innervation.

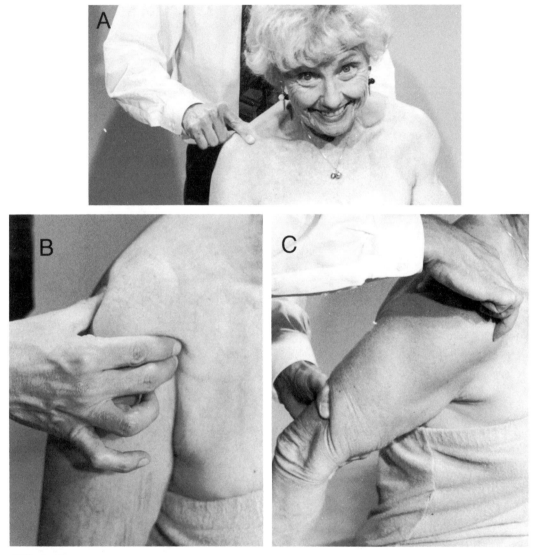

FIG 9–3.
A, palpation of the acromioclavicular joint. **B,** palpation of the greater tuberosity at the insertion site of the rotator cuff. **C,** palpation of the biceps tendon in the bicipital groove.

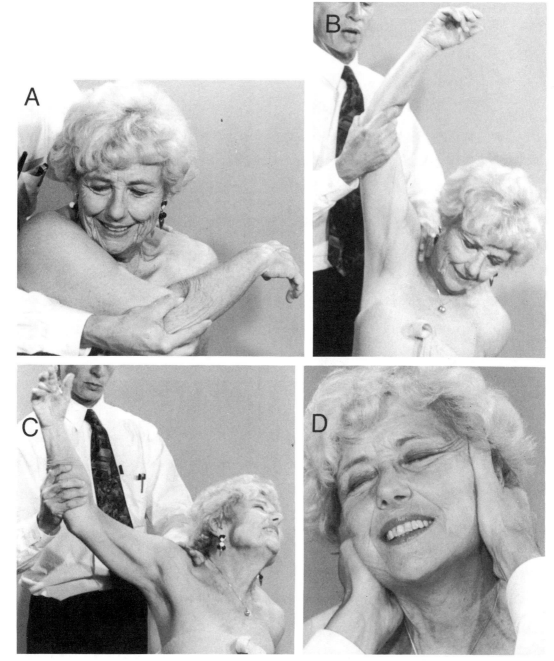

FIG 9–4.
A, Galle maneuver to elicit acromioclavicular joint tenderness. **B,** impingement maneuver to elicit impingement pain. **C,** apprehension maneuver to elicit glenohumeral instability. A positive test result will produce pain and apprehension. **D,** posterolateral extension of the neck to reproduce radicular pain.

ment syndrome commonly occurs, and this is usually associated with degenerative changes in the rotator cuff. Classically, impingement syndrome is described as stage I, stage II, or stage III.[5] Stage I consists of hemorrhage and edema, and usually occurs in an individual who is under the age of 35 years. This usually responds well to conservative treatment. It may or may not be associated with an impingement lesion and spurring of the anterior portion of the acromion or degenerative spurring of the acromioclavicular joint (Fig 9–5,A).

Stage II impingement is seen more commonly in patients in the age range of 35 to 50 years. Evidence of degeneration and fibrosis of the supraspinatus

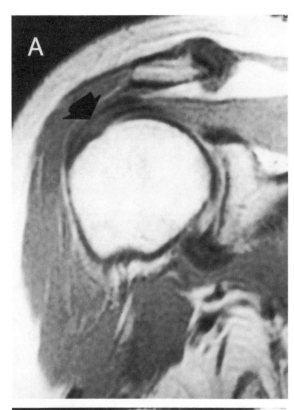

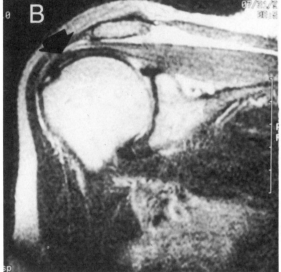

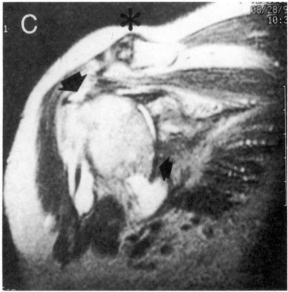

FIG 9–5.
A, normal magnetic resonance image (MRI) of the shoulder. **B,** MRI of the shoulder showing a partial rotator cuff tear. **C,** MRI of the shoulder showing a complete rotator cuff tear *(large arrow)*, degenerative joint disease of the glenohumeral joint *(small arrow)*, and the acromioclavicular joint *(star).*

tendon and biceps tendon are noted (Fig 9–5,B). Impingement lesions with spurring of the anterior aspect of the acromion and acromioclavicular joint degenerative changes are common. Conservative treatment takes longer to obtain a good result in these patients. Some will require operative intervention consisting of decompression of the subacromial space by removing the inferior portion of the acromion and possibly debridement of a partial rotator cuff tear.[3, 4, 12, 13, 15, 16]

Stage III impingement involves a complete tear of the rotator cuff, most commonly the supraspinatus tendon (Fig 9–5,C), less commonly the subscapularis tendon. Complete rotator cuff tears can progress over time to also include the biceps tendon with rupture and disruption of the infraspinatus and teres minor from their insertions on the greater tuberosity of the humerus.

Impingement syndrome can occur secondary to repetitive overhead activity, a sudden fall or jerk on the shoulder, or attempts to lift a heavy weight with an outstretched arm. The most consistent positive

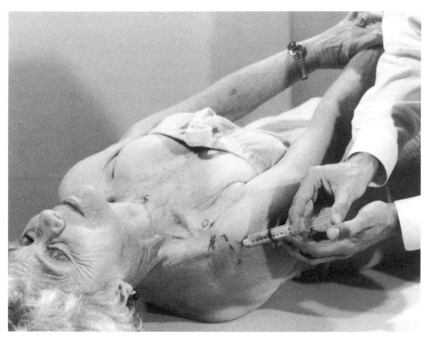

FIG 9-6.
Injection site for the subacromial space.

findings in impingement syndrome are a limitation of internal rotation (see Fig 9–1,B), a positive impingement maneuver (see Fig 9–4,B), and weakness of the external rotators (see Fig 9–2,D). Injection of the subacromial space with lidocaine will relieve pain (Fig 9–6). MRI is extremely helpful in determining the diagnosis of a complete vs. a partial tear of the rotator cuff as well as evaluating the size and extent of the impingement lesions and the extent of arthritis in the acromioclavicular joint. Complete tears of the rotator cuff require operative repair with an anterior acromioplasty and, if symptoms merit and radiographic examination shows evidence of acromioclavicular arthritis, partial or complete resection of the distal end of the clavicle.[15] This is followed by a progressive physical therapy program for gaining range of motion followed by strengthening exercises. Impingement syndrome with rotator cuff pathology is the most common cause of pain in the active geriatric population.

GLENOHUMERAL JOINT

Instability

The second anatomic site for shoulder pain in the geriatric population is the glenohumeral joint. The most common athletic injury in this area is a dislocation or subluxation of the glenohumeral joint with a sprain or tear of the glenohumeral ligaments. In the geriatric population such injuries are more commonly associated with a fracture of one of the tuberosities where the rotator cuff muscles attach or a rupture of the supraspinatus tendon. Shoulder dislocations need to be reduced immediately. If a fracture is present and is minimally displaced, treatment with immobilization until early healing of the fracture is noted followed by range of motion and subsequent strengthening programs is the recommended treatment and usually yields good results.[2] If significant displacement of the tuberosity with the rotator cuff attached has occurred, operative repair may be necessary. Likewise, torn supraspinatus tendons require repair. Recurrent dislocations of the shoulder are a common problem in young athletes; however, this is very rare in older athletes, and the older an individual gets, the less likely he is to have a recurrent dislocation of the shoulder.

Osteoarthritis

Degenerative arthritis of the glenohumeral joint (see Fig 9–5,C) is not as common as degenerative arthritis of the hip or knee.[6] Clinical signs and symptoms are pain with progressive limitation of motion, morning stiffness, and symptomatic changes with the weather. On examination the patient will show a limitation of internal and external rotation with some limitation of active elevation. Power testing usually shows normal strength. On x-ray evaluation, narrowing of the glenohumeral joint is found. Range of motion and strengthening exercises with nonsteroidal anti-inflammatory medicine will yield improvement in most patients. In severe cases joint replacement is performed, followed by an intensive physical therapy program for range of motion and strengthening exercises. The results of total-shoulder arthroplasty are very rewarding for most patients and allow resumption of recreational sports. Long-term results of total-shoulder arthroplasty are good, and longevity is expected to be high.[8] Large stresses are put through the shoulder joint with sports, but they are not as severe as the stresses put through the weight-bearing joints of the hip and knee.

Frozen Shoulder Syndrome

Frozen shoulder syndrome, or adhesive capsulitis, is another source of pain emanating from the glenohumeral joint. This is most common in women aged 40 to 55 years and can occur bilaterally. The diagnosis is made by examination when the patient exhibits a limitation of motion in all planes. X-ray findings are usually negative. Most causes of frozen shoulder are idiopathic. Diabetics and patients with renal disease seem especially susceptible. Underlying pathology such as calcification of the supraspinatus tendon or a rotator cuff tear can contribute to a frozen shoulder. However, with a rotator cuff tear, in addition to limitation of motion in all planes, weakness of the external rotators is also noted.[9] Treatment for frozen shoulder syndrome consists of an intensive rehabilitation program including range of motion exercises three times a day, as well as supervised rehabilitation with a physical therapist for range of motion and progressive strengthening exercises. Most patients are treated successfully with a conservative treatment plan.[10] If stiffness persists after an aggressive physical therapy program, manipulation of the shoulder under anesthesia followed by an intensive physical therapy program is of benefit.

ACROMIOCLAVICULAR JOINT

Degenerative Arthritis

The third anatomic location for shoulder pain in active older adults is the acromioclavicular joint (see

Fig 9–5,C). Degenerative arthritis of the acromioclavicular joint is the most common cause of pain in this region of the shoulder. The diagnosis is made by radiographic evidence of degenerative arthritis of the joint. On clinical examination patients with acromioclavicular symptoms will have tenderness to palpation over the acromioclavicular joint (see Fig 9–3,A) and pain in the acromioclavicular joint upon adduction of the shoulder, a Galle maneuver (see Fig 9–4,A). Treatment consists of nonsteroidal anti-inflammatory medicine and avoidance of compressive loads on the acromioclavicular joint such as lifting heavy objects overhead or pushups. An injection with a corticosteroid in the acromioclavicular joint is sometimes helpful (Fig 9–7). For patients who do not improve with conservative treatment, surgery with partial or complete resection of the acromioclavicular joint is recommended. This is followed by a period of rest to allow healing of the trapezius and deltoid muscles and later a range of motion and strengthening program for the shoulder.

Acromioclavicular Separation

A fall on the posterior aspect of the shoulder drives the scapula distally while the clavicle, which is still attached to the sternum, remains in place. The annular ligaments of the acromioclavicular joint and the coracoclavicular ligaments, which stabilize the distal end of the clavicle, are torn by this force, with ensuing upward elevation of the distal portion of the clavicle. This injury is more common in the younger athlete.[14] Most can be treated symptomatically with rest and ice followed by a range of motion and subsequent strengthening program for the shoulder with avoidance of abduction of the shoulder and compressive loads. It is rare for a separation of the acromioclavicular joint in the geriatric patient to be so severe that it requires surgery. However, with severe displacement, the clavicle can herniate through the muscles and be irreducible. This requires operative repair and stabilization followed by a range of motion and strengthening program when the repair is satisfactorily healed.

Osteolysis

A third cause of pain in the acromioclavicular joint is an entity called osteolysis. This was originally seen in weight lifters, but is very rare in the geriatric population. Significant inflammation develops in the acromioclavicular joint with progressive resorption of the distal end of the clavicle. Again, con-

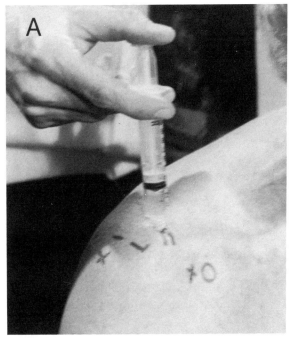
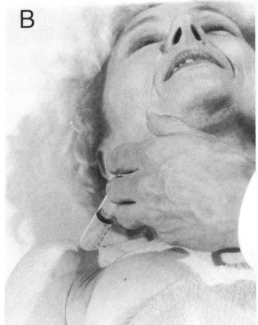

FIG 9–7.
A and **B**, injection site for the acromioclavicular joint.

servative treatment is usually of benefit, with injection of the acromioclavicular joint if nonsteroidal anti-inflammatory medicine is unsuccessful. Rarely is resection of the distal portion of the clavicle required for symptomatic improvement. Following healing of the suture line, a progressive range of motion and strengthening program is instituted.

ELSEWHERE

Degenerative Joint Disease of the Cervical Spine With Radiculopathy

Degenerative changes in the cervical spine with narrowing of the disc space and progressive spurring of the bone can result in impingement of the cervical nerve roots as they exit the spine. With narrowing of the neuroforamen, pinching of the nerve roots can occur and cause pain to radiate down the arm, sometimes in association with numbness in the fingers and hand. The most common level is the C6 nerve root, which classically causes symptoms of numbness to the thumb and weakness to the wrist extensors and biceps. Another common level for cervical radiculopathy is the C5 nerve root, compression of which causes pain radiating to the shoulder

and associated weakness of the deltoid. On examination, pain originating from the cervical spine should be suspected when the pain can be reproduced by extending and laterally flexing the neck (see Fig 9–4,D). This maneuver pinches the nerve as it exits the cervical spine and will reproduce pain along the course of the cervical nerve root. Abnormalities are also usually noted on neurologic examination of the upper extremities, with changes in strength, sensation, and reflexes commonly observed. Most cervical radiculopathies are improved with a conservative treatment program consisting of nonsteroidal anti-inflammatory medicine, a neck rehabilitation program consisting of range of motion and strengthening exercises, and cervical traction. Surgical decompression of the nerve root and/or spinal cord is indicated if the patient is not improved after a reasonable conservative program or if there is evidence of progressive neurologic deficit or spinal cord compression.

Lungs

A lung mass can refer pain to the shoulder (Fig 9–8). Most common is a Pancoast tumor. An index of suspicion should be present in individuals who are in their 50s and 60s and have a history of smoking and diffuse shoulder pain often associated with pain radiating into the chest and neck. These pa-

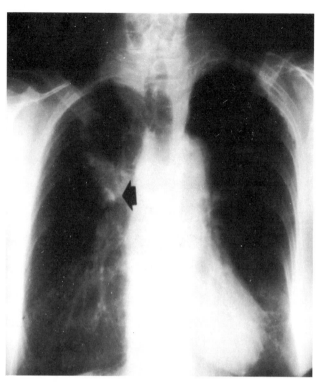

FIG 9–8.
Radiograph showing a lung tumor causing shoulder pain.

tients often have normal findings on shoulder and neck examination.

Abdomen

Occasionally, irritation of the diaphragm and cholecystitis can cause referred pain to the shoulder.

Reflex Sympathetic Dystrophy/Shoulder-Hand Syndrome

Occasionally, a pathology or trauma distal to the shoulder can result in stiffness and pain in the shoulder. This is called shoulder-hand syndrome or reflex sympathetic dystrophy, an entity that is not completely understood but can occur after carpal tunnel syndrome, hand trauma, elective hand surgery, or chronic tendinitis. Joint stiffness is a significant part of this entity, and treatment consists of modalities to gain control of the pain with intensive physical therapy for range of motion and subsequent strengthening exercises. Sympathetic blocks have been used to help the pain and may be helpful.

SUMMARY

When examining a painful shoulder in an older active adult, the clinician should keep in mind the positive findings on examination as they relate to a specific pathology, and the yield of successful diagnoses will improve. The right diagnosis yields the most appropriate treatment plan and the greatest chance for success.

To summarize, the most common causes for shoulder pain are as follows:

1. Impingement, which is associated with a positive impingement maneuver and weakness of the external rotators.
2. Acromioclavicular arthritis, which is associated with pain upon palpation over the acromioclavicular joint and acromioclavicular pain with adduction of the arm.
3. Degenerative arthritis of the glenohumeral joint, which is associated with a limitation of motion in all planes and positive x-ray evidence of narrowing of the glenohumeral joint.
4. Frozen shoulder syndrome, which is associated with a limitation of motion in all planes but normal power testing and radiographic findings.
5. Cervical spine pathology, which is associated with radicular pain, positive findings on a neurologic examination, and radicular pain with posterolateral extension of the cervical spine.

Combinations of the above pathology occur in clinical practice and can give a confusing picture. Noting positive findings with a logical and simple approach is most helpful in determining which combination exists.

REFERENCES

1. Bigilioni LU, Kimmel J, McCoon PD: Repair of rotator cuff tears in tennis players. *Am J Sports Med* 1992; 20:112–117.
2. Burkhead WZ, Rockwood CA: Treatment of instability of the shoulder with an exercise program. *J Bone Joint Surg [Am]* 1992; 74:890–986.
3. Ellman H: Arthroscopic subacromial decompression: Analysis of one-to-three years results. *Arthroscopy* 1987; 3:173–181.
4. Gortsman GM: Arthroscopic acromioplasty for lesion of the rotator cuff. *J Bone Joint Surg [Am]* 1990; 72:169–280.
5. Neer CS II: Anterior acromioplasty for the chronic

impingement syndrome in the shoulder. A preliminary report. *J Bone Joint Surg [Am]* 1972; 56:41–50.

6. Neer CS II: Replacement arthroplasty for glenohumeral osteoarthritis. *J Bone Joint Surg [Am]* 1974; 56:1–13.

7. Neer CS II, Foster CR: Inferior capsular shift for involuntary inferior and multidirectional instability of the shoulder. A preliminary report. *J Bone Joint Surg [Am]* 1980; 62:897–908.

8. Neer CS II, Watson KC, Stanton FJ: Recent experience in total shoulder replacement. *J Bone Joint Surg [Am]* 1982; 64:319–337.

9. Neviaser RJ: Adhesive capulitis of the shoulder: Study of pathological findings in periarthritis of the shoulder. *J Bone Joint Surg [Am]* 1945; 27:211–222.

10. Neviaser RJ, Neviaser TJ: The frozen shoulder. Diagnosis and management. *Clin Orthop* 1987; 223:59–65.

11. Neviaser RJ, Neviaser TJ, Neviaser JS: Concurrent rupture of shoulder in the rotator cuff and primary anterior dislocation in the older patient. *J Bone Joint Surg [Am]* 1988; 70:1308–1311.

12. Norlin R: Arthroscopic subacromial decompression versus open acromioplasty. *Arthroscopy* 1983; 5:321–323.

13. Paulos LE, Franklin JL: Arthroscopic shoulder decompression development and application. A five year experience. *Am J Sports Med* 1990; 18:235–244.

14. Rockwood CA Jr: Injuries to the acromioclavicular joint, in Rockwood CA Jr, Green D (eds): *Fractures in Adults*, ed 2. Philadelphia, JB Lippincott, 1984, pp 860–910.

15. Snyder SJ, et al: Partial thickness rotator cuff tears: Results of arthroscopic treatment. *Arthroscopy* 1991; 7:1–7.

16. Von Holsbeck E, et al: Subacromial impingement: Open versus arthroscopic decompression. *Arthroscopy* 1992; 8:173–178.

Chapter 10

Shoulder Injuries: A Rehabilitation Perspective

Janet Sobel, P.T.

The shoulder complex is subject to extraordinary stresses in meeting the challenge of balancing the stability and mobility demands over an individual's life span. Effective management of shoulder pathology begins with thorough knowledge of its anatomy and biomechanics, as well as the normal and pathologic effects of aging on its function.

ANATOMY

Bones and Joints of the Shoulder Complex

There are five major joints that make up the shoulder complex: sternoclavicular, acromioclavicular, glenohumeral (all of which are synovial joints), scapulothoracic (a muscular joint), and humerocoracoclavicular joints.[99] The S-shaped clavicle is thicker and cylindrical medially and flat and narrow laterally.[39] The sternoclavicular joint is incongruent and planar, and acts like a ball-and-socket joint. A fibrocartilaginous disc increases the congruity between the clavicle and manubrium, thus stabilizing the joint. This disc also acts as a buffer, protecting the joint from degenerative changes.[27] Movements at this joint include elevation, depression, protraction, retraction, and rotation. The scapula itself consists of a body, spine, acromion, neck, the glenoid fossa, and the coracoid process. The body covers the second through seventh ribs and is oriented approximately 30 to 45 degrees anterior to the coronal plane of the body.[39] The costal surface is concave, forming the subscapular fossa. The dorsal convex surface is divided into supraspinous and infraspinous fossas by the scapular spine. On the superior border of the supraspinous fossa is the supraspinous notch, through which travels the suprascapular nerve. The suprascapular ligament closes the notch and the supraspinous artery travels above the ligament. The suprascapular nerve may become entrapped here by thickening of the ligament or by ganglion formation. The coracoid process is a bony projection off the scapula medial to the scapular neck.[39] Bigliani and co-workers[7] describe three variations in acromion shape: type 1 has a flat surface with high angulation, type 2 has a downwardly curved undersurface with less angulation, and type 3 has a hook-shaped configuration anteriorly, with the least angulation. These classic variations become significant in rotator cuff pathology, which will be discussed later.

The acromioclavicular joint is also incongruent, with a fibrocartilaginous disc. The anterior-posterior stability of this joint is controlled by the acromioclavicular ligaments, while the vertical stability is controlled by the coracoclavicular ligaments.[89] DePalma[27] describes the acromial variations in terms of the joint itself, where type 1 is vertically oriented, type 2 more oblique with the clavicle sloping medially at the inferior surface and type 3 has an almost horizontal angulation between the clavicle and the acromion. He found that most patients with degenerative changes at the acromioclavicular joint had type 1 clavicles.[26]

The glenoid fossa is shaped like an inverted comma and is normally retroverted from 2 to 12 degrees.[39] There is considerable disagreement in the literature as to the effects of variations in this positioning. Saha describes patients with anterior instability as tending to have more anteversion of the glenoid.[85] Some feel posterior instability is more prevalent in patients with increased posterior retroversion.[39] The humerus consists of the head, neck, and the greater and lesser tuberosities. The greater tuberosity is more lateral, projecting superiorly and posteriorly. The lesser tuberosity lies along the anterior margin of the proximal humerus. The tuberosities are separated by the intertubercular groove, through which the biceps tendon passes.[41] According to Neer et al,[64] a shallow intertubercular groove makes the tendon of the long head of the biceps and its overlying ligaments more prominent and thus more vulnerable to impingement injury. The major blood supply to the humeral head, the ascending branch of the anterior humeral circumflex artery, enters the humerus in this intertubercular groove.[41] Hurley[39] describes the glenohumeral joint as a golf ball sitting on its tee. Because of the positional relationship and the incongruity of contact, only about one third of the humeral head makes contact with the glenoid at any one time.[29, 75] The labrum increases the contact to about three quarters, thus enhancing the stability of the glenohumeral joint. Mosely and Overgaard[58] describe the labrum as a redundant fold of capsular tissue with a small fibrocartilaginous component.

Joint Capsule and Ligaments

The acromioclavicular joint is reinforced by surrounding ligaments anteriorly, posteriorly, superiorly, and inferiorly, as well as by the coracoclavicular, conoid, and trapezoid ligaments. Distraction of the acromioclavicular joint is limited by the acromioclavicular ligaments; compression is limited by the trapezoid ligament. The conoid ligament is the primary restraint to anterior and superior displacement of the clavicle.[31, 92] The coracoclavicular ligaments also help to rotate the clavicle on its long axis in overhead activities.[75]

The capsule of the glenohumeral joint attaches around the perimeter of the glenoid and spans across to attach to the anatomic neck of the humerus except inferiorly, where its attachment is about 1 cm distal to the articular margin. At the upper end of the biceps groove, the capsule is the transverse humeral ligament.[62]

A study by Clark et al[18] found that the capsule is thickest anteriorly, in the interval between the subscapularis and the supraspinatus. It is also thick where it is most firmly attached to the tendons of the rotator cuff, adjacent to their insertions onto the tuberosities. It is thinnest where it has no attachments: posteroinferiorly along the margins of the glenoid and on portions with tendinous insertions; and inferiorly, adjacent to the glenoid and where it is continuous with the bursal sacs between the glenohumeral ligaments. Clark et al[18] found that at least half of the capsular surface receives an insertion of muscle or tendon from the rotator cuff and that some of the tension of the rotator cuff muscles may be distributed into the capsule. Thus the capsule reinforces the rotator cuff and tears of the rotator cuff may alter the anatomy of other structures around the shoulder joint.[17]

The glenohumeral joint capsule has a medial recess that allows large arcs of unrestricted movement, as well as anterior capsule thickenings referred to as the glenohumeral ligaments. These ligaments statically help reinforce the anterior capsule.[29] The capsule is extremely strong, with great stretching capacity.[43] The glenohumeral ligaments are thickenings of the anterior joint capsule and play an important role in the stability of the glenohumeral joint.[39, 74] The anterior ligaments may insert directly onto the labrum or further medially along the scapular neck, forming synovial recesses above and below the middle glenohumeral ligament and above the inferior glenohumeral ligament.[25, 58] The superior glenohumeral ligament lies under the coracohumeral ligament and provides passive resistance to inferior subluxation or dislocation of the humerus. The middle glenohumeral ligament lies under the subscapular muscle and tendon and is considered to be the major constraint to anterior humeral displacement. The inferior glenohumeral ligament, the thickest of the ligaments, reinforces the inferior capsule. It is considered by many to be the primary stabilizer against anterior and posterior inferior glenohumeral instability.[56, 72, 74] Superiorly, the coracohumeral ligament also provides shoulder stability. It extends from the base of the coracoid to the top of the biceps groove, and provides stability when the arm is dependent.[4, 74] The posterior labrum is loosely attached to the surrounding capsule, which is thin posteriorly. There appears to be no direct posterior ligamentous reinforcement.[87]

The coracoacromial arch is formed by the coracoacromial ligament and the acromial process. The coracoacromial ligament is a triangular band whose role has been widely discussed. It appears to function in protecting the humeral head from trauma, providing some constraint against superior migration of the humeral head. The subacromial bursa lies between the coracoacromial ligament and the rotator cuff. It extends from the coracoid process medially to the greater tuberosity laterally.[39]

Musculature

The shoulder is unique in its constant dynamic interplay of stability and mobility. The muscles of the shoulder complex are called upon to generate motion and provide dynamic stability. They can be divided into five groups: the axioscapular group, the axiohumeral group, the scapulohumeral group, the scapuloradial, and the scapuloulnar group. The muscles of the axioscapular group run from the trunk to the scapula. They include the trapezii, the rhomboids, the serratus anterior and the levator scapula. Movement of the scapula is created by the combined action of these muscles. The upper trapezius elevates the outer border of the spine of the scapula, causing inward pivoting around the acromioclavicular joint. The middle trapezius fixes the medial border of the scapula to the thorax and the lower trapezius depresses the medial border of the spine of the scapula, pulling it down and in. The serratus anterior protracts the scapula and contributes significantly to scapular stability. Jobe[42] found the serratus anterior to be active in all movements of the humerus. The combined action of the lower trapezius, the upper trapezius, and the serratus anterior upwardly rotates the scapula around the axis center of the acromioclavicular joint, depressing the vertebral border and elevating the glenoid fossa,[13] thus rotating the acromion away from the humeral head in forward flexion of the arm. The rhomboids and the levator scapula retract the scapula and rotate it downward. The serratus, trapezii, and rhomboids stabilize the scapula to the thorax, providing a base for shoulder activities.

The muscles of the axiohumeral group run from the trunk to the scapula. This includes the pectoralis major and the latissimus dorsi. The pectoralis major adducts and internally rotates the arm; the latissimus adducts, internally rotates, and extends the arm.

The muscles of the scapulohumeral, scapuloradial, and scapuloulnar groups include the teres major, deltoid, rotator cuff, biceps, triceps and coracobrachialis. The upper borders of the teres major, the lower border of the teres minor, and long head of

the triceps form the triangular space, the scapular circumflex arteries travel. The ... eral or quadrangular space is lateral to this. It is formed by the lower border of the teres minor, the upper border of the teres major, the lateral border of the long head of the triceps, and the medial border of the humerus. The axillary nerve and posterior humeral circumflex arteries travel through this quadrilateral space.[39]

The long head of the biceps originates at the superior border of the labrum and passes through the shoulder joint into the bicipital groove. It acts as a humeral head depressor when the arm is externally rotated.

The rotator cuff is made up of the supraspinatus, infraspinatus, teres minor, and subscapularis. The supraspinatus arises from the supraspinous fossa of the scapula, passes beneath the acromion and acromioclavicular joint and attaches to the upper aspect of the greater tuberosity. The infraspinatus arises from the infraspinous fossa of the scapula and attaches to the posterolateral aspect of the greater tuberosity. The teres minor arises from the lower lateral aspect of the scapula and attaches to the lower aspect of the greater tuberosity. The infraspinatus and teres minor externally rotate the arm. The subscapularis arises from the anterior aspect of the scapula and attaches over much of the lesser tuberosity.[53] The subscapularis internally rotates the arm. In addition to their independent motions, the muscles of the rotator cuff work together to stabilize the glenohumeral joint, compressing it and preventing upward displacement of the humeral head by the pull of the deltoid. According to Saha,[85] if a healthy relationship exists, a locking of the greater tuberosity against the acromion never occurs in active forward flexion or abduction, because of this rolling down, or caudal glide, of the humeral head in the glenoid fossa.

Colachis et al[23, 24] found that the supraspinatus and infraspinatus provide 45% of shoulder abduction and 90% of external rotation strength. Codman[20] and Clark[17] each described an interlacing of the fibers of each of the rotator cuff tendons with its neighbor tendon, so that the tendons of the four muscles flare out and interdigitate as they insert onto the humerus. The role of the rotator cuff then involves stabilizing the shoulder, rotating the arm, and adding power to elevating the arm, and possibly enhancing nutrition to the articular cartilage by containing the synovial fluid.[53]

The vascularity of the rotator cuff has been discussed extensively.[13, 20, 49, 57, 79, 83] Several arteries provide the blood supply to the rotator cuff:

- Anterior humeral circumflex artery (subscapularis, humeral head, and long head of the biceps)
- Posterior humeral circumflex artery (teres minor, infraspinatus)
- Suprascapular artery (teres minor, infraspinatus)
- Thoracoacromial artery (subscapularis, supraspinatus)
- Suprahumeral artery (subscapularis, lesser tuberosity of the humerus)
- Subscapular artery (subscapularis)

The first three arteries are present in all individuals; the last three are present in decreasing order of frequency.[83]

There is considerable disagreement about the vascularity of an area near the insertion of the supraspinatus known as the critical zone of the rotator cuff.[47, 49, 52, 57, 71, 83] This critical zone, which seems most prone to degenerative changes and calcium deposits, is also thought to be the area of greatest tensile force on the supraspinatus. Lindblom,[47] Rothman and Parke,[83] and McMasters[52] describe it as an area of relative avascularity. McMasters concluded that since this area of avascularity coincides with the area most prone to degeneration, blood supply must be considered strongly as an important factor in degenerative lesions.[52]

According to Mosely and Goldie,[57] as well as Nixon and deStefano,[71] the critical zone is rich in anastamoses between the osseous and tendinous blood vessels. Rathburn and McNab[79] found the filling of the rotator cuff to be dependent on the position of the arm: there was poor filling when the arm was adducted and good filling when abducted. They concluded that rotator cuff tendon failure may result from the constant pressure of the humeral head, which tends to wring out the blood supply to the tendon when the arm is held in adduction. Lohr and Uhthoff[49] saw a relative hypovascularity of the deep surface of the supraspinatus insertion as compared with the superficial aspect. They describe a layering in the supraspinatus tendon: the bursal side has an abundance of blood vessels and the articular side is sparsely supplied, with almost no blood vessels distally. This articular side with its decreased vascularization is thus more susceptible to failure. They attribute their observation of little inflammatory response in partial tears on the articular side to this absence of vessels.[49]

BIOMECHANICS OF THE SHOULDER COMPLEX

Full clavicular motion at both the sternoclavicular and the acromioclavicular joints is essential for full scapulothoracic motion.[35] The glenohumeral joint has extraordinary range of motion because of the complex interplay of the articular, capsular-ligamentous and dynamic stabilizers.[56] The articular surfaces themselves impart virtually no inherent stability; most of this is provided by the soft tissues (ligaments and rotator cuff).[42]

Codman first described the scapulohumeral rhythm in 1934.[20] For each 15 degrees of abduction, 10 degrees occur at the glenohumeral joint and 5 degrees are the result of scapular rotation against the chest wall. The scapula can rotate 90 degrees actively and 120 degrees passively. For shoulder elevation, the scapula rotates upwardly, preserving optimal muscle length and increasing stability by keeping the glenoid cavity directly under the humeral head and removing the acromion from the path of the humeral head. The humerus must externally rotate fully to move the greater tuberosity posterior to the acromion, thus preventing soft-tissue impingement.[13]

The capsular-ligament complex is the major static stabilizer of the shoulder. The ligaments function in a coordinated manner to resist joint translation in two ways: first, in that their presence resists displacement and second, by increased joint contact pressure opposite the direction of displacement.[56]

With the arm at the side in a neutral position the subscapularis muscle and the middle glenohumeral ligament provide the major stability. With the arm abducted beyond 45 degrees, the subscapularis is positioned above the humeral head, thus uncovering it anteriorly and superiorly and providing little stability. Here, the superior band of the glenohumeral ligament is the major stabilizer of the glenohumeral joint.[90] There is no direct posterior ligamentous reinforcement, but when the arm is flexed, adducted, and internally rotated, the anterior capsule winds up like a cord, preventing posterior subluxation and dislocation.[13] The middle glenohumeral ligament is thought to become taut in the extremes of internal and external rotation.[56] Saha[84] described the "zero position" of the shoulder, at approximately 165 degrees of elevation and 45 degrees anterior to the coronal plane. Here, shear and compression forces of the rotator cuff and deltoid are equally balanced. Here, too, the rotator cuff muscles are ineffective and active rotation is lost.

The force couples acting at the shoulder are of tremendous significance. Ellenbecker and Derscheid[29] described a force couple as two equal but oppositely directed forces not acting along the same line. The deltoid muscle and the rotator cuff act to elevate the humerus. The rotator cuff provides caudal glide and glenohumeral compression throughout elevation and all four rotator cuff muscles are active throughout forward flexion and abduction. The deltoid muscle, because of poor leverage and low angular pull, creates a shear force in early elevation. This force tends to upwardly displace the humeral head and is greatest to 90 degrees, especially when inadequately opposed by rotator cuff compression and caudal glide. Above 90 degrees, the deltoid pull passes through the glenohumeral joint, providing additional stability.[40, 96] Fatigue, poor tension generation, or intrinsic tension overload may cause failure of this force couple, so that elevation of the humerus could lessen the acromiohumeral interval.[68] The other force couple at the shoulder involves the trapezius and serratus anterior muscles. They work together to hold the scapula against the thorax, thus preventing winging, and to track the scapula anteriorly, laterally, and superiorly for upward rotation of the glenoid fossa.[20]

THE EFFECTS OF AGING

Menard summarizes physical aging as "a gradual impairment of our organ systems such that their functional reserves are eroded to the point that we are gradually less able to compensate for environmental stresses, metabolic disturbance, and disease processes."[55] Although aging does seem to affect all aspects of our being, it is critical in working with aging patients that we begin to discern what extent of physiologic decline is affected by aging versus inactivity.

One skeletal change occurring with age is loss of bone mass, which is generally more extensive in women than in men. Men achieve a higher peak skeletal mass than women and after age 50 lose bone mass at a rate of approximately 0.4% per year. Women start to lose bone mass much earlier and experience a much higher rate of loss.[6] Connective tissue (e.g., ligaments and tendons) undergoes a reduction in water content, resulting in decreased shock absorption capacity and loss of tissue compliance. Furthermore, the molecular stability of collagen improves, thus lessening collagen fiber compliance, and elastin fibers get more brittle and more susceptible to injury.[93] Because of decreased water content and decreased compliance of collagen fibers, articular cartilage also suffers with age, becoming a less effective shock absorber.[55] There is a loss of neurons with age, so that fewer neurons activate more muscle fibers.[14]

A number of studies have found a decrease in skeletal muscle strength with age. Borges[9] found a significant inverse correlation between age and isokinetic thigh muscle torque with age. She attributed this to decreased fiber areas in old age, loss of total muscle fibers between the ages of 30 and 70, and changes in the neuromuscular system, with progressive decrease in the trophic function of the nerve cell in old age.[9] She found the changes in isokinetic torque at all velocities. Aniansson[2] found a decrease in maximum isometric strength with age. In a study of 118 people ages 62 to 102, Rice et al[81] found age to be the most important variable with respect to loss of strength. Although muscle does undergo changes with age, it does seem to remain biochemically stable and to maintain its capillary density.[2, 30, 33] There is, however, a decrease in muscle strength beyond age 50,[3] a decrease in muscle fiber area, and an increase in stiffness as a result of increased collagen content.[1]

Finally, Eagleston[28] explains the age-dependent slowing of healing in each stage of the healing process: the inflammatory stage is dampened, the proliferative stage is altered by the decreased cellular activity with age and the remodeling stage is affected because collagen is laid down more slowly, in smaller volumes, and with different binding patterns. It has been shown, however, that these undesirable effects of aging, however, are alterable with activity.[3, 4, 5, 55, 82, 88] It is expected that as our aging population grows and becomes more active, the positive effects of exercise and activity will, to some extent, overshadow the negative effects of aging.

Thus aging does involve a decrease in the body's resilience and efficiency in compensating for the stresses imposed upon it and in returning to its healthy, balanced state. The effect of age does appear to be altered by genetics and lifelong activity levels.

The Effects of Aging on the Shoulder Complex

A number of degenerative changes are known to occur at the shoulder with age. An exaggeration of the normal dorsal kyphosis, often a result of disc degeneration and postural inadequacies, results in an altered position of the scapula. As some postural muscles often weaken and opposing muscles shorten, an imbalance of the muscle forces of the shoulder complex results and self-perpetuates. The acromioclavicular joint normally begins to undergo a degenerative process as early as in the second decade, so that degenerative changes of the disc and articular cartilage of the acromioclavicular joint are more common than not in the 40 and older age group.[27] The acromions of people over 50 often have degenerative spurs and excrescences.[41] In the 60s the articular disc may be gone.[27] Interestingly, degenerative changes are not often noted in the sternoclavicular joint until the seventh decade.[27] Mechanical stress tests have shown that the strength of the joint capsule decreases with age and is considerably weaker in later decades.[43] De Palma found that with age, the superior portion of the labrum disassociates from the underlying glenoid.[27] Reeves[80] reported that while the weakest point of the glenohumeral capsule in young people is at the labral side, a dislocated shoulder of an older person will more likely show tearing of the capsule and subscapularis tendon.

The aging of the rotator cuff appears to be a chronologic progression, the rate and extent of which are determined by its ability to handle the physiologic and biomechanical demands placed upon it in the individual's activities. The inherent nature of this degeneration is somewhat based on its progressive physical and chemical degradation and on an increasingly compromised vascular supply. With time, the rotator cuff undergoes a loss of cellularity and resilience, fragmentation, disarray, and disorganization of the tendon fibers, and loss of vascularity.[12, 52, 63, 76] Codman[20] found a histologically normal rotator cuff tendon to be a rarity in older people. The degeneration of the rotator cuff commonly begins in the third decade and continues with age. In the fifth decade, many rotator cuffs are noted to be pulling away from their insertion sites and showing signs of thinning and defibrillation. This thinning has been most commonly noted in the so-called critical zone.[12, 76] This finding of progressive degeneration of the rotator cuff has been supported by a number of postmortem studies.[48, 97]

Interestingly, shoulder disorders often appear to be less symptomatic in the elderly than in the middle-aged population.[15, 37, 45] In a study by Chard and co-workers[16] of 664 persons older than 70 years, 21% had identifiable shoulder dislocations (more common in women); 26% had a complaint of current shoulder pain, 70% of which involved the rotator cuff. Fewer than 40% of the subjects sought medical attention for their symptoms. Upward subluxation of the humeral head and decreased space between the acromion and humeral head has been a common finding in the abnormal shoulder joints of the elderly and often is associated with failure of the rotator cuff.[12, 96] Age-induced changes at the shoulder, then, may include[12, 13, 20, 27, 43, 52, 62, 76]

- Weakening of the shoulder capsule
- Thickening and distention of the walls of the subacromial bursa
- Loss of cellularity and fragmentation of the bone, cystic degeneration, and irregularity of the greater tuberosity
- Absorption of the tuberosities of the humerus, resulting in shallowing and distortion of the bicipital grooves and compression of the biceps tendon
- Eburnation and thickening of the undersurface of the acromion, with spur and osteophyte formation further contributing to rotator cuff degeneration with increasing age
- Decreased vascularity and progressive degeneration of the rotator cuff
- Altered position of the scapula and dorsal kyphosis
- Upward subluxation of the humeral head with abnormal joint mechanics

Aging also has been found to impair joint range of motion owing to trauma from mechanical stresses, disuse, arthritis, altered scapular position, and increased dorsal kyphosis. Flexion-extension motion was found to decrease about 50 degrees, from 240 degrees in the young to 190 degrees at age 70. Abduction decreased from 180 degrees in the young to 116 degrees at age 70.[78] After age 60, a University of Pennsylvania study found flexion and abduction ranges to average 150 to 165 degrees in shoulders with no identifiable pathology, although some did achieve 180 degrees.[10]

Aging, however, is only one factor in these changes. Genetics, lifestyle, occupation, sports when young, and ongoing exercise tremendously affect the degree of these changes. Study after study shows the importance of ongoing exercise in minimizing, delaying and often offsetting strength, flexibility, and degenerative changes.[19, 60, 78, 81]

Before turning to treatment principles it is important to look at some specific pathologies of the shoulder in the elderly population and findings associated with these pathologies.

Arthritic Changes of the Glenohumeral Joint

Arthritis in the glenohumeral joint may be primary, with no apparent antecedent cause, or secondary. Causes of secondary arthritic changes include:

1. An old fracture or fracture-dislocations. In a study of 74 shoulders by Samilson and Prieto,[86] no relationship was found between the number of dislocations and the severity of joint disease. These researchers did find, however, that shoulders with posterior instability had a higher incidence of arthritis. In chronic dislocations, the humeral head may be indented and worn; cartilage may be replaced with scar tissue, and joint surfaces may be incongruent from weakening of the subchondral bone.[44]

2. Iatrogenic conditions from previous surgery in which internal fixation devices affected the joint surface.[21]

3. "Cuff tear arthropathy," as described by Neer and co-workers. Nutritional changes from massive rotator cuff tearing result in loss of articular cartilage, humeral head collapse, glenohumeral instability, and bone loss.[64]

4. Systemic diseases such as hematologic disorders, kidney failure, gout, and rheumatoid arthritis. Shoulder involvement seems to be common in rheumatoid arthritis and involves many pathologic changes, including inflammation, fibrosis, thinning, and instability of the shoulder capsule; inflammation, fibrosis, and hypertrophy of the synovial lining; inflammation and fibrosis of the subdeltoid bursa; erosion, resorption, sclerosis, cystic changes, and fracture of the bone; loss of articular cartilage; and rotator cuff disease. These pathologic findings vary in involvement and extent in each case.[21]

The pathologic findings of osteoarthritis of the shoulder joint are also likely to be multiple. At the humeral, there may be cartilage loss, sclerosis, os-

teophyte formation (usually inferiorly), erosion, subchondral cysts, and often central flattening. The bony surface irregularities are more common at the capsule and tendinous attachments. Glenoid changes include osteophytes, especially inferiorly, sclerosis, and erosion.[44] Degeneration of the joint may result in posterior wearing of the glenoid and posterior positioning of the humerus.[11] The capsule may be enlarged and develop anterior contractures. Loose bodies may be present in the joint or in the subscapularis bursa.[21] The major complaint of the patient with degenerative joint disease of the shoulder is usually pain and some resultant limitations of function. Often the patient will complain of pain on overhead activities and bringing the arm across the midline, pain if side-lying on that side, a generalized aching, and feeling of shoulder fatigue. Although activity exacerbates the pain and rest relieves it, the patient will often complain of night pain, especially when supine or side-lying on the involved side. In more severe situations, the patient will have given up on sleeping in bed and sleeps better in an easy chair. Objective findings may include significantly limited forward flexion and abduction range of motion, markedly limited rotations and internal rotation contractures, atrophy of the infraspinatus and supraspinatus, weak external rotation, and crepitus or grinding on shoulder elevation. Often the tenderness and crepitus are palpable posteriorly. Manual muscle testing is often inaccurate because of pain and grinding interference. The normal shoulder contours may be altered so that the anterior shoulder appears flattened and the posterior aspect more protruding.

Treatment usually involves some form of anti-inflammatory medication, exercise, and activity modification. Range-of-motion exercise must be gradual and gentle to avoid exacerbation or extension of symptoms. The goal is to maintain, rather than increase, the patient's range of motion. Isometrics and placing exercises are extremely effective for strengthening within the pain-free motion arcs. Unlike with rotator cuff tendinitis problems, the patient is usually very willing to modify activities to avoid pain. At the same time, he or she needs to be reminded of the importance of continuing to use the arm as much as possible. Emphasizing the need to keep the shoulder warm at all times is very helpful.

In more severe cases, where pain and loss of functional arm use are unacceptable, total shoulder arthroplasty may be desirable. The designs of currently available prostheses vary in terms of degree of constraint. Those that constrain minimally require a normally functioning rotator cuff. With increasing degrees of constraint, there is a decreasing need for a functional rotator cuff but increased chance of long-term dysfunction and failure.[21, 63, 64, 94] Some physicians recommend cuff repair before joint replacement to maximize postoperative functional potential. Postoperatively patients usually experience marked pain relief. If the rotator cuff is deficient, the patient is still likely to enjoy pain relief but only partial strength and motion gains. Postoperative rehabilitation programs vary widely, depending on the quality of the tissue (muscle and/or bone), the stability of the implant, and the surgeon's philosophy. Those who feel early motion is desirable may recommend a continuous passive motion device in addition to physical therapy. Generally, early passive motion (starting 1 to 2 days postoperatively) in flexion and external rotation is followed by pendulum, extension, and internal rotation. At about 3 to 6 weeks isometrics and abduction are added, then active exercise, progressing to resisted strengthening. Extensive postoperative guidelines are well covered by Neer.[63, 64]

Adhesive Capsulitis

Adhesive capsulitis, or frozen shoulder, describes the presentation of a shoulder with limited active and passive glenohumeral motion.[61] Adhesive capsulitis may present idiopathically or in association with other problems, such as cardiovascular accident, angina, or upper extremity injuries. Bateman indicates that adhesive capsulitis is much more common in the older population, usually after the age of 50 years.[5] Postmenopausal women appear to be most susceptible.[72] The onset is usually insidious, with a progressive loss of motion. Neviaser[65] describes a contracted, thickened joint capsule drawn tightly around the humeral head with a relative absence of synovial fluid. He found cellular changes of chronic inflammation with fibrosis and perivascular infiltration in the subsynovial layer of the capsule comparable to a reparative inflammatory reaction.[65] With progression of the capsulitis, there may be contracture with inelasticity of the rotator cuff muscle bellies and involvement of the bicep tendon sheath.[5, 51] Many authors report that frozen shoulder is most common in the 40- to 70-year-old population.[50, 61] It is more common among diabetics (10% to 20% incidence) than in the general population (2% to 5% incidence).[49, 60] It is more common in women than in men, but men usually present with less motion than women. There is considerable variation in the literature as to what actually are the criteria for making the diagnosis of adhesive capsulitis, in terms of degree of motion restriction, planes of motion restriction, duration of the problem, and functional limitations. Table 10–1 reviews some of these variations.

Patients with frozen shoulder often present with a very similar history. The patient describes a period of progressively worsening shoulder pain, which decreased the less the shoulder was moved. Often, patients are unable to sleep on the involved side. Following the painful period, the patient notices the shoulder becoming progressively stiffer over a pe-

TABLE 10–1.

Diagnostic Criteria for Frozen Shoulder

Author	Flexion	Abduction	Internal Rotation	External Rotation	Other
Murnaghan	<130 degrees	<120 degrees combined	Variable	<30 degrees	Painful shoulder with no other identifiable cause
Lundberg	<135 degrees combined	<135 degrees combined			Loss of motion restricted to glenohumeral joint
Rizk et al	<140 degrees combined	<100 degrees combined	<70 degrees	<50 degrees	
Neviaser & Kay		<90 degrees combined			
Quigley		<45 degrees glenohumeral	<85 degrees combined		
Bruckner & Nye		<20 degrees glenohumeral	<40 degrees		Pain at night
Binder et al				<50%	All movements restricted somewhat; duration >1 month; pain at night
Lioyd-Roberts et al				<50%	Duration >3 months; unable to lie on involved side

riod of several months. With this stiffening, patients become more aware of functional limitations, e.g, inability to reach behind themselves, reach overhead, or use that arm for activities of daily living. This is often the point at which patients seek out medical attention. Physicians seem to vary extensively in their approach to treatment. Many emphasize physical therapy, with medications to assist in its effectiveness, while others wait until the pain is under control before starting therapy; still others rely on medications, injections, and manipulation. Of the orthopedic problems with which this author has worked, adhesive capsulitis is the most painful to resolve, and it has been my experience that the combination of pain medications and physical therapy is generally most effective.

Physical therapy treatment should involve some modalities, extensive exercise, and patient education. Patients seem to vary widely in terms of what works best for them. In our experience, the modalities of choice include heat and ultrasound or electrical stimulation before exercise, and ice afterwards. Sensory high-voltage electrical stimulation can be useful to control pain and inflammation. Ultrasound should be effective for increasing tissue extensibility and its thermal effect. In general, the ultrasound–heat–exercise–ice combination is most effective; however, a study by Quin[77] in 1969 found ultrasound no more effective than combined heat and exercise in terms of pain and recovery time.

The exercise program depends greatly on the extent of motion limitation. An accurate diagnosis is critical to treatment effectiveness. Very often, adhesive capsulitis will be diagnosed while the symptoms of rotator cuff tendinitis are overlooked. If this happens when the patient actually has both tendinitis and adhesive capsulitis, stretching alone will be likely to exacerbate symptoms. If the patient's range of motion is less than 80 degree of abduction, 100 degrees of forward flexion, and 45 degrees of external rotation, it is essential to achieve this range of motion as a first step. Once beyond these motion goals, the therapist must determine—through the patient's history, subjective complaints, and strength limitations—if there is an element of rotator cuff tendinitis. If so, the tendinitis must be addressed first, to avoid worsening the tendinitis and not helping the capsulitis. All too often, a patient with this combination of lesions is perceived as having poor pain tolerance when he or she finds the stretching is just making the pain worse. If the rotator cuff is inflamed and weak, it cannot perform its role in humeral head depression; thus,

stretching will cause painful impingement-like symptoms. At this point in therapy, then, it is effective to work on strengthening the rotator cuff in protected positions while maintaining the achieved range of motion. Once some rotator cuff strength has been restored stretching can again be emphasized, but rotator cuff strengthening must continue. In patients with rotator cuff tendinitis, it is critical that the tendinitis be controlled and to some extent resolved before addressing internal rotation and extension motion limitations. Motion exercises should include some combination of passive stretch, proprioceptive neuromuscular facilitation (PNF), and mobilization, depending on the extent of pain motion limitation, the patient's response both subjectively and objectively, and the therapist's comfort with each. In this author's experience, the use of these techniques must be constantly reassessed and modified for each patient at each treatment session. There is a wide variety of mobilization techniques applicable to the frozen shoulder in terms of force, direction, and amplitude. In a study by Nicholson[66] using active exercise vs mobilization with active exercise, improvement in the mobilization group was only found in abduction. All other motions showed no significant difference between the two groups. In addition to the physical therapy sessions, a home exercise program to maintain the motion achieved is critical to treatment progress. The patient's comfort with and ability to trust the therapist is a major factor in the success of this approach. If therapy fails, many patients need to undergo closed manipulation. If this is necessary, they must understand clearly in advance that this is by no means simple or pain-free and that all other measures should be exhausted before manipulation is considered. Once the problem has resolved, the patient should be aware that he or she needs to recheck motion daily at first, then less frequently but nevertheless consistently to avoid any recurrence.

Rotator Cuff Disease and Failure

The literature is replete with discussion of rotator cuff pathology.* Among the many problems involved are inflammation, degeneration, calcification, partial tears, rupture, and disease. In the older person, rotator cuff pathology is rarely an isolated condition. Associated factors may include[62, 67, 73, 94]:

---

*References 12, 13, 17, 18, 22, 34, 36, 38, 42, 45, 49, 53, 54, 68, 76, 91, 94, 95, and 97.

- Glenohumeral instability and subluxation
- Capsular and glenohumeral ligament laxity
- Labrum deficiency and/or tear
- Osteoarthritis of the acromioclavicular joint and glenohumeral joint
- Subdeltoid bursitis
- Biceps tendinitis
- Subacromial osteophytes
- Erosion or exostosis of the greater tuberosity

There is tremendous disagreement as to the cause-and-effect relationships that exist among these factors. According to Nirschl,[68] the causative factor is tension overload to the rotator cuff, especially the supraspinatus. The rotator cuff tendons are subjected to tension from intrinsic muscle contraction (especially eccentric), compression, and shear. The supraspinatus is a small muscle upon which enormous demands are placed during a lifetime. Furthermore, glenohumeral instability is not uncommon. Tensile overload of the supraspinatus results in fatigue, weakness, and avascularity, which are followed by changes within the tendon. The rotator cuff then fails in its role of humeral head stabilization, especially in overhead activities, and a secondary impingement syndrome results, with bony changes, coracoacromial arch compromise, and joint dysfunction.[67]

Warren[94] described a process wherein, with repeated overuse, inflammation, and edema develop in the rotator cuff. These progress and eventually cause an altered vascularity in the cuff and dysfunction of the rotator cuff, with degenerative changes in the fibers and tearing. The bursa thickens, the humeral head migrates superiorly, and the acromion loses its normal convexity; scarring and degeneration are seen in the coracoacromial ligament.[94] According to Jobe,[42] instability and impingement are on a continuum of shoulder abnormalities: overuse stretches and breaks down the static stabilizers and thus allows the anterior subluxation of the humeral head; at the same time, this overuse results in disruption of the balanced interaction of the rotator cuff and scapular rotators as they now try to provide stability. Several authors have reported increased frequency of subluxation and instability in the elderly owing to muscular laxity and joint abnormalities.[40, 94] The result is a syndrome and cycle of impingement and dysfunction. Neer attributed the syndrome to a combination of mechanical factors (e.g., instability), nutrition, vascularity, and hereditary variations in acromial slope and shape.[62] As the discussion goes on, its seems evident that the rotator cuff problems of youth are generally different and distinct from those of old age. While the remainder of this discussion will be limited to rotator cuff problems of the elderly population, it is critical that any therapist dealing with these problems gain a thorough history from the patient to identify problems that occurred in youth.

With age, human tissue tends to weaken. The rotator cuff of most older people has been subject to some trauma, loss of vascularity, and attrition. The reasons for this may vary widely:

- History—if the patient participated seriously in throwing, racquet sports, or swimming when young, it is likely that some weakening of the rotator cuff developed from its overload. A history of dislocation or subluxation in youth is also indicative of long-term damage to the cuff.
- Degenerative joint changes from disease or mechanical alterations
- Inadequacy of the soft tissue stabilizers, e.g., muscles, tendons, ligaments
- Vascular changes with age
- Variations in anatomy, such as acromial design, positioning of the glenoid

Many authors have noted that rotator cuff tears begin in the deep surface, where the fibers insert onto the greater tuberosity, and then extend upward.[25, 51, 53, 54] According to DePalma,[25] this tearing of the innermost fibers normally begins in the fifth decade. Matsen and Arntz[53] summarize the process of failure very effectively. Each instance of fiber failure increases the load on the neighboring fibers, resulting in detachment of the fibers from the bone and weakened performance of the rotator cuff. The anatomy of the vascularity also becomes distorted; thus, the rotator cuff becomes less vascular. The rotator cuff gets weaker, more prone to additional failure, and less able to heal. With failure of the rotator cuff in its performance as a humeral head depressor, the mechanics of the glenohumeral joint become altered in overhead activities with unchecked upward migration of the humeral head under the pull of the deltoid, development of subacromial spurs, additional load on the biceps tendon, more avascularity and nutritional deficiency to the cuff, loss of articular cartilage, and softening of the subchondral bone of the humeral head with the eventual potential for "cuff tear arthropathy," as described by Neer.[64] Petersson and Gentz[76] describe this process as "creeping tendon ruptures," in which repeated failure of small groups of fibers results in symptoms and progressive weakening, which then makes the rotator cuff more susceptible to damage by lesser loads.

Since people under 50 years old ordinarily subject their shoulders to more trauma than those over 50, age-related inelasticity and weakening seem to be prerequisite to rotator cuff tear and the subsequent pathology in the elderly.[53, 76] It is most interesting that many patients present with age-related soft tissue changes without significant symptoms.[34, 53, 64] The effect of the age-related changes is compounded by steroid injections, major injuries, minor trauma, and genetic or constitutional predisposition.[57, 66]

In treating the elderly shoulder with rotator cuff pathology a few distinctions are helpful; assuming that there is some degree of tearing and degeneration:

1. Is the tear acute, chronic, or both? The acute tear is sudden, resulting from an injury, as opposed to the chronic tear, which is degenerative in nature, often insidious, and has a history of least 3 months. An injury to a chronically degenerated tendon may, with failure of additional fibers, result in an acute extension.[53] In general, tears in the older population are more likely to result from a degenerative process as opposed to trauma alone.[32, 94, 99]

2. Is it a partial or full-thickness tear? A partial tear involves the supraspinatus tendon and perhaps others of the rotator cuff, but the defect involves only the deep, midsubstance, or superficial fibers. A full-thickness tear extends through from the articular to the bursal surface of the rotator cuff.[53]

3. Is calcification present? In calcific tendonitis, the inflammatory process results in calcium deposition in the substance of the tendon. Two presentations are described[72]: the chronic phase, in which the calcification appears well-circumscribed, gritty, and sandlike (here the pain is of a chronic nature); and the resorptive phase, in which there is an amorphous deposit of toothpastelike consistency (the pain here is often exquisite).

4. Is the pathology isolated to the rotator cuff or extensive, involving other shoulder structures? Pathology isolated to the rotator cuff is rare in the older shoulder complex, whose parts are so closely interrelated and interdependent in their actions that isolated age-related pathology in any one part would be remarkable.

Common associated problems include:

- Subacromial impingement, involving the coracoacromial arch, the subacromial bursa, the long head of the biceps, and/or the humeral head; pathology, structural variations, or injury in any of these may be contributory
- Constitutional factors that may predispose the patient to tendonitis; Nirschl[67] describes mesenchymal syndrome, in which systemic constitutional factors result in multiple sites of tendon pain and/or alteration
- Cervical arthritis and/or radiculopathy
- Weakness and/or tightness of the joint capsule

An overall treatment approach to the shoulder will be discussed later in this chapter. Treatment considerations specific to rotator cuff failure in the elderly must depend on a careful, thorough assessment of what structures are involved. Patients often present with visible atrophy of the infraspinatus and supraspinatus and weakness on rotator cuff muscle strength tests. Painful positions include internal rotation with hyperextension (e.g., closing a brassiere, putting on a coat, putting hand in back pocket); holding the arm in the 90-degree to 120-degree range (e.g., driving); adduction across the midline; the extremes of external rotation; and side-lying on the involved side.[27] Partial-thickness tears may show decreased range of motion, while full-thickness tears may show quite good motion. Elevating the arm may result in pain, crackling, crepitus, or popping. The course of treatment must be based on the patient's stated goals, needs, and his or her objective findings. Pain relief, restoration of function, and prevention of progression are usually realistic. If these goals cannot be reached conservatively, surgery may be indicated. Surgical procedures, rehabilitation, and prognosis will vary widely depending on the extent of rotator cuff tear, associated pathologies, and the surgeon's technique. While some surgeons routinely resect the coracoacromial ligament, others avoid this unless damage to this structure is apparent. Some rotator cuff tear procedures may only involve the pathologic tissue, others involve repairs, while some large tears may involve a graft to enhance the quality of the repair.[67] These factors and the surgeon's philosophy most affect the postoperative rehabilitation, which may involve extensive immobilization or immediate motion and may take anywhere from 6 weeks to 6 months.

Shoulder Instability

Subluxation, dislocation, and instability are not uncommon in the older population.[13, 15, 32] These instabilities are usually entirely different from those seen in the younger athletic population. They may be caused by generalized muscle laxity, a history of fracture or some abnormality of the glenohumeral joint structure, rupture or deterioration of the rotator cuff, bone degeneration, osteoarthritis, or rheumatoid arthritis. The two most common types are upward subluxation, usually associated with rotator cuff failure,[13, 15] and posterior subluxation, often associated with arthritis.[31, 32] The physical therapy approach is based on the causative factors, functional limitations, and restorative potential.

Biceps Tendinitis, Subluxation, and Rupture

The long head of the biceps tendon originates at the superior and posterior aspects of the glenoid and labrum and runs an intraarticular course until it enters the bicipital groove. It is a two-joint muscle, inserting into the bicipital tuberosity of the radius and the bicipital aponeurosis. In its course, it passes directly under the supraspinatus tendon.[99] It is subject to pathologic change from tension (as a humeral head stabilizer), compression (from upward migration of the humeral head as in rotator cuff failure or from impingement in a shallow or osteophytic groove), and shear if it subluxes from the groove.[69] Warren[94] indicates that slow, progressive ruptures are fairly common in the older population but do not require treatment. These occur at the proximal aspect, unlike the sudden distal ruptures occurring in the younger population.[62, 72, 94] Ruptures in the older population are attributed to tendon degeneration and/or disorders of the bicipital groove.[62]

The long head of the biceps tendon is subject to constant wear and tear from movement of the glenohumeral joint and from its roles in humeral head stabilization, elbow flexion, and forearm supination. Overload of the biceps is more likely in a patient with rotator cuff failure or with a history in the throwing sports. According to Bateman[5] this wear will eventually result in laxity and fraying. With an extension injury such as a backward fall, the weakened tendon may rupture.

According to Nirschl,[67] rotator cuff tendinitis is often misdiagnosed as biceps tendinitis because of the location of the long head under the supraspinatus tendon. On palpation, the patient's extreme tenderness is elicited and misinterpreted as a biceps problem. The differential diagnosis can be made using the Yergason test[98] (resisted supination in a flexed elbow) rather than tests of the rotator cuff tendon. Therapy involves a progressively graduated strengthening program to restore function.

CLINICAL EVALUATION OF THE SHOULDER

When a patient begins physical therapy, it is a great advantage for the therapist to have access to all test results, such as radiographs and magnetic resonance images. The potential for multiple areas of involvement at the shoulder is great, and offering the most effective possible treatment must begin with obtaining the most accurate information available about the patient.

Subjective Evaluation

It is helpful to begin the subjective evaluation with a form that the patient has filled out in advance. This can then be reviewed and clarified in a discussion between the patient and therapist. The following information should be covered with respect to the shoulder.

Shoulder History

History of Shoulder Pain, Injury, Dysfunction.—This should go back as far as the patient can remember.

Sports, Occupations, and Activities When Younger.—With recent advances in sports medicine, a significant rotator cuff weakness has been found in the asymptomatic shoulders of tennis players, swimmers, and those involved in the throwing sports. Rotator cuff strength deficits early on may alter joint mechanics and predispose the shoulder complex to pathological changes. Furthermore, the knowledge available 50 years ago about conditioning exercise and injury prevention was minimal, and as a result, many who participated in sports did excessive sport participation but no support work. Injuries were not rehabilitated, deficits often went uncorrected, and were carried into old age.

Present Problem

Present Complaints.—What is the chief complaint? What are secondary complaints?

History of Present Problem.—How did the present problem start? Was there a trauma; overuse? Did the patient have a chronic problem? Was there any significant change in activities? A chronic shoulder problem is likely to present with pain, instability, weakness, functional limitations, and possibly crepitus. An acute shoulder problem in the older patient is likely to have some history of chronicity.

Nature and Site of Pain (Be Specific).—Radiation; factors that relieve the pain; activities that aggravate the pain; positions that aggravate the pain; type of pain (deep, searing, sharp, burning); presence of clicking, snapping, catching in association with pain or independent of pain; stiffness; weakness or feeling of a dead arm; presence of paresthesias?

Behavior.—In what ways and to what extent is the problem interfering with the patient's daily activities? Does it hurt, click, pop, catch, grind, with overhead motions, lifting, lying on that side, crossing the midline, reaching behind back; is there a painful arc?

Pain Phases.—It is helpful to categorize the pain level based on the following[70]:

1. Temporary soreness after activity
2. Soreness (more than 12 hours) resolved with warm-up
3. Pain with activity (sports or occupation) that does not cause a change in activity level
4. Pain with activity (sports or occupation) that causes a change in activity level
5. Pain during activities of daily living
6. Pain at rest
7. Pain that disrupts sleep

This offers the therapist a clinical picture of the extent of the pathology. Pain phases 1 and 2 represent a problem that is likely to respond quickly and fully to treatment. Phases 3 to 5 indicate the need to modify activities and undertake a fairly extensive treatment program, but also have a good prognosis. Phases 6 and 7 indicate a more serious problem whose prognosis with a conservative approach is questionable.[67]

Visual Analog Scale.—It is informative and useful later in the program to have the patient rate his or her pain by marking an X on a horizontal line:

0	10
No pain	Impossible pain

The pain phases and the visual analog scale can be used throughout the rehabilitation program to reassess the patient's status and monitor progress.

Medications.—How much and what kind of medicines are used? What are their effects on the patient's problem?

Treatment History.—It is important to know if the patient has had any cortisone injections. If so, how many and when? Multiple cortisone injections may well affect the tissue's healing potential. Other treatments include physical therapy, surgeries, and any other medical approach.

Medical History

It is essential in working with this population, or any other, to know what other illnesses the patient has had and is dealing with now and what treatment he or she is receiving. A number of medical problems can alter the presentation of the shoulder problems, including cervical problems, renal disease, gastric disease, lung pathology, and other diseases such as rheumatoid arthritis.

Objective Evaluation

In order to effectively evaluate the shoulder, the therapist needs to begin with a clearing test of the cervical region to rule out or to identify any neck problems that may cause or contribute to the problems at the shoulder. Unfortunately, both strengthening and stretching of the shoulder can cause flareup of a preexisting neck problem.

Inspection

The following features should be observed.

Posture and Attitude.—Head position should be noted; exaggerated dorsal kyphosis, commonly seen in the older population, alters the scapulothoracic and glenohumeral musculature and joint biomechanics. Protracted scapulae in association with or independent of kyphosis results in stretch weakening of the posterior scapular muscles and tightening of the anterior muscles. Rounded, collapsed shoulders may compromise the subacriomial joint space, enhancing the symptoms and possibly leading to further degeneration. Actual shoulder asymmetry (such as a high-riding clavicle), alterations in contour (posterior position of the humerus, bulging biceps), and carriage (e.g., holding one shoulder higher) should be noted.

Muscle Atrophy.—Careful investigation here is very helpful to the therapist and is often a very effective tool in helping the patient understand the extent of his or her problem. Since the involved side is often the dominant arm, muscle wasting is often all the more dramatic. Posterior wasting of the infraspinatus and supraspinatus may be apparent in and of itself or may be seen as excessive prominence of the spine of the scapula. Deltoid wasting can be seen as a squaring off of the shoulder in the anterior view.[36]

Scapular Winging.—This may be a result of muscle and/or nerve dysfunction. According to Hawkins and Bokor,[36] a high-riding scapula with medial protrusion of the inferior angle indicates serratus anterior deficiency; a downwardly migrated scapula with lateral drifting of the inferior angle indicates trapezius deficiency.

Swelling.—Swelling around the glenohumeral joint is unusual; however, in a massive defect of the rotator cuff, synovial fluid may leak through so that the patient presents with swelling in the bursa area of the shoulder.

Scars and Surgical Incisions.—Note should be made of signs of previous surgery or trauma.

Palpation

Palpation is useful to identify or rule out tenderness, swelling, malalignment, or joint displacement. Starting at the sternoclavicular joint the therapist can move laterally along the clavicle to the acromioclavicular joint, at the distal end of the clavicle. The coracoid, approximately 1 cm below the lateral end of the clavicle, is tender even in normal shoulders. At the proximal humerus, the lesser tuberosity, where the subscapularis inserts, is palpable. The arm is internally rotated for access to the greater tuberosity and biceps groove, then extended for access to the supraspinatus. Tenderness here may indicate tendinitis. While passively rotating the arm, palpation for crepitus in the subacromial area (which may indicated bursa thickening) or clicking (which may indicate rotator cuff tear) can be accomplished.

Range of Motion Testing

With each motion tested, the therapist should note active motion, available passive motion and end feels, and any clicking, snapping, catching, grinding, popping, slipping, or pain. If pain is present, it is important to identify whether or not it is the cause of motion limitation. The range of motion of the shoulder involves contributions from the sternoclavicular, acromioclavicular, glenohumeral, and scapulothoracic joints. By feeling the movement

of the inferior angle of the scapula, assessment of the scapulohumeral rhythm can be made in flexion and abduction. A frozen shoulder or osteoarthritis may alter the glenohumeral versus the scapulothoracic contribution so that the scapulothoracic joint compensates for glenohumeral limitations. Lack of smoothness of active motion may indicate rotator cuff pathology. It is recommended by some that the total elevation (somewhere between flexion and abduction) be measured instead of isolating abduction and flexion, as this is more functional information.[36] In the older patient, it is probably not advisable to measure internal and external rotations with the arm abducted. Measuring the hands behind the low back (the thumb should reach T_6) and hands behind head (should at least reach T_3) is functionally very useful. In the former, it is important to note scapular winging. Accessory motion testing of all the joints can often identify crepitus, pain, and clicking.

Muscle Strength Tests

In addition to cardinal motions, muscle strength tests should evaluate all the force couple components, e.g., upper and lower trapezii; supraspinatus (empty can[59] or Blackburn[8] test), serratus anterior (*Note:* this author has yet to find an accurate serratus anterior strength test); scapular retractors, latissimus dorsi, subscapularis, teres minor, infraspinatus, biceps, and triceps. Since Blackburn's test for supraspinatus strength[8] and the lower trapezius strength test require placing the arm in motion extremes, they may not be possible in this population. Isokinetic testing of the shoulder rotators may or may not be indicated, depending on the nature of the problem, the patient's activity level, and functional demands. If tested, the external rotation to internal rotation ratio at 60 degrees/sec (in modified neutral position) should be 66% to 75%.

Neurologic.—Dermatomes and reflex testing should be performed bilaterally, including the biceps (C_5), brachioradialis (C_6), and triceps (C_7).

Additional Tests.—Some specific clinical tests that may also be helpful are:

1. Neer impingement sign test.—The arm is passively flexed forward while downward pressure is applied to the scapula. Pain in the end range is considered positive. Another impingement test involves internally rotating the arm at 90 degrees forward flexion. *Note:* While these test results may be

positive, they do not indicate the *cause* of impingement.

2. Drop arm test.—With the arm passively flexed to beyond 120 degrees the patient tries slowly to lower the arm. If patient is unable to do this, or if the arm suddenly drops at approximately 100 degrees to 70 degrees, it may indicate a rotator cuff tear.

3. Yergason's test.—With the elbow flexed to 90 degrees, forearm pronated, the patient supinates against the therapist's resistance. If there is a problem with the long head of the biceps, pain may be felt in the bicipital groove.[98]

4. Speed's test.—With the elbow in full extension and forearm supinated, the therapist resists shoulder forward flexion to approximately 60 degrees. Pain in the biceps groove indicates biceps pathology.[36]

5. Glenohumeral translation tests.—Glenohumeral translation tests to assess stability of the joint are important but often are not indicated or not informative in the older population because of the limitations of pain, multiple pathologies, and positioning requirements. One effective test is the "load and shift test," described thoroughly by Hawkins and Bokor.[36] To test the right arm, the patient is seated with the arm at his or her side. While standing behind and to the side of the patient, the examiner stabilizes the scapula with the left hand while grasping the humeral head with the right hand, then stresses it anteriorly and posteriorly, noting the extent of translation and any clunking. Then the examiner grasps the elbow, applies inferior stress, and notes inferior translation, noting any dimpling adjacent to the acromion ("sulcus sign").[36]

TREATMENT AND REHABILITATION

The central and overriding feature of rehabilitation must be specific individualization with constant reevaluation and modification of the treatment program. Initially, the goal of treatment is to control pain and inflammation and to eliminate abusive activities. In many cases, the patient has been prescribed an oral inflammatory medication and may have had a cortisone injection. It has been our experience at Virginia Sportsmedicine Institute that a brief, early course of anti-inflammatory medications in conjunction with therapeutic modalities helps to speed the rehabilitation process. *Note:* It has also been our experience that an arm that has had several cortisone injections is significantly more difficult to rehabilitate.

We have found several modalities to be effective. High-voltage electrical stimulation decreases pain, enhances circulation, and controls inflammation. It is also very effective postoperatively in muscle reeducation and lessening muscle disuse atrophy. Its role in stimulating the biologic healing process is unclear at this time.

Ultrasound is also helpful to increase circulation and decrease pain. It is thought to increase cell membrane permeability, resulting in better transport of metabolic products. It may help enhance connective tissue extensibility by enhancing collagen fiber separation. Ultrasound is thus helpful before exercise, because it makes the tissue more susceptible to remodeling by tensile forces.

Moist heat promotes vascular supply and relieves pain.

Ice is helpful after exercise or aggravating activity. Ice is indicated as long as the signs of inflammation persist, which may mean throughout all rehabilitation and activity return. It encourages local vasoconstriction, lessens the inflammatory response, slows local metabolism, and helps to relieve pain and muscle spasm through counterirritation and slowed nerve conduction velocity.

Phonophoresis and transverse friction massage are commonly used modalities; however, we at Virginia Sportsmedicine Institute have generally found these to be ineffective in this patient population. Steroids have been found to lessen collagen and ground substance production and decrease the tensile strength of tendons, and they may lead to failure of tissue under stress. In this author's opinion, the potential benefits of phonophoresis cannot justify its use in view of these dangers, especially where cortisone injections have already been tried. Transverse friction massage is considered by many to be an effective way of increasing circulation to tissue and lessening excessive or abnormal scar tissue formation. As there is no experimental or clinical research available at this time to substantiate the value of transverse friction massage, and as it is generally very painful, it is rarely a modality of choice at the shoulder.

Active rest is another important aspect of the effort to minimize pain and inflammation. Absolute rest (e.g., immobilization) should be avoided if medically reasonable. Although it undoubtedly helps to eliminate abuse, absolute rest also encourages atrophy, deconditions tissue, lessens vascular supply to the area because of reduced demand, and is detrimental to the healing process. With most shoulder problems, patients should be advised to avoid sleeping or lying on the side of the involved shoulder, activities that require holding the arms fully overhead or across the body for prolonged periods, and hyperextension with adduction or internal rotation. Beyond this, pain is the best guide as to what to avoid.

Postural correction is essential and needs to be addressed at the patient's first visit. The patient needs to be made aware of the effect of slumped posture on collapsing the shoulder joint and on creating muscle imbalance.

The remainder of rehabilitation is largely dependent on the diagnosis, extent of pathology, and the patient's needs and goals. To promote healing, rehabilitation exercise is added to the anti-inflammatory measures. The goals of these early exercises are to enhance oxygenation and tissue nutrition, to prevent or minimize neurophysiologic reflex inhibition (thus minimizing unnecessary atrophy), to align collagen fibers along the lines of stress and inhibit excessive scar formation, and to stimulate the joint mechanoreceptors, all while protecting the healing fibers against excess stress or reinjury.

These exercises involve very low-intensity, submaximal effort and progress gradually and methodically, primarily based on our knowledge of biologic healing time factors and patient's pain. As the exercises progress, the goals become reconditioning and restoration of strength, endurance, and flexibility for functional performance. Flexibility exercises should probably include some combination of the pendulum, active and passive stretch, proprioceptive neuromuscular facilitation techniques (without stressing the pathologic structures), and gentle mobilization, in keeping with the diagnostic and age-related limitations. The selection of strengthening exercise forms and equipment may include UBE (upper body ergometer, Lumex Corporation, Ronkonkoma, NY); isometrics, isotonics, isokinetics, or rubber tubing, depending on the patient's problems and pain. Biceps and trapezius strengthening is initiated early on. In patients with identified rotator cuff weakness, it is essential to restore the strength of the rotator cuff through exercise in a protected position before beginning overhead motions that depend on the integrity of the cuff to prevent humeral head translation (Table 10–2). The scapular stabilizers and rotators must be addressed to place the glenoid in its optimal position. The combination of rotator cuff and scapular rotator exercise is essential to restore the desirable scapulohumeral rhythm and provide stability to the joint.

Depending on the patient's personality and the physical therapist's impression of the problem and

TABLE 10–2.

Basic Rehabilitation Exercises for Rotator Cuff Muscles

Side-lying internal rotation	
Exercise benefits:	Subscapularis
Starting position:	Lie on involved side with involved arm just in front of body, elbow bent 90 degrees.
Exercise action:	Slowly rotate arm upward and inward toward abdomen, then slowly rotate back out again.
Side-lying external rotation	
Exercise benefits:	Infraspinatus, teres minor
Starting position:	Lie on uninvolved side; hold involved elbow bent to 90 degrees with pillow between arm and side. Involved hand holds weight on stomach.
Exercise action:	Holding elbow close to side, externally rotate arm so that hand points to ceiling. Hold 2 seconds and then slowly lower.
Empty can	
Exercise benefits:	Supraspinatus
Starting position:	Sitting or standing, raise arm out to side and forward 30 degrees in front of body (arm just below shoulder height). Internally rotate shoulders so that thumb points down as in emptying a can.
Exercise action:	Keeping elbow straight, slowly lower arm to thumb at waist level. Hold 2 seconds and then raise to starting height.
Biceps curl	
Exercise benefits:	Biceps
Starting position:	Stand or sit, palm facing up.
Exercise action:	Slowly raise hand to shoulder level by bending elbow up. Slowly lower.

rehabilitation potential, it may be helpful to explain to the patient some of the probable differences between injury rehabilitation at this time of life and when he or she was young. There is a likely chronicity to shoulder pathology in these patients; they may heal less quickly; they may have more osteoarthritic changes and tendon degeneration; they may have more frequent and/or longer plateaus; strength and/or motion gains may require more effort and time; there may be long-term functional and motion limitations. When the conservative approach does not adequately resolve the patient's problem, surgery may be considered. In the older person, at least two additional factors must be considered. Because many older people have disorders that are neither highly symptomatic nor functionally impairing, the patient should consider whether the need for surgery exists. Also, in view of other medical problems that are more prevalent in older persons, it should be determined whether the potential benefits outweigh the risks of surgery. Tremendous gains in shoulder surgeries, both arthroscopic and open, are being made at this time. The rehabilitation time and potential benefit from each type depend on the extent of the problem, the quality of the repair, the surgical procedure, and the patient's healing capabilities.

At the time of this writing, the knowledge of the shoulder complex is constantly changing and growing. The current changes in the makeup of the elderly population and the emphasis on lifetime fitness compound the challenge of effective treatment and rehabilitation. The key to accomplishing those goals is a highly individualized approach and constantly modified treatment program based on ongoing reassessment of objective findings and patient input. With this, we can expect to help each patient and gain insight into shoulder pathomechanics in the elderly population for future application.

REFERENCES

1. Alnaqeeb MA, Alzrid NS, Eoldspink E: Connective tissue changes and physical properties of developing and aging skeletal muscle. *J Anat* 1984; 139:677–689.
2. Aniansson A, et al: Muscle fiber composition and fiber area in various age groups. Muscle and Nerve. 1980; 2:271–272.
3. Astrand PO: Exercise physiology of the mature athlete, in Sutton JR, Brock RM (eds): *Sports Medicine for the Mature Athlete*. Indianapolis, Benchmark Press, 1986.
4. Basmajian JV, Bazant FJ: Factors preventing downward dislocation of the adducted shoulder joint. *J Bone Joint Surg (Am)* 1959; 41:1182.
5. Bateman JE: *The Shoulder and Neck*. Philadelphia, WB Saunders, 1972, pp 195–292.
6. Beyer RE: Regulation of connective tissue metabolism in aging and exercise: A review, in Borer KT, Edington DW, White TP (eds): *Frontiers in Exercise Biology*. Champaign, Ill, Human Kinetics Publishers, 1983.
7. Bigliani L, Morrison DS, April EW: Morphology of the acromion and its relationship to rotator cuff tears. *Orthop Trans* 1986; 10:228.
8. Blackburn TA: Personal communication, 1987.
9. Borges O: Isometric and isokinetic knee extension and flexion torque in men and women aged 20–70. *Scand J Rehab Med* 1989; 21:45–53.
10. Boyle S: (thesis) Philadelphia, University of Pennsylvania, 1988.
11. Brems JJ: Degenerative joint disease of the shoulder, in Nicholas J, Hershman E (eds): *The Upper Extremity in Sports Medicine*. St Louis, Mosby-Year Book, 1990, pp 23–40.
12. Brewer B: Aging of the rotator cuff. *Am J Sports Med* 1979; 7:102–110.
13. Calliet R: *Shoulder Pain*. Philadelphia, FA Davis, 1982.
14. Campbell M, McComas A, Petito F: Physiological changes in aging muscles. *Neurol Neurosurg Psychiatr* 1973; 36:174–182.
15. Carpenter GI, Millard MB: Shoulder subluxation in elderly patients. *J Am Geriatr Soc* 1982; 30:441–446.
16. Chard MD, Hazelman R, Hazelman BL, et al: Shoulder disorders in the elderly: A community survey. *Arthritis Rheum* 1991; 34:766–769.
17. Clark JC: Fibrous anatomy of the rotator cuff (abstract). Presented to the American Academy of Orthopaedic Surgeons, 1988.
18. Clark J, Sidles JA, Matsen FF: The repair of the glenohumeral joint capsule to the rotator cuff. *Clin Orthop* 1990; 254:29–34.
19. Clarkson PM, Dedrick ME: Exercise-induced muscle damage, repair and adaptation in old and young subjects. *J Gerontol* 1988; 43:91–96.
20. Codman EA: *The Shoulder*. Boston; Thomas Todd, 1934.
21. Cofield R: Degenerative and arthritic problems of the glenohumeral joint, in Rockwood C, Matsen F (eds): *The Shoulder*. Philadelphia, WB Saunders, 1990, pp 678–749.
22. Cofield RH: Tears of the rotator cuff. *AAOS Instr Course Lect* 1981; 30:373.
23. Colachis SC, Strohm BR: The effect of suprascapular and axillary nerve blocks and muscle force in the upper extremity. *Arch Phys Med Rehabil* 1971; 52:22–29.
24. Colachis SC, Strohm BR, Brechner VL: Effects of axillary nerve block on muscle force in the upper extremity. *Arch Phys Med Rehabil* 1969; 50:647–654.
25. DePalma AF: *Surgery of the Shoulder*. Philadelphia, JB Lippincott, 1983.
26. DePalma AF, Callery G, Bennett G: The variational anatomy and degenerative lesions of the shoulder joint. *Instr Course Lect* 1949; 6:255.
27. DePalma AF: Degenerative Changes in the Sternoclavicular and Acromioclavicular Joints in Various Decades. Springfield, Ill, Charles C Thomas, 1957.
28. Eagleston WH: Wound healing and aging. *Clin Geriatr Med* 1989; 5:183–188.
29. Ellenbecker TS, Derscheid GL: Rehabilitation of over-

use injuries of the shoulder. *Clin Sports Med* 1989; 8:583–603.

30. Essen-Eustausson B, Borees O: Histochemical and metabolic characteristics of human skeletal muscle in relation to age. *Acta Physiol Scand* 1986;126:107–114.

31. Fukuda K et al: Biomechanical study of the ligamentous system of the acromioclavicular joint. *J Bone Joint Surg (Am)* 1986; 68A:434.

32. Ganel A, Horoszowski H, Helm M, et al: Persistent dislocation of the shoulder in elderly patients. *J Am Geriatr Soc* 1980; 28:282–284.

33. Green HJ. Characteristics of aging human skeletal muscles, in *Sports Medicine for the Mature Athlete.* Indianapolis, Benchmark Press, 1986.

34. Ha'erl GB: Ruptures of the rotator cuff. *Can Med Assoc J* 1980; 123:620–627.

35. Halbach JW, Tank R: The shoulder, in Gould JA, Davies GJ (eds): *Orthopedic and Sports Physical Therapy.* St Louis, Mosby-Year Book, 1985, pp 497–517.

36. Hawkins R, Bokor D: Clinical evaluation of shoulder problems, in Rockwood C, Matsen F (eds): *The Shoulder.* Philadelphia, WB Saunders, 1990, pp 149–177.

37. Hazelman BL: The painful stiff shoulder. *Rheumatol Phys Med* 1972; 2:413–421.

38. Howell AB et al: Role of the supraspinatus muscle in shoulder function, *J Bone Joint Surg (Am)* 1986; 68A:398.

39. Hurley J: Anatomy of the shoulder, in Nicholas J, Hershman E (eds): *The Upper Extremity in Sports Medicine.* St Louis, Mosby-Year Book, 1990, pp 23–40.

40. Inman VT, Saunders JB, Abbott LC: Observations on the function of the shoulder joint. *J Bone Joint Surg (Am)* 1944; 26A:1–30.

41. Jobe C: Gross anatomy of the shoulder, in Rockwood C, Matsen F (eds): *The Shoulder.* Philadelphia, WB Saunders, 1990, pp 34–97.

42. Jobe FW: Impingement problems in the athlete. *Instr Course Lect* 1989; 38:205–209.

43. Kaltasas DS: Comparative study of the properties of the shoulder joint capsule with those of other joint capsules. *Clin Orthop* 1983; 173:2–26.

44. Kerr R, Resnick D, Pineda C, et al: Osteoarthritis of the glenohumeral joint. *AJR* 1985; 144:967–972.

45. Kessel L: *Clinical Disorders of the Shoulder,* New York, Churchill Livingstone, 1982.

46. Knortz KA: Muscle physiology applied to geriatric rehabilitation. *Top Geriatr Rehabil* 1987; 2:1–12.

47. Lindblom K: Arthrography and roentgenography in ruptures of the tendon of the shoulder joint. *Acta Radiol* 1939; 20:548.

48. Lindblom K: On the pathogenesis of rupture of the tendon aponeurosis of the shoulder joint. *Acta Radiol* 1937; 20:563–577.

49. Reference deleted in proofs.

50. Lundberg BJ: The frozen shoulder. *Acta Orthop Scand (Suppl)* 1969; 119:1–59.

51. McLaughlin HL: The frozen shoulder. *Clin Orthop* 1961; 20:126–131.

52. McMasters P: Tendon and muscle ruptures. *J Bone Joint Surg* 1933; 15:705–721.

53. Matsen F, Arntz C: Rotator cuff failure, in Rockwood C, Matsen F (eds). *The Shoulder.* Philadelphia, WB Saunders, 1990, pp 647–677.

54. Matsen F, Arntz C: Subacromial impingement, in Rockwood C, Matsen F (eds): *The Shoulder.* Philadelphia, WB Saunders, 1990, pp 623–646.

55. Menard D: The aging athlete. *Top Geriatr Rehab* 1991; 6:1–16.

56. Morrey BF, An K: *Biomechanics of the Shoulder.* Philadelphia, WB Saunders, 1990, pp 208–245.

57. Moseley H, Goldie I: The arterial pattern of the rotator cuff of the shoulder. *J Bone Joint Surg (Br)* 1983; 45:780–789.

58. Moseley H, Overgaard B: The anterior capsular mechanism in recurrent anterior dislocation of the shoulder. *J Bone Joint Surg (Br)* 1962; 44:913.

59. Moynes DA: Prevention of injury to the shoulder through exercise and therapy. *Clin Sports Med* 1983; 2:413–422.

60. Munns K: Effects of exercise on the range of joint motion in elderly subjects, in Smith EL, Serfass RC (eds): *Exercise and Aging: The Scientific Basis.* Hillside, NJ, Enslow Publishers, 1981.

61. Murnaghan JP: Frozen shoulder, in Rockwood C, Matsen F (eds): *The Shoulder.* Philadelphia, WB Saunders, 1990, pp 837–862.

62. Neer CS II: Impingement lesions. *Clin Orthop* 1983; 173:70–77.

63. Neer CS, Brems JJ: Shoulder replacement in the active and athletic patient, in Jackson W (ed): *Shoulder Surgery in the Athlete.* Rockville, Md, Aspen Press, 1985, p 93.

64. Neer CS II, Craig EV, Fukuda H: Cuff tear arthropathy. *J Bone Joint Surg (Am)* 1983; 65:1232–1244.

65. Neviaser JS: Adhesive capsulitis of the shoulder. *J Bone Joint Surg (AM)* 1945; 27:211–222.

66. Nicholson GG: The effects of passive joint mobilization on pain and hypomobility associated with adhesive capsulitis of the shoulder. *Orthop Sports Phys Ther* 1985; 6:238–246.

67. Nirschl R: Mesenchymal syndrome. *Va Med Month* 1969; 96:659.

68. Nirschl RP: Rotator cuff tendinitis. *Instr Course Lect* 1989; 38:447–462.

69. Nirschl RP: Personal communication, 1990.

70. Nirschl RP, Sobel J: *Tennis Elbow: Prevention and Treatment.* Arlington, Va, Medical Sports, in press.

71. Nixon JE, DiStefano: Ruptures of the rotator cuff. *Orthop Clin North Am* 1975; 6:423–447.

72. Norris T: Treatment and physical examination of the shoulder, in Nicholas J, Hershman E (eds): *The Upper Extremity in Sports Medicine.* St Louis, Mosby-Year Book, 1990, pp 41–90.

73. Norwood L, Barrack R, Jacobson K: Clinical presentation of complete tears of the rotator cuff. *J Bone Joint Surg* 1989;:499–505.

74. Ovsen J, Nielsen S: Stability of the shoulder joint. *Acta Orthop Scand* 1985; 56:149, 1985.

75. Perry J: Anatomy and biomechanics of the shoulder in throwing, swimming, gymnastics and tennis. *Clin Sports Med* 1983; 2:247.

76. Petersson CJ, Gentz CF: Ruptures of the supraspinatus tendon. *Clin Orthop* 1983; 174:143–148.

77. Quin EH: Humeroscapular periarthritis. Observations on the effects of x-ray therapy and ultrasonic therapy in cases of "frozen shoulder." *Ann Phys Med* 1969; 10:64–69.

78. Raab DM, Agre JC, McAdam M, et al: Light resistance and stretching exercise in elderly women. *Arch Phys Med Rehabil* 1988; 69:268–272.
79. Rathburn J, McNab J: The microvascular pattern of the rotator cuff. *J Bone Joint Surg (Br)* 1970; 52B:540.
80. Reeves B: Anterior capsular strength of the shoulder. *J Bone Joint Surg (Br)* 1968; 50B:858.
81. Rice CL, Cunningham DA, Paterson D, et al: Strength in an elderly population. *Arch Phys Med Rehabil* 1989; 70:391–397.
82. Rikli R, Busch S: Motor performance of women as a function of age and physical activity level. *J Gerontol* 1986; 41:645–649.
83. Rothman RH, Parke WW: Vascular anatomy of the rotator cuff. *Clin Orthop* 1985; 41:176–186.
84. Saha AK: Mechanism of shoulder movements and a plea for the recognition of "zero position" of glenohumeral joint. *Indian J Surg* 1950; 12:153.
85. Saha AK: Dynamic stability of the glenohumeral joint. *Acta Orthop Scand* 1971; 42:491.
86. Samilson RL, Prieto V: Dislocation arthropathy of the shoulder. *J Bone Joint Surg (Am)* 1983; 65A:456–460.
87. Sciatczynski P, unpublished data, January 1989.
88. Reference deleted in proofs.
89. Sobel J, Pettrone F, Nirschl R: Prevention and treatment of upper extremity sport injuries, in Nicholas J, Hershman E (eds): The Upper Extremity in Sports Medicine, St. Louis 1990, CV Mosby, 843–860.
90. Turkel SJ, et al: Stabilizing mechanisms preventing anterior dislocation of the glenohumeral joint. *J Bone Joint Surg (Am)* 1981; 63:1208.
91. Uhthoff H, Sarkar K: Calcifying tendinitis, in Rockwood C, Matsen F (eds): *The Shoulder*. Philadelphia, WB Saunders, 1990, pp 774–790.
92. Urist MR: Complete dislocation of the acromioclavicular joint: The nature of the traumatic lesion and effective methods of treatment with an analysis of 41 cases. *J Bone Joint Surg (AM)* 1946; 28:813.
93. Viidik A: Connective tissues: Possible implications of the temporal changes for the aging process. *Mech Ageing Devel* 1979; 9:267–285.
94. Reference deleted in proofs.
95. Wasilewski SA, Frankel U: Rotator cuff pathology. Clin Orthop 1991; 267:65–70.
96. Weiner DS, MacNab I: Superior migration of the humeral head. *J Bone Joint Surg (AM)* 1970; 52:524–527.
97. Wilson CL, Duff GL: Pathological study of degeneration and rupture of the supraspinatus tendon. *Arch Surg* 1943; 47:121–135.
98. Yergason RM: Supination sign. *J Bone Joint Surg (AM)* 1931; 13:160.
99. Zuckerman JD, Frankel VH: Geriatric shoulder pain. *Geriatrics* 1987; 42:43–58.

Chapter 11

Elbow Injuries: A Rehabilitation Perspective

Janet Sobel, R.P.T.

ANATOMY

Osteology and Arthrology

The elbow is made up of three joints—the humeroradial joint, the humeroulnar joint, and the proximal radioulnar joint. The distal humerus is flattened anteroposteriorly and projects anteriorly from the shaft at a 45-degree angle.[17] There are three concavities, or fossae, on the distal humerus: the coronoid and radial fossae anteriorly and the olecranon fossa posteriorly. The coronoid fossa, just proximal to the capitellum, receives the radial head in flexion. The olecranon fossa, just superior to the trochlea, receives the olecranon process in extension. The trochlea covers the anterior, inferior, and posterior aspects of the medial humeral condyle. The medial lip of the trochlea is more prominent than the lateral lip. The trochlea forms a sellar surface (concave in the frontal plane, convex in the sagittal plane). It is marked by a deep central groove that lies not exactly vertically, but in an oblique plane.[35] The capitellum, on the lateral aspect of the humerus, is hemispherical and lies on the anterior aspect of the humerus (e.g., is in front of the humerus). It forms an ovoid articular surface that is convex in all planes. Unlike the trochlea, the capitellum does not extend posteriorly and it stops short of the lower end of the humerus.[17]

The medial epicondyle is the point of origin for the flexors and the medial collateral ligament. The ulnar nerve runs in a groove on its posterior aspect.

The lateral epicondyle is the point of origin for the extensors and the lateral collateral ligament.[35] The proximal ulna contains two processes, the coronoid and olecranon. The olecranon is the most proximal part of the ulna. It also contains two notches, the trochlear notch and the radial notch. The radial head has a cupped surface with a cylindrical rim, covered by articular cartilage.[4] Motions available at the elbow joint are flexion-extension and pronation-supination, although pronation-supination also involves the distal radioulnar joint.[2]

The pulleylike trochlea of the humerus articulates with the semilunar notch of the ulna to form the humeroulnar joint. It is a highly congruent joint and thus its continuous joint cartilage is very thin. This joint is responsible for the elbow's carrying angle and variations in the obliquity of the trochlear groove cause variations in the carrying angle.[2, 17] The trochlear groove dictates the path of the ulna in flexion-extension. The humeroulnar joint acts like a hinge joint, allowing flexion and extension.[19] At the humeroradial joint, the cupped rim of the head of the radius articulates with the capitulotrochlear groove, and the radial head rides in this groove during flexion-extension and pronation-supination. Since the capitellum does not extend posteriorly, the radial head does not fit congruently with the capitellum in full extension. Here, only the anterior half of the proximal surface of the radial head articulates with the capitellum. In full flexion, the rim of the radial head extends beyond the capitellum and enters the radial fossa, which is much more shallow than the coronoid fossa.[2, 4]

The axis of motion of the elbow is approximated by a line connecting the center of the trochlear groove with the center of the capitellum. This line makes a 94 to 98 degree angle with the humeral shaft, declining from lateral to medial. The position of the axis is also internally rotated 3 to 8 degrees with respect to the humeral epicondyles.[19]

Pronation and supination occur at the proximal and distal, or superior and inferior, radioulnar joints. In supination, the radius and ulna are parallel to each other, in pronation, they cross each other, with the radius lateral to the ulna proximally and medial to the ulna distally.[2] The superior radioulnar joint is made up of the radial head, which is covered by articular cartilage, and a fibro-osseus ring. This ring consists of the radial notch of the ulna, covered by articular cartilage, and the annular ligament, which consists of strong fibrous bands and is attached by its ends to the anterior and posterior margins of the radial notch of the ulna. It is internally lined with cartilage, which is continuous with the lining of the radial notch.[20] The primary movement is rotation of the radial head about its axis in the fibro-osseus ring. This movement is limited by tension in the quadrate ligament. The axis of rotation is at the center of the curve of the fibro-osseus ring.[2]

Static Supports.—The fibrous capsule is thin anteriorly and posteriorly and is thickened at the sides to form the collateral ligaments. All the elbow joints are encased in one capsule, so that with injury there may be effusion into the entire capsule. The anterior capsule is a thin, broad, pliable structure. It is very sensitive to injury and alterations in its anatomy can significantly affect the flexion-extension range of motion. It is attached to the anterior surface of the humerus just above the radial and coronoid fossae. It attaches inferiorly to the anterior surface of the coronoid process and to the annular ligament of the superior radioulnar joint. It blends with the collateral ligaments on the sides.[4, 35] The posterior capsule is also thin and loose, attached superiorly to the humerus just behind the capitellum and the lateral margin of the trochlea. It extends around the rim of the olecranon fossa and onto the posterior aspect of the medial epicondyle. Inferiorly, the posterior capsule attaches to the olecranon process at its superior and lateral margins. Laterally, it is continuous with the capsule of the superior radioulnar joint, deep to the annular ligament.[4]

The elbow ligaments function to keep the articular surfaces in apposition and to prevent sideways movements. As in most hinge joints, the strong ligaments are found along the sides. The medial collateral ligament, or ulnar collateral ligament, provides the major ligamentous contribution to elbow stability. It arises from the medial epicondyle of the humerus and fans out to insert on the coronoid process and olecranon of the ulna. Its three distinct bundles are continuous with each other.[20] The anterior oblique band is, anatomically and mechanically, the major ligamentous support of the elbow. It passes downward and anteriorly from the front of the medial epicondyle to the medial edge of the coronoid process. It becomes taut in extension. The posterior oblique band is weaker than the anterior oblique. It is fan shaped and passes from the back of the medial epicondyle to the posterior and medial aspects of the olecranon process. It becomes taut in flexion. The transverse band, or ligament of Cooper, originates from the inferior medial epicondyle and its base is attached to an oblique band that extends between the distal ends of the anterior and posterior bands. It contributes little or nothing to elbow stability.[20, 30]

The lateral ligament complex is not as strong as the medial collateral ligament. It consists of three major components: the lateral collateral ligament, the accessory lateral collateral ligament, and the annular ligament. The lateral collateral ligament, or radial collateral ligament, originates on the lateral epicondyle and terminates on the annular ligament. It is a poor stabilizer against varus stresses. It is taut throughout flexion and extension. The supinator muscle originates from its superficial aspect.[30] The accessory lateral collateral ligament blends with the annular ligament proximally and inserts into the supinator tubercle of the ulna. It is taut only when varus stress is applied to the elbow and functions to stabilize the annular ligament during varus stress. It is not altered with flexion, extension, pronation, or supination and has little length variation.[30] The annular ligament forms four fifths of a circle (the remaining fifth is the radial notch). The ligament and notch form a cup-shaped socket, wide above and narrow below, thus preventing distal malalignment of the radial head. It functions (1) as a ligament, binding the radial head to the ulna, and (2) as an articular surface, in contact with the radial head.[20] The interosseus membrane, sometimes referred to as the middle radioulnar joint, binds the shafts of the radius and ulna. The anterior fibers run obliquely downward and medially from the radius to ulna. It functions to attach the radius and ulna, to transmit force, and to prevent proximal displacement of the radius on the ulna.[35]

The synovial membrane extends from the margin of the articular surfaces of the humerus, lines the fossae and covers the medial nonarticular, flattened surface of the trochlea. It is then reflected over the deep surface of the fibrous capsule and attaches inferiorly to the margins of the trochlear notch of the ulna and to the radial neck. It forms a saclike pouch below the radial head, which permits rotation of the radius without tearing the membrane.[4, 20]

There are three fat pads inside the fibrous capsule and outside the synovial membrane; the largest is over the olecranon fossa. During flexion, it is pressed into the fossa by the triceps tendon. On extension, it is displaced from the fossa. Anteriorly, there are two smaller fat pads over the radial and coronoid fossae. These are pressed into their fossae in extension and displaced during flexion.[35]

There are three bursae at the elbow: the superficial bursa separates the superficial fascia from the olecranon; a small, thick-walled bursa separates the triceps tendon from the posterior capsular ligament; the bicipitoradial bursa separates the biceps tendon from the anterior surface of the radial tuberosity.[2, 35]

Musculature.—Elbow flexion is accomplished by the brachialis, the brachioradialis, and the biceps brachii. The brachialis acts only as an elbow flexor and is considered to be the workhorse of elbow flexion. It is one of the few muscles of the body with only one function. It is strongest on a pronated forearm but can flex from all positions.[20] The brachioradialis is strongest on a neutral forearm and when the elbow is flexed 100 to 110 degrees. It assists in pronation and supination to neutral. The biceps flexes most efficiently when the elbow is at 80 to 90 degrees of flexion. On a pronated forearm, it acts as a supinator. The long head also functions in shoulder flexion and stability.[17, 20] The overall most advantageous position for the elbow flexors is at 90 degrees of elbow flexion where the muscle pull is perpendicular to the axis of the lever arm. On a straight elbow, the direction of forces of the elbow flexors is almost parallel to the lever arm axis. The triceps is the major extensor of the elbow. It is strongest when both the shoulder and elbow are simultaneously extending. The triceps is most efficient at 20 to 30 degrees of elbow flexion. The anconeus stabilizes the elbow joint.[17] The supinator is actually a weaker supinator than the biceps, but its effectiveness is not altered by the position of elbow flexion. The pronator teres pronates but is actually less of a force than the pronator quadratus.[20]

The shape of the radius is like a crank with three segments: The upper segment, to the neck of the ra-

dius, runs obliquely distally and medially. The middle segment, including the upper half of the shaft, runs obliquely distally and laterally. At the level of the radial tuberosity, it forms an obtuse angle with the upper segment. This is the supinator bend of the radius. The lower segment runs distally and medially. At the level of the pronator teres insertion, it forms an obtuse angle with the middle. This is the pronator bend of the radius.[17]

Two mechanisms are available to move this crank: that of unwinding a cord coiled around one of the arms of the crank and that of pulling on the apex of one of the bends. In each mechanism, there is a short, flat muscle that acts by unwinding, e.g., the supinator and pronator quadratus; and a long muscle inserted into the apex of the bend, e.g., the biceps and pronator teres. Bowing of the radius affects pronation-supination range of motion, so that with forearm fractures, angular malunion will significantly limit this range.[17]

Neurology.—The nerve roots supplying the elbow come from C5 to T1. The major nerve components are the ulnar nerve, C8-T1; the radial nerve, C6-8; the musculocutaneous nerve, C5-8; and the median nerve, C5-T1. The median nerve, from the medial and lateral cords of the brachial plexus, passes in front of the elbow joint, medial to the biceps tendon and to the brachial artery and provides innervation to the pronators. It passes between the two heads of the pronator teres and travels under the flexor digitorum superficialis. It can be compressed at any of these locations. The radial nerve, from the posterior cord of the brachial plexus, travels down the radial groove of the humerus. It pierces the intermuscular septum as it passes from the posterior compartment to the anterior, then descends in front of the lateral epicondyle behind the brachioradialis and brachialis. In the antecubital space, the radial nerve divides into the superficial radial nerve (superficial to the supinator, covered by the brachioradialis) and the posterior interosseus nerve (motor). It supplies the triceps and brachoradialis. The ulnar nerve, from the medial cord of the brachial plexus, passes from the anterior to the posterior compartments in the arm, through the intermuscular septum and the arcade of Struthers. It supplies the flexors of the wrist and fingers. Owing to its course through the groove on the posterior aspect of the medial condyle, it is highly vulnerable to injury. The musculocutaneous nerve, from the lateral cord of the brachial plexus, splits the coracobrachialis muscle then travels between the biceps and the brachialis. It supplies the flexors of the elbow and terminates lateral to the biceps tendon.[20, 35]

Vascularity.—The brachial artery and its branches provide the only vascular supply to the elbow, forearm, and hand. The brachial artery lies anterior to the brachialis muscle, courses into the antecubital fossa, and divides into the radial and ulnar arteries just distal to radioulnar joint. In addition, there are many collateral branches around the elbow. These provide abundant circulation to the region, but are also at high risk for injury owing to the proximity of the vessels to the bones in the elbow.[20, 35]

BIOMECHANICS OF THE ELBOW

Carrying Angle

During elbow extension, the posterior aspect of the trochlear groove contacts the trochlear notch of the ulna and its obliquity is matched by a similar obliquity in the forearm. Thus, the forearm has a slight obliquity inferiorly and laterally and its axis (which is out of line with that of the arm) forms an obtuse angle with that of the arm. This angle is the carrying angle of the elbow. Variations on this obliquity of the trochlear groove cause variations in the carrying angle. The normal carrying angle is 10 to 15 degrees in men and 15 to 20 degrees in women. It appears to change with flexion-extension, but there is considerable controversy as to whether it actually does.[2, 19]

The elbow joint is essentially a hinge joint owing to the congruity of the humeroulnar articulation. However, the axis of motion deviates in a rotatory plane near the extremes of flexion. Thus, the ulna internally rotates in full flexion and externally rotates 5 degrees in full extension. This ulnar rotation occurs regardless of pronation-supination. It is noteworthy that the axis of rotation for elbow flexion does not coincide with the line through the epicondyles or with the flexor crease: it is 1 to 2 cm distal. During elbow movement, the muscle moment arm imposes multiple stresses on the integrity of the joint. When the elbow is extended and axially loaded, the distribution of stress across the joint is 40% across the humeroulnar joint and 60% across the humeroradial joint.[2]

Elbow extension is limited primarily by the impact of the olecranon in the olecranon fossa. It is also limited by tension of the anterior capsule and resistance of the flexor muscles (biceps, brachialis, supinator). If the end range of extension is surpassed, then (1) the muscles are intact but the brachial artery is damaged; (2) the olecranon is fractured and the capsule is torn; or (3) the olecranon is not fractured but the capsule and ligaments are torn and the elbow is dislocated posteriorly.

Active elbow flexion is limited primarily by contact of the soft tissue on the anterior arm and forearm. Thus, owing to the relative incompressibility of actively contracting muscle, active elbow flexion is usually approximately 135 degrees. Passive elbow flexion, which usually goes to approximately 150 degrees, is checked by the impact of the radial head against the radial fossa and the coronoid process against the coronoid fossa, by tension of the posterior capsule and by passive tension in the triceps.[11, 16] In the frontal plane, the collateral ligaments provide the primary restraint to motion. In extension, valgus stress is checked equally by the joint configuration, the medial collateral ligament, and the anterior capsule. In flexion, valgus stress is checked by the medial collateral ligament with the common flexor origin as a backup. Varus stress is checked in extension equally by the joint configuration and the soft tissue (lateral collateral ligament and anterior capsule). Varus stability is provided primarily by the joint itself.[16, 30]

In the forearm, the radius rotates in relation to the ulna about an axis that passes through the axes of both the superior radioulnar and the inferior radioulnar joints. The shift in the axis of motion occurs through a concomitant movement of the ulna. The distal ulna moves laterally (abducts) during pronation and medially (adducts) during supination. Supination is limited by the quadrate ligament at the superior radioulnar joint, the anterior ligament and capsule of the inferior radioulnar joint, and the pronators.[17] Pronation is limited by the quadrate ligament at the superior radioulnar joint, the posterior capsule, and the triangular ligament of the inferior radioulnar joint. Its primary restraint is soft tissue compression as the two bones cross. In full pronation and supination, the articular disk is relaxed. The ligaments of the inferior radioulnar do not function in limiting movement.[17]

Several accessory joint movements, not under voluntary control, are present at the elbow. While it is not possible to perform these movements in an isolated fashion, they do occur in combination with other movements.[35] Accessory movements at the humeroulnar joint are abduction, adduction, medial

TABLE 11–1.
Close-Packed and Resting Positions

	Close-Packed	Resting Position
Humeroulnar joint	Full extension	80 degrees elbow flexion
Humeroradial joint	80 degrees elbow flexion	Full extension
	Neutral forearm	Neutral forearm
Superior radioulnar joint	Neutral	70 degrees elbow flexion, 35 degrees supination
Inferior radioulnar joint	Neutral	10 degrees supination

glide, lateral glide, and distraction of the ulna; distraction, compression, ventral glide, and dorsal glide of the radius occur at the humeroradial joint. Accessory movements at the superior radioulnar joints are ventromedial and dorsolateral glide of the radius.[4, 35]

In the close-packed position, the joint surfaces are most congruent, the major ligaments are maximally taut, and there is minimal intracapsular space. In the loose-packed, or resting position, the major ligaments and supporting tissues are most lax and there is maximal intracapsular space.[4]

The close-packed and resting positions of the humeroulnar joints and humeroradial joints coincide (Table 11–1). This relationship becomes significant in the Monteggia fracture, since a joint excessively stressed in its close-packed position is prone to fracture while a joint stressed in its resting position is prone to dislocation.[4, 16]

Power at the elbow is greater with the forearm pronated; this varies with shoulder position so that it appears that the strength relationships support its design for climbing. With the shoulder overhead, the elbow flexion to extension strength ratio is 3:2. With the shoulder at 90 degrees, elbow flexion strength is greater than extension in a 3:2 ratio, while with the arm alongside the body, flexion and extension strength are about equal. These positional relationships must be taken into consideration during strength tests of the arm.[17]

FACTORS RELATED TO AGE

The elbow joint and its surrounding tissues are more independent of the age-related changes seen in many other parts of the body. As pointed out by Brems, "the elbow is remarkably resistant to progressive degenerative joint disease."[5] Thus, injuries and problems of the elbow are more likely to be re-

lated to the individual's life-style, types of activities, and history than they are to aging. Of course, quality of soft tissue changes that occur throughout the body will also occur at the elbow, but these changes do not appear to significantly alter its function, stability, mobility, or pathoanatomic vulnerability. At the same time, the limitations in healing potential that are true of the aging body are also true at the elbow. Furthermore, certain factors characteristic of this joint render full functional return from major trauma a formidable challenge to the physician, the patient, and the therapist. These factors include:

1. The congruency of the joint surfaces which, when altered, often cause major alterations of the elbow's biomechanics. Alterations at the humeroulnar joint may limit the elbow's extension motion; the mechanical alterations of the radiohumeral joint will alter flexion motion; and pronation-supination, essential to normal elbow function, can be limited by mechanical dysfunction of the inferior and/or superior radioulnar joints.

2. The sensitivity of the joint capsule and soft tissue to trauma with resultant increased potential for pain and motion limitations from fibrosis and scarring.

3. The relationship of the muscles and ligaments to the joint surface. The medial ligaments, which are the primary stabilizers of the elbow, are vulnerable to rupture, calcification, and contracture.[27] Because the brachialis crosses the joint as a muscle more than as a tendon, myositis ossificans is a significant problem at the elbow.

4. The potentially deforming forces of the muscles with fractures and dislocations may well result in significant functional deficits.

5. The positioning of the nerves and blood vessels can result in significant deficits in traumatic fractures and dislocations. In the case of the ulnar nerve, it is vulnerable to dysfunction in trauma as well as in inflammatory reactions in and around the medial epicondylar groove.

Cervical osteoarthritis, common in the older population, must certainly be considered as a contributing factor and/or as a complicating factor whenever an elbow problem presents. Age-related factors in treating the elbow can be broken down into three areas: traumatic fractures and dislocations; rheumatoid arthritis, and musculotendinous overuse injuries.

EVALUATION OF THE ELBOW

The physical therapist's evaluation of the elbow must begin with knowledge of all relevant test results and surgical factors so as to provide the best possible environment to establish the pathomechanics and dysfunction in the patient's arm. The patient is then asked to describe the history of the problem, identifying whether the onset was sudden or insidious and if there was a past history of relevant injury or dysfunction. The subjective evaluation then needs to identify what caused the patient to seek medical attention: was it pain, dysfunction, and/or trauma? If pain is a primary factor, the clinician first locates the pain's origin, or epicenter, and its pattern of radiation. It is very useful to objectify the pain information by using two scales: pain phases[31] (Table 11–2) and the visual analog scale (Fig 11–1). Here, the patient rates on a blank line with "0" at one end, "10" at the other, the intensity of pain with activity *(A)*, at rest *(R)*, and to palpation *(P)*. The nature of the pain (e.g., superficial vs dull, deep, sharp, throbbing, sensory changes) and behavior (e.g., constant vs intermittent; what causes it and what relieves it; duration) are then discussed. The extent of and type of dysfunction are then explored. The elbow's role in the use of the arm is likely to create significant limitations in daily living if a problem exists here. The dysfunction may present in weakness, loss of motion, and/or clumsiness in using the hand. Finally, other medical problems and treatment history of the problem should be discussed including medications, cortisone shots, and therapy.

TABLE 11–2.

Pain Phases

Phase I: Soreness after activity, usually gone in 24 hr
Phase II: Mild soreness and stiffness before activity, which disappears once warmed up; mild soreness after activity
Phase III: Stiffness before and mild pain during activity but not enough to alter activity
Phase IV: Pain during play that alters ability to perform
Phase V: Constant pain, even at rest

The objective evaluation begins with a clearing examination of the neck and shoulder. As the elbow is the major link in the entire upper extremity kinetic chain, it may well appear to be the problem spot when it is not. The upper extremity is inspected (evaluating both arms) for skin appearance, signs of previous incisions, swelling, muscle asymmetries and/or atrophy, and overall alignment. Changes in the carrying angle indicate previous trauma or abnormal growth. Laterally, shiny, thin skin over the lateral epicondyle is likely an abnormal response to cortisone injections. Loss of the normal recess below the lateral condyle may mean synovitis, joint effusion, or a problem in the radial head. Posteriorly, the inverted triangular relationship of the epicondyles and olecranon at 90 degrees of elbow flexion and their linear relationship on a straight elbow will be altered if there has been uncorrected trauma to the distal humerus.[32]

Range-of-motion tests include passive, active, and accessory movements. The normal elbow passive range of motion is flexion about 150 degrees, extension to 0 degrees, pronation 75 degrees, and supination 85 degrees. Although these are the normal physiologic ranges, they represent about 20 degrees more motion in each direction than is needed for normal function.[3, 23] With each movement, the therapist should also address the nature of the motion barrier, or end-feel, and the relationship of pain to each motion barrier. The normal motion barriers are bony approximation in elbow extension; soft tissue compression in pronation and flexion; capsular end feel in supination. Pathologic barriers include bony end-feel before full extension, which may indicate

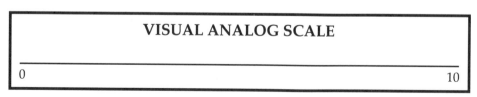

FIG 11–1.
Visual analog scale. Patient marks rating of pain intensity on scale as described in text.

arthritic changes; a springy block may be a loose body; muscle guarding is indicative of an acute inflammation in the joint or surrounding tissues.[11] The goal of identifying these problems is to help establish an effective treatment approach. Loose bodies and bony changes cannot be altered but the patient's pain, inflammation, and function can be improved. In most situations, passive stretching into elbow extension carries great potential harm, especially where there is a springy or muscle-guarding barrier to motion. If accessory and passive movements are limited, mobilization of the accessory movements is likely far more effective in overcoming capsular or ligamentous restrictions.[4] Crepitus should be explored during passive and active movements. Palpation should include all the bony landmarks statically as well as the radial head as the forearm and pronated and supinated. Soft tissue palpation is best carried out by starting in a nonpainful area and progressing toward the pain. Medially, the ulnar nerve feels tubular and is easily palpable in the ulnar notch. Occasionally it can be felt to dislocate from its groove.[32] Laterally, the "mobile wad of 3," consisting of the brachioradialis, extensor carpi radialis longus (ECRL), and extensor carpi radialis brevis (ECRB) is easily palpated with the arm at rest, forearm neutral.[3] It is important to note that extensor tendinitis presents with tenderness just anterior and distal to the lateral epicondyle, not directly on it.[26] Further down the extensor forearm, there may be tenderness to palpation where the posterior interosseus nerve passes through the heads of the supinator. These two areas of tenderness indicate entirely different problems.

Strength can be evaluated through manual muscle testing (Table 11–3), grip testing, and isokinetic testing if indicated (although this author has rarely found isokinetic testing indicated on initial evaluation). Grip testing should be performed with the elbow bent and straight. Significant differences in results between the two positions may indicate extensor tendinitis, flexor tendinitis, wrist and/or shoulder involvement. Dominant arm grip strength should normally be about 10% to 20% greater than that of the nondominant arm. If measured with the elbow bent at 90 degrees and the forearm neutral, elbow extension strength should be 65% to 75% of flexion and supination should be slightly stronger than pronation, approximately 10% to 20%.[32]

Structural integrity of the elbow is best evaluated with the elbow slightly bent (about 15 to 20 degrees) to remove the olecranon from its fossa and relax the anterior capsule.[32] Stabilizing the humerus is critical: the humerus should be stabilized in full internal rotation for testing varus stability and in full external rotation for testing valgus stability.[3] Reflex and sensory testing are summarized in Table 11–4. Finally, a few special tests are useful to evaluate specific problems. For extensor tendonitis, it is useful to test wrist extension isometrically using third-finger extension and wrist extension with the wrist and fingers each in 90 degrees of flexion. These should be tested with the elbow at 90 degrees of flexion where the extensors are on slack and in extension where the extensors are more stressed, to determine the extent of the problem. If the patient's pain is significant when these tests are performed on a bent elbow, the problem is more severe. At the medial elbow, ulnar nerve symptoms can often be reproduced by a positive Tinel sign, where tapping the nerve in its groove creates sensory disturbances into the forearm, hand, and sometimes up the arm, and/or the elbow flexion test, where the elbow is held fully flexed for 5 minutes.

TABLE 11–3.
Manual Muscle Tests*

Elbow flexion:
  If biceps involved, there will also be pain on supination
  If brachioradialis involved, there will be pain on resisted supination in full pronation and/or resisted pronation in full supination.
  If brachialis is involved, there will be no pain in supination or pronation.
Elbow extension: triceps
Supination: Biceps, supinator, brachioradialis (full pronation to neutral)
Pronation: Pronator teres, quadratus, brachioradialis (full supination to neutral)
Wrist extension: ECRL, ECRB, ECU, EDC
Wrist flexion: FCR, FCU, FDS, palmaris longus
*ECRL = extensor carpi radialis longus; ECRB = extensor carpi radialis brevis; ECU = extensor carpi ulnaris; EDC = extensor digitorum communis; FCR = flexor carpi radialis; FCU = flexor carpi ulnaris; FDS = flexor digitorum superficialis.

TABLE 11–4.
Reflex and Sensory Testing

Reflexes:
  Biceps reflex: C5
  Brachioradialis reflex at distal radius: C6
  Triceps reflex: C8
Sensations:
  C5: Lateral arm; sensory branches of the axillary nerve
  C6: Lateral forearm; sensory branches of the musculocutaneous nerve
  C8: Medial forearm; anterbrachial cutaneous nerve
  T1: Medial arm; brachial cutaneous nerve

The evaluation can be concluded by asking the patient for any other positions or actions that reproduce symptoms, or for information on other functional limitations not yet covered.

TRAUMATIC FRACTURE AND DISLOCATIONS

Most fractures and dislocations about the elbow in the older population are related to a fall on the outstretched arm or other similar type of direct trauma.[7, 8, 18, 21, 25,] Older patients with osteoporotic bones are likely candidates. The slower healing rates characteristic of the older population often necessitate prolonged immobilization, which can greatly complicate the elbow's rehabilitation potential. Fractures of the distal humerus are often very difficult to treat because of the nature of the elbow as described above. Those that cross the joint surfaces may, in addition to demonstrating displacement into the frontal and sagittal planes, involve rotational deformity.[7] These are more likely to result in injury to any of the three nerves, long-term predisposition to arthritic changes, and greater functional deficits. Their treatment is quite controversial[7, 9, 34] and possible complications to be considered by the therapist include soft tissue fibrosis, especially if the anterior capsule is damaged; articular malalignment with limitations of motion; myositis ossifications; and problems related to placement of internal fixation devices. Instability is rarely an issue in these fractures.[7] Motion limitations often result from problems in realignment, callus formation into the fossae, and/or the placement of the fixation device. Early treatment with ice and electrical stimulation can facilitate pain and edema control. The patient should be encouraged to exercise uninvolved proximal and distal joints. Exercises to regain motion and strength can begin once there is radiographic evidence of solid union (Table 11–5). Bryan and Morrey[7] compared the reported results of several treatment approaches in terms of stability, motion, pain, deformity, and function. It is reasonable to expect limited but functional strength and motion (at least 90 degrees of flexion-extension and somewhat more rotation).

Radial head fractures, not common in the older population, are far more likely to result in instability, especially if the surgeon excised the radial head and/or the integrity of the lateral collateral ligaments

TABLE 11–5.

Traumatic Fracture and Dislocation

Evaluative findings
  Usual history of a fall on outstretched arm
  Positive x-ray findings
  Some loss of strength but functional range of motion
Treatment suggestions
  Pain and edema control (ice or cool packs)
  Initially active range of motion of any moveable joint
  Strengthening exercises when radiographs show solid union

is altered. Excision of the radial head is likely to create an increased valgus at the elbow, with greater potential for ulnar nerve irritation. Some loss of strength but a functional range of motion should be expected.[21]

Monteggia fractures involve a fracture of the ulna with dislocation of the radial head. Myositis ossificans is more common here than in fractures without dislocation and posterior interosseus nerve neuropathy may also result.[8] Dislocations of the elbow are second in frequency only to those of the shoulder in the adult population, according to Linscheid. They usually involve extensive soft tissue damage and swelling and may be extremely slow in restoration of full potential, sometimes up to 18 months.[18]

One elbow injury in which age is a factor is the rupture of the distal biceps. Preexisting tendon degeneration at its attachment to the radial tuberosity seems to predispose the biceps to rupture here.[12, 22] The long term results vary greatly based on whether the tendon is surgically reattached to the radial tuberosity immediately, late, or not at all. Morrey[22] reports on return to almost normal flexion and supination strength with early reattachment and a loss of about 40% of flexion and supination strength if untreated. The decision as to how to treat this injury must be based on the patient's life-style, needs, and other medical problems which might factor into the desirability for elective surgery.

RHEUMATOID ARTHRITIS

Rheumatoid arthritis has a 20% to 50% incidence of elbow involvement,[13, 15] often presenting here within the first 5 years of its onset.[13] The painful synovitis and distention of the joint capsule may cause the patient to hold the elbow flexed, resulting in a flexion contracture.[15] With time, erosion of the cartilaginous articular surfaces, then cystic and osteophyte formation in the subchondral bone, result in loss of joint space, weakness, and instability.[2] The olecranon bursa may become painfully distended. The synovitis may also weaken the elbow ligaments with further instability. Finally, muscular, vascular and ulnar nerve dysfunctions may also result from distortion of the synovium and joint capsule.[15]

In addition to the medical and pharmacologic treatments for rheumatoid arthritis, rest (sometimes splinting), active motion, muscle conditioning, and patient education are among the conservative aspects of treatment. Surgery may include synovectomy with radial head resection for pain relief and to prevent further joint destruction; however, its success will be limited if the synovitis progresses.[14, 28, 29, 33] Advanced destruction of the elbow joint cause by rheumatoid arthritis is the primary indication for a total elbow joint replacement.[24] Currently, the available types are the semiconstrained prosthesis, the resurfacing arthroplasty, and the unconstrained design. All seem to offer good pain relief. Semiconstrained devices offer stability by a mechanical locking of the components, but also allow some play at the humeroulnar articulation. Resurfacing arthroplasty is an attempt to replicate the normal anatomy, and stability is derived from the joint congruency. The possibility of dislocation is greater with this type and a considerable flexion contracture may result.[24] The unconstrained design overall offers a better result, but its potential stability and success require good soft tissue support preoperatively. The elbow is splinted for several days postoperatively and thereafter while not exercising. Gentle passive motion is initiated about three to five days postoperatively followed by active exercises at three weeks, then functional strengthening (Table 11–6).

TABLE 11–6.
Rheumatoid Arthritis

Evaluative findings
  Painful synovitis
  Distention of joint capsule, causing flexion posture and possible
    flexion contracture
  Positive laboratory tests for rheumatoid arthritis
Treatment suggestions
  Pharmacological and surgical management
  Rest, sometimes splinting
  Active motion
  Patient education

MUSCULOTENDINOUS OVERUSE (INJURY)

Tendinitis about the elbow may occur laterally, medially, or much less commonly, posteriorly. Although Nirschl reported in 1985[26] that the average age of patients with this condition is 41 years, it is becoming more prevalent in the older population. As older people continue to enjoy an active life-style with considerable participation in sports such as tennis, golf, and fishing; and with their greater ability to continue to use equipment that stresses these tendons (e.g., hammers, screwdrivers, saws, axes, computers) than that of previous generations, tendinitis about the elbow is likely to continue to present more frequently in this population. Lateral elbow tendinitis primarily involves the origin of the extensor carpi radialis brevis, sometimes the extensor communis and extensor carpi radialis longus, and rarely the extensor carpi ulnaris.[26] In tennis, it is commonly associated with inappropriately using the arm instead of the body to generate power, especially in the backhand and with oversized racquets. In golf, it generally presents in the nondominant arm. Tendinitis of the medial elbow involves the common flexor origin but ulnar nerve neuropraxia is a common complication.[26] Poor form and overuse in golf and tennis are often causes. In any age group, the rehabilitation potential depends on a variety of factors, including nature of onset (acute trauma eg, hitting the epicondyle generally has much more difficulty than does overuse); duration and intensity of symptoms; hereditary and physical variables (individual variations in anatomic design, chemical makeup, tissue quality); and ability to modify lifestyle to lessen the stresses on the tendon.[31]

Treatment

As with any tendon, age is a factor in the healing potential of this problem. The treatment program is best approached as a series of components based on the individual's response to each step. Inflammation and pain control are achieved through a combination of protected activity, oral antiinflammatory medications, ice, and physical therapy modalities. It has been this author's experience that electrical stimulation, heat, and ice are most effective at the elbow. Most importantly, this phase should involve using the arm actively but avoiding stressful overload to the tissues. Although absolute rest, as in splinting, obviously eliminates abuse, it also deconditions tissue, hastens atrophy, lessens the vascular supply, and is thus detrimental to healing. Pain is the best guide for determining the ideal balance of rest and activity: reproducing the elbow pain, for which the patient sought medical attention, is to be avoided. In many cases, the patient can carry out most activities but with the elbow bent at least 80 degrees (thus relieving intrinsic stress on the tendon) and for briefer time periods than normal. Transverse friction massage, although widely used in treating tendinitis about the elbow, has not been found helpful in this author's experience—and in more cases than not, creates more pain, tissue trauma, and slows the rehabilitation process. Once the pain and inflammation have been controlled, promotion of healing is addressed through a methodically graduated strengthening exercise program to all the muscles involved. The exercises begin with no or minimal resistance in order to facilitate the healing response, then gradually resistance is added based on the patient's tolerance for muscle strengthening and endurance. Lastly, flexibility exercises are introduced once 75% of normal strength has been regained. Patient education is essential to avoid injury recurrence. A summary of evaluative findings and treatment suggestions appears in Table 11–7.[31]

Most problems at the elbow, whether resulting from overuse or trauma, and whether localized or systemic in origin, take on greater significance because of the important role of the elbow as the link between the mobile shoulder and the functional hand. While its design makes it less vulnerable to

many of the degenerative processes of aging and allows for some limitation of strength and motion without compromised function, it also presents a great challenge in injury to minimize involvement of the closely interacting components.

A treatment plan can be established based on these findings and the individual's needs. Modalities, medications, therapeutic exercise, and activities are reevaluated and upgraded based on the patient's response and progress. Medications and modalities are decreased and eventually discontinued as exercise and activity tolerance are increased. Once full functional potential is achieved and maintained for several weeks, the exercises can be phased out gradually. To minimize recurrence potential, the patient is advised to periodically reassess his/her strength and motion and to modify activities as needed. This general approach, with attention to individual variations, needs, and response, is applicable to any problem in the elbow. In this author's experience, greatest success is achieved when patient and therapist focus fullest attention on the tissue's response to treatment with appropriate modifications. This assures the most efficient route to restoring maximal functional potential.

REFERENCES

1. Amiss AA, et al: A functional study of the rheumatoid elbow. *Rheum Rehabil* 1982; 21:151.
2. An KN, Morrey BF: Biomechanics of the elbow, in BF Morrey (ed): *The Elbow and its Disorders*, Philadelphia, WB Saunders, 1985, pp 43-61.
3. Anderson TE: Anatomy and physical examination of the elbow in Nichols J, Hershman E (eds); *The Upper Extremity in Sports Medicine*. St Louis, Mosby-Year Book, 1990, pp 275–290.
4. Bowling R, Rockar P: The elbow complex, in Gould J and Davies G (eds), *Orthopedic and Sports Physical Therapy*. St Louis, Mosby-Year Book, 1985.
5. Brems JJ: Degenerative joint disease of the elbow, in Nicholas J, Hershman E (eds): *The Upper Extremity in Sports Medicine*, St Louis, Mosby-Year Book, 1990, pp 349-350.
6. Brumfield, RH, Resnic CT: Synovectomy of the elbow. Rheumatoid Arthritis. *J Bone Joint Surg [AM]* 1987; 67:16–20.
7. Bryan RS, Morrey BF: Fractures of the distal humerus, in BF Morrey (ed): *The Elbow and Its Disorders*, Philadelphia, WB Saunders, 1985, pp 302–339.
8. Cabanela ME: Fractures of the proximal ulna and olecranon, in Morrey BF (ed): *The Elbow and Its Disorders*, Philadelphia, WB Saunders, 1985, pp 382–399.
9. Conn J, Wade PA: Injuries of the elbow: A ten year review. *J Trauma* 1961; 1:248.
10. Coventry M: Ectopic ossification about the elbow, in Morrey BF (ed): *The Elbow and Its Disorders*, Philadelphia, WB Saunders, 1985, pp 464–471.

TABLE 11–7.

Tendinitis

Evaluative findings
  Pain laterally or medially (rare posteriorly)
  Precipitated by overactivity (overuse of the arm or poor form in tennis or golf)
  Significant differences in grip strength (i.e., greater than 20%) from dominant to nondominant hand.
  Pain in resisted movements
Treatment suggestions
  Inflammation and pain control (electrical stimulation, heat and ice)
  Encourage protected activity
  Avoid reproducing elbow pain; do all daily activities with at least 80% of elbow flexion
  Once pain and inflammation are gone, graduated strengthening to all involved muscles
  Begin flexibility exercises once 75% of strength has been regained

11. Cyriax J: *Textbook of Orthopedic Medicine,* vol 1, ed 5. Baltimore, Williams & Wilkins, 1969.

12. Davis WM, Yassine Z: An etiologic factor in the tear of the distal tendon of the biceps brachii. *J Bone Joint Surg (Am)* 1956; 38A:1368.

13. Ellison MR, Kelly KJ, Flatt AE: The results of surgical synovectomy of the digital joints in rheumatoid disease. *[Am] J Bone Joint Surg [Am]* 1971; 53:1041.

14. Ferlic DC, Clayton ML, Parr PL: Surgery of the elbow in rheumatoid arthritis. *J Bone Joint Surg (Am)* 1976; 58A:726.

15. Inglis AE: Rheumatoid arthritis, in Morrey BF (ed): *The Elbow and Its Disorders,* Philadelphia, WB Saunders, 1985, pp 638–655.

16. Kaltenborn FM: *Manual Therapy for the Extremity Joints,* ed 2. Oslo, Olaf Norlis Bokhandel, 1980.

17. Kapandjii IA: *The Physiology of the Joints,* vol 1. *The Upper Limb.* London, E & S Livingstone, 1970.

18. Linscheid RL: Elbow dislocations, in Morrey BF (ed): *The Elbow and Its Disorders,* Philadelphia, WB Saunders, 1985, pp 414–432.

19. London JT: Kinematics of the elbow. *J Bone Joint Surg [Am]* 1981; 63(4):529.

20. Morrey BF: Anatomy of the elbow joint, in Morrey BF (ed): *The Elbow and Its Disorders,* Philadelphia, WB Saunders, 1985, pp 7–42.

21. Morrey BF: Radial head fractures, in Morrey BF (ed): *The Elbow and Its Disorders,* Philadelphia, WB Saunders, 1985, pp 355–381.

22. Morrey BF: Tendon injuries about the elbow, in Morrey BF (ed): *The Elbow and Its Disorders,* Philadelphia, WB Saunders, 1985, pp 452–463.

23. Morrey BF, An KN, Chao EYS: Functional evaluation of the elbow, in Morrey BF (ed): *The Elbow and Its Disorders,* Philadelphia, WB Saunders, 1985, pp 73–91.

24. Morrey BF, Bryan RS: Total joint replacement, in An KN, Chao EYS: *The Elbow and Its Disorders,* Philadelphia, WB Saunders, 1985, pp 546–569.

25. Netter F: *Injuries to the Elbow.* Summit, NJ, CIBA, 1969.

26. Nirschl RP: Muscle and tendon trauma: Tennis elbow, in Morrey BF (ed): *The Elbow and Its Disorders,* Philadelphia, WB Saunders, 1985, pp 481–496.

27. Nirschl RP, Morrey BF: Rehabilitation, in Morrey BF (ed): *The Elbow and Its Disorders,* Philadelphia, WB Saunders, 1985, pp 147–152.

28. Porter BB, Park N, Richardson C, et al: Rheumatoid arthritis of the elbow: The results of synovectomy. *J Bone Joint Surg (Br)* 1974; 56B:427–437.

29. Schlein AP: Semiconstrained total elbow arthroplasty. *Clin Orthop* 1976; 121:222–229.

30. Schwab GH et al: Biomechanics of elbow instability. *Clin Orthop* 1980; 46:42.

31. Sobel J, Pettrone FP, Nirschl R: Prevention and rehabilitation of racquet sports injuries, in Nicholas J, Hershman E (eds): *The Upper Extremity Sports Medicine.* St Louis, Mosby-Year Book, 1990, pp 843–860.

32. Volz RG, Morrey BF: The physical examination of the elbow, in Morrey BF (ed): *The Elbow and Its Disorders,* Philadelphia, WB Saunders, 1985, pp 62–71.

33. Weiland A et al: Capitellocondylar total elbow replacement. *J Bone Joint Surg (Am)* 1989; 71A:1989.

34. Wickstrom J, Meyer PR: Fractures of the distal humerus in adults. *Clin Orthop* 1967; 50:43.

35. Williams PL, Warwick R (eds): *Gray's Anatomy,* ed 36. Philadelphia, WB Saunders, 1980.

Chapter 12

The Aging Wrist: An Orthopedic Perspective

Leo M. Rozmaryn, M.D.

ANATOMY AND BIOMECHANICS OF THE WRIST

The wrist is the most complex and least understood joint in the human body. It is the final adjusting unit of prehension in the upper extremity. It acts as a mechanical transducer and shock absorber for both extrinsic stress to the hand on one side and the action of the fingers on the other. Its boundaries are somewhat nebulous. Distally, the region of the wrist consists of an area bounded by the five metacarpals, eight carpal bones, and proximally by the distal end of the radius and the ulna. There is a bewildering array of articulations whose movements are governed by interlocking three-dimensional geometric constraints as well as a myriad of intrinsic and extrinsic powerful restraining ligaments.[9] Curiously, the wrist has no intrinsic musculature; rather, its complex movement is governed by muscle tendon units that cross it at its periphery.

For purposes of this discussion, the wrist will "begin" at the junction of the diaphysis and the metaphysis of the distal radius and ulna.

In the adult, this represents a rather abrupt transition from bone that is primarily tubular and cortical to cancellous bone with a thin cortical shell (the significance of this will be apparent later). The dorsal aspect of the radius has prominences that form tunnels for the extrinsic tendons, as well as attachments for the extensor retinacular. The radius fans into a triangular structure bearing essentially three articular surfaces: the scaphoid fossa, which tapers radially by the radial styloid; the lunate fossa; and the sigmoid notch for the articulation with the distal ulna. The ulna caput has nearly a circular cross section with articular cartilage covering a 300-degree arc, which allows for the extensor carpi ulnaris groove and the ulnar styloid. The distal end of the ulna is covered by articular cartilage, except for the styloid, which forms an attachment site for the numerous intercarpal ligaments and the triangular fibrocartilage. The articular disc of the triangular fibrocartilage stretches over the distal ulna and inserts on the ulnar side of the lunate fossa of the distal radius. This complex also has a myriad of vertical ligaments that connect the articular disc with the distal ulna and the ulnar carpus.

Distally, the proximal carpal row consists of the scaphoid, lunate, triquetrum, and pisiform. The scaphoid is considered to be a functional bridge between the proximal and distal carpal rows, comprising the trapezium, trapezoid, capitate, and hamate. These, in turn, articulate with the metaphyseal bases of the metacarpals (Fig 12–1). Curiously, the trapezium joins with the bases of the thumb and index metacarpals; the trapezoid with the ulnar half of the second metacarpal; the hamate with the fourth and fifth metacarpal; and the capitate with an exclusive third metacarpal articulation. In cross section, the carpus forms the shape of a Roman arch with the lunate capitate axis as the keystone. The long axis of the hand begins at the distal radius and continues through the third metacarpal, providing the wrist and hand with longitudinal stability and the mobil-

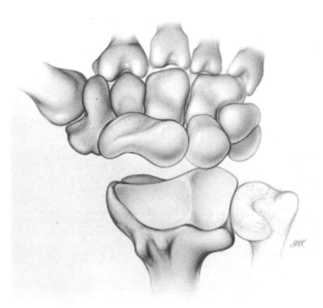

FIG 12–1.
An exploded view of the radiocarpal articulation illustrating the scaphoid and lunate fossa on the distal radius, the distal radioulnar joint articulation, the proximal carpal row with the scaphoid on the left, midcarpal row, and the carpal-metacarpal joints.

ity required for prehension. The scaphoid spans both rows anatomically and functionally and the pisiform is a sesamoid bone that enhances the mechanical advantage of the wrist's most powerful motor, the flexor carpi ulnaris, and also its own joint with the triquetrum. The two main moving articulations in the wrist are the radiocarpal and the midcarpal joints.

Ligaments

The wrist is interlaced with a complex array of intrinsic and extrinsic interosseous ligaments that are capable of inducing bony displacements and transmitting energy at a distance.[14] The palmar ligaments are far thicker and stronger than the dorsal ones. The extrinsic ligaments run from the radius to the carpals and from the carpals to the metacarpals. The interosseous ligaments insert between the carpal bones. The palmar extrinsic ligament system consists of the radial collateral ligament, the palmar radiocarpal ligaments, and the ulnar carpal ligaments. These are divided up into the superficial and deep layers. Superficial layers are V-shaped and provide support during radial and ulnar deviation. Deep ligaments include the radioscaphoid capitate, radiolunate, radioscapholunate, the ulnocarpal com-

plex (including the triangular fibrocartilage complex), the ulnar lunate ligament, and the ulnar collateral ligament. The dorsal extrinsic system is thinner and weaker than the palmar ligaments and connect the radius to the proximal carpal row. The intrinsic ligaments are short, strong fibers that, under most circumstances, connect the carpal bones into a fixed unit and dictate the stereotyped interosseous movement associated with wrist flexion, extension, and radial and ulnar deviation.

Muscles and Tendons

Ten forearm muscles control flexion, extension, pronation, and supination. Six are direct flexors or extensors whose tendons cross the joint over the wrist. The extensor carpi radialis longus and brevis, the extensor carpi ulnaris, the flexor carpi ulnaris, and the flexor carpi radialis insert at the metacarpal bases. Pronation is governed by the pronator teres and the pronator quadratus, and supination by the supinator and the biceps muscles. Six extrinsic tendon compartments cross over the dorsum of the wrist and these tendons effect all finger, wrist, and thumb extension. On the volar side, all the digital flexors cross the wrist in the carpal tunnel and the two wrist flexors cross in their own compartments.

Kinematics

The epicenter of movement instability of the wrist resides at the proximal pole of the capitate. The longitudinal column of the wrist, as previously indicated, consists of the third ray, the capitate, the lunate, and the radius axis. The radial and ulnar columns come off this central axis and provide the mobility required for hand function. Normal wrist flexion is approximately 85 degrees, extension is 75 degrees, with 55% of flexion occurring at the midcarpal joint and 45% at the radiocarpal joint. Total radial deviation is 15 degrees and ulnar deviation is approximately 35 degrees. In radial deviation, the proximal carpal row moves ulnarly and the distal carpal row moves radially. The scaphoid flexes and turns the lunate to a flexed position.[5] The triquetrum moves dorsal to the hamate and disengages it. In ulnar deviation, the scaphoid extends, the lunate extends, and the triquetrum rides up dorsally on the hamate.

There have been several studies to define the range of motion necessary for the activities of daily living. Voltz[16] in 1980 found that as long as the wrist achieves 15 degrees of extension, there is a minimal disturbance of the activities of daily living. Any disruption of the wrist ligaments, e.g., the scapholunate ligament, can cause a serious disability because of the development of instability patterns. These instability patterns occur in two broad categories in a predictable fashion: one is called a dorsal intercalated segment instability, the other is called a volar intercalated segment instability. There is also a predictable pattern of degeneration of the wrist that occurs as a result of the disruption between the scaphoid and the lunate.[8] This is called scapholunate advanced collapse, and results in a painful loss of motion of the wrist.

Wrist-Hand Synergy

Wrist position is critical in augmenting the fine motor control of the hand. Wrist extension allows digital flexors to obtain maximal functional length. Conversely, wrist flexors place the finger in extension. However, digital flexors have little effect on wrist flexion because of their close proximity to the center of rotation of the wrist in the carpal canal. Wrist flexors and extensors cross at the periphery of the wrist and are at an increased mechanical advantage. Voltz[15] in 1975 found that grip strength is maximized at 20 degrees of wrist extension at neutral rotation. Ulnar deviation of approximately 10 to 15 degrees would also maximize grip strength.

THE AGING WRIST

Fundamentally, there are two changes that occur in the wrist with aging: osteopenia and articular degeneration. The latter can occur as a result of wrist trauma earlier in life owing to primary degenerative arthrosis or as a result of an inflammatory process such as rheumatoid arthritis or mineral deposition disease. The former is important because it renders the wrist area extremely vulnerable to a host of classic injury patterns that, unless treated appropriately, can cause severe disability with marked inability to perform even the simple tasks of daily living without constant pain. The other category of dysfunction around the wrist relates to a sequela of neurologic events causing contractures about the wrist, rendering prehension impossible.

Osteoarthritis

The trapezial metacarpal joint is the pivotal interface between the wrist and the thumb, without whose function thumb opposition and apprehension would be impossible. This is a complex saddle joint that allows thumb flexion/extension, abduction, adduction, and circumduction for opposition. There is a complex interplay between the mobility and the stability necessary for power grip. The main static restraint of this joint is the volar oblique ligament, which prevents adduction and proximal migration of the metacarpal owing to deforming forces of the extrinsic and intrinsic musculature about the thumb. The geometry of the carpometacarpal joint with the restraining ligaments forms stable anchors through which extrinsic and intrinsic muscles of the thumb can operate. It is the balance of the muscle forces that ultimately gives the joint its stability. The compressive forces across the carpometacarpal joints are ten times the force generated at the fingertips and proper functioning depends on maintenance of a smooth, congruent joint surface.[3] Anything that renders the joint unstable or incongruent will hasten articular cartilage degeneration. This can occur as a result of major trauma or chronic overuse.

Osteoarthritis in the carpometacarpal joint is common in middle-aged women, predominantly those in their 50s and 60s. Clinically, this condition has been accompanied by joint subluxation. Whether this is a cause or an effect of the degenerative arthritis is unknown. Subluxation is usually radial at the metacarpal base, with formation of large bone spurs in the ulnar side of the trapezium that limit movement (Fig 12–2). The metacarpophalangeal joint may be hyperextended. Onset of pain may be vague and can take months or even years to become clinically evident. Osteoarthritis presents with pain and crepitus, and the characteristic deformity of the radial aspect at the base of the metacarpal at the carpometacarpal joint is visible. Any compressive or rotatory movement becomes very painful. Curiously, there is a poor correlation between the radiologic appearance of the joint and the degree of symptomatology. Patients gradually become unable to perform even the most simple tasks of daily living.

Conservative Management

The initial treatment of CMC arthrosis consists of splinting, rest, heat, ice, and use of anti-inflammatory medications. Joint protection splints that keep the thumb in 45 degrees of abduction but allow

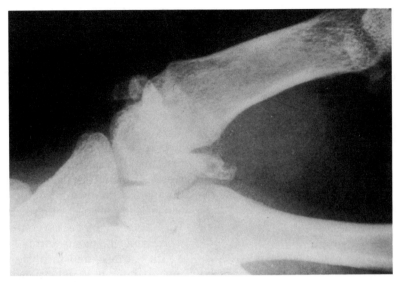

FIG 12–2.
End-stage osteoarthritis of the trapezial metacarpal joint of the thumb. Note the large radial and ulnar osteophytes with complete obliteration of the joint space.

the interphalangeal joint to move are recommended and will effect stabilization of the thumb in a functional position, allowing easier grasp with less discomfort. Intraarticular injections of a water-soluble corticosteroid solution can be helpful in selected cases but repeated injections should be avoided as they may hasten articular cartilage degeneration.

Surgical Management

The author generally recommends surgery to patients who have had unremitting pain in a splinted wrist to the extent that there is disruption in the activities of daily living, or with patients who are unwilling or unable to wear the splints but cannot function without them. Deformity without pain is a poor indication for surgery. At the present time, there are two categories of procedure for the salvage of the carpal metacarpal joints: arthroplasty and arthrodesis. In general, each of these procedures fulfills one of the requisites for good carpal metacarpal joint function. Arthroplasty, while allowing excellent movement, may not provide sufficient stability and could result in a weak pinch measured objectively, although the patient may actually experience an improved pinch depending on the level of preoperative morbidity. Arthrodesis on the other hand will provide excellent stability, but the patient will lose the ability to move the carpometacarpal joint, which will lead to arthritis at the thumb metacarpophalangeal joint and the scaphoid trapezoid joint.

Arthroplasty.—Over the years, there have been many approaches to treating carpometacarpal arthrosis. The range from a simple resection of the trapezium to interposition arthroplasty using various materials from rolled tendon graft (palmaris longus or fascia latae to synthetic materials, rolled Goretex to a total joint replacement with metal and polyethylene components). These allow for improved pinch with relatively painless movement. However, such procedures may be unsuitable for patients with very high occupational or life-style demands. Complications of total joint replacements include disarticulation, loosening, or fracture. Silastic implants have been associated with a late synovitis, which can cause cystic degeneration of the surrounding bone necessitating later removal and debridement.[10] Some recent modifications of the rolled tendon arthroplasty have been proposed to further stabilize the base of the carpometacarpal joint. One such modification is to include the use of one half of the flexor carpi radialis or abductor pollicis brevis securing the base of the thumb in a functional position and stabilizing this with a smooth percutaneous pin for internal fixation. This has shown to improve pinch and lessen metacarpophalangeal joint subluxation and swan-neck deformity of the thumb. This procedure is known as a suspensionplasty and is the procedure of the author's choice.

Arthrodesis.—Using the same surgical approach as the arthroplasty of the thumb interposition, the thumb is fused at 25 degrees of palmar abduction, 25 degrees of extension, and slight circumduction. Internal fixation is used to secure the fusion; occasionally, bone graft may be necessary to affect union. Thorough preoperative planning is necessary, if union is achieved, it will give the patient a stable, painless articulation, although the loss of movement is clearly evident.

CARPAL OSTEOARTHRITIS

Degenerative arthritis in the wrist is the final common pathway to destruction, usually stemming from previous injury. Such injuries may include fractures of any of the articular surfaces, ligamentous disruptions, and articular cartilage destruction. This may occur at the moment of impact or there may be a slow wear and tear on the articular surface caused by articular incongruity from fracture or by carpal ligament disruption in the wrist.

Characteristic findings of joint space narrowing, subchondral sclerosis, osteophyte formation, and degenerative cysts occur in two patterns, both described by Watson[17] and others. These are scapholunate advance collapse and triscaphe arthritis. Scapholunate

advance collapse of the wrist occurs usually as a late sequela of scaphoid fracture malunion or scapholunate dissociation. Radioscaphoid arthritis begins at the styloid and progresses proximally (Fig 12–3). The radiolunate articulation is curiously spared. The scapholunate dissociation of these two bones widens and the capitate pushes down as a wedge between them, eventually reaching the radius. This results in severe radial-side pain and loss of movement. The best treatment is prevention. Timely treatment of scaphoid fractures and subluxations can forestall this process, although there is no guarantee of success. Radial styloidectomy as described by Barnard and Stubbins in 1948,[2] i.e., the removal of part of the radial styloid is a treatment for the radial-sided wrist pain. This technique can work quite well if radial scaphoid arthrosis is limited to the tip of the styloid, and can effect pain relief with preservation of motion. However, it will not arrest the progression of scapholunate advance collapse. Silastic carpal implants have been plagued by silicone synovitis and cannot be recommended at this time.

Selective limited intercarpal arthrodesis, i.e., radial scaphoid or capitolunate, can forestall the ultimate demise of the wrist, requiring total wrist fusion. Proximal row carpectomy can offer temporary pain relief and should be recommended for older people with lower wrist demands, although this, too, can degenerate.

Triscaphe arthritis pain is located at the base of

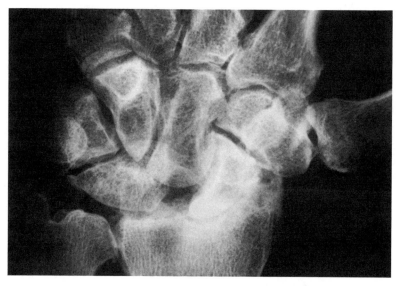

FIG 12–3.
Scapholunate advance collapse secondary to an old scapholunate dissociation with a rotatory subluxation of the scaphoid. Note the radioscaphoid joint space narrowing, sparing of the radiolunate articulation. Also evident is the proximal migration of the capitate through the old scapholunate diastasis.

the thumb. This can occur as an end result of local trauma and is expressed as pain and weakness to grip and pinch. It is best treated by splinting and local cortisone injection. Recalcitrant cases are treated by a local intercarpal fusion between the scaphoid, trapezium, and trapezoid.

INFLAMMATORY ARTHRITIS

There are many inflammatory disorders, but the prototype and most common disorder is rheumatoid arthritis. This is a slowly progressive disorder that affects virtually any joint in the body and can have a profound affect on the hand. Rheumatoid synovitis releases lytic substances in clearly defined patterns that destroy articular cartilage, as well as joint, capsule, bone, or tendon sheath. An understanding of these patterns will dictate the timing and indication for surgical and nonsurgical treatment. It is important to realize that the underlying disease can take three different forms—monocyclic, polycyclic, and progressive—but it is difficult to predict which pattern the patient will follow. One must also never forget that the primary treatment for this is medical, and surgery should be reserved for cases of progressive deformity, failure of medical treatment to stem synovitis, or impending tendon rupture. Barring these indications, a simple splint may be all that is necessary. One must also avoid being judgmental with these patients, as many of them, despite apparent severe deformity, retain function and may not require any surgical reconstruction.

Synovitis

In the wrist, hypertrophic rheumatoid synovium may invade the radiocarpal compartment, the distal radioulnar joint, the dorsal extensor compartment, or the flexor tendons across the carpal tunnel. Synovitis is easier to detect on the dorsum of the wrist as the skin in that area is subcutaneous tissue or thinner than on the volar aspect. This tenosynovitis begins beneath the extensor retinaculum on each of the extensor compartments and extends distally over the dorsum of the hand and envelops the extensor tendons of the wrist and the fingers (Fig 12–4). Lysosomal enzymes are released that digest and weaken the dorsal tendons and wrist ligaments and directly invade the tendons themselves, mechani-

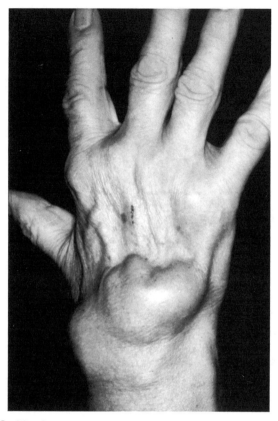

FIG 12–4.
Dorsal tenosynovitis, commonly seen as an early manifestation of rheumatoid arthritis.

cally weakening them. If left unchecked, the synovitis can cause tendon rupture and loss of dorsal support for the wrist, creating a collapse deformity as the dorsal suspensory ligaments of the wrist fail. Involvement of the distal radioulnar joint with infiltrative rheumatoid synovium will weaken the restraining ligaments around the distal ulna and also the extensor carpi ulnaris, causing the carpus and the distal radius to sublux volarly creating a relative dorsal subluxation of the distal ulna. The synovitis will also sculpt the distal ulna into a sharp point dorsally (Fig 12–5). This is known as caput ulnae syndrome, and will now be discussed in greater detail.

Tenosynovitis

The extrinsic extensor tendons of the wrist and hand cross the carpus but do not insert into it. Dorsally, each tendon goes in its own compartment; volarly, all the finger flexors course along with the median nerve and the flexor pollicis longus through the carpal tunnel and are covered by the transverse carpal ligament. All these tendons are covered by a ten-

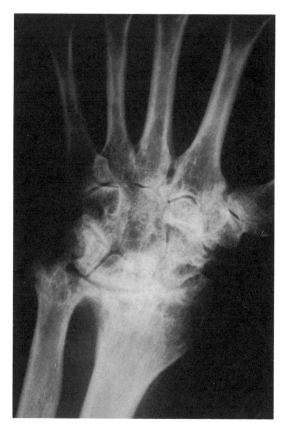

FIG 12–5.
Classic presentation of a caput ulnae syndrome in moderately advanced rheumatoid arthritis. Note the osteophytes emanating from the distal ulnar head. The joint collapse affecting both radiocarpal and midcarpal joints are evident. Note the ulnar carpal impingement and the generalized osteopenia.

don sheath, which assists in nutritive and gliding functions of the tendon. Rheumatoid arthritis causes proliferation of the synovial tissue with copious amounts of synovial fluid, rich in lysosomal enzymes, which fill the synovial sheaths. Eventually, this hypertrophic synovium assumes the texture of "sticky rubber" and invades the tendon tissue itself, resulting in tendon rupture if left unchecked. Dorsally, the process is usually obvious, as the skin is quite thin. The protuberances, which are easily seen and palpated, have been occasionally mistaken for ganglion cysts early in the disease. Volarly, the process is more insidious and one may not be aware of the presence of the disease until the tendon rupture has already occurred. A high index of suspicion is necessary to avoid disaster. Interestingly, tenosynovectomy can be curative even though the tendons are grossly attenuated. Tendon ruptures are uncommon after tenosynovectomy.[12] On the volar side,

tenosynovectomy is accomplished with the release of the carpal tunnel. This is frequently necessary because the patients present with concomitant carpal tunnel syndrome.

Tendon Ruptures.—Flexor and extensor tendons crossing the wrist are all-too-frequent victims of the relentless tenosynovitis that slowly destroys them. This may occur as a result of direct invasion by rheumatoid pannus or through lysosomal enzymes that digest them. Sharp bony prominences, such as of the ulnar head, Lister's tubercle, or the scaphoid tubercle, form a mechanical shearing device that assist in this process. Digital extensor tendons crossing over the caput ulnae are affected most commonly. Ruptures usually affect the ulnar digits first and progress radially. Clinically, this can manifest suddenly and without pain. The extensor pollicis longus can be affected independently.

Treatment.—The best treatment is prevention. Tenosynovectomy can be curative and is of an urgent nature especially if the patient has begun to rupture some of these tendons. Such tendon ruptures must be distinguished from tendon subluxation and from the possibility of a radial nerve palsy secondary to rheumatoid tissue infiltration around the radial nerve. This can be evaluated the "tenodesis effect." If the digits cannot be extended at the metacarpophalangeal joints by flexing the wrist, then chances are the tendons have been ruptured.

In the early stages of the disease, the tendons can be repaired in a side-to-side fashion to intact extensor tendons. Direct end-to-end repair may work in very early stages but will become impossible later on. If all the extensor tendons have ruptured on the dorsum, reconstruction becomes increasingly difficult and will require a tendon transfer from the volar side, usually a digital flexor. Flexor tendon ruptures are much more difficult to deal with. Tendon transfers or grafts or secondary reconstructions may be necessary as direct repair is usually impossible. Fusions of distal interphalangeal joints may be required where a profundus tendon rupture becomes irreparable. Again, prevention is key here.

Wrist Architecture

Collapse of wrist architecture occurs in characteristic patterns in rheumatoid arthritis. These patterns are governed by the close proximity of the synovial pouches to the supporting wrist ligaments. Collapse of the joint is also a result of articular cartilage and subchondral bone erosion, which may also be significant. These concepts are well illustrated by the distal radioulnar joint. Synovitis in the distal radioulnar joint destroys the joint capsule, thinning it distally, and grossly distending and thinning the triangular fibrocartilage complex. In caput ulnae syndrome, the head of the ulna becomes grossly deformed by the destruction of the articular surfaces, and as indicated previously, a relative dorsal subluxation of the ulna occurs, exposing a razor-sharp surface dorsally to the extensor tendons coursing over it. Volar subluxation and relative supination of the carpus on to the distal radioulnar joint occurs, which increases the dorsal prominence of the ulna. Pain, weakness, and loss of function with loss of rotation are common, as is limitation of wrist dorsiflexion.

Other areas of involvement include the radiocarpal joint where the intercarpal collapse patterns predominate. Destruction of articular cartilage in the radioscaphoid and radiolunate articulation will result in joint space narrowing, as evident on x-ray studies. Insufficiency of the radioscapholunate ligament can cause rotatory subluxation of the scaphoid and carpal malalignment. This will eventually lead to bony ankylosis, which may or may not be painful to the patient. In addition, the distal carpal row rotates radially along with the metacarpals giving rise to the "zig-zag" deformity of the digits. The carpus can migrate ulnarly as the radio lunate ligament and radial triquetral ligaments fail. Subchondral collapse of the scaphoid fossa of the distal radius can cause proximal migration of the scaphoid as well (Fig 12–6). Volar collapse of the wrist in a unidirectional fashion can be seen as a result of failure of all the volar radial carpal ligaments. Proximal migration of the capitate through a scapholunate diastasis is a direct result of weakening of the interosseous scapholunate ligament. Erythema, pain, and swelling are the predominant physical symptoms. Loss of grip and dexterity follow. At one end of the spectrum, stiffness with painful ankylosis, crepitation, and loss of flexion/extension may result. At the other end, gross instability can accompany volar collapse.

Reconstruction

Reconstructive options can be divided into two groups: soft tissue and bone-joint procedures.

In the soft tissue procedure, the first option is synovectomy. This is usually considered in patients early in the course of the disease who, after a period of about 6 months of medical therapy, have persis-

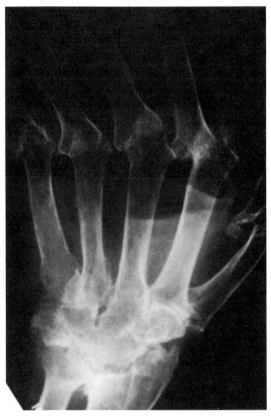

FIG 12–6.
Advanced rheumatoid arthritis in the wrist and the metacarpal phalangeal joints with the classic zig-zag deformity of the metacarpal phalangeal joints and the complete collapse of the wrist joint, most pronounced in the radiocarpal articulation. Note the massive destruction of the distal radius.

tent pain, swelling, and loss of function as a result of inflammation. There is usually little or no joint or bony collapse. Removal of inflammatory synovium is not a permanent solution, but a synovectomy may bring about pain relief and delay the joint collapse associated with capsular distention and weakening. The procedure is performed through a dorsal approach in conjunction with a tenosynovectomy. In closure, the dorsal wrist capsule can be augmented by a slip of extensor retinaculum to reinforce these ligaments.[7] Patients usually regain a strong sense of security and grip and do not mind the relative increase in stiffness after the procedure. The bowstringing of the extensor tendons that may follow surgery can be limited by retaining approximately one third of the extensor retinaculum. Recently, the arthroscope has been employed to effect a synovectomy of the wrist with minimal distortion of the soft tissue envelope. This can be helpful if there has been no tendon involvement. Volar synovectomy of the wrist is more difficult but may be used in conjunction with carpal tunnel and volar tenosynovectomy.

The use of tendons to reconstruct intercarpal articulation has only fair results. This is because of two reasons. First, unlike in posttraumatic situations, the carpal bones themselves are extremely osteopenic, lessening the hold of soft tissue restraints on the bone; second the progressive nature of the disease will ultimately cause a weakening of these transplanted tendons.

Despite the progressive appearance of joint destruction seen on x-rays, patients with rheumatoid wrist involvement retain excellent function for a long period of time, mainly because the process occurs so slowly that the patients are able to adapt their activities of daily living. Early on, bony procedures will focus on the distal ulna. Surgical attempts to relocate the distal ulna are fraught with problems because the carpus may be contracted so that pulling it out is impossible. In this setting, shortening of the ulna, hemiexcision of the radial side of the ulna leaving the ulnar styloid intact, or excision of the distal 1 cm of ulnar head may be considered (Darrach procedure).[13] Although the Darrach procedure has lost favor in the reconstruction of post-traumatic radial ulnar joint problems especially in younger patients, in older rheumatoid patients the Darrach procedure will afford the patient increased movement and less pain, and remove the risk of extensor tendon ruptures. There have been many attempts to reconstruct the ulnar head with a Silastic prosthesis to support the ulnar carpus. While theoretically this is sound, and some patients can achieve good results, the technique has had its problems with fragmentation and silicone synovitis. In general, a well-performed Darrach procedure is all that is necessary in this setting to achieve good results.

Arthroplasty/Arthrodesis

As wrist disease progresses and the pain and instability become more prominent, one needs to consider performing an arthroplasty or an arthrodesis. Arthrodesis will create a strong, painless wrist devoid of motion. This can be problematic if the patient has another ankylosed joint in that extremity, a contralateral wrist fusion or ankylosis, or a desire to maintain wrist movement. Such patients may be candidates for arthroplasty. This has been performed with varying degrees of success with either soft interposition or Silastic endoprosthesis. Short-term results appear promising with these techniques. However, over the long term they have proven to be quite problematic. Silastic endoprosthesis can fracture and cause silicone synovitis. Arthrodesis is a final common pathway in these patients although many techniques have been described. The use of one or two intermedullary pins with or without the use of bone grafts has been advocated. The pins may be placed into the space between the 2–3 and 3–4 intermetacarpal spaces or a single stout Steinmann pin may go up the axis of the third metacarpal and up the intermedullary space of the radius (Fig 12–7). An oblique pin is placed temporarily to control rotation. These procedures force the wrist into a neutral position with respective flexion-extension axis. This is the best position for a single-wrist arthrodesis. In a bilateral case, a person may have his wrist flexed 5 to 10 degrees to facilitate hygiene. Fusion is readily achieved and pseudoarthrosis is rare. If there is concern about bilateral arthrodesis, a Swanson wrist arthroplasty may be performed on the dominant side.[1]

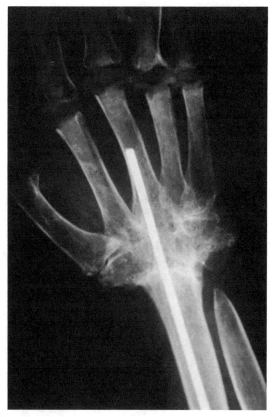

FIG 12–7.
A well-fused radiocarpal articulation. Note the excision of the distal ulna and the metacarpal phalangeal implant arthroplasties.

FRACTURES OF THE DISTAL RADIUS

Perhaps the most prominent hallmark of the aging wrist is osteopenia resulting from osteoporosis. This age-related thinning out of cortical and cancellous bone is an entity whose etiology remains obscure. It is well known that this disorder is probably an accelerated resorption of bone over time in the face of a normal rate of bone formation. This affects cancellous bone more profoundly than cortical bone and as such, the cancellous metaphyses of bone are more susceptible to fracture that the diaphyseal regions. This explains the preponderance of fractures in the proximal and distal femur, humerus, vertebral body, and in the distal radius of this age group. Injuries to the distal radius were described over 100 years ago by Abraham Colles, who felt that these deformities—once developed—were essentially incurable, but some function could be achieved regardless over time. These assumptions have been held to be true until very recently as better reporting brings to light the true nature of the long-term problems associated with these injuries. Until recently, the classifications of injuries to the distal radius have simply been relegated to eponyms, i.e., Colles', Barton's, and Smith's. These classifications have significant problems. Over the past 25 years, there have been multiple attempts to classify these injuries based on angulation, displacement and position of the fracture, displacement of the articular surface, the mechanism of injury, the number of fracture parts, and the axis of displacement (either on anteroposterior or the lateral planes). Recently, most useful classifications by Melone[11] and the AO group[4] clearly define the location and position of articular fragments, and will help predict a method of treatment and prove useful for prognosis.

Prognostic Factors

It has been clear that the following factors play a key role in determining a poor prognostic outcome[6]: (1) reversal of the normal palmar tilt of 11 degrees; (2) joint incongruity greater than 3 mm; (3) radial shift of the distal radial fragment greater than 2 mm; (4) flattening of the normal articular shape of the distal radius seen on the anteroposterior x-ray. Al-

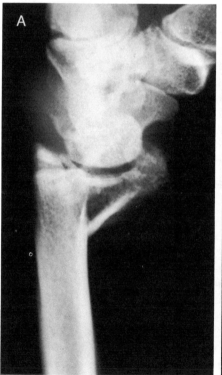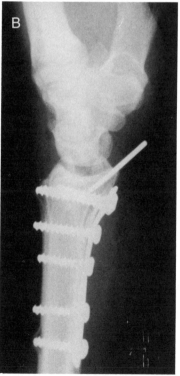

FIG 12–8.
A, comminuted fracture of the distal radius. Note the volar cortex of the distal radius and the volar displacement of the carpus. **B,** after open reduction internal fixation with a volar plate and screws and a K-wire, with reduction of the radiocarpal articulation.

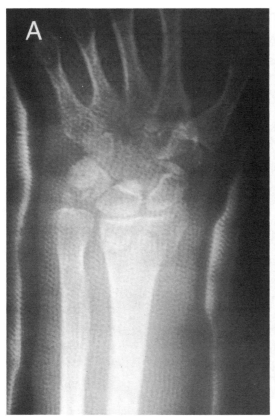
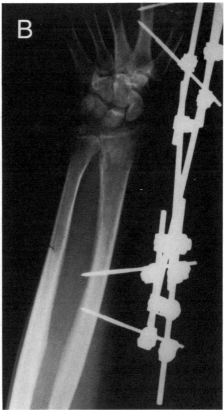

FIG 12-9.
A, comminuted fracture of the distal radius with persistent shortening as a result of settling of the fracture. If left untreated, this patient would develop an ulnar carpal impingement. **B,** after external skeletal fixation of this fracture, length of the distal radius has been maintained; however, open reduction internal fixation is still required because of persistent articular incongruity of the distal radius.

though these concepts have been used to treat high-energy fractures of the distal radius in young patients, similar patterns exist in osteopenia fractures of the elderly. However, the demands of these patients are low, and long-term problems of osteoarthritis are less of an issue.

Treatment

Treatment in a long- and short-arm cast or sugar tong splint will suffice in extraarticular, noncomminuted, or nondisplaced fractures. However, if any of these conditions are not met, redisplacement after closed reduction is common and will require further treatment such as percutaneous pinning, pins and plaster, external skeletal fixation, or open reduction internal fixation with pins, screws, or plates and screws. Occasional combinations of the above techniques are necessary to achieve a stable reduction. Recently, there has been an increasing trend towards external skeletal fixation and/or open reduc-

tion internal fixation (Fig 12-8). External fixation has the advantage of counteracting muscle forces that tend to compress the fracture. Also, the distraction tends to pull the comminuted fragments into place by tightening up the joint ligaments and soft tissues sleeve around the bone (Fig 12-9). Pin tract infections and injury to the radial nerve are known complications of this technique, but with attention to detail, this can be avoided. Other complications include postoperative long-term stiffness, median neuropathy, flexor tendon rupture, and tendon adherence, as well as posttraumatic arthritis.

STROKE AND BRAIN INJURY

A myriad of clinical features can be seen with patients who are hemiplegic owing to a stroke or brain injury. The wrist is an active participant in this disease complex. It must be kept in mind that hemiplegic patients retain nearly normal sensitivity on the affected side; however, this affected side may be partially insensate but can still be used as a helper hand. Depending on degree of neurologic injury, patients may have variable use of their affected hand. Ultimately, sensibility of the hand will determine what kind of use there will be. The hand surgeon is frequently called upon to intervene in these patients because of spasticity and contracture that may ensue. Frequently, in these patients the hand is balled into a tight fist and there may be marked flexion contractures in the wrist of greater than 70 degrees. This frequently can interfere with hygiene. Hand function may be absolutely impossible. One also needs to consider that elbow contractures are also quite common and need to be considered in the comprehensive care of the patient. Furthermore, prolonged flexion of the wrist will cause pain owing to joint contracture and median nerve compression. Surgical procedures to lengthen or cut tendons across the wrist will afford patients pain relief. Sometimes stretch therapy can be useful in early stages if the wrist can be brought out into extension easily; however, if a firm contracture has already developed, this will not be helpful. Occasionally, a procedure known as the flexor origin slide—where the origin of the flexor tendons can be sectioned at the elbow, and the shortened muscle tendon units allowed to drift into the forearm—can be helpful. This flexor origin slide has been useful in the management of wrist contractures in stroke patients.

REFERENCES

1. American Academy of Orthopaedic Surgeons: *Orthopaedic Knowledge Update III,* chap 30. Park Ridge, Ill, AAOS, 1990, p 373.
2. Barnard L, Stubbins SG: Styloidectomy of the radius in the surgical treatment of nonunion of the carpal navicular. *J Bone Joint Surg (Am)* 1948; 30:98.
3. Cooney WP, Chao EY: Biomechanical analysis of static forces in the thumb during hand function. *J Bone Joint Surg* (Am) 1977; 59A:27–36.
4. Heim U, Pfeiffer KM: Internal Fixation of Small Fractures, ed 3. Berlin, Springer-Verlag, 1988, pp 152–153.
5. Johnston JM: Varying positions of the carpal bones in the different movements at the wrist. I. Extension, ulnar and radial flexion. *J Anat* 1907; 41:109.
6. Knirk JL, Jipeter JB: Intraarticular fractures of the distal end of the radius in young adults. *J Bone Joint Surg* (Am) 1986; 68A:647–659.
7. Kulick RG, De Fiore JC, Straub LR, et al: Long term results of dorsal stabilization in the rheumatoid wrist. *J Hand Surg* 1981; 6:272–280.
8. Linscheid RL, Dobyns JH, Beabout JU, et al: Traumatic instability of the wrist. Diagnosis, classification, and pathomechanics. *J Bone Joint Surg* (Am) 1972; 54:1612–1632.
9. Mayfield JK: Wrist ligamentous anatomy and pathogenesis of carpal instability. *Orthop Clin North Am* 1984; 15:209–216.
10. McGrath MH, Watson HK: Arthroplasty of the carpometacarpal joint of the thumb in arthritis—an emphasis of bone configuration. *Orthop Rev* 1979; 8:127–131.
11. Melone CPjr: Articular fractures of the distal radius. *Orthop Clin North Am* 1984; 15:217–236.
12. Millender H, Nalebuff EA: Preventive Surgery—tenosynovectomy and synovectomy. *Orthop Clin North Am* 1975; 6:765–792.
13. Smith-Peterson, Au Franc OE, Larson CB, et al: Useful surgical procedures for rheumatoid arthritis involving joints of the upper extremity. *Arch Surg* 1943; 46:764–770.
14. Taleisnik J: The ligaments of the wrist. *J Hand Surg* 1976; 1:110.
15. Voltz RG: The development of a total wrist joint. *Clin Orthop* 1976; 116:209–214.
16. Voltz RG, Lieb M, Benjamin J: Biomechanics of the wrist. *Clin Orthop* 1980; 149:112–117.
17. Watson HK, Ryu J: Degenerative disorders of the carpus. *Orthop Clin North Am* 1984; 15:337–353.

Chapter 13

The Aging Wrist: A Rehabilitation Perspective

Janet Jensen, P.T.

The wrist is an important junction between the forearm and the hand that offers stability for the hand and enhances finger function with its ample range of motion. The aging wrist and the pathologies that occur are significant because of the importance this joint has on the function of the hand when performing activities of daily living (ADL). For success in the evaluation and treatment of the wrist, the anatomy and biomechanics of this joint first must be understood.

ANATOMY AND BIOMECHANICS

Anatomy

The wrist region comprises the distal ends of the radius and ulna and two rows of carpal bones. As shown in Figure 13–1, the proximal carpal row consists of the scaphoid, lunate, and triquetrum. The distal row contains the trapezoid, capitate, hamate, and trapezium. The pisiform is a sesamoid bone that articulates with the triquetrum anteriorly and enhances the mechanical action of the flexor carpi ulnaris. The radiocarpal joint, which is the intersection of the lunate and scaphoid with the distal radius, is a vulnerable portion of the wrist in the elderly. The articulation between the proximal and distal carpal rows is called the midcarpal joint and is more precise in its articulation than the radiocarpal joint.[21]

The radiocarpal joint capsule is loose, allowing for extensive movement between the concave radius articulating with the convex structure of the lunate and scaphoid. Distally, the ulna joins with a complex of structures called the triangular fibrocartilage and the lateral border of the radius, forming the distal radioulnar joint. The ulna does not articulate with the carpus. The triquetrum and ulna are separated from the the radiocarpal joint by an articular disc. The triangular fibrocartilage located between the distal end of the ulna and the carpus was found by Palmer and Werner to be a complex of structures consisting of the articular disc, the dorsal and volar radioulnar ligaments, the meniscus homologue, the ulnar collateral ligament, and the sheath of the extensor carpi ulnaris. This complex functions as a cushion or support for the lunate, triquetrum, and ulnar carpus and provides stability for the distal radioulnar joint.[11, 16]

Ligaments of the wrist are multidirectional, connecting the distal ends of the radius and ulna to each other and to the carpal bones. This complex network of ligaments stabilizes 21 separate joints.[9] The carpal tunnel is formed in the wrist by the concave structure of the anterior carpal bones and the flexor retinaculum, which is attached to the anterior aspect of the carpal bones medially and laterally. This tunnel is completely filled with tendons and the median nerve.[14]

Biomechanics

The radiocarpal joint has two degrees of freedom, which allows for flexion and extension and radial-ulnar deviation of the wrist. In the normal wrist, 70 degrees of wrist extension and 75 to 90 de-

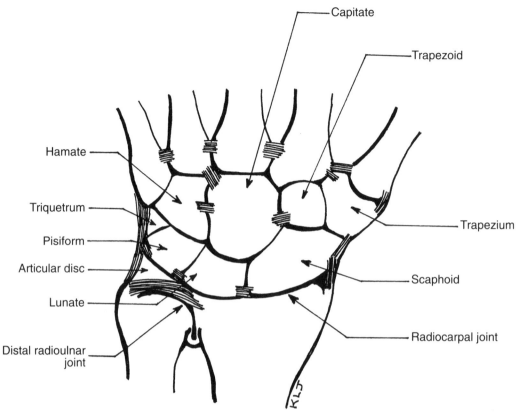

FIG 13–1.
The proximal and distal carpal rows. The midcarpal joint is formed by the articulation of these two rows. The radiocar- pal joint is the articulation of the distal radius with the scaph- oid and lunate.

grees of flexion are present.[11] Flexion range of motion exceeds extension by 10 degrees on average owing to the slight volar tilt of the distal radial plates.[21]

The axis of wrist motion during wrist flexion and extension changes. It has been acknowledged that there is a variation in the contribution of the proximal and distal carpal rows in the total arc of flexion and extension. Radiographic views of a normal wrist have shown that flexion occurs mainly at the radiocarpal joint, with the midcarpal joint contributing more to wrist extension.[13] Other authors have concurred with this finding and have found that 50 degrees of flexion occurs at the radiocarpal joint with 35 degrees of movement at the midcarpal joint.[11] However, other studies have shown the opposite.[21] In this chapter the radiographic findings will form the basis for determining the axis of motion during evaluation goniometrically, and when applying joint mobilization techniques.

The axis of motion for ulnar and radial deviation is located within the proximal pole of the capitate.[21] Norms for these motions are 20 degrees of radial deviation and 30 degrees of ulnar deviation.[11] The proximal and distal carpal rows function as separate segments; however, they possess an integrated relationship with one another. During radial deviation, the proximal carpal row moves ulnarly with radial displacement of the distal row. Movement of the carpal rows is reversed during ulnar deviation, giving the appearance of the carpal rows moving in one plane (coronal) as linked segments.[21]

Three muscles flex the wrist and three perform extension. Given their contralateral position these muscles work in opposition regarding flexion and extension, but are capable of working in unison. For example, the extensor carpi ulnaris and flexor carpi ulnaris share the same insertion at the base of the fifth metacarpal and work together to perform ulnar deviation.[9] The flexors and extensors also function as dynamic stabilizers for the carpal bones, aiding in the prevention of subluxations and dislocations. Lunate dislocations and scapholunate dissociation may occur with the disruption of important intracapsular and intercapsular ligaments.[21]

Kinematic studies by Klopsteg have shown that the angular position of the wrist most frequently used during activities of daily living is 0 to 10 degrees of extension and a neutral position (0 degrees) for radial-ulnar deviation with the forearm slightly pronated (30 to 40 degrees).[11] Knowledge of these movement patterns helps the physical therapist and the elderly patient set appropriate goals during rehabilitation to maximize function without being too preoccupied with returning the patient to the norms of range of motion.

Changes With Aging

Osteoporosis is one of the age-related changes that affect the wrist and is characterized by skeletal bone reduction. This thinning of the bone mass makes the wrist more vulnerable to fractures and disability. Osteoporosis may be idiopathic in nature, but in most instances it is caused by a combination of metabolic bone diseases, for example osteopenia, which is the decreased rate of osteoid synthesis. One possible cause of osteopenia in the elderly is dietary deficiencies of proteins such as meats, which the older person may avoid owing to dental problems.[1]

Another change in the wrist with aging is joint degeneration; this may be a result of an acute trauma or minor repetitive traumas, which are usually occupational. When progressive, this disease leads to a painful joint with limited range of motion reducing function during daily tasks.[1]

Appearance of interosseous muscle wasting is a common change with aging and is caused by subcutaneous tissue loss. Often, elderly persons complain of nonspecific weakness, grip loss, or numbness.[5] Skeletal muscle undergoes functional and structural changes with age characterized by a loss of strength and a change in contractile quality. It has been observed that the muscle takes a longer period of time to reach peak tension and relax after contraction in an older person. A decrease in cross-sectional area of muscle as well as the number of type II fibers present was also reported.[15] Narici and co-workers studied isometric contractions of the adductor pollicis muscle and found aged muscle is weaker and slower and tetanizes at a lower fusion frequency but is more resistant to static fatigue.[15]

FRACTURES

Given the high incidence of falls in the elderly population, the wrist is particularly vulnerable to fracture, since the outstretched hand usually absorbs the impact. The distal radius is the most commonly fractured bone in the body as well as the most common wrist injury in the elderly, especially in women.[14] The initial contact area with small compressive loads is between the scaphoid, lunate, and distal radial plate. As the load increases, the contact area extends to the triangular fibrocartilage complex overlying the distal ulna.[21] A fracture that occurs in the distal radius 1 to 2 inches above the carpus with displacement of the radial fragments posteriorly and upward has been classified as a Colles' fracture. Depending on the magnitude of the force, this may or may not include a fracture of the ulnar styloid or dislocation of the distal radioulnar joint. There is a 51% incidence of an associated fracture of the ulnar styloid and it is believed that this injury has a poor prognosis because of the loss of integrity of the distal radioulnar joint.[20] The immediate management of a Colles' fracture is either an open reduction with insertion of pins or a closed reduction under anesthesia followed by a period of immobilization in both cases.[22]

Fracture of the scaphoid can also result from a fall in which the force is directed through the palm of the hand with the wrist abducted. Clinical signs of this fracture are tenderness in the "snuff box region" (which is the depression formed between the abductor pollicis longus and the extensor pollicis brevis anteriorly and the extensor pollicis longus posteriorly) or on the anterior aspect of the wrist over the tubercle of the scaphoid. A fracture of the scaphoid is easy to overlook and is often misdiagnosed as a wrist sprain.[14]

It is important to provide fixed traction during immediate management of the Colles' fracture to prevent shortening of the radius. Cole and Obletz have shown that an 8-week immobilization period is necessary for the comminuted fracture to prevent radial shortening. Because of this prolonged immobilization, it is critical for the patient to have function of the hand.[4]

A classic immobilization position for a Colles' fracture is with the elbow set in flexion and the forearm pronated with the wrist in extension and ulnar deviation. This technique of immobilization places the brachioradialis in a position to exert a deforming force on the fracture fragment and is the main reason for recurrence of the original deformity. Sarmiento et al. achieved good functional results by placing the patient in a supinated position with a hinged wrist brace. In this position the individual can compensate for loss of pronation with humeral abduction.[17] Ledingham et al also observed better results on radiographs and better wrist function with the use of a functional plaster brace allowing full range of motion at the radiocarpal joint compared with a standard Colles' plaster brace.[10] Because of the differences in the outcome of different immobilization techniques, it is helpful to determine the position of the forearm and wrist during immobilization prior to physical therapy management.

Evaluation

A reliable subjective and objective evaluation is necessary in order to set appropriate goals for the patient as well as assess the patient's progress at a later date. During evaluation, the patient may report pain in the distal radius region. The patient may also complain of pain in the ulnar region if triangular fibrocartilage damage or an ulnar styloid fracture is present. Bearing weight on the wrist and hand may be painful and avoided by the patient. A numerical pain scale can be utilized for documentation of the initial evaluation and subsequent reevaluations. Patients may not complain about loss of grip strength, even though it is present, unless the clinician inquires about specific functional activities the patient has difficulty performing.

The clinician begins functional assessment when the patient enters the clinic by observing how the patient removes his or her coat, or the way personal possessions are lifted and carried. A checklist of functional activities can be devised by the therapist to help the patient identify the activities that are compromised. The patient may have difficulty holding moderately heavy objects as well as performing fine motor tasks. A function board that includes activities such as locking and unlocking bolt, chain, and key locks, and manipulating doorknobs, buckles, zippers, etc., can be fabricated. This function board can serve as a valuable assessment tool as well as a therapeutic one during treatment.

Upon examination edema may be present, depending on the patient's stage of recovery. A distortion at the wrist called a "dinner fork" deformity may be observed; this results from the posterior tilt of the distal radial fragments accompanying a Colles' fracture.[14] A 3-year study by Villar et al showed that the presence of a persistent dorsal tilt, radiocarpal joint involvement, and an ulnar styloid fracture were associated with reduced range of motion but had no effect on grip strength. However, the presence of radial shortening 1 week after reduction had a detrimental effect on grip strength after 3 years.[20] During evaluation, the physical therapist can determine if radial shortening is present by palpating the radial and ulnar styloid to see if they appear to be at the same level, instead of the radial styloid being positioned distally to the corresponding ulnar process.[14]

The gross movement of the wrist should be evaluated goniometrically progressing to assessment of movement limitations of the radiocarpal joint and individual carpal joints. A gross evaluation of shoulder movement is important to assess since the patient may have lost range of motion while immobilized. Joint play of the wrist should only be assessed if the fracture site is well healed and stable. It is necessary for the clinician to have good palpation skills and anatomic knowledge in order to be proficient in determining specific joint limitations as well as to apply mobilization techniques. Important bony landmarks include the scaphoid bone, which is located distal to the radial styloid process and becomes prominent with ulnar deviation; the capitate, which is centrally located in line with the third digit where there is a slight depression in the wrist; and finally the lunate, which can be palpated just proximal to the capitate and becomes prominent when the wrist is passively flexed and recedes when the wrist is extended.[11]

A reliable and valid evaluation of grip strength is necessary to determine the success of surgical and treatment procedures. The best strength measurement tool was found to be the Jamar dynamometer, which had the highest calibration accuracy. The American Society of Hand Therapists concluded that upper extremity position might influence grip strength measurements and has therefore suggested a standardized arm position for hand strength tests. It was recommended that the patient be seated with the shoulder abducted and neutrally rotated, the elbow flexed 90 degrees, and the forearm and wrist in a neutral position.[12]

Normative grip strength data for different age groups were collected by Mathiowetz et al using a Jamar dynamometer set at the second handle position. These data can be used as a basis of comparison when assessing grip strength after a Colles' fracture. For example, the mean grip strength of men 70 to 74 years of age was 75.3 pounds on the right hand and 64.8 on the left. For women in this age group, the mean was 49.6 with the right hand and 41.5 with the left.[12] Weakness of the wrist extensors, flexors, and radial deviators may also be found by manual muscle testing and should be documented using a 0/5 to 5/5 number scale.

The demerit point system shown in Table 13–1 uses numerical values to evaluate residual deformity, subjective complaints of pain, range of motion, grip strength, and various complications. It is a good objective tool to use to evaluate the end results

TABLE 13–1.

Demerit Point System Used to Evaluate End Results of Healed Colles' Fractures*

	Points
Residual deformity	
Prominent ulnar styloid	1
Residual dorsal tilt	2
Radial deviation of hand	2–3
Point range	0–3
Subjective evaluation	
Excellent: no pain, disability, or limitation of motion	0
Good: occasional pain, slight limitation of motion, no disability	2
Fair: occasional pain, some limitation of motion, feeling of weakness in wrist, no particular disability if careful, activities slightly restricted	4
Poor: pain, limitation of motion, disability, activities more or less markedly restricted	6
Point range	0–6
Objective evaluation†	
Loss of dorsiflexion	5
Loss of ulnar deviation	3
Loss of supination	2
Loss of palmar flexion	1
Loss of radial deviation	1
Loss of circumduction	1
Pain in distal radio-ulnar joint	1
Grip strength—60% or less of opposite side	1
Loss of pronation	2
Point range	0–5
Complications	
Arthritic change	
Minimum	1
Minimum with pain	3
Moderate	2
Moderate with pain	4
Severe	3
Severe with pain	5
Nerve complications (median)	1–3
Poor finger function due to cast	1–2
Point range	0–5
End-result point ranges	
Excellent	0–2
Good	3–8
Fair	9–20
Poor	≥21

*From Sarmiento A et al: *J Bone Joint Surg (Am)* 1975; 57:311–317. Used by permission.
†The objective evaluation is based on the following ranges of motion as being the minimum for normal function: dorsiflexion, 45 degrees; palmar flexion, 30 degrees; radial deviation, 15 degrees; ulnar deviation, 15 degrees; pronation, 50 degrees; and supination, 50 degrees.

TABLE 13–2.

Summary of Evaluation Findings After Fracture

Subjective complaints of pain and stiffness in the wrist joint
Edema in the wrist and hand
Radial shortening with posterior tilt of distal radius ("dinner fork deformity")
Decreased wrist joint range of motion
Decreased grip and wrist strength
Decreased function holding objects and performing fine motor tasks

and pain control application of ice, electrical stimulation, massage, and instruction in elevation of the limb may be implemented. Heat is effective in improving the blood supply to and from the wrist in the absence of acute edema and promotes physical relaxation, which is beneficial prior to mobilizing a stiff joint. Functional electrical stimulation can be used to facilitate strength as well as range of motion.

Joint mobilization techniques are essential in order to evaluate and address joint limitations present after a Colles' fracture. The following mobilization techniques, described in Kaltenborn's book, *Mobilization of the Extremity Joints,* are recommended in order to restore functional range of motion.[6]

Limited Wrist Flexion (posterior glide of radiocarpal or midcarpal joint)

1. Patient sits with the dorsal forearm placed on a wedge or towel roll with the palm up and the hand extended over the edge. The therapist stands facing the radial side of the hand.
2. The therapist's left hand stabilizes the patient's distal forearm or proximal row of carpal bones from the ventral side.
3. The therapist's right hand holds the metacarpal bones and all the carpal bones (or just the distal carpal row if mobilizing the midcarpal joint) and exerts a dorsal movement (Fig 13–2).

Limited Wrist Extension (anterior glide of the capitate on the lunate)

1. Patient sits with the hand held forward and the palm facing down. The therapist stands facing the hand.
2. With both hands the therapist holds the patient's thenar and hypothenar eminences with the three ulnar fingers producing a slight separation at the wrist. Both index fingers are placed on the anterior surface of the lunate.
3. The therapist places both thumbs on the dorsal surface of the patient's capitate and applies an

of a healed Colles' fracture.[17] Evaluation findings in a wrist fracture are summarized in Table 13–2.

Treatment

Initial physical therapy treatment after a Colles' fracture should address edema and pain, if present, as well as range-of-motion limitations. For edema

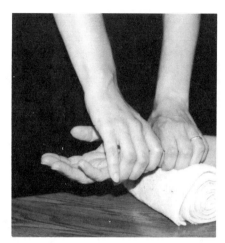

FIG 13–2.
Posterior glide of the proximal carpal row on the distal radius or the distal carpal row on the proximal row for limited wrist flexion.

anterior glide (towards the palm) of the capitate (Fig 13–3).

If wrist extension is the result of decreased movement between the lunate and the radius, the lunate is moved in an anterior direction in relation to the radius by using the same hand placement shown in Figure 13–3, fixating the radius with the index fingers, placing the thumbs on the dorsal surface of the lunate, and applying an anterior glide. When wrist flexion is limited by decreased posterior gliding of the capitate on the more proximal lunate or the lunate on the radius, the same position may be used as shown in Figure 13–3, but the fixation pro-

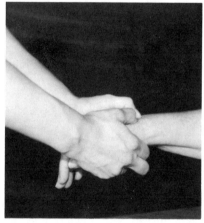

FIG 13–3.
Anterior glide of the capitate on the lunate or the lunate on the distal radius for limited wrist extension. The fixation provided by the index fingers is proximal to the bone being moved.

vided by the index fingers is always distal to the bone being mobilized as shown in Figure 13–4. By moving the more proximal lunate on the capitate anteriorly, a posterior glide of the capitate on the lunate is achieved.[6]

Long Axis Distraction (distal forearm on proximal carpal row or between proximal and distal carpal row)

This technique is effective for stretching the capsule, ligaments, and muscles on both sides of the joint. It is used only as a therapeutic maneuver and not as an evaluation procedure.

1. Patient sits with arm abducted and the therapist stands facing the ulnar side of the hand.
2. The therapist's left hand stabilizes the distal forearm or, if midcarpal joint distraction is desired, the proximal row of carpal bones. The patient's forearm is fixated against the therapist's body.
3. The therapist's right hand is placed around the metacarpal and all the carpal bones or only the distal carpal row, and a distal pull is applied to cause a separation of the joint surfaces (Fig 13–5).

Limited Radial Deviation (ulnar glide of proximal carpal row on distal forearm)

1. The patient sits with the ulnar side of the forearm placed on a wedge or towel roll with the

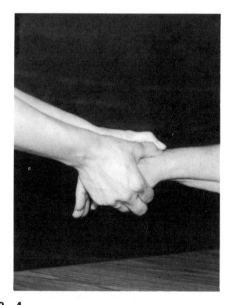

FIG 13–4.
Posterior glide of the capitate on the lunate or the lunate on the radius for restricted wrist flexion. The lunate is being mobilized anteriorly, which causes a relative posterior glide of the capitate. In this mobilization the fixation by the index fingers is distal to the bone being moved.

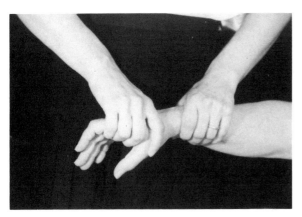

FIG 13–5.
Long axis distraction of the distal forearm and the proximal carpal row or between the carpal rows.

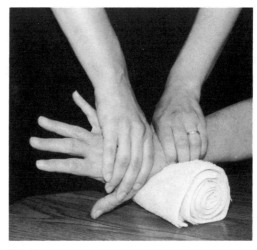

FIG 13–7.
Radial glide of the proximal carpal row on the distal forearm for restricted ulnar deviation.

hand extending over the edge of the roll. The therapist stands facing the dorsal surface of the hand.

2. The therapist's left hand stabilizes the distal forearm.

3. The therapist's right hand holds the metacarpals and carpal bones and applies force in an ulnar direction (Fig 13–6).

Limited Ulnar Deviation (radial glide of proximal carpal row on distal forearm)

1. The patient sits or lies supine with the arm abducted and the radial side of the hand placed on a wedge or towel roll. The therapist stands facing the volar side of the hand.

2. The therapist's left hand stabilizes the distal forearm or proximal carpal row.

3. The therapist's right hand holds the metacarpals and all the carpal bones or only the distal row for midcarpal deviation, and a radial force is applied (Fig 13–7).

The patient can be instructed in self range of motion techniques in order to increase wrist flexion and extension. To increase wrist flexion, the patient places his or her wrist over the edge of a table with a straight elbow and the palm down and stretches the wrist into flexion using the opposite hand as shown in Figure 13–8. The same exercise can be used to increase wrist extension by placing the palm up and exerting the same downward force. The patient

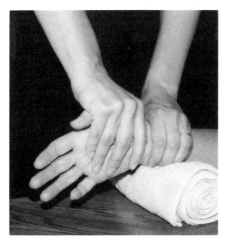

FIG 13–6.
Ulnar glide of the proximal carpal row on the distal forearm for restricted radial deviation.

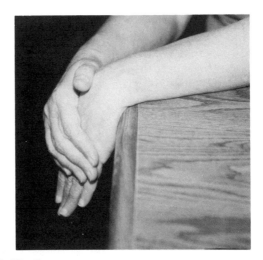

FIG 13–8.
Self range of motion to increase wrist flexion. The patient can perform the same exercise with the palm facing up to increase wrist extension.

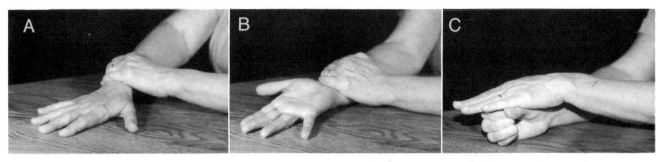

FIG 13–9.
Isometric exercises for strengthening of the wrist. **A,** flexors; **B,** extensors; **C,** radial deviators.

should hold the stretch for a period of 10 seconds and repeat 5 to 10 times. This stretch can be performed before and/or after strengthening exercises.

Strengthening exercises for the wrist and hand can be initiated early by utilizing isometric techniques, especially if pain and limited range of motion are still present. The patient can strengthen the wrist extensors and flexors isometrically by pressing the wrist and hand against a table and holding the contraction for 5 to 10 seconds. The radial deviators can be strengthened isometrically by placing the ulnar side of the hand on a table and resisting the movement with the opposite hand. These exercises are demonstrated in Figure 13–9.

Wrist curls, which strengthen the extensors, flexors, and radial deviators, are demonstrated in Figure 13–10. These exercises can be initiated as range-of-motion exercises by starting without a weight. When the patient is able to perform five sets of ten repetitions comfortably, progressive resistive exercises may be implemented by adding 1 pound. Begin each set of exercises with 1 set of 10 repetitions and progress to 5 sets as tolerated. When 5 sets can be performed easily with the 1 pound, the weight can be progressed. Resistive exercise for the forearm supinators and pronators can be performed by resting the entire forearm and hand holding a hammer on a table in a neutral position. The patient slowly supinates and pronates the forearm, lowering the hammer towards the table (see Fig 13–10).

TABLE 13–3.
Summary of Treatment Techniques After Fracture

Modalities to decrease pain, edema and joint stiffness (i.e., heat, ice, electrical stimulation, massage, ultrasound)
Joint mobilization techniques and instruction in self range of motion
Strengthening beginning with active range of motion progressing to resistive exercise with free weights or tubing
Functional exercises to improve gripping and fine motor activities

Strengthening of the supinators can also be achieved by holding a piece of rubber tubing with the hands in a neutral position resting on a table about 6 in. apart. The patient supinates both forearms simultaneously against the resistance of the tubing. Tubing can also be an effective tool for strengthening the wrist flexors and extensors.

To improve use of the wrist and hand during ADL, a function board can be used, as mentioned previously. The patient can practice writing tasks if the dominant wrist was the one fractured. Limitations of finger function during fine motor tasks can be addressed by having the patient pick up marbles

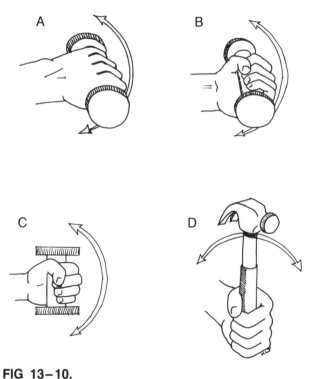

FIG 13–10.
Progressive resistive exercises for the wrist. **A,** extensors; **B,** flexors; **C,** radial deviators. **D,** resistive strengthening of the forearm supinators and pronators.

or work with push pins. The therapist can be creative in addressing functional limitations by tailoring the tasks to the individual and specific needs of the patient. Treatment techniques are summarized in Table 13–3.

RHEUMATOID ARTHRITIS AND OSTEOARTHRITIS

Rheumatoid Arthritis

Rheumatoid arthritis is a systemic disease of the connective and skeletal, as well as the lymphatic and circulatory, systems. The incidence of rheumatoid arthritis is two to three times greater in females than males and often begins during the third decade of life, but can occur after age 50. The usual course is one of exacerbations and remissions of symptoms ultimately resulting in disability and deformity in the elderly patient. The onset is often sudden, affecting a single joint initially and spreading to other joints as the disease progresses.[1] Early involvement of the hands is common, with the distal radioulnar joint and carpal joints affected. Because of the devastating functional effects of this disease, proper physical management should be instituted as early as possible. The collapse of the wrist structures may severely compromise hand function since hand placement and stability depend on the more proximal joints. In addition, the wrist position affects the functional length of the finger muscles and their ability to generate force. Given the high incidence of limited finger function in a person with rheumatoid arthritis, good wrist mobility may play an important role.[22]

Evaluation

Even though rheumatoid arthritis is a systemic disease affecting connective tissue throughout the body, the chief complaint by the patient is of joint pain, stiffness, and fatigue. During an exacerbation phase, the joint may feel warm to the touch, with edema present.

The most common form of wrist deformity observed is wrist flexion, radial deviation, and palmar subluxation. Radial deviation of the wrist and carpometacarpal joints may produce a corresponding ulnar deviation of the fingers in order to maintain alignment of the fingers with the forearm. Dorsal subluxation of the ulnar head can occur leading to a disruption of the distal radioulnar joint and displace-

ment of the extensor carpi ulnaris tendon palmarly. Ulnar stability during wrist extension, thumb abduction, and finger flexion are compromised with the displacement of this tendon. Ankylosis of the intercarpal and carpometacarpal joints may occur as well, producing an inability to cup the hand.[22]

During an exacerbation phase wrist range of motion, particularly at the end range, is extremely painful, and is accompanied by an inability to tolerate resistance of the wrist musculature. Severe limitation of the finger flexor strength will occur if the wrist spontaneously fuses in flexion.[22] During remission when the acute inflammation subsides, the patient may be able to perform movement with less pain. At this point the patient may be more tolerant of a manual muscle testing of the wrist musculature and grip strength testing.

Treatment

When initiating treatment of the rheumatoid wrist, the therapist should be aware of the patient's exacerbation status since management in the acute and chronic stage is different. During the acute or postoperative phase, the use of ice may be appropriate to decrease pain, swelling, and inflammation. Heating modalities, such as ultrasound, paraffin, and whirlpool, can be effective in increasing circulation and mobility as well as controlling pain in the chronic phase. Splints such as the "cock-up" splint help prevent deformity at the early stages of the disease by maintaining proper alignment of the joints and providing relief of pain and swelling. During an exacerbation, gentle range-of-motion exercise should be performed to prevent joint stiffness while avoiding the painful ranges. The therapist should be careful not to overstretch the joint, as this can cause tissue damage. Active assistive range-of-motion exercises are appropriate but again, painful ranges of motion should be avoided. Strengthening should be limited to isometric exercise while the joint is inflamed. When inflammation subsides, isotonic exercises may be initiated to promote movement and function. Strengthening of the wrist extensors may help to counteract the flexion deformity at the wrist. Heavy resistive exercises are not recommended at any phase for the rheumatoid patient because of the destructive effect they may have on the weakened tissues.[22] The patient should be encouraged to perform as much functional activity as he or she can tolerate in order to help prevent deformity; however, fatigue should be avoided by including frequent rests during exercise and daily activity. When home exercises are prescribed, the patient should be instructed to perform short periods of exercise throughout the day rather than one long period of exercise. The evaluation and treatment of rheumatoid arthritis are summarized in Table 13–4.

Osteoarthritis

Osteoarthritis or degenerative joint disease is a progressive functional and structural deterioration of the joint and is the most common of all joint ailments. The disease most often occurs in middle-aged and elderly persons for various reasons, but it is most often the result of the demand for excessive function at a time when the efficiency of the circulatory system is deteriorating. Osteoarthritis is initially evident in a large weight-bearing joint but is rarely confined to one joint. The distal phalangeal joints of the fingers most commonly become involved. Laboratory finding are not conclusive since, unlike rheumatoid arthritis, degenerative joint disease is not a systemic illness. The degree of deformity depends on the joints involved but is less severe than in rheumatoid arthritis.[1]

Evaluation

The patient goes through a pain cycle with complaints of pain and stiffness, particularly after inactivity, which decreases as the patient begins to move the joint. However, the pain increases again with continued use and fatigue, which is subsequently decreased with rest. Joint deformity or subluxation may be observed, but ankylosis does not occur.[1]

Joint inflammation with edema may be present. The patient is more likely to experience pain at the extremes of movement rather than throughout the entire range. The presence of limited wrist flexion and/or extension depends on whether the radiocarpal or midcarpal joint is involved. Decreased wrist flexion will tend be present with a greater involvement of the radiocarpal joint, whereas the involvement of the midcarpal joint will produce extension range of motion limitations. Decreased wrist and grip strength may be present upon testing owing to the presence of pain at the joint rather than deterioration of skeletal tissue. Unlike rheumatoid arthritis, the osteoarthritic joint usually remains functional even though painful.

Treatment

Palliative treatment for osteoarthritis includes application of heat via paraffin, ultrasound, or whirlpool. Electrical stimulation, such as with a transcutaneous electrical nerve stimulation (TENS) unit, may be used for pain control as well. Cryotherapy may be used when edema is present for the control of inflammation after exercise, depending on the patient's tolerance to the cold. Splints may be helpful by providing stability for the wrist and thus allowing the patient to function with less pain.

Active assistive and passive range of motion may be initiated immediately, being careful to avoid the painful ranges. The joint mobilization techniques described previously may be performed gently to increase mobility, but should not be performed if painful. Strengthening should be initiated isometrically

TABLE 13–4.

Summary of Evaluation Findings and Treatment of the Rheumatoid Wrist

Evaluation findings:
  Complaints of joint pain and stiffness
  Deformity with the wrist set in flexion, radial deviation and
    palmar subluxation
  Joint feels warm to the touch with edema present
  Severely limited and painful range of motion in all directions
  Severe limitation of finger flexor strength secondary to fusion of
    the wrist in flexion
  Limited function cupping hand secondary to ankylosis of the
    intercarpal and carpo metacarpal joints
Treatment
  Modalities such as ice during the acute phase, and paraffin,
    ultrasound, whirlpool during the chronic phase
  Splinting to prevent deformity and control pain
  Gentle range of motion passively and actively through pain-free
    ranges
  Isometric strengthening of wrist musculature in the acute phase
    progressing to isotonic exercises in the chronic phase
  Performance of functional activities avoiding excessive levels of
    fatigue and pain.

TABLE 13–5.

Summary of Evaluation Findings and Treatment of Osteoarthritis

Evaluation findings:
  Wrist pain that increases with activity and subsides with rest
  Joint stiffness particularly after immobility
  Decreased range of motion of wrist flexion and/or extension
  Decreased wrist muscle strength and grip strength with joint
    pain with resistance
  Decreased function during daily activities secondary to pain
    rather than joint deformity
Treatment
  Modalities (heat, ultrasound, electrical stimulation, and ice) to
    decrease pain, inflammation and edema, and increase
    mobility
  Active range of motion exercises, passive stretching, and joint
    mobilization techniques through pain-free ranges of motion
  Strengthening of wrist musculature and grip beginning with
    isometric exercises and progressing to isotonic and resisted
    movement
  Functional activities in the clinic and at home to facilitate range
    of motion, grip function, and fine motor coordination

progressing to isotonic and resistive exercise as tolerated. Unlike the management of rheumatoid arthritis, progressive resistive exercises may be performed as long as the patient does not complain of pain before or after the exercise. The weight should be progressed slowly as described in the treatment of fractures of the wrist. Performing functional activities helps to maintain available range of motion and should be encouraged. Evaluation and treatment of osteoarthritis are summarized in Table 13–5.

NERVE COMPRESSION DISORDERS

Radial, ulnar, and median nerve compressions in elderly people cause dysfunction in the hand. It is important to be able to distinguish among these three disorders in order to implement appropriate physical management.

Radial Nerve Compression.—The radial nerve is commonly injured in the upper arm where it winds around the humerus. Compression at this site leads to weakness of the finger extensors and forearm flexors while the forearm is in a supinated position. Weakness of the forearm extensors occurs as well, causing wrist drop. Because actions of the intrinsic muscles in the hand, such as gripping, cannot be accomplished with the wrist in flexion, the presence of a radial nerve lesion may give a false impression of total hand weakness. If the wrist is placed and supported in a neutral position, the clinician will see that there is no true weakness present.[5]

Ulnar Nerve Compression.—Ulnar nerve compression may occur in elderly people because of inappropriate gripping of a cane or crutch as well as alteration in carpal bone alignment as the result of a fracture or inflammatory process. Distal lesions of this nerve generally produce a pure motor disorder involving the intrinsic hand musculature. Compression at the pisohamate tunnel or proximally to it produces weakness of all the ulnar intrinsic muscles and variable sensory loss over the distal palm and dorsal surface of the fourth and fifth digits.[5]

Median Nerve Compression.—Carpal tunnel syndrome, which is the compression of the median nerve as it passes through the carpal tunnel, is the most common of the three nerve impingement syndromes and will be discussed in terms of evaluation and treatment. The median nerve supplies the extrinsic and intrinsic hand muscles, including the short and long flexors of the first two digits and the long flexor of the thumb. Its sensory distribution is the radial two thirds of the palmer aspect of the hand and dorsal distal phalanges of the index and third finger.[5]

Any increase in the contents of the carpal tunnel may produce median nerve compression. In elderly people, the cause of carpal tunnel syndrome may be a bone spur resulting from degenerative joint disease, rheumatoid arthritis, or the presence of an old fracture.[5] The median nerve tends to be more vulnerable in the elderly and as shown by Seror the denervation is much more severe in patients over 70 years old presenting with carpal tunnel syndrome.[19] For reasons that are not obvious, increasing age has also been associated with an increase in thenar atrophy and sensory abnormalities as well as with failure of treatment. The increased incidence of stenosing tenosynovitis in the elderly population may be one explanation: however, this alone does not explain the strong effect age has on these conditions. Another explanation: may be the increased sensitivity to pressure that exists in the peripheral nerves in an older person. This increased sensitivity may be the result of decreased reparative ability, alteration in the microcirculation, or an increased incidence of proximal nerve compression.[7]

Surgical intervention (carpal tunnel release) is indicated when carpal tunnel syndrome has been present for over a year with tactile sensory changes or thenar atrophy. Surgery is also appropriate when continuous intense pain is present, with no symptom relief from a steroid injection (a common initial management technique). However, carpal tunnel release does not always produce good results and surgical techniques have an important influence on the quality of the outcome. If compression of the median nerve was severe or the surgery performed too late, sensory and motor impairment may persist indefinitely.[19]

Evaluation

The patient with carpal tunnel syndrome usually complains of tingling, burning, and painful paresthesias in the hand that become worse at night. Hand paresthesias may wake the patient up during the night and the patient often shakes or massages the hand to relieve the symptoms. Sometimes the deep, aching pain extends to the forearms and shoulders. The patient usually complains of nonspecific hand weakness and decreased grip.[5]

During evaluation, the patient may be found to

have edema over the volar aspect of the wrist. Sensory loss during light touch and pinprick testing in the median distribution of the hand may be present. Motor weakness in the abductor pollicis and thenar opponens muscles can be present in persons with the syndrome.[5] In a study done by Phalen, thenar atrophy was present in 36% of the subjects tested. A positive Tinel's sign, that is, inducing tingling by tapping over the wrist, was found in 60% of the patients. The Phalen's sign, which measures the amount of time it takes for sensory changes to occur with extreme flexion of the wrist, was present in 80% of the individuals. In 24% of patients with carpal tunnel syndrome there was a decreased nerve conduction velocity.[22] According to a study done by Kaplan et al there was a correlation between the amount of time taken to elicit a positive Phalen's sign and the severity of the carpal tunnel syndrome. The Phalen's sign was more likely to occur sooner in subjects with constant paresthesia, thenar atrophy, a positive Tinel's sign, and altered two-point discrimination.[7]

Again, the measurement of grip strength using the Jamar grip dynamometer can be a good objective tool in determining the patient's functional status and clinical course of progression or deterioration. It is also a useful guide in determining when a patient can return to a previous level of function without fear of injury. Gellman et al found that it may take up to 3 months after a carpal tunnel release for grip strength to return to preoperative levels.[3]

A common early postoperative finding is the presence of pain at the base of the hypothenar region, which is associated with decreased grip strength. This is the result of changes in the pisotriquetral joint alignment and tracking of the pisaform caused by the release of the transverse carpal ligament. In most cases this pain resolves; however, in some patients persistence of these symptoms may require excision of the pisiform to provide permanent relief.[18]

Treatment

Splinting is a common initial treatment method since immobilizing the wrist in a neutral position maximizes available space in the tunnel, decreasing compression and providing symptomatic relief. It has been found that patients with carpal tunnel syndrome have elevated intracanal pressure with active wrist flexion and extension, causing a pressure three to six times greater than the pressure found in the wrist in a neutral position. Extension results in a greater increase in pressure than flexion, particularly

in the distal portion of the tunnel. A study by Kruger et al suggested that splinting will yield optimal results if used within the first 3 months of onset, with a more favorable outcome in individuals with no structural damage.[8]

Preoperatively, modalities may be used to manage pain, inflammation, and edema. Mobilization of the fingers may be necessary if finger tightness is present owing to the tendency of the patient to remain immobile to avoid the pain. If thenar atrophy is not present, exercise may be beneficial in preventing or delaying muscle wasting. If atrophy is already present, active and resistive strengthening should be initiated and can be performed while wearing the splint, which will help maintain a neutral position at the wrist. Isometric exercises with the wrist in a neutral position can be initiated as long as they do not reproduce symptoms. Progression to active range of motion and progressive resistive strengthening for the wrist should be performed with caution since repetitive flexion-extension can contribute to carpal tunnel syndrome. Because an increase in the intracanal pressure is not desired, these exercises should be avoided if tingling, burning, or pain occurs. Helping the patient function with less pain can be achieved by educating the patient about wrist positions that should be avoided. These include pinching or holding objects with the wrist in a flexed position.

Postoperatively, paresthesias usually disappear immediately, while sensory and motor impairments continue over a longer period of time. This is important to explain to the patient. Utilization of splints after a carpal tunnel release is common. It has been shown by Chaise that patients managed with postoperative splinting recovered faster with a greater return of grip strength to preoperative levels.[19] After surgery, a bulky compression dressing is usually applied and the hand is elevated for 3 to 4 days. After the dressing is removed initial treatment includes controlling edema with modalities and early active range of motion while wearing the splint. The use of the splint while performing active movement has been recommended until the seventh postoperative day.[22] Isotonic and isometric strengthening of the wrist may be initiated 8 weeks after surgery. The patient should be careful not to overexercise as it may cause tenosynovitis.[2]

The nerve gliding exercises shown in Figure 13–11 were developed by James Hunter, M.D., to facilitate gliding of the medial nerve through the carpal tunnel. These exercises incorporate a passive stretch of the thumb into extension to prevent adhesions from forming along the palmar cutaneous and

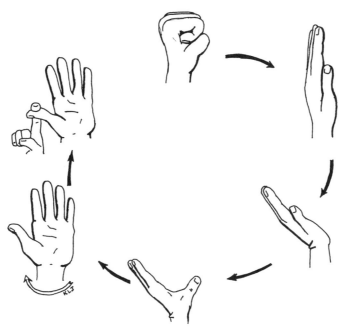

FIG 13–11.
Nerve gliding exercises developed by James Hunter, M.D., to
facilitate proper gliding of the median nerve in the carpal tunnel.

motor branch of the median nerve. This exercise was described by Julie Belkin, O.T.R., who designed a home program. The patient starts the exercise by making a fist with the wrist in a neutral position. Next, the patient extends the fingers and thumb with the wrist still neutral. The wrist is then extended with the thumb in a neutral position after which the thumb is extended. The forearm is then supinated with the thumb still extended and a gentle stretch of the thumb into further extension is applied by the patient.[2] Evaluation and treatment of carpal tunnel syndrome are summarized in Table 13–6.

TABLE 13–6.

Summary of Evaluation Findings and Treatment for Carpal Tunnel Syndrome

Evaluation findings:
  Subjective complaints of burning, tingling, weakness, and painful
    paresthesias in the hand that are worse at night
  Presence of edema in the volar aspect of the wrist
  Presence of thenar atrophy, a loss of strength of the abductor
    pollicis and thenar opponens muscle and decreased grip
    strength
  A positive Tinel's sign and Phalen's test
Treatment:
  Early splinting of the wrist in a neutral position preoperatively
    and postoperatively
  Modalities preoperatively and postoperatively to decrease pain,
    inflammation, and edema
  Preoperatively, initiate isometric and thenar strengthening
    without reproducing symptoms. Isotonic exercises should not
    be performed if they illicit pain burning or tingling in the hand.
  Postoperatively, initiate active range of motion 3–4 days with a
    splint, which may be removed after the seventh day. Nerve
    gliding exercises to facilitate proper movement of the median
    nerve through the carpal tunnel. Isometric and Isotonic
    strengthening 8 weeks after surgery.

CONCLUSION

Radial fractures, arthritis, and carpal tunnel syndrome are all common in the elderly population. When managing the wrist, physiologic changes that occur with aging, such as osteoporosis, joint degeneration, and skeletal changes, should be considered. Functional assessment is of utmost importance and should be the focus when contemplating a treatment plan. Returning the wrist joint to a functional status is essential given that this joint provides the stability and movement necessary for the hand to function optimally.

REFERENCES

1. Aegerter E, Kirkpatrick JA: *Orthopedic Diseases,* ed 4. Philadelphia, WB Saunders, 1975.
2. Baxter-Petralia PL: Therapist's management of carpal tunnel syndrome, in Hunter JM, Schneider LH,

Mackin EJ, et al (eds): *Rehabilitation of the Hand*, ed 3. St. Louis, Mosby-Year Book, 1990, pp 640–646

3. Gellman H, Kan D, Gee V, et al: Analysis of pinch and grip strength after carpal tunnel release. *J Hand Surg (Am)* 1989; 14A:863–864.

4. Green DP: Pins and plaster treatment of comminuted fractures of the distal end of the radius. *J Bone Joint Surg (Am)* 1975; 15A:304–310.

5. Harrell LE, Massey EW: Hand weakness in the elderly. *J Am Geriatr Soc* 1983; 31:223–227.

6. Kaltenborn FM: *Mobilization of the Extremity Joints.* Oslo, Olaf Norlis Bokhandel, 1980.

7. Kaplan SJ, Glickel SZ, Eaton RG: Predictive factors in the non-surgical treatment of carpal tunnel syndrome. *J Hand Surg (Br)* 1990; 15B:106–108.

8. Kruger VL, Kraft GH, Deitz JC, et al: Carpal tunnel syndrome: objective measures and splint use. *Arch Phys Med Rehabil* 1991; 72:517–520.

9. LaCroix E: *Geriatric Orthopaedics.* Gaithersburg, Md, Aspen, 1990.

10. Ledingham WM, Wytch R, Goring CC, et al: On immediate functional bracing of Colles' fracture. *Injury* 1991; 22:197–201.

11. Lehmkuhl LD, Smith LK: *Brunnstrom's Clinical Kinesiology*, ed 4. Philadelphia, FA Davis, 1983.

12. Mathiowetz V, Kashman N, Volland G, et al: Grip and pinch strength: Normative data for adults. *Arch Phys Med Rehabil* 1985; 66:69–74.

13. Mennell JM: *The Musculoskeletal System.* Gaithersburg, Md, Aspen, 1992.

14. Moore KL: *Clinically Oriented Anatomy.* Baltimore, Williams & Wilkins, 1980.

15. Narici MV, Bordini M, Cerretelli P: Effect of aging on human adductor pollicis muscle function. *J Appl Physiol* 1991; 71:1277–1281.

16. Palmer AK, Werner FW: The triangular fibrocartilage complex of the wrist—anatomy and function. *J Hand Surg (Am)* 1981; 6:153–162.

17. Sarmiento A, Pratt GW, Berry NC, et al: Colles' fractures. *J Bone Joint Surg (Am)* 1975; 57A:311–317.

18. Seradge H, Seradge E: Piso-triquetal pain syndrome after carpal tunnel release. *J Hand Surg (Am)* 1989; 14A:858–862.

19. Tubiana R: Carpal tunnel syndrome: Some views on its management. *Ann Hand Surg* 1990; 9:325–330.

20. Villar RN, Marsh D, Rushton N, et al: Three years after Colles' fracture. *J Bone Joint Surg (Br)* 1987; 69B:635–638.

21. Volz RG, Lieb M, Benjamin J: Biomechanics of the wrist. *Clin Orthop* 1980; 149:112–117.

22. Wadsworth CH: The wrist and the hand, in Gould JA, Davies GJ (eds): *Orthopaedic and Sports Physical Therapy*, vol 2. St Louis, Mosby-Year Book, 1985, pp 437–475.

Chapter 14

Hand Injuries: An Orthopedic Perspective

William Garvin, M.D.

Hand injuries in the geriatric patient do not result in the magnitude of morbidity and mortality that certain other orthopedic injuries such as hip fractures represent.[11] Many hand injuries, however, lead to significant periods of disability for patients affected by them. The hand should be thought of as a sensory organ. From early childhood we explore our environment and learn from the sensory input of the hand by touching, feeling, and manipulating objects. To quote the father of hand surgery, Sterling Bunnell, "The brain developed the hand but it is also true that in each one of us many of our mental processes have developed from the feeling and movement of our hands."[5] Bunnell in his preface to the first edition of his textbook *Surgery of the Hand* further goes on to state, "Although the hand is composed mainly of tough material it also includes exact machinery of much refinement and tissues of great delicacy and specialization. Such a mechanism is readily wrecked by trauma and infection, and it is little wonder that hands mangled by trauma or those infiltrated and gutted by infection later present difficult problems in reconstruction."[5]

We come to depend upon hand function to button a shirt, feed ourselves, and recreate. When hand function is lost even temporarily, adjustments must be made in our activities of daily living (ADL). Although specific local problems in the hand will be addressed, it is worth remembering that the hand functions as a unit and when part of that unit is lost the rest of the hand and the remainder of the organism must make the necessary adjustments. In approaching the problem of hand injuries in the geriatric patient, one must carefully consider the patient's functional status at the time of the injury in formulating the treatment plan. The goal of treatment must be to restore the maximum degree of function possible for the injured patient.

Studies have suggested that hand function as measured by the Williams manual test serves as a predictive factor with respect to which elderly patients will require formal services. It was shown that those elderly people who took longer to perform the gross and fine motor skills required by this test were more likely to need additional formal long-term care services than their counterparts who took less time to perform the same maneuvers.[27] It therefore behooves all caregivers to optimize hand function in elderly people as it is so important to the individual's ability to function independently.

The evaluation and treatment of an injury to the hand of an elderly person must take into consideration the general health and activity status of the patient. Coexisting disease processes have a major impact on the patient's ability to respond to treatment and heal the injury. Systemic diseases such as diabetes mellitus may have significant impact on the wound-healing ability of the soft tissue or bone. Vision loss may prevent the patient from identifying certain early warning signs of impending problems following an injury, such as redness, swelling, or unusual discoloration. The same is true for sensory loss in the hand itself. Hearing loss may prevent a patient from understanding instructions, thus leading to a less-than-optimal result for a particular problem. Not only does osteoarthritis cause joint deformity, but it and other connective tissue diseases result in considerable stiffness in the joints of the hand and wrist. When these joints are injured further, particular care must be given to adequate mobilization in an effort to prevent further deformity. Circulatory disturbances, whether associated with atherosclerotic disease, connective tissue diseases, or disorders affecting the small blood vessels, are an obvious cause for concern in the elderly person with a hand injury. The thin cortices and the wide medullary canal associated with osteoporosis may lead to problems with fracture union and with maintaining fixation devices within the bone if such method of treatment is decided upon.

In this chapter we shall explore various injuries to the hand of the elderly patient, demonstrate some methods of treatment, and illustrate problems encountered as well as complications. This chapter will present selected cases from a clinical practice in hand surgery, emphasizing principles felt to be important in managing hand injuries in the elderly. Since this is not intended to be an exhaustive review of hand injuries, the reader is referred to any of the many excellent reference textbooks for hand surgery.[3, 5, 9, 13, 18]

HAND COMPLICATIONS OF WRIST FRACTURES

Although wrist fractures have been addressed in another chapter, some sequelae of wrist fractures, such as the stiff hand, carpal tunnel syndrome, and extensor tendon ruptures, often cause considerable morbidity in the population long after the fracture has solidly healed. The management of the stiff hand and associated problems such as reflex sympathetic dystrophy and pain dysfunction syndrome have been addressed in great detail in other publications.[1, 18] Every effort should be made to prevent these problems by avoiding traumatic manipulations of the wrist, insisting upon elevation and early motion of the digits, and paying proper attention to casts and/or dressings so that the hand is not placed in extreme positions of flexion or extension at the wrist, as these extreme positions make it very difficult if not impossible for the patient to achieve full metacarpophalangeal joint and proximal interphalangeal joint motion.

If external fixation is chosen as a method of treatment, it is often helpful to ensure that the patient is fully cognizant of the complications of this treatment and is referred to a hand therapist in an effort to encourage motion and maintain good hygiene of the hand and forearm pin sites. A tight cast resulting in swelling of the hand may lead to 1 or more years of significant disability.

Median Nerve Compression

Forceful positions such as the full wrist flexion or Cotton-Loder position decrease the potential space within the carpal tunnel and thus lead to increased compression on the median nerve.[10, 24] A patient with a history of prior fractures and of mild symptoms of carpal tunnel syndrome presented with a comminuted displaced intraarticular fracture of the distal radius (Fig 14–1). She complained of burning dysesthesias and paresthesias in the thumb, index, and long finger and radial side of the ring finger. In addition to reduction and external fixation of the fracture (Fig 14–2), a carpal tunnel release was accomplished and a physical therapy program was instituted. Her numbness resolved, her finger motion was maintained, and her fracture healed with only mild deformity (Fig 14–3). Her functional disability was short term. It cannot be emphasized enough that prevention of the hand complications of wrist fractures is much better than trying to treat the established complications themselves.

Extensor Tendon Rupture

Because of the anatomy of the wrist and hand it is important to carefully assess tendon and neurovascular function at the time of fracture. The extensor tendons are held tightly against the bone of the distal radius by the extensor retinaculum. The problem of extensor tendon ruptures, most com-

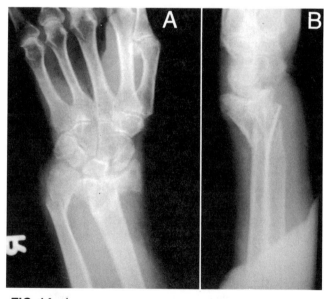

FIG 14–1.
Comminuted displaced intra-articular fracture of the distal radius with fracture of the distal ulna in posterior anterior **(A)** and lateral **(B)** views.

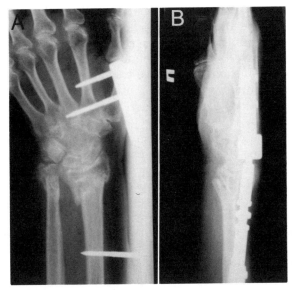

FIG 14–2.
An external fixator has been applied in order to maintain alignment of the fracture in posterior anterior (**A**) and lateral (**B**) views.

monly the extensor pollicis longus, may not be easy to prevent. In fact, the literature suggests that the rupture of the extensor pollicis longus at Lister's tubercle is likely the result of local ischemia from the swelling of fracture hematoma and tenosynovium within the third extensor compartment in addition to an attrition process from the roughened dorsal radial cortex. The rupture of the extensor pollicis longus is often associated with a relatively simple distal radius fracture rather than a more complex one.[28]

The treatment of extensor pollicis longus tendon rupture at the level of Lister's tubercle on the dorsum of the wrist is best accomplished by transfer of the extensor indicis proprius rather than by attempting direct repair of the ruptured tendon or by the use of a bridge graft.[28] Direct repair carries the risk of not regaining correct muscle-tendon unit length as it is generally necessary to resect a portion of the "zone of injury," i.e., the necrotic segment of tendon on either side of the rupture. Bridge graft requires the healing of two tendon junctures with its inherent problem of slowed rehabilitation until one is confident that the tensile strength has been regained. The advantage of the tendon transfer includes a much more rapid rehabilitation and much earlier return of function. The donor muscle-tendon unit is one that is in phase and has presumably been functioning normally up to the time of its transfer. The viability of the tendon is good and a secure juncture can be accomplished through the interweave technique (Fig 14–4), thus allowing relatively early mobilization of the muscle-tendon unit.

Failure of Bone Healing in Correct Alignment

Other complications of distal radius fracture in the elderly include failure of the bone as a result of

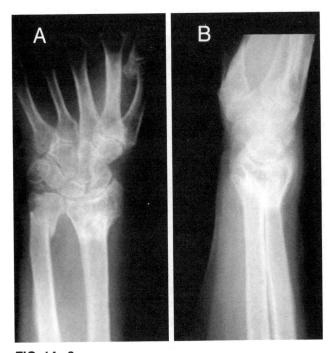

FIG 14–3.
The fractures have healed with some loss of length of both the radius and the ulna in posterior anterior (**A**) and lateral (**B**) views.

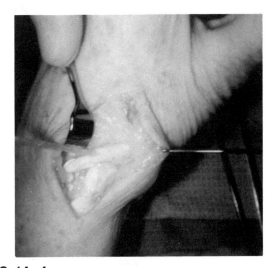

FIG 14–4.
The tendon of the extensor indicis proprius is woven through the distal portion of the ruptured extensor pollicis longus and is sutured with interrupted nonabsorbable material.

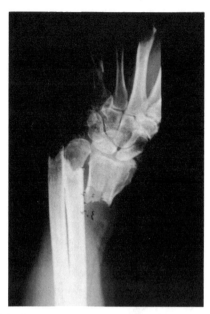

FIG 14–5.
Completely displaced fractures of the radius and ulna.

osteopenia if an internal fixation device is chosen or inappropriately applied. A 68-year-old woman with a history of diabetes tripped on a crack in a sidewalk and fell, landing on her left forearm. She sustained a comminuted distal radius fracture in addition to a type 1 open fracture of the ulna (a 1-cm open wound) and was noted to have a moderate amount of paresthesia in the ulnar nerve distribution (Fig 14–5). She underwent irrigation and debridement of the open ulnar fracture as well as exploration of the ulnar nerve, which was found to be in continuity. Open reduction and internal fixation of the distal radius fracture was carried out as well through a separate incision (Fig 14–6). Her initial x-rays showed satisfactory position; however, subsequent x-rays demonstrated progressive apex dorsal angulation at the radius (Fig 14–7) fracture site. This angulation progressed to the range of 65 degrees. Because of continued pain and deformity, corrective osteotomy of the distal radius and a bone graft from the left iliac crest was carried out. The patient regained excellent wrist motion, and subsequent x-rays showed the fractures to be healed (Fig 14–8). She did not however, regain normal sensitivity in the ulnar nerve distribution. Electrodiagnostic studies demonstrated a moderate ulnar neuropathy proximal to the wrist at the level of the fracture where the nerve was contused. There was, as well, a peripheral neuropathy with primarily sensory deficit possibly related to her diabetes. She regained good function of her upper extremity despite her persisting neurologic deficit in sensation.

Two issues come to mind in reference to this case. The first is possibly a technical concern in that the hardware placed on the apparent tension side of the bone failed when the screws pulled out of the

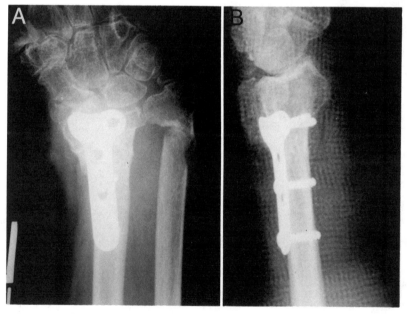

FIG 14–6.
A, posterior anterior view, which shows a T-plate and screws on the distal radius with an ununited fracture of the distal ulna. Note the ununited fracture of the ulnar styloid suggesting previous injury to the wrist. **B,** alignment in the lateral view with the hardware in position.

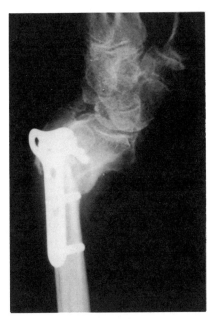

FIG 14–7.
The fracture is angulated to a significant degree following loss of fixation on the distal fragment as the screws have pulled out of the bone of the distal fragment.

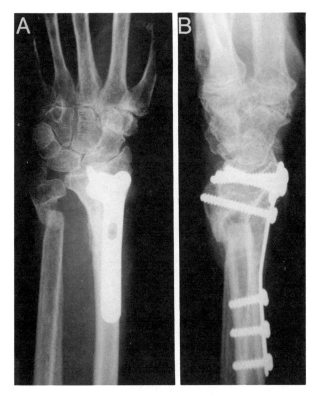

FIG 14–8.
A, posterior anterior view of the fixation and bone graft. **B,** lateral view of the healed fracture of the distal radius with intercalated segment bone graft.

osteoporotic bone, even though the operating surgeon noted that the fixation appeared quite rigid at the time of the initial surgery. The second issue is the question of a chronic ulnar nerve injury predating the traumatic event and the inability of this patient to heal the injury despite adequate external support and no demonstrable localized compression of the nerve.

Infection

A 66-year-old man who was actively involved in farming had a history of rheumatoid arthritis under treatment with nonsteroidal anti-inflammatory medications (NSAIDs). He sustained a closed fracture of his left distal radius after he tripped and fell. The fracture was reduced initially but the reduction was lost (Fig 14–9) and internal fixation with K-wires was carried out. Since the position was again felt to be unacceptable, an open reduction and internal fixation using a T-plate through a dorsal approach was carried out. Some 6 weeks following the open reduction he presented with redness about the wound but no numbness or tingling in the fingers. X-rays demonstrated a persistent collapse deformity with loss of length of the radius and exaggeration of the normal palmar tilt of the distal radius (Fig 14–10). Bone lysis was noted about the screw holes. Surgery for removal of the retained hardware, extensor tenosynovectomy of the second and third compartments,

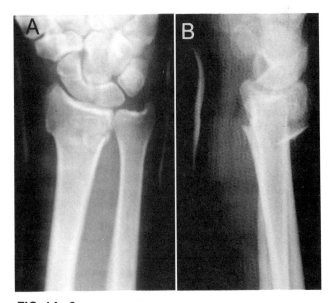

FIG 14–9.
A, posterior anterior view, which shows nonarticular fracture of the distal radius with some loss of length. **B,** dorsal displacement of the fracture on the lateral view.

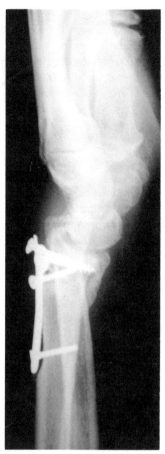

FIG 14–10.
Lateral x-ray shows loss of fixation of the fracture fragments and lysis of cortical bone about proximal screw hole beneath plate.

along with debridement of the distal radius (Fig 14–11) and application of an external fixator were carried out (Fig 14–12). Cultures from the tissue and wound showed the presence of coagulase-negative *Staphylococcus*. Antibiotic therapy was continued for some 4 weeks using vancomycin. An antibiotic-impregnated methyl methacrylate spacer was inserted, and oral antibiotics were continued under the direction of an infectious disease consultant. A segmental bone graft for reconstruction of the distal radius was done using autogenous iliac crest graft. External fixation was continued with the complication of a pin tract infection, which was treated locally and with oral antibiotics. The external fixator was removed 10 weeks after its application. The most distal pin in the radius had broken but no infection was noted in the area of the broken pin. The left wrist continued to have aching and pain; however, the wounds had healed and there was no drainage. Subsequent x-rays demonstrated the fracture of the distal radius remained nonunited and the

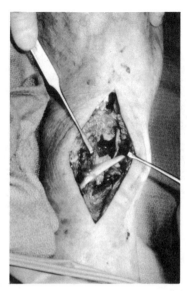

FIG 14–11.
At surgery, marked tenosynovitis as well as loss of bone of the distal radius was present. The tendon running obliquely across the field of view is the extensor pollicis longus.

bone graft had resorbed (Fig 14–13). The patient was returned to the operating room 18 months following his initial injury for another segmental reconstruction of the distal radius with an interposition bone graft from the right iliac crest and fixation with a plate and screws. This bone graft healed successfully. At 34 months following the patient's initial injury he was back to his usual job driving a tractor. He complained of moderate aching at the level of

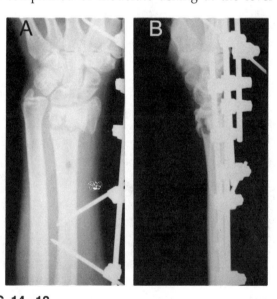

FIG 14–12.
A, the external fixator could not correct for all of the loss of length that was present. Note the extent of bone lysis about the screw hole on the proximal fragment of the distal radius. **B,** lateral view demonstrates satisfactory alignment.

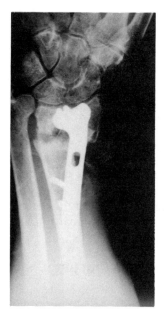

FIG 14–13.
Posterior anterior view of the ununited distal radius fracture following insertion of bone graft.

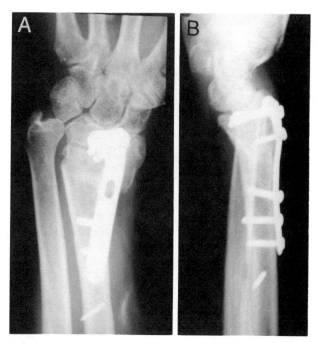

FIG 14–14.
A, the posterior anterior view illustrates the presence of the corticocancellous graft in the distal radius with internal fixation using plate and screws. **B,** lateral view demonstrates the incorporation of the bone graft with satisfactory alignment.

the wrist but had no evidence of recurrent infection. His grip strength averaged 66 pounds on the right and 54 pounds on the left. The wrist had a range of motion of 35 degrees flexion, 28 degrees extension, 7 degrees ulnar deviation, and 30 degrees radial deviation. His forearm motion showed supination of 40 degrees and pronation of 60 degrees. X-rays demonstrated the bone graft was incorporated; the hardware remained in position with a collapse deformity and early degenerative change at the radiocarpal joint along with a positive ulnar variance (Fig 14–14). The patient declined any further attempts at reconstruction as he was quite satisfied with his functional level and he continues to actively participate in farming at a moderately intense level.

This case illustrates the problems involved with the aggressive invasive treatment of a fracture in a patient with rheumatoid arthritis, a disease process that may not only affect the immune system and the patient's ability to handle infection but whose treatment may have some effect upon healing of the bone; i.e., the nonsteroidal anti-inflammatory medication that was required for his treatment of rheumatoid arthritis may inhibit new bone formation and possibly fracture healing.

Although it has been stated[32] that patients over 55 years of age may not be candidates for external fixation, it has been this author's experience that external fixation of wrist fractures does have a place in the treatment of older people. It is true that the bone quality in the metacarpals and the distal radius in some cases may be rather poor, but in carefully selected patients external fixation has been an excellent means to maintain adequate position of the fracture and allow considerable functional activities without the need for large and heavy casts. As a general rule, an ulnar gutter splint or a sugar-tong Orthoplast splint (Johnson and Johnson, Raynham, Mass) is utilized. This allows good functional use of the extremity and minimizes the potential for stiffness. In addition, those patients who have median neuropathy can easily have the carpal tunnel decompressed at the same time that the external fixator is applied or later in the course of fracture treatment if symptoms persist. Patients with open wounds and more complex fractures also benefit from this method of treatment. The combination of internal plus external fixation of the wrist and hand has provided the surgeon with the ability to maintain excellent flexibility in the approach to this problem.

HAND FRACTURES

Fractures in the hands may not be as common as the wrist fracture in the elderly population but

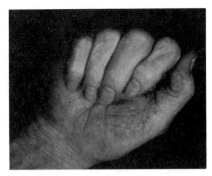

FIG 14–15.
The flexed fingers normally point toward the tubercle of the scaphoid, an anatomic landmark at the base of the palm. The flexor carpi radiolis tendon passes directly over the tubercle of the scaphoid.

still can lead to significant problems. Nonunion, malunion, stiffness of adjacent joints, and progression of arthritis are all-too-frequent sequelae of fractures in the hands of elderly patients. Therefore, it behooves us to address these problems in our treatment plans. Complicated devices including heavy splints, casts, and/or external fixators may not be well tolerated because of coexisting medical problems such as arthritis, neuromuscular disorders, and diabetes. Fragile bone may not hold fixation devices as well as a younger person's bone, so methods of fixation may need to be adjusted. For example, screws may not be as likely to hold in soft bone, so one may opt to consider one of the many variations of intraosseous wiring techniques either with tension bands or Kirschner wires. Functional bracing techniques with the supervision of a hand therapist is often quite helpful if a nonsurgical approach is chosen.[23]

In the assessment of closed and open injuries to the hand it is very important to note the appearance and posture of the hand in addition to palpating for areas of tenderness. If the examiner is not familiar with x-ray evaluation or even if he or she is a radiologic expert, significant findings are available from a physical examination. Rotational deformities can be assessed by having the patient flex the fingers into the palm. As a general rule, the fingertips should point toward the tubercle of the scaphoid (Fig 14–15), an anatomic landmark that is readily palpable and usually visible on the palmar radial aspect of the wrist. If one of the four digits does not point toward this scaphoid tubercle (Fig 14–16), one must suspect a significant injury to bone or ligament structure even if x-rays appear normal.

Hamatometacarpal Fracture Dislocation

Fractures of the carpal bones are relatively rare in the elderly population although when they occur they might easily be missed, as is the case in a patient who sustained a fall on his hand with an axial compressive load directed to the little and ring fingers.[7] His hand was rather thick and heavy. On presentation to the emergency room the rotational deformity and shortening of the little finger were not noted. X-rays were obtained and were interpreted as normal. He was treated with a splint for some six weeks but because of persistent pain and swelling he sought further opinions. Clinical examination showed a significant rotational deformity of the little finger in addition to a very stiff hand. The x-rays were reviewed and showed a fracture of the hamate with a dislocation of the base of the fifth metacarpal on the hamate (Fig 14–17,A). Note the presence of the base of the small finger metacarpal adjacent to the triquetrum. This injury was treated by means of an open reduction and internal

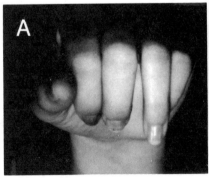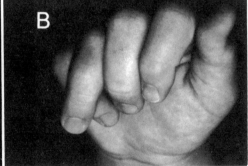

FIG 14–16.
A, appearance of the digits flexed into the palm in a patient with a fracture of the metacarpal. **B,** appearance of the hand of a patient with a fracture of the proximal phalanx. The overlapping of the little finger by the ring finger is quite obvious here but in other cases it may be somewhat more subtle and manifested simply by a rotational deformity of the tip of the fingernail.

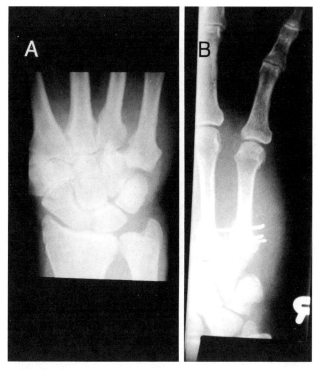

FIG 14–17.
A, note the proximal displacement of the base of the little finger metacarpal relative to that of the ring finger metacarpal. Also note the little finger metacarpal is displaced in an ulnar direction and no longer articulates fully with the adjacent hamate facet. **B,** note the alignment of the base of the little finger metacarpal relative to the hamate facet. Multiple Kirschner wires were used for fixation.

fixation with the requirement for significant mobilization of the soft tissues and removal of heterotopic bone that had formed in response to the injury (Fig 14–17,B). Although the patient still has some stiffness, he is able to make a fist well enough to hold a golf club and participate in his activities of daily living.

Scaphoid Fracture

While fractures of the scaphoid are not common in the elderly population, they can occur. The initial diagnosis can often be missed on x-ray so again, attention must be directed to the specific site of tenderness on physical examination, which is typically the snuff box or region of the wrist between the extensor pollicis longus and abductor pollicis longus–extensor pollicis brevis tendons.[14]

Metacarpal Fracture

Metacarpal fractures that result in shortening of more than 4 mm and have evidence of rotation are often treated with internal fixation. The patient whose x-ray is shown in Figure 14–18 was afflicted with advanced Alzheimer's disease and had a habit of tearing off all dressings and splints, as well as having some evidence of minor self-destructive behavior after previous surgical procedures when he attempted to remove the sutures from the wound before it was healed. Although the ideal treatment for this fracture might be internal fixation, it is not the appropriate treatment in this patient. After an initial attempt at using a splint failed because the splint was removed within 2 hours of its application, the patient was treated with a short arm cast with a dorsal extension block. The extensor tendons acted as a tension band to prevent significant apex dorsal angulation of the fracture. He was allowed to move his fingers to the limits of comfort. Rotational control was provided by a buddy strap and the fracture healed without difficulties. His resultant range of motion was good (Fig 14–19).

Although it is generally agreed that the restoration of normal anatomy tends to result in optimal function, the amount of soft-tissue dissection required to provide a rigid internal fixation may in fact

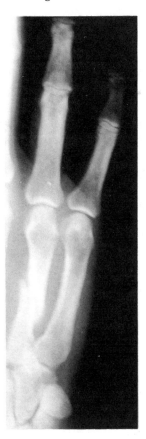

FIG 14–18.
A spiral oblique frature of the ring finger metacarpal with displacement and shortening was noted.

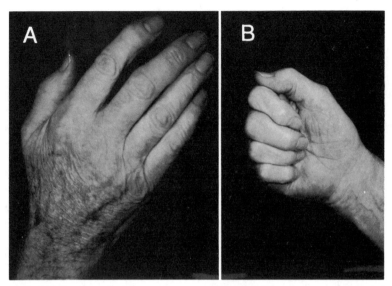

FIG 14–19.
A, alignment in extension. **B,** rotation is well maintained.

result in increased stiffness, swelling, and thus poor function in the hand of an elderly person whose existing disease processes, bone quality, and capacity for rehabilitation are limited. An attempt should be made, however, to provide satisfactory alignment, particularly in the rotational plane, and to avoid excessive shortening. These goals can usually be achieved by means of closed treatment methods along with a rehabilitation program.

Since the metacarpal fracture generally angulates in an apex dorsal position owing to the pull of the interosseous muscles (Fig 14–20), a tension band effect can be created by providing a dorsal splint with the metacarpophalangeal joints in flexion and allowing the patient to actively flex the interphalangeal joints. Angular deformities are relatively rare but minor rotational problems can frequently be overcome by techniques such as "buddy strapping" or providing rubberband traction through garment hooks glued to the fingernails (Fig 14–21). If one chooses the rubberband technique in an effort to try to correct rotation, great care must be taken to avoid proximal interphalangeal joint stiffness and, specifically,

flexion contractures (Fig 14–22). In cases where the rotational deformity simply cannot be corrected, internal fixation may still be the optimum technique depending upon the individual patient. Methods of internal fixation can vary from interfragmentary screws and plates to tension band wiring techniques or Kirschner wires. Closed methods have been described whereby intramedullary pins can be inserted to provide an internal splint but external protection with splint or cast is still necessary. Treatment must be tailored to the individual fracture and patient.

These considerations are illustrated by the case of a 74-year-old woman who sustained a fracture of her metacarpal shaft after a relatively minor fall on her hand (Fig 14–23). She also had injured her adjacent proximal interphalangeal joint, with a stable fracture of the base of the proximal phalanx. This patient had a history of osteoporosis with some increased risk factors owing to her small size. Since there was no rotational deformity and no significant amount of soft-tissue injury it was felt that internal fixation would not be necessary and that a functional bracing technique would provide the best

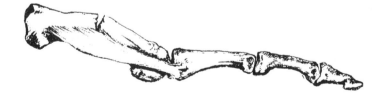

FIG 14–20.
The interosseous muscle has its origin on the proximal fragment of the fracture of the metacarpal. Its insertion is distal to the metacarpal. The resultant deformity is apex dorsal angulation.

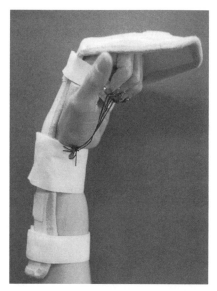

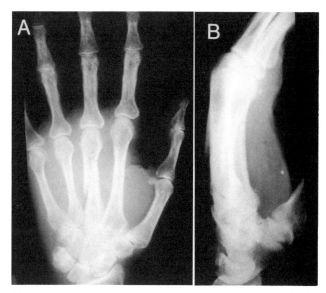

FIG 14–21.

A dorsal block splint made of thermoplastic material allows the patient to fully flex the fingers while providing a dorsal "tension band" created by the extensor tendons, thus holding the fracture in position.

treatment for this patient. Although the treatment program was splinting and not internal fixation, she developed significant flexion contractures of the proximal interphalangeal joints of the injured and adjacent fingers. It was evident that she suffered from osteoarthritis but the symptoms of such in her oppo-

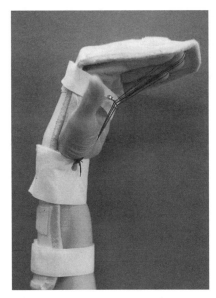

FIG 14–22.

It is essential that the patient be instructed in frequent exercises to provide full extension of the proximal and distal interphalangeal joints to prevent flexion contractures of these joints.

FIG 14–23.

A, posterior anterior x-ray shows the spiral oblique fracture of the long finger metacarpal, as well as a fracture of the ring finger metacarpal neck. An undisplaced fracture of the long finger proximal phalanx is also noted. **B,** the lateral view shows slight dorsal displacement of the distal fragment of metacarpal.

site, uninjured hand were relatively minimal while at the same time the injured hand showed evidence of significant swelling, redness, and local tenderness about her joints at the interphalangeal level. Despite the best efforts of a hand therapy program, a very significant pain dysfunction syndrome developed. This patient was very reluctant to move her hand despite analgesics and anti-inflammatory medications. As a result, she developed contractures in her fingers that required long-term physical therapy and splinting. Her fracture healed without deformity (Fig 14–24).

Intra-articular Fractures of the Base of the Thumb Metacarpal

Intra-articular fractures of the base of the thumb metacarpal, often known as a Bennett's fracture, can only be reduced if the distracting force of the abductor pollicis longus is neutralized either by internal fixation or external fixation techniques (Fig 14–25). While it is generally felt important to try to reestablish the joint surface in an anatomic fashion as shown in Figure 14–25,C, this may not be possible because of problems with preexisting osteoarthritis or because of the severe amount of comminution of the articular surface. Fractures with a marked amount of comminution are sometimes known as

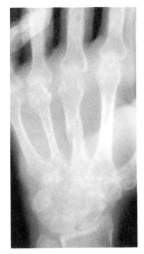

FIG 14–24.
Posterior anterior view shows the fractures of the metacarpals and proximal phalanx to be healed in satisfactory position.

Rolando fractures (Fig 14–26). Although an open reduction and internal fixation using K-wires or screws may be possible, an alternative technique, particularly in the more severely comminuted fracture, that has worked well in the older patient is that described by Breen.[4] In this technique a K-wire is drilled obliquely through the metacarpal shaft and is attached to an outrigger device to provide traction.

This traction allows maintenance of reduction of the dislocation of the metacarpal fragment on the trapezium and allows molding of the fracture fragment (Fig 14–27) through ligamentotaxis (Fig 14–28). The cast and pin can remain in position for some 6 weeks. This technique has proven to be quite helpful in patients who have had burn or abrasion injuries in the area of the thumb base that prevented an open reduction and internal fixation.

For patients who have had unreduced Bennett's fractures and an incongruous joint the resultant posttraumatic arthritis and deformity may lead to significant pain. Treatment options might include an arthrodesis of the metacarpotrapezial joint or arthroplasty. If arthroplasty of the metacarpotrapezial joint is to be considered, stability is quite important. This stability can be achieved by reconstruction of the ligament by means of a tendon. This author's experience with the technique described by Burton and Pelligrini has been good.[6] The x-rays in Figure 14–29 represent an example of such a technique; however, other tendon reconstructions are possible. Some authors have had good experiences with silicone interposition. There have, however, been recent concerns with respect to "silicone synovitis" or particulate debris that may be associated with silicone and the resultant foreign body reaction leading to increased pain and swelling postoperatively.[22, 29]

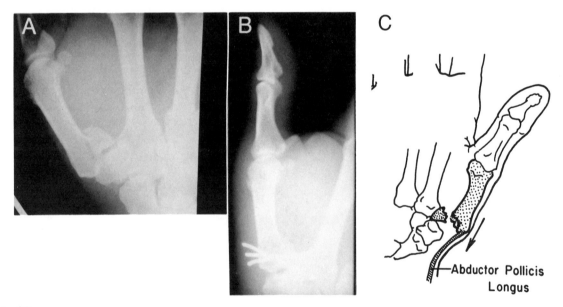

FIG 14–25.
A, lateral view of a Bennett fracture demonstrating the proximal and dorsal migration of the major portion of the thumb metacarpal as a result of the deforming force of the abductor pollicis longus. **B,** the fracture has been anatomically reduced in an open fashion. Multiple Kirschner wires have been used to maintain the position of the fracture fragment as well as the joint. **C,** the abducor pollicis longus is attached to the distal fragment of metacarpal, providing the deforming force to hold the fracture fragments separated.

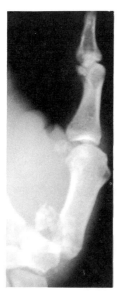

FIG 14–26.
Lateral x-ray of the thumb shows a comminuted displaced intra-articular fracture of the base of the thumb metacarpal.

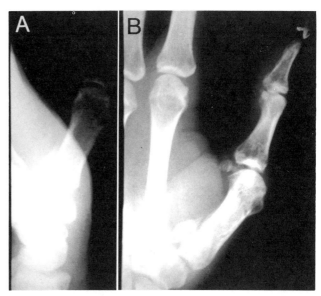

FIG 14–28.
A, posterior anterior view following removal of the traction and cast shows the early healing of the fracture fragments. **B,** note the maintenance of the reduction of the thumb metacarpal relative to the trapezium but the continued presence of the comminuted segments. These radiographs were taken one week following removal of the traction device and cast.

Proximal Phalanx

Metaphyseal fractures of the proximal phalanx base that are nonarticular typically angulate in a radial or ulnar plane and often involve the ulnar digits. Diaphyseal fractures generally angulate in an apex palmar direction owing to the pull of the intrinsic muscles as well as the extrinsic flexor and extensor mechanical action (Fig 14–30). More distal fractures of the proximal phalanx often involve the condyles at the proximal interphalangeal joint and are very unstable. These more distal fractures can have a rotational component and generally benefit from internal fixation, either percutaneously or in an open fashion. Again, if open reduction is necessary, there is a high risk of stiffness at the proximal interphalangeal joint so mobilization is indicated as soon as possible. If these unstable fractures are allowed to heal with depression of the joint surface, a significant angular deformity as well as posttraumatic arthritis is likely to be the result.

The diagnosis of phalangeal fractures can be compromised by inadequate x-rays. All too often x-rays of the hand are requested for evaluation of an injured finger. The result is that the injured part is not in the central beam of the x-ray and the fracture cannot be adequately evaluated. Not infrequently,

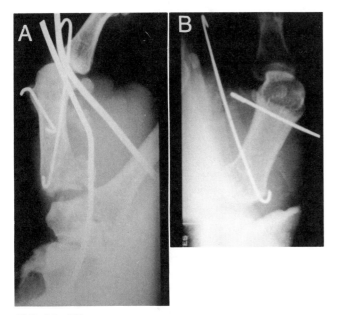

FIG 14–27.
A, lateral view of a thumb metacarpal through which two Kirschner wires have been inserted to provide distraction at the fracture site. Note the presence of the comminuted fragments but the dorsal subluxation of the base of the metacarpal has been corrected through the traction technique. The larger metal wire on this view represents the coathanger wire that was used to provide the outrigger for the short arm cast. **B,** posterior anterior view of the same patient shows the traction wires in place. The hooked end of the wire at the base of the thumb metacarpal provides the grasping force on the bone to allow the traction to be applied.

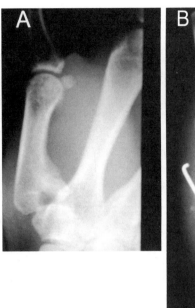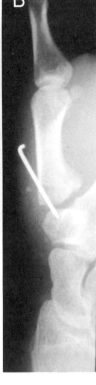

She did have a history of osteoarthritis, and Bouchard's nodes were evident at the proximal interphalangeal joints. Closed reduction of the right little finger was accomplished; however, subsequent x-rays showed loss of reduction with rotational deformity of the finger. Open reduction and internal fixation (Fig 14–33) was carried out. Her postoperative course was marked by significant stiffness in the finger. The hardware was removed 7 months following the initial surgery, and capsulotomy and extensor tendolysis was carried out. Despite obtaining good passive range of motion at the time of surgery and a well-supervised hand therapy program, her 6 month postoperative follow-up showed only 20 degrees of active motion at the proximal interphalangeal joint and 10 degrees at the distal interphalangeal joint. Her joints remained swollen and painful. This case represents a good example of some of the difficulties encountered in dealing with treatment of fractures in a patient with established osteoarthritis. Despite anatomic reduction and adequate healing of the fracture her functional result is poor. These issues should be discussed with the patient preoperatively so that the goals of the treatment program may be clearly understood.

Distal Phalanx

Fractures of the distal phalanx may be articular or nonarticular. The nonarticular fractures are often associated with crushing injuries to the distal phalanx and need attention directed toward the soft tissue component of the injury and the resultant wound.

Nail Bed

Frequently a nail bed laceration will be involved (Fig 14–34). In order to assess the nail bed laceration it is often necessary to block the finger, elevate the fingernail, and repair the nail bed.[25] Unless the nail plate is irretrievably damaged it is best that the plate be inserted back under the eponychial fold after the repair of the nail bed has been performed with a fine

FIG 14–29.
A, lateral view of thumb metacarpal shows a healed Bennett fracture with dorsal subluxation of the metacarpal on the trapezium. **B,** following removal of the base of the thumb metacarpal, interposition of the flexor carpi radialis tendon, and insertion of a Kirschner wire as a temporary fixation device, the relationship of the thumb metacarpal base to the trapezium has been improved.

the injury is missed because of this. Thus, x-rays of the hand are not an acceptable means of evaluating digital injuries. The use of dental film forces the careful radiographic evaluation of the injured area in addition to providing excellent detail of bone and soft tissues. Figure 14–31 demonstrates the injury well and allows planning of the repair.

The patient was a 69-year-old woman who sustained a fracture of the proximal phalanx of her right little finger after striking it on the dashboard of a car that had been involved in an accident (Fig 14–32).

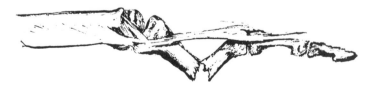

FIG 14–30.
The proximal phalanx fracture is pulled into an apex palmar angular deformity through the deforming force of the intrin-sic muscles, in this case the interossei and lubricals, which make up the lateral band mechanism of the digit.

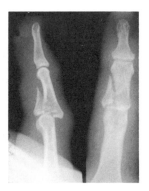

FIG 14–31.
Anterior posterior as well as lateral view of the injured proximal interphalangeal joint allow for adequate assessment of the bony injury. On the left side or lateral view the dorsal displacement of the base of the middle phalanx is noted relative to the proximal phalanx.

catgut suture. If a transverse displaced fracture has lacerated the nail bed, consideration must be given to internal fixation of the fracture in order to provide good stability for healing of the nail bed. The techniques of evaluation and treatment of nail bed injuries have been well described by Van Beek[34] and Zook.[35]

Articular

Articular fractures of the distal phalanx may present as a mallet finger with the patient having been struck by an object with an axial load. Although some authors have recommended closed treatment for all such injuries,[33] others have felt that

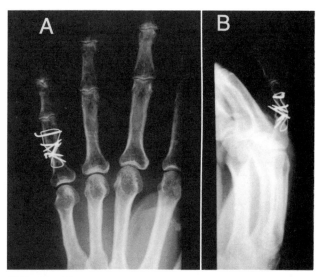

FIG 14–33.
A, the fracture of the proximal phalanx has been reduced and internally fixed by means of multiple Kirschner wires and a tension band technique. **B,** lateral view shows the hardware in position and the alignment restored.

those fractures involving the distal phalanx that have palmar subluxation of the distal fragment are best treated with an open reduction and internal fixation in an effort to establish a congruous joint and decrease the risk of arthritic change. In the elderly population it is important to exercise appropriate judgment with due consideration to the vascular status of the finger as well as the ability of the bone to accept internal fixation.

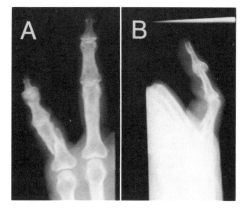

FIG 14–32.
A, posterior anterior view of the little finger demonstrates the angulation of the proximal phalanx fracture and the presence of arthritis at the proximal as well as distal interphalangeal joints. **B,** a lateral view of the same finger shows the marked hypertrophic bone formation at the distal interphalangeal joint (Heberden's node).

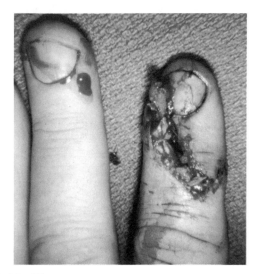

FIG 14–34.
Power saw injury to the distal and middle phalanges of the index finger. The nail bed has been damaged with this open injury.

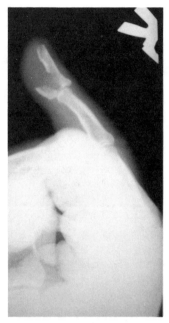

FIG 14–35.
Lateral x-ray shows the fracture of the distal phalanx. Palmar fragment is attached to the flexor digitorum profundus tendon. The dorsal fragment that is displaced dorsally is still attached to the extensor tendon.

Profundus Tendon Avulsion

A somewhat unusual injury is represented by the case of a 77-year-old man who was pulling a lawn mower and felt his ring finger "pop." He noted swelling and pain. Examination showed no distal in-

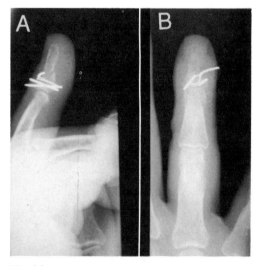

FIG 14–36.
A, this x-ray shows anatomic reduction of the articular surface of the distal phalanx with reduction of the joint subluxation as well. **B,** the lateral view confirms satisfactory alignment.

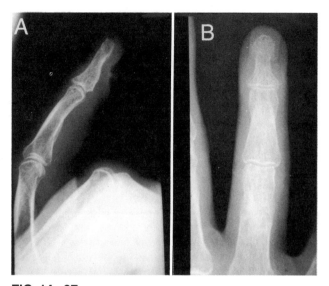

FIG 14–37.
A, following hardware removal, the fracture line is no longer visible and the joint remains well reduced. **B,** posterior anterior view demonstrates satisfactory healing and alignment of the distal interphalangeal joint.

terphalangeal joint motion and only 30 degrees of active proximal interphalangeal joint motion. Despite his age this man was very active, he enjoyed gardening and some sports activities. The x-rays demonstrated a complete palmar avulsion of the distal phalanx associated with avulsion of the flexor digitorum profundus tendon (Fig 14–35). He was treated by reattachment of the avulsed profundus tendon and bone to the distal phalanx with reduction of the dislocated interphalangeal joint and internal fixation of the intra-articular fracture of the distal phalanx of his ring finger (Fig 14–36). His postoperative course included passive flexion and active extension, as would be carried out following a flexor tendon laceration. His wound healed well and good motion was regained. The result showed a 20-degree flexion contracture at the proximal interphalangeal joint and further flexion to 106 degrees, full extension to 40 degrees flexion at the distal interphalangeal joint. The follow-up x-rays are shown in Figures 14–37,A and B.

OPEN FRACTURES

The treatment of open fractures in the elderly patient demands the same meticulous wound care that is provided to any patient with an open fracture. Tetanus toxoid immunization must be current, if not, consideration must be given to human immunoglobulin treatment. The wound debridement must be thorough with removal of all foreign bodies through mechanical means including lavage. Antibiotics appropriate for the type of wound are indicated. Although *Staphylococcus aureus* is a common organism on the skin, soil-contaminated wounds often have gram-negative enteric organisms, which may be best treated by the administration of an aminoglycoside. Due consideration must be given to renal status of the patient. Computerized aminoglycoside monitoring programs are available in many hospitals and it is often helpful to consult with an infectious disease specialist regarding specifics of antibiotic treatment. The duration of treatment depends on the nature of the wound and its response to the initial and subsequent debridements.

A particularly troublesome type of wound is the human bite wound, which requires the same thorough debridement and irrigation. As a general rule, no attempt should be made to close human bite wounds. Anaerobic organisms are often present in the saliva and the antibiotics must be adjusted accordingly. Cat and dog bites are often contaminated with *Pasteurella*, which is adequately covered by penicillin. Although newer antibiotics are available orally for gram-negative coverage, it has been this author's practice that the more difficult type of wounds be treated initially with intravenous antibiotics so as to insure adequate blood levels in the early phases following the injury.

Many older patients in farm communities continue to be very actively involved in their business endeavors and accordingly are subject to mutilating injuries in the upper extremity, for example, when the hand is caught in a piece of farm equipment such as an auger, corn picker, or the pulley of a V-belt. These complex injuries demand immediate attention as they often have a significant crushing and tearing component in addition to severe contamination with grain or silage. There are often major neurovascular injuries. The goals in approaching these problems should be to first stabilize the patient, then obtain a clean wound, and finally achieve the best function possible with the remaining tissues about the extremity. The use of distant pedicle flaps can be fraught with multiple problems, including severe stiffness and involvement of other uninjured joints with stiffness and subsequent pain. Thus, a patient with a badly mangled hand may not only be left with a significant loss of function in the hand and forearm but may develop significant stiffness in the

shoulder as well which would limit him from using a prosthesis if such might be necessary at a later date. Microvascular reconstruction may also be fraught with significant pitfalls, as the arteries in the upper extremity are frequently involved with an atherosclerotic process in the elderly patient and may not be suitable for anastomosis into a microvascular tissue transfer.

Replantation would seem to have very limited application in the elderly population in view of the risks not only of the surgery but also in terms of time for anesthesia as well as potential complications of anticoagulation. One must be careful to see that technology does not overcome reason in the approach to some of these more difficult problems of reconstruction.

LIGAMENT INJURIES

Ligament injuries are not common in the geriatric population; however, they do occur and one must be mindful of them when a patient presents with complaints of pain and clicking in the wrist. The x-rays may not show any bone abnormality, but tenderness can generally be elicited over the specific intracarpal joints that are involved. The treatment of carpal ligament instability seems to be in an evolutionary phase and the reader is referred to many of the excellent recent publications for diagnosis and possible treatment recommendations.[20, 31] Treatments have included immobilization for short periods followed by an exercise program for strengthening, ligament reconstruction possibly with augmentation by tendons, or limited intracarpal arthrodeses.

A 65-year-old woman fell onto her right wrist when she was walking with the Senior Striders. Examination demonstrated specific tenderness over the proximal carpal row and a distinct click as she moved her wrist from ulnar to radial deviation. Standard wrist x-rays were normal (Fig 14–38,A). Imaging studies that can assist in a diagnosis of these problems include the use of MRI as well as videofluoroscopic evaluation and wrist arthrography. In this patient a triple-compartment wrist arthrogram demonstrated a lunotriquetral tear as well as a triangular fibrocartilage complex tear (Fig 14–38,B). This patient declined further aggressive surgical treatment as she felt her functional demands were limited and the injury did not significantly interfere with her everyday activities.

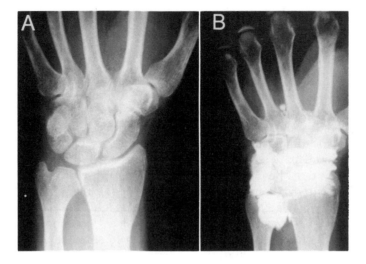

FIG 14-38.
A, posterior anterior view of the wrist shows no evidence of fracture with normal alignment of the carpal bones. **B,** this wrist arthrogram after injection of dye into the radiocarpal joint shows the presence of dye in the distal radioulnar as well as midcarpal and carpometacarpal joints.

In approaching problems of carpal instability resulting from intracarpal ligament tears in the older population both the provider and the patient must be fully aware of the potential complications of treatment. There is the risk of stiffness in the hand that already has osteoarthritic change when major reconstructive surgery is performed on the wrist. It is also important to recognize that with our increasing dependence on technology for diagnosis some of the changes in the structures may not be truly posttraumatic but may be the consequences of the aging process. For example, it has been shown there is an increasing incidence of tear of the triangular fibrocartilage complex with increasing age.[21] In a study of 180 wrist joints, triangular fibrocartilage complex perforation was present in 53 percent of patients over the age of 70 years, compared with an incidence of 7.6 percent in patients in the third decade of life.

As the population ages, it is necessary to identify some problems that may be peculiar to aging so that we may manage them more effectively. With the elderly making up an increasingly larger percentage of our population it is necessary to treat those conditions of the hand and upper extremity which lead to increasing disability.

SKIN

Skin in the elderly is easily subject to injury owing to the loss of subcutaneous fat and fibrous septa associated with the aging process. Sometimes injury is related to other factors, such as collagen vascular diseases, medications, and chronic trauma. Even minor trauma may result in marked ecchymosis and swelling. Patients who receive tissue plasminogen activator, streptokinase, heparin, warfarin, and other varieties of anticoagulants are subject to very significant swelling, ecchymosis, and even skin loss as a result of sometimes minor injuries or insults. Following the swelling comes stiffness, so edema control and range of motion exercises are very important in these patients.

COMPARTMENT SYNDROMES

It is important also to be on guard for compartment syndromes. Compartment syndromes are the result of increased pressure in a closed space. They may occur as the result of an externally applied pressure such as from a cast or tight dressing. This syndrome may also be caused by increased compartment pressure as a result of bleeding from a crush injury or fluid infusion, as might occur from a deep intravenous needle infiltration. The diagnosis is suggested by increased pain complaints out of proportion to the nature of the injury. The pain is exacerbated by passive stretch of the involved compartment muscles. The pulses may remain normal but tissue ischemia can occur because the end organ (muscle) is deprived of its blood supply owing to increased pressure within the specific fascial com-

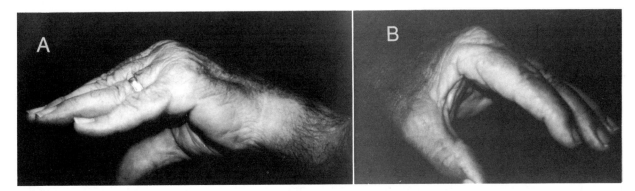

FIG 14–39.
A, this x-ray is a view of the left hand of a very physically active man in his 70s with intrinsic plus deformity. **B,** this x-ray shows the position of the hand as viewed from the lateral side Note the flexed position of the metacarpophalangeal joints and relatively extended positions of the proximal interphalangeal joints.

partment. In addition to the palmar and dorsal forearm, the interosseous compartments are at risk with any type of crush injury to the hand. In the unconscious patient it may be very difficult to establish the diagnosis. The diagnosis can be established by intracompartmental pressure measurements. The treatment involves relieving the source of the pressure and may include a surgical fasciotomy of the involved compartments.

CONTRACTURES

The problem of contractures in the elderly patient following a hand injury may adversely affect the outcome. The contracture may simply be a result of the posttraumatic scarring process or may be associated with progression of a local disease process such as fibromatosis. Systemic disorders such as diabetes are known to lead to rather significant stiffness about joints. Osteoarthritis with its inherent tendency to form bone will also result in local stiffness. It is well known that preexisting osteoarthritis is exacerbated by injury to the joint or surrounding bone adjacent to the joint. This leads to increased scar formation, as is frequently seen with check-rein ligament contractures at the proximal interphalangeal joint. Central nervous system (CNS) disorders of the basal ganglia can lead to intrinsic contractures of the hand with a neurogenic basis (Fig 14–39). Just as with the hand of a child with cerebral palsy, very specific goals must be outlined prior to surgery for intrinsic contractures caused by CNS disease, as the practitioner is not addressing the under-

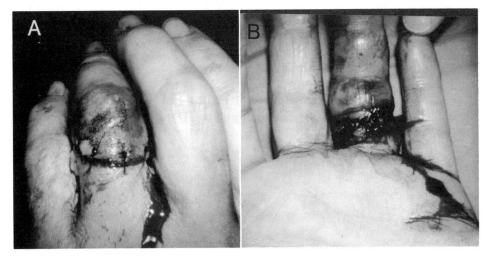

FIG 14–40.
This elderly woman sustained a ring avulsion injury of her finger when her wedding band was caught on a hook as she was trying to grasp with her left hand during an episode of falling. **A,** appearance of the dorsum of the finger. **B,** palmar surface of the digit prior to repairing the neurovascular structures.

lying cause but is operating on the effect of the problem. Associated disease processes that impair function, cooperation, and judgment need to be considered in plans for management of a particular hand injury.

Ethical dilemmas can arise in approaches to treatment within orthopedics and hand surgery. Is it appropriate to perform a highly technical reconstruction in a patient with limited functional potential? These decisions should not necessarily be age related but function related. Elderly patients often live alone in small apartments with limited access to transportation and rehabilitation facilities. Availability of technical expertise to perform a procedure should not necessarily dictate that such a procedure should be carried out. For example, the elderly widow or widower with a ring avulsion injury may be best treated by amputation rather than revascularization even though the latter procedure might be successfully performed (Fig 14–40). One must certainly consider risks of prolonged anesthesia, anticoagulants, and possibility of a worse result after the surgery with significant pain and cold intolerance in the digit. The surgeon should discuss the options for treatment fully with the patient and the family and then recommend the simplest procedure to accomplish the goals that have been established. For some patients this is to return to an independent living status; for others, it may involve nursing home or custodial care. For other patients of the same age it may be a full, active life-style.

TUMORS

There seems to be little dispute that certain types of tumors, specifically squamous cell carcinoma and melanoma, are related to exposures of noxious agents. The incidence of melanoma has tripled in the past 4 decades. Approximately 32,000 Americans will be found to have melanoma in 1991, and 6,500 will die of it.[17]

The median age at diagnosis of melanoma is 53 years. It is generally accepted that the early diagnosis of melanoma and thus early treatment will decrease the morbidity and mortality of this disease. In fact, the 5-year survival rate of melanoma has increased from 49 percent in the 1950s to 81 percent today.[17]

A particularly difficult type of melanoma that is seen on the hand is that of the acral-lentiginous mel-

anoma, which can present on the palmar surface or subungual area of the digit. These lesions can often have a somewhat indolent appearance; however, they are frequently a full thickness or Clark's stage 5 lesion, which carries a rather poor prognosis. The lesion is visible on the skin; thus, visual examination remains the most reliable means of identification.[30]

Acral-lentiginous melanoma occurs more frequently in blacks and Asians than Caucasians. Although benign pigmentation within the nail plate is not uncommon, particularly in blacks, a dark subungual area or periungual spread of pigmentation in any patient should suggest the possibility of acral-lentiginous melanoma. Acral-lentiginous melanoma accounts for about 2% to 8% of melanoma in whites but 25% of melanoma in blacks. Sunlight does not seem to be involved in causing this subtype.[17]

BURNS AND FROSTBITE

Thermal burns of the hand in the elderly population require aggressive management. Blood flow to the extremities can be compromised owing to peripheral vasoconstriction associated with hypovolemia because of the burn injury, and the problem may be remedied by adequate fluid resuscitation. Decreased perfusion to the digits can also be related to eschar formation and in such a case surgical or chemical (enzymatic) escharotomy is indicated. Compromised blood flow may be associated with peripheral vascular disease in the upper extremities of the elderly patient. Although controversies have existed regarding timing of wound excision and closure, it is the opinion of many burn surgeons that early debridement and skin grafting within the first few days of injury are indicated for treatment of the deep burn injury in the elderly. Fibrin glue techniques may be used to increase adherence of the skin graft and allow early motion.[12] Elevation and protective splinting between exercise sessions is important.

Burn care is a highly specialized area and any patient with significant hand burns should be referred to a burn treatment center where a team of physicians, nurses, therapists, psychologists, and social workers can provide for the many specialized needs of the patient. In some cases an extended posthospital rehabilitation unit may allow the patient a better transition to home life. The elderly patient with a hand burn may lack the strength and joint mobility to maintain proper position of the hands and thus is predisposed to stiffness and joint contractures. Early motion programs are very helpful to these patients.[2]

The effects of frostbite on the hand may be made more severe by peripheral vascular disease, in addition to smoking or previous frostbite injury. The treatment of frostbitten digits is rapid rewarming of the frozen extremity at 40° to 44° C. These treatments may include whirlpool baths. It is recommended that early amputation be avoided and that the resection of dead tissue be carried out only after clear demarcation has occurred. The digit may be painful and hypersensitive for an extended period following the initial insult.[15]

TENDONS

Flexor Tendons

Flexor tendon lacerations in the elderly are diagnosed by history and physical examination (Fig 14–41). The penetrating wound may on occasion need to be explored in order to confirm the presence of a partial tendon laceration. As a general rule, if over 50% of the tendon has been divided a repair is best done in order to prevent delayed tendon ruptures.[26] On occasion the partial flexor tendon laceration may present as a "trigger finger" owing to the presence of a flap of tendon catching on the pulley mechanism. In this latter situation a "tendoplasty" or trimming of the frayed tendon edge may be done if only a minor portion of the tendon is involved.

Flexor tendon lacerations in zone 2 or the zone of pulleys—that is, the area between the distal palmar crease and the middle of the middle phalanx— are known to be at risk for the development of adhesions with subsequent limitation of motion in the digit. This propensity for scarring is increased in the elderly population, with associated osteoarthritis or fibromatosis. Elevation in an effort to prevent edema and subsequent fibrosis is important. Early controlled motion of the digit with passive flexion and active extension of the metaphalangeal and interphalangeal joints is helpful in preventing scar. When rubber bands are used to maintain the proximal interphalangeal joints in flexion, great care must be taken to insure that the patient understands the need to provide full extension of the proximal interphalangeal joint at frequent intervals or the result will be a fixed proximal interphalangeal joint con-

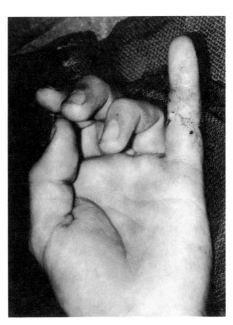

FIG 14–41.
Note the extended posture of the little finger with the hand at rest. The adjacent digit with intact flexor tendons show the normal flexed posture of the digits with the hand at rest. Note the healed scar at the proximal phalanx level of the little finger. This patient had presented to an emergency room some ten days previously with a laceration, but the diagnosis of flexor tendon injury was not made at the time of the emergency room visit.

tracture, which in itself can be very disabling. Frequent follow-up with the surgeon or hand therapist is very beneficial in preventing this complication.

Extensor Tendons

Extensor tendon lacerations of the dorsum of the hand and wrist can result in significant scarring. Adherence of the tendon to the bone as well as tendon to the skin can occur and result in limitation of joint motion. Recent reports have demonstrated the benefits of early dynamic splinting (Fig 14–42).[8] Chapter 15 offers specific guidelines regarding dynamic splinting of flexor and extensor tendon injuries.

Mallet finger, in which an extensor lag at the distal interphalangeal joint occurs because of avulsion of the distal insertion of the extensor tendon from the bone of the distal phalanx, commonly results from a direct blow to the tip of the outstretched finger against a firm object. The patient may not notice the deformity initially as there is often no pain, swelling, or ecchymosis. Treatment may thus be delayed. It is important to obtain good AP and lateral x-ray views of the distal phalanx in order to make certain that a significant intra-articular fracture of the

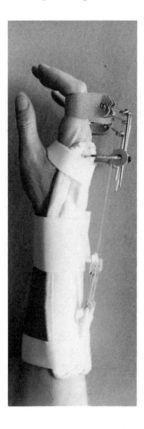

FIG 14–42.
The patient for whom this splint was fabricated had lacerated multiple extensor tendons at the level of the metacarpals. This splint was applied early in the postoperative period.

distal phalanx has not occurred. If a large fragment of bone has been broken off and displaced from the articular surface and palmar subluxation of the distal phalanx occurs, function may well be improved by means of an open reduction and internal fixation of the fracture.

For pure avulsion of the extensor tendon insertion without significant associated fracture, splinting of the distal interphalangeal joint in full extension is

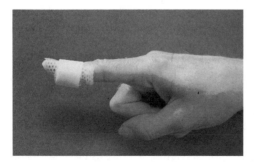

FIG 14–43.
This patient had an extensor tendon avulsion at the level of the distal phalanx. A custom-made orthosis was utilized.

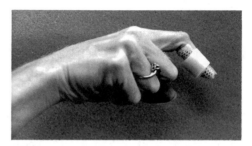

FIG 14–44.
Since only the distal interphalangeal joint requires immobilization it is important to be certain the patient has the ability to flex the PIP joint, to prevent stiffness of that joint.

successful provided that the extended position at the distal interphalangeal joint is maintained full time for 8 weeks (Fig 14–43). A slow weaning process from the splint is begun. Failed treatment of mallet finger, as may occur in osteoarthritis of the distal interphalangeal joint, is most predictably treated by arthrodesis of the joint, as soft-tissue procedures for this injury have been unreliable in the elderly patient in most cases. It is frequently beneficial to have a splint custom-made for the patient (Fig 14–44), as the incidence of skin problems with foam-backed metal splints or ready-made plastic splints can be high, particularly in warm, humid climates. The patient or a designated assistant is allowed to remove the splint on a daily basis provided full extension of the distal interphalangeal joint is maintained. The digit is cleansed with alcohol, which allows drying as well as toughening of the skin. This method of treatment is not effective for the noncompliant patient.

INFECTIONS

Infections in the hand of an elderly patient can have disastrous consequences. A simple puncture with a contaminated needle, rose thorn, or splinter into the flexor tendon sheath can result in a florid flexor tenosynovitis. The diagnosis of this condition can be made by Kanavel's four cardinal signs, including symmetrical swelling of the digit, proximal interphalangeal joint flexion contracture, pain with passive extension of the digit, and tenderness along the flexor tendon sheath.[16] Depending on the location, some of these infections can break into the midpalmar or thenar spaces, thus resulting in another area of closed space infection. As a general rule, closed space infection either within a fascial en-

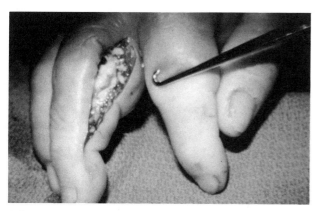

FIG 14–45.
This elderly patient with a history of diabetes mellitus sustained a puncture wound to the palmar aspect of her long finger. At the time of surgery a midaxial incision was made in the finger. A moderate amount of purulent material poured forth from the flexor tendon sheath.

velope or within the joint capsule (septic arthritis) is treated by surgical drainage. The edema and scar from the residual of infection can lead to significant stiffness, so early range-of-motion exercises can be of benefit in preventing a loss of motion. The use of resting splints between exercise sessions is helpful. In this setting the therapist is responsible for ensuring that the wound care instructions are followed in addition to supervising the splinting and exercise program. In the case of flexor tenosynovitis, for example, the patient may have an incision and drainage of the closed space (Fig 14–45), then 24 hours of catheter irrigation of the flexor tendon sheath followed by a visit to the therapist for exercises, wound care, and splinting. Antibiotics, either parenteral or oral, are indicated and may need to be adjusted depending upon the antibiotic sensitivities noted after identification of the organism by culture.

A felon is a pulp space infection on the distal palmar aspect of the digit. It is quite painful and the diagnosis is made on the basis of swelling and tenderness over the tip of the finger. These infections typically occur from a penetrating wound with a contaminated object. A felon requires surgical drainage as continued infection in the pulp space carries the risk of an osteomyelitis of the distal phalanx.

SUMMARY

In summary, the evaluation and treatment of injuries of the hand in an elderly person present a unique set of challenges for the provider of care. The effects of aging on the whole person should be considered in addition to the functional status and demands of the individual patient prior to establishing a treatment plan. Certain techniques suitable for a younger or middle-aged individual may not be appropriate for an elderly person.

REFERENCES

1. Amadio PC: Current concepts review: Pain dysfunction syndromes, *J Bone Joint Surg (Am)* 1988; 70A:944–945.
2. Boswick JA: Management of the burned hand. *Hand Clinics* 1990; 6:298.
3. Boyes JH: *Bunnell's Surgery of the Hand*, ed 5. Philadelphia, JB Lippincott, 1970.
4. Breen TF, Gelberman RH, Jupiter JB: Intraarticular fractures of the basilar joint of the thumb. *Hand Clinics* 1988; 4:491–501.
5. Bunnell S: Preface to First Edition in Boyes JH: *Bunnell's Surgery of the Hand*, ed 5. Philadelphia, JB Lippincott, 1970, p vii.
6. Burton RI, Pelligrini VD: Surgical management of basal joint arthritis of the thumb. II. Ligament reconstruction with tendon interposition arthroplasty. *J Hand Surg (Am)* 1986; 11A:324–332.
7. Cain Jr. JE, Shepler TR, Wilson MR: Hamatometacarpal fracture-dislocation: classification and treatment. *J Hand Surg (Am)* 1987; 12A:762–767.
8. Evans RB: Therapeutic management of extensor tendon injuries. *Hand Clinics* 1986; 2:157–169.
9. Flynn JE: *Hand Surgery*, ed 3. Baltimore, Williams & Wilkins, 1982.
10. Gelberman RH, Hergenroeder PT, Hargens AR, et al: The carpal tunnel syndrome: A study of carpal canal pressures. *J Bone Joint Surg (Am)* 1981; 63A:380–383.
11. Gerhart TN: Fractures in the elderly, in Rowe JW, Besdine RW (eds): *Geriatric Medicine*. Boston, Little, Brown, 1988.
12. Gillespie RW: personal communication, 1991.
13. Green DP: *Operative Hand Surgery*, ed 2. New York, Churchill Livingstone, 1988.
14. Herbert TJ: *The Fractured Scaphoid*. St Louis, Quality Medical Publishing, 1990.
15. House JH, Fidler MO: Frostbite of the hand, in Green DP (ed): *Operative Hand Surgery*, New York, Churchill Livingstone, 1988, pp 2165–2174.
16. Kanavel AB: *Infections of the Hand*, ed 7. Philadelphia, Lea & Febiger, 1943, pp 241–242.
17. Koh HK: Cutaneous melanoma. *N Engl J Med* 1991; 325:171–182.
18. Lamb DW, Kuczynski K: *The Practice of Hand Surgery*. London, Blackwell Scientific, 1981.
19. Lankford LL: Reflex sympathetic dystrophy, in Green DP: *Operative Hand Surgery*, ed 2. New York, Churchill Livingstone, 1988, pp 633–663.
20. Lichtman DM: *The Wrist and Its Disorders*, Philadelphia, WB Saunders, 1988.
21. Mikic Z: Age-related changes in the triangular fibro-

cartilage complex of the wrist joint, *J Anat* 1978; 126:367–384.

22. Peimer CA, Medige J, Eckert BS, et al: Destructive synovitis following silicone arthroplasty. *J Hand Surg (Am)* 1986; 11A:624–638.

23. Reyes FA, Latta LL: Conservative management of difficult phalangeal fracture. *Clinical Orthop* 1987; 214:23–30.

24. Richman JA, Gelberman RH, Rydevik BL, et al: Carpal tunnel syndrome: Morphologic changes after release of the carpal ligament. *J Hand Surg (Am)* 1989; 14A:852–857.

25. Scher RK, Daniel CR: *Nails: Diagnosis and Therapy.* Philadelphia, WB Saunders, 1990.

26. Schneider LH: *Flexor Tendon Injuries.* Boston, Little, Brown, 1985.

27. Scholer SG, Potter JF, Burke WJ: Does the Williams manual test predict service use among subjects undergoing geriatric assessment?. *J Am Geriatr Soc* 1990; 38:762–772.

28. Smith RJ: Tendon transfers following trauma or ischemic necrosis, in Smith RJ (ed): *Tendon Transfers of the Hand and Forearm,* Boston, Little, Brown, pp 263–285.

29. Smith RJ, Atkinson RE, Jupiter JB: Silicone synovitis of the wrist. *J Hand Surg (Am)* 1985; 10A:47–60.

30. Sober AJ, Fitzpatrick TB, Mihm MC: Early recognition of cutaneous melanoma. *JAMA* 1979; 242:2795–2799.

31. Taleisnik J: *The Wrist.* New York, Churchill Livingstone, 1985.

32. Weber ER: A rational approach for the recognition and treatment of Colle's fracture. *Hand Clinics.* 1987; 3:1.

33. Wehbe MA, Schneider LA: Mallet fractures. *J Bone Joint Surg (Am)* 1984; 66A:658–669.

34. Van Beek AL, Kassan MA, Adson MH, et al: Management of acute fingernail injuries. *Hand Clinics* 1990; 6:23–35.

35. Zook EG: Discussion of "management of acute fingernail injuries." 1990; 6:37–38.

Chapter 15

Hand Injuries: A Rehabilitation Perspective

Sam Dovelle, O.T.

Patricia K. Heeter, M.S., O.T.

ANATOMY

Volumes have been dedicated to describing the anatomy of the hand; often, separate chapters are required to describe the individual complexities of its anatomic structures. This chapter provides a brief review of hand anatomy and highlights the individual structures altered by the aging process. Anatomic structures both intrinsic and extrinsic to the hand are described to provide the reader with a practical understanding of the hand anatomy. The reader is urged to consult other references for more extensive information.

The hand normally functions to grasp, manipulate, stabilize, and release objects. These activities are carried out through a complex interplay of bones, joints, muscles, tendons, ligaments, and nerves. With age, prolonged use, and continuous demands, this finely tuned interplay becomes disrupted. The muscles lose strength, the bones become brittle, the joints become worn and narrowed, ligaments become less elastic, and nerves may become less tactilely discriminate.

The Thumb

The thumb consists of the first metacarpal and two phalanges (proximal and distal). The thumb functions as a separate unit from the other digits. Its most important function is its ability to oppose the fingers. The carpometacarpal joint of the thumb is classified as a saddle joint with reciprocal convex and concave surfaces formed by the trapezium and the base of the first metacarpal. Motions at this joint include flexion (+30/15 degrees), palmar and radial abduction, and opposition. The metacarpophalangeal joint of the thumb is a condylar joint formed by the head of the metacarpal, the base of the proximal phalanx, and two sesamoid bones. This joint is capable of extension and flexion (0 to 60 degrees). The metacarpophalangeal joint also exhibits some lateral movement produced by the adductor pollicis brevis. This lateral movement and collateral ligament flexibility is markedly restricted in the aged. The interphalangeal joint of the thumb is a hinge joint formed by the head of the proximal phalanx and the base of the distal phalanx. This joint is capable of extension and flexion (0 to 80 degrees).[1, 22, 37]

The Fingers

Each of the four fingers consists of one metacarpal, three phalanges, and four joints. The finger joint capsules function as a unit, which allows for a variance in the range of motion. With prolonged use and excessive demand, as often seen in aging, the joint capsules change. The articular surfaces can become irregular and the ligaments can retract or stretch.[55]

The carpometacarpal joints of digits 2 to 4 are plane joints and allow for flexion and extension. The degree of motion noted in these individual joints is dependent on the articulating surfaces between the metacarpals and carpals. This explains the restricted movement in the second and third carpometacarpal joints and the increased mobility of the fourth and fifth carpometacarpal joints. The carpometacarpal joint of the fifth digit has an articulating surface similar to that of the first carpometacarpal joint and also allows for some rotation of the metacarpal as well as flexion and extension.

The finger's metacarpophalangeal joints are condylar and are formed by the irregular spheroid head of the metacarpal and the base of the proximal phalanx. Joint stability is provided by the radial and ulnar collateral ligaments and the volar plate. Owing to the irregular shape of the metacarpal head and the eccentric placement of the collateral ligaments, the metacarpophalangeal joint is most stable and is at its greatest length when at approximately 70 degrees of flexion. This provides the rationale for splinting the metacarpophalangeal joint in flexion during prolonged periods of immobilization. Normal motion in the metacarpophalangeal joint is extension and flexion (0 to 90 degrees) as well as adduction and abduction.

The finger's interphalangeal joints are bicondylar joints. The proximal interphalangeal joint is formed by the head of the proximal phalanx and the base of the middle phalanx. The proximal interphalangeal joint allows for extension and flexion (0 to 100 degrees). The distal interphalangeal joint is formed by the head of the middle phalanx and the base of the distal phalanx. The distal interphalangeal joint allows for extension and flexion (0 to 70 degrees). Stability of these joints is provided by the concentric bony attachment of the radial and ulnar collateral ligaments. The volar plate of the proximal interphalangeal joint with its bony attachment provides further stability of the joint by preventing proximal interphalangeal joint hyperextension. The volar plate of the distal interphalangeal joint has a capsular attachment that allows for hyperextension of the joint.[1, 37, 55]

Muscles of the Hand

Muscles that act on the hand or digits are classified in two categories: intrinsic and extrinsic. Intrinsic muscles are those 18 muscles that originate and insert within the hand and/or digits. The nine extrinsic muscles have their point of origin and muscle bellies proximal to the hand. The delicate balance of both the intrinsic and extrinsic muscles allows for in-

tricate performance of the hand for a variety of gross and fine motor tasks. Both cross-sectional and longitudinal studies report grip strength declines beginning after 50 years of age. Contributing factors for this decline in strength include chronic disease, osteoarthritis of the hand, decreased physical activity, decreased motivation, and changes in the muscle tissue itself.[30]

Intrinsic Muscles.—The thenar muscle group consists of four intrinsic muscles that act on the thumb and hand: the abductor pollicis brevis, the flexor pollicus brevis, the opponens pollicis, and the adductor pollicus. These muscles act to adduct and abduct the thumb's CMC joint, rotate the first metacarpal into opposition, and flex the thumb's MCP joint. The four dorsal and three palmar interosseous muscles are located between the metacarpals. These are numbered in the radial-to-ulnar direction. The palmar interossei act to adduct the second, fourth, and fifth metacarpals; The dorsal interossei radially abduct the second and third metacarpals as well as ulnarly abduct the third and fourth metacarpals.

There are four lumbrical muscles, which are numbered in a radial-to-ulnar direction. The lumbricales act to moderate the extension and flexion forces on the fingers via their origination on the flexor digitorum profundus tendons and their insertion on the extensor hood mechanism.

The last three intrinsic muscles of the hand are the hypothenar muscles. The hypothenar eminence affects the fifth digit and hand. The abductor digiti minimi, the flexor digiti minimi, and the opponens digiti minimi comprise the hypothenar muscle group.

Table 15–1 presents specific origins, insertions, innervations, and actions of the thenar muscle group, the interosseous muscles, and the hypothenar muscle group.

Extrinsic Muscles.—There are four extrinsic muscles originating in the forearm, which act on the thumb. The flexor pollicis longus, extensor pollicis longus, extensor pollicis brevis, and the abductor pollicis longus. The extensor pollicis brevis, extensor pollicis longus, and abductor pollicis longus originate in the deep dorsal musculature of the forearm. The extensor pollicis brevis and abductor pollicis longus pass through the first dorsal compartment prior to inserting on the thumb. The flexor pollicis longus originates in the deep volar musculature of the forearm and passes through the carpal canal to its insertion point on the thumb. Prior to its distal insertion on the thumb, the extensor pollicis longus

TABLE 15–1.

Intrinsic Muscles of the Hand*

Muscle	Origin	Insertion	Innervation	Action
Abductor digiti minimi	Pisiform bone, tendon of ulnar flexor muscle of wrist	Medial side of base of proximal phalanx of little finger	Ulnar	Abducts little finger
Abductor pollicis brevis	Tubercles of scaphoid and trapezium, flexor retinaculum of hand	Lateral side of base of proximal phalanx of thumb	Median	Abducts thumb
Adductor pollicis	Oblique head second metacarpal, capitate, and trapezoid; transverse head front of third metacarpal	Medial side of base proximal phalanx of thumb	Ulnar	Adducts, opposes thumb
Flexor digiti minimi brevis	Hook of hamate bone transverse carpal ligament	Medial side of proximal phalanx of little finger	Ulnar	Flexes little finger
Flexor pollicis brevis	Tubercle of trapezium, flexor retinaculum	Lateral side of base of proximal phalanx of thumb	Median, ulnar	Flexes, adducts thumb
Interossei dorsales	Each by two heads from adjacent sides of metacarpal bones	Extensor tendons of second, third, and fourth fingers	Ulnar	Abduct, flex proximal, extend middle and distal phalanges
Interossei palmares	Sides at first, second, fourth and fifth metacarpal bones	Extensor tendons of first, second, fourth and fifth fingers	Ulnar	Adduct, flex proximal, extend middle and distal phalanges
Lumbricales	Tendons of deep flexor muscle of fingers	Extensor tendons of four lateral fingers	Median ulnar	Flex MCP joints extend middle and distal phalanges
Opponens pollicis	Tubercle of trapezium flexor retinaculum	Lateral side of first metacarpal	Median	Opposes, flexes thumb
Opponens digiti minimi	Hook of hamate bone	Front of fifth metacarpal	Ulnar	Abducts, flexes, rotates fifth metacarpal

*From *Dorland's Pocket Medical Dictionary*, ed 24. Philadelphia, W. B. Saunders, 1989. Used by permission.

passes through the third dorsal compartment, taking a 45 degree turn at Lister's tubercle (Table 15–2).[2, 36]

There are two extrinsic flexors of the fingers. The flexor digitorum profundus and the flexor digitorum superficialis tendons originate in the middle and deep layers of the volar musculature of the forearm (see Table 15–2). The muscle bellies of each divide into four bundles at the level of the distal third of the forearm and pass through the carpal canal to insert in the fingers. These two flexor tendons, along with the flexor pollicis longus, glide through individual flexor sheaths. At specific intervals, the sheaths thicken and form pulley systems that hold the tendon close to the bones and joints of the digits (Fig 15–1). There are five anular pulleys beginning at the metacarpophalangeal joint and three cruciate pulleys.[20, 31] The flexor tendons (and flexor tendon injuries) are often associated with five defined zones in the hand and wrist. Zone 1 originates distal to the flexor digitorum superficialis tendon insertion at the middle phalanx and includes the entire distal pha-

lanx. Zone 2 includes the A1 pulley and extends distally to include the insertion of the flexor digitorum tendon. This zone is commonly referred to as "no man's land" owing to the reported unfavorable postoperative results following tendon reconstruction in this zone. Zone 3 begins at the distal border of the transverse carpal ligament and extends distally not to include the A1 pulley. Zones 4 and 5 are in the wrist and forearm. Zone 4 includes the carpal canal and zone 5 lies proximal to the canal.

There are three long extensors of the fingers, which originate in the superficial and deep layers of the forearm's dorsal musculature (see Table 15–2). The extensor digitorum communis splits into four tendons prior to passing through the fourth dorsal compartment and inserting on the fingers. The extensor digiti minimi passes through the fifth dorsal compartment and inserts on the fifth finger. The extensor indicis proprius also passes through the fourth dorsal compartment with the extensor digitorum tendons and inserts on the second finger.[35]

TABLE 15–2.

Extrinsic Muscles of the Hand*

Muscle	Origin	Insertion	Innervation	Action
Abductor pollicis longus	Posterior surface of radius and ulna	Lateral side of base of first metacarpal bone and trapezium	Posterior interosseous	Abducts, extends thumb
Extensor digitorum	Lateral epincondyle of humerus	Extensor expansion of four medial fingers	Deep branch of radial	Extends wrist joint and phalanges
Extensor indicis	Posterior surface of ulnar interosseous membrane	Extensor expansion of index finger	Posterior interosseous	Extends index finger
Extensor digiti minimi	Lateral epincondyle of humerus	Extensor aponeurosis of little finger	Deep branch of radial	Extends little finger
Extensor pollicis longus	Posterior surface of ulnar and interosseous membrane	Back of distal phalanx of thumb	Posterior insterosseous	Extends, adducts thumb
Extensor pollicis brevis	Posterior surface radius	Back of proximal phalanx of thumb	Posterior interosseous	Extends thumb
Flexor digitorum superficialis	Humeroulnar head-medial epincondyle of humerus, coronoid process of ulna; radial head-anterior border radius	Sides of middle phalanges of four medial fingers	Median	Flexes middle phalanges
Flexor digitorum profundus	Shaft of ulna, coronoid process interosseous membrane	Bases of distal phalanges of four medial fingers	Anterior interosseous ulnar	Flexes distal phalanges
Flexor pollicis longus	Anterior surface of radius, medial repincondyle of humerus, coronoid process of ulna	Base of distal phalanx of thumb	Anterior interosseous	Flexes thumb

*From *Dorland's Pocket Medical Dictionary*, ed 24. Philadelphia, W. B. Saunders, 1989. Used by permission.

Nerves of the Hand

The innervations of the hand originate from the anterior horn cells of the seventh cervical to the first thoracic spinal cord levels. The median, radial, and ulnar nerves are the three peripheral nerves that innervate the intrinsic and extrinsic muscles of the hand. These three peripheral nerves also provide sensory innervation to the hand. The median nerve is derived from the fifth through eighth cervical root levels of the brachial plexus. At the forearm level, the median nerve provides motor function to the flexor digitorum superficialis and the flexor digitorum profundus to the index and middle fingers. Distally, the median nerve passes through the carpal tunnel in the wrist providing motor function to the flexor digitorum superficialis and the flexor digitorum profundus to the index and middle fingers. Distally, the median nerve passes through the carpal tunnel in the wrist providing motor function to the opponens pollicis, superficial head of the flexor pollicis brevis, abductor pollicis brevis, and the first and second lumbrical muscles. Sensory innervation from

the median nerve extends from the palmar aspect of the tips of the thumb, index and long fingers, and the radial aspect of the ring finger proximally to the wrist, as well as the dorsal tips of the same fingers.[58, 61]

The ulnar nerve is derived from the eighth cervical and first thoracic roots. Extrinsically, it provides motor function to the flexor digitorum profundus of the ring finger and small finger. Distally, the ulnar nerve passes through Guyon's canal at the wrist and provides intrinsic motor innervation to the hypothenar muscles, the third and fourth lumbricales, palmar and dorsal interossei, and the adductor pollicis. Sensory innervation from the ulnar nerve extends from the palmar and dorsal aspects of the tips of the small finger and the ulnar half of the ring finger proximally to the wrist.[58, 61, 62]

The last of the three peripheral nerves to the hand, the radial nerve, is derived from the fifth through the eighth cervical roots. Extrinsically, the radial nerve provides motor innervation to the extensors of the thumb, the abductor pollicis longus, and the extensors of the fingers. There is no intrinsic

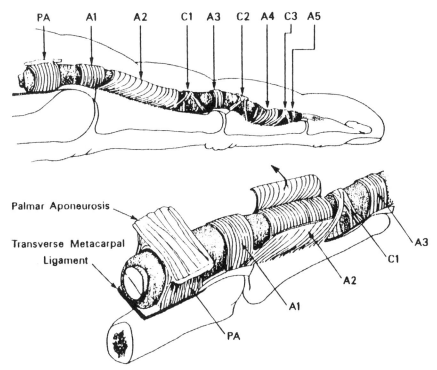

FIG 15–1.
The finger flexor tendon sheath and pulley system. (From Doyle JR: *J Hand Surg (Am)* 1988; 13A:473. Used by permission.)

motor innervation supplied by the radial nerve. Sensory innervation from the radial nerve involves the dorsum of the thumb and extends proximally from the distal interphalangeal joint level on the dorsal aspect of the radial three quarters of the hand.[58, 61]

Blood Supply of the Hand

The radial and ulnar arteries provide the blood supply to the hand through the superficial and deep palmar arches. The superficial palmar arch is a continuation of the ulnar artery and is completed by the palmar or digital branches of the radial artery. This superficial arch provides the blood supply to the thumb, index and middle fingers, and radial aspect of the ring finger via the digital arteries. The deep palmar arch is a continuation of the radial artery and provides the blood supply to the ulnar aspect of the ring finger and to the small finger via the digital arteries.[61, 62, 68, 69]

Two sets of veins provide the venous drainage system for the hand. One set of veins lies superficially on the dorsum of the hand and the other travels with the arteries. An interruption in the venous system via disease or injury can result in marked edema of the hand, which may ultimately affect hand function.

EVALUATION OF THE HAND

The thorough assessment of hand function is the foundation for all treatments. Prior to evaluating the hand, it is important to gather baseline information to appreciate the demands placed on the hand and the level of present hand function. These data, which directly impact on future treatment planning, should include patient's age, hand dominance, past medical history of injury or disease, vocational and avocational interests, as well as the patient's present life-style and habits.[2, 3, 5, 38, 64] The therapist must also critically observe the patient's hand posturing, joint and skin integrity, and functional movement patterns during each phase of the evaluation and treatment process.[4, 38]

When evaluating a patient postoperatively or posttraumatically, it is important to identify when the surgery was performed or when the accident occurred. Understanding the mechanism of injury and how the trauma occurred is helpful in realizing the extent of the injury and the biologic state of the tissues. This is critical in deciphering the approximate stage of wound healing and the formulation of a rehabilitation regimen that correlates with each stage of wound healing. A good, working knowledge of the stages of healing is fundamental in determining the appropriate time frames for rest and immobilization, controlled motion, or functional training of the involved digit or hand.

In evaluations associated with nontraumatic pathologies a knowledge of when the symptoms began and any changes in the symptomatology is helpful in pinpointing chronic or acute problems as well as forecasting responses to therapeutic intervention. Understanding the patient's perceptions of any resultant functional limitations resulting from pain, swelling, loss of motion, or changes in neurovascular status is also important in setting goals and developing the most appropriate and effective therapeutic intervention.[8, 38, 56]

The physical examination of the hand should take into account the integrity of the cervical spine and the entire upper extremity. Specific evaluations of and assessment recommendations for the cervical spine, shoulder, elbow, and wrist are discussed in detail in other chapters. When examining the hand, note any scars, lesions, swelling, muscular atrophy, abnormal bony prominences, decreased joint mobility, and presence of deformities. If only one hand is injured, compare the injured hand to the uninvolved hand.

Skin Integrity, Color, and Temperature

Begin by inspecting the skin integrity, color, and temperature. Palpate the skin. Note thickness, mobility, callus formation, and presence of fluid accumulation. The palmar skin is typically more durable, irregular, and thick than the dorsal skin, allowing traction for prehension. The dorsal skin of the hand is loose and mobile. The subcutaneous tissues on the dorsum of the hand contain the majority of the hand's lymphatic drainage system; it is important, therefore, to assess fluid accumulation in the dorsum of the hand, as this may be indicative of impaired lymphatic drainage system.[61] Prolonged fluid accumulation may result in an interruption in the overall functional mobility of the hand.[13, 40, 47, 59] Edema of the hand is assessed and monitored periodically using either a volumeter or tape measure. The volumeter allows for assessment of overall hand mass whereas the circumferential tape measurement technique quickly assesses individual joint swelling.[32, 38, 40, 59]

Skin color and temperature are indicative of the vascular integrity of the hand. Specific tests are used to evaluate blood supply of the hand. The more sophisticated Doppler and arteriographic tests allow

accurate monitoring of the vascular status of the hand. The Allen's test, however, can be easily performed during the primary clinical evaluation to assess blood flow to the hand. This test is performed by pressing both the ulnar and radial arteries to occlude blood flow to the hand. The blood remaining in the hand is removed by instructing the patient to repeatedly flex and extend the digits until the hand is blanched. The patient then opens the blanched hand and pressure on one of the two arteries is released. The flow of blood into the hand and refill time are observed and compared with those of the other artery.[3] Assessment of the skin viability, color, and temperature should be performed periodically during the course of treatment to ensure that the treatment techniques, exercise program, or splinting regimens are not compromising the vascular integrity of the hand.

Range of Motion

Active motion is assessed to determine if there is weak or absent motion secondary to a disease process or injury. A differentiation must be made between loss of motion resulting from joint and capsular pathology vs. musculotendinous problems. In the elderly, joint and capsular problems secondary to an articular disease process are often associated with ligamentous instability, subluxations, dislocations, and loss of joint mobility.[62] Musculotendinous problems are often associated with a disruption in length or of gliding or contractile capability of a musculotendinous unit.[48, 54]

Manual muscle tests are performed on any hand in which a loss of motor function is suspected. Evaluation of muscle tightness in the hand can be performed via the intrinsic and extrinsic muscle tightness tests.

The intrinsic muscle tightness test is performed by holding the involved digit's metacarpophalangeal joint in hyperextension while passively flexing the proximal interphalangeal joint of the same digit. The degree and relative tightness of proximal interphalangeal joint passive flexion is noted. This is compared with the degree and relative tightness of proximal interphalangeal joint passive flexion when the digit's metacarpophalangeal joint is held in flexion. Intrinsic muscle tightness is present when there is greater ease in proximal interphalangeal joint passive flexion with the metacarpophalangeal joints held in flexion.[3]

Extrinsic muscle tightness is tested by holding the involved digit's metacarpophalangeal joint in flexion while passively flexing the proximal interphalangeal joint of the same digit. The degree and relative tightness of proximal interphalangeal joint passive flexion is noted. This is compared with the degree and relative tightness of proximal interphalangeal joint passive flexion when the involved digit's metacarpophalangeal joint is held in extension. Extrinsic muscle tightness is present when there is greater ease in proximal interphalangeal joint passive flexion with the metacarpophalangeal joints held in extension.[3]

Since active and passive range of motion of the hand is often limited in the elderly, normal motion values may not accurately reflect a patient's normal functional arc of motion. It is important, therefore, whenever possible, to compare active range of motion measurements of the injured or diseased joint(s) to the contralateral uninjured side.

A universal standard goniometer designed for the hand is used to measure both active and passive range of motion. The initial measurements serve as a baseline to assess response to treatment. Active range of motion is measured first.[29] If full motion is attained, there is no need to assess passive range of motion. If there are limitations in active range of motion, passive range of motion is measured to assess the maximum motion available at each specific joint.

In the literature there are a variety of standardized techniques described for evaluating the active range of motion of the hand.[1, 11, 29] Typically, active range of motion is measured either on the dorsal or lateral aspect of the joint being measured. Each method is an accurate means of measuring the arc of joint motion. The measuring technique used and the method of recording must be consistent. This not only allows accurate documentation of the patient's response to subsequent treatments, but also allows other health care providers to interpret evaluation findings.[11, 24, 25] The arc of motion measured in the joints of the hand are recorded in degrees of extension (E) and flexion (F) and documented as E/F. Normal extension in the joints of the hand is 0 degrees; any hyperextension is recorded as a positive. For example, 10 degrees of hyperextension in the joint is recorded as +10 degrees. Refer to the literature[1, 11] for detailed information on measuring techniques of evaluation of the active and passive ranges of motion of specific joints of the hand.

Sensation

Sensation of the hand is a critical factor in evaluating function. Much of the hand's function is dependent on sensation. When sensation is limited,

function becomes disrupted and the patient risks further injury to the hand.[10, 14] A variety of tools is available for evaluating hand sensation. The capability of each tool is limited and is dependent to a certain degree on subjective interpretation.

One of the more accurate sensory tests is the Semmes-Weinstein aesthesiometer monofilament test. This test is used to assess single-point, light-touch discrimination of the hand. The test consists of 20 nylon monofilaments with calibrated force sensitivities ranging from 1.65 mg to 6.65 mg. Each monofilament bends at a specific force, thus lending to testing consistency and reproducibility. With the patient's hand fully supported and vision occluded, the patient is asked to identify areas of the hand that are stimulated by the monofilament. The ability of the patient to accurately identify the area of light-touch discrimination on two nonsuccessive trials is recorded. The following grading scale is used to interpret test results: normal sensation (1.65 to 2.83 mg), diminished light touch (3.22 to 3.61 mg), diminished protective sensation (3.84 to 4.31 mg), loss of protective sensation (4.56 to 6.65 mg), and unresponsive (above 6.65 mg).[10, 14, 15, 25, 42, 67]

Static and moving two-point discrimination tests are widely used to assess a patient's ability to discriminate between two stimuli. These tests are correlated to the patient's ability to perform fine manipulative tasks.[10, 14, 15] There are several commercially available aesthesiometers or blunt-tipped calipers that can be used to test this level of sensitivity. Paper clips are not recommended for these tests since their ends have differing levels of sharpness which can skew the interpretation results.[14] Both the static and moving two-point discrimination tests are performed with the patient's hand fully supported with vision occluded. For the static two-point discrimination test, the calipers are aligned longitudinally on the volar distal tip, each digit is lightly stimulated on the radial and then ulnar side of the finger with either one or two points. Seven out of ten consistent responses is considered an accurate test result. The ability of the patient to differentiate between stimuli at increments ranging from 2 to 15 mm is recorded using the following grading scale: normal two-point discrimination, 1 to 5 mm; diminished, 6 to 10 mm; poor, 11 to 15 mm, protective, one point perceived; anesthetic, no points perceived.[10, 14] For the moving two-point discrimination test the calipers are aligned over the longitudinal axis of the finger and the two ends moved lightly, proximally to distally, over the digit. The distance between the caliper ends is increased until seven out of ten consistent responses are made. Recognition of stimulation of a distance of

2 mm between the caliper ends is considered to be normal two-point discrimination.[10]

Phalen's test (wrist flexion test) is performed to assess the possibility of median nerve compression at the carpal tunnel. This test is performed with the forearms held vertically and the wrists dropped into full flexion for 1 minute. A positive test result is recorded if the patient complains of numbness, tingling, or aching of the thumb, index, middle, or ring fingers.[3] The amount of time between initiation of the test and onset of dysesthesias is recorded and used as a comparison with future assessments.

Tinel's test is performed by tapping distally to proximally along a nerve pathway. Any paresthesias in the nerve distribution are referred to as Tinel's sign. This sign may be an indication of regeneration of sensory axons (repair of nerve lacerations) or of partial nerve lesions or compressions (e.g., peripheral neuropathies). The location of the Tinel's sign is measured from a consistent anatomical landmark. Subsequent measurements are to be compared to the initial measurement to annotate advancement of the level of Tinel's sign.[10]

When evaluating functional sensibility following nerve injuries, other subjective tests are also helpful in determining the presence of protective sensation, temperature perception, light touch, deep pressure, and tactile gnosis. These include: sharp-dull, hot-cold, nongraded material stimulation (e.g., cotton, feather, eraser, etc.), and localization of touch.

Grip and Pinch Strength

The gross grasp strength of the hand serves as a baseline for assessing a patient's response to treatment. A variety of instruments are available to assess grip strength but the Jamar dynamometer is the most commonly used tool (Fig 15–2). Since this dynamometer is adjustable to five different grip-size settings, several techniques for evaluating grip strength are used. Normative data are available for comparison when testing a patient using either the second or third grip setting.[44–46, 57] Typically, this test is performed using either the average of three trials using the same handle position or a single measurement for each of the five handle positions.[3] The right and left hands are measured alternately to diminish fatigue factors and to have bilateral measurements as a basis of comparison. Maximal effort can also be assessed using all five dynamometer settings. A normal bell-shaped curve is exhibited when a patient is eliciting maximal effort. A flat curve is noted when a patient is exerting less than maximal effort.[3, 59, 60]

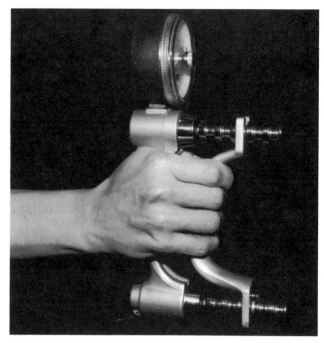

FIG 15–2.
The Jamar dynamometer, used for the evaluation of grip strength in the hand.

When evaluating the grip strength of an elderly person with significant hand impairment, it may be impossible to obtain baseline data using a dynamometer. A sphygmomanometer is an alternate means of obtaining grip strength measurements. The sphygmomanometer is rolled to 5 cm in diameter and then inflated to 50 mm Hg. The patient is instructed to maximally squeeze the cuff and the therapist records the change in millimeters of mercury from the original 50 mm Hg as the strength measurement.[64]

Pinch strength is evaluated using commercially available pinch meters. A variety of pinch prehensions are evaluated to provide the evaluator with a general understanding of the patient's potential for hand function. The pinch prehensions most often evaluated include: lateral/key, tip-to-tip, and three-jaw chuck pinch (Fig 15–3).[3] Lateral/key pinch is performed with the pad of the thumb against the radial aspect of the distal two thirds of the index finger. Tip-to-tip pinch is performed with the tip of the thumb's volar pad against the volar tip of the index finger. Three-jaw chuck pinch is performed with the volar tip of the thumb against the volar tips of the index and middle fingers. Each pinch prehension is repeated three times and the average of the three trials is recorded in pounds or kilograms.[26]

During the initial evaluation and subsequent assessments of both gross grasp and pinch prehension, the patient is to be in a standardized posi-

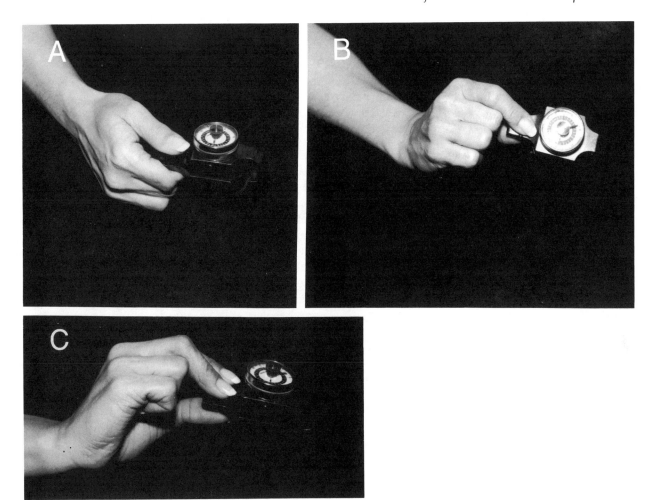

FIG 15–3.
Evaluation of pinch strength. **A,** assessment of lateral/key pinch; **B,** tip-to-tip pinch; **C,** chuck pinch.

tion.[65] The most commonly used position is with the patient seated and the arm unsupported and adducted with the elbow flexed to 90 degrees. Appropriate rest intervals between trials should also be considered an important variable in interpreting the evaluation results.[45, 65]

Dexterity

Hand dexterity evaluations provide the examiner with information regarding the patient's ability to combine strength, active motion, and sensation for successful completion of a task. Standardized tests to assess hand dexterity are available. Normative data for these test instruments are based on standardization of administration and equipment. When comparing a patient's performance with a specific set of norms, it is imperative that the examiner ensure that the testing conditions were the same as those outlined in the test instructions. If there is a deviation in any aspect of the test, the normative information is invalid for documentation purposes.[5, 24] The most commonly used dexterity tests include the Minnesota rate of manipulation test (MRMT), the Jebsen hand function test (JHFT), the Purdue pegboard test (PPT), the Crawford small parts dexterity test and the Bennett hand-tools dexterity test.

The Minnesota rate of manipulation test measures manual dexterity for unilateral turning, placing, displacing, turning and placing, and for bilateral turning and placing.[50] This test provides limited information on a patient's endurance, coordination, and functional sensibility. It cannot be used, however, as a predictor of job performance or successful completion of activities of daily living (ADL). Another disadvantage of the MRMT is that successful completion of this test is dependent upon mobility of the entire upper extremity and trunk.[4]

The Jebsen hand function test consists of **seven**

timed subtests that measure the ability to perform unilateral manipulative tasks with common objects. The test materials are collected and assembled by the therapist. Standardized instructions are used for administration of the test. The JHFT measures a person's ability to write, turn pages, pick up, release, and stack objects (pennies, paper clips, bottle caps, checkers, cans), and manipulate a spoon.[34] Normative data are based solely on task completion time and do not take into account coordination of movement, substitution patterns or bilateral manipulative ability.[4, 5] As with the MRMT, successful completion of the JHFT requires trunk stability and upper extremity coordination and mobility.

The Purdue pegboard test assesses unilateral and bilateral fine manipulation of small washers, pins, and collars. There are four subtests for the PPT: right-hand prehension test, left-hand prehension test, prehension test with both hands, and assembly test. Each subtest is timed and a score is derived from either a single trial or three repetitions of each subtest.[66] Information regarding fingertip sensibility and fine prehension ability can be obtained using this test. A disadvantage of the PPT is that the norms are based on a select population of factory workers, college students and veterans. Normative data for the PPT therefore cannot be generalized to the elderly population.[4, 5]

The Crawford small parts dexterity test and the Bennett hand-tools dexterity test assess a patient's ability to manipulate small objects with tools. The patient is required to use both hands simultaneously for completion of these tests.[7, 12] For both tests the normative data are limited to a specific population. The tasks measured in these tests can be equated to many job skills, but the results alone cannot be used as a predictor of successful job performance.[4, 5]

Other observational and nonstandardized activities can be used to assess hand function. These include physical capacity evaluations and performance of specific vocational tasks, avocational tasks, and activities of daily living. The selection of these activities is based on the patient's individual life-style and daily performance activities as well as the treatment goals jointly established between the patient and the therapist. Performance of nonstandardized assessments must be reproducible and documented in measurable terms. This serves as a basis of comparison for future assessments and allows for a more objectively verifiable annotation of progress.

TREATMENT OF THE HAND

Arthritis

Of the many hand injuries and diseases associated with the geriatric population, one of the most predominant is osteoarthritis. Osteoarthritis has been characterized as joint failure.[56] It is a degenerative joint disease in which there is a progressive loss of articular cartilage accompanied by new bone formation and capsular fibrosis. The etiology and pathophysiology of this degenerative joint process are not fully understood. Symptoms may be associated with repetitive stressful use of the hand or may be secondary to a specific joint injury, infection, or metabolic deficit.[39, 56, 62] In the hands, the most commonly affected joints are the distal and proximal interphalangeal joints of the fingers, and the thumb carpometacarpal and metacarpophalangeal joints. Nodule formation at the distal interphalangeal joint (Heberden's nodes) and the proximal interphalangeal joints (Bouchard's nodes) is common. Cystic lesions may also form just beneath the joint surface.[62] Other complications of osteoarthritis are joint instability, pain, inflammation, and stiffness. There is a loss of active or passive range of motion resulting in decreased function and ultimately in deformity.[39, 56, 62]

Although the incidence of osteoarthritis is much more prevalent, rheumatoid arthritis is a disease process that also frequently affects the elderly population. Rheumatoid arthritis is an inflammatory process that affects the synovium and leads to joint destruction. The disease is progressive and its severity is highly variable. The onset of symptoms may be acute and rapidly progressive or there may be a slow and gradual progression of symptoms. The main symptoms include morning stiffness, muscle fatigue, and hot, swollen, painful joints. Joint contractures and deformities often are secondary complications of rheumatoid arthritis.[48] Since this a systemic polyarthritic condition, the patient with rheumatoid arthritis requires a very time-intensive and thorough occupational therapy treatment regimen.

Hand involvement by rheumatoid arthritis follows a characteristic pattern. The disease process affects all joints of the hand with the exception of the distal interphalangeal joints. The main hand deformities secondary to rheumatoid arthritis are ulnar drift and subluxation of the metacarpophalangeal joints swan-neck deformities and boutonnière deformity of the fingers, "Z" deformities of the thumb, and spontaneous tendon ruptures.[48, 54]

Therapeutic intervention for conservative, nonoperative treatment of osteoarthritis and rheumatoid arthritis begins with resting the involved joints.[56] Activities that stress the joints should be identified and modified or discontinued. Instruction in joint protection and work simplification techniques is helpful in encouraging the patient to perform routine tasks more proficiently and with less stress to the joints. Specific principles of joint protection should be reviewed with the patient. These principles are as follows:

1. Respect pain. The patient must learn to distinguish between a debilitating pain that can exacerbate symptoms vs an uncomfortable pain associated with a particular activity. Activities are to be modified based on the level and extent of pain experienced.

2. Balance activity and rest. A patient's daily activity schedule must be outlined and modified to ensure the proper planning, pacing, and prioritization of activities. Daily routines must incorporate adequate time for rest of involved joints.

3. Employ work simplification techniques. Patients are encouraged to use proper body mechanics, and to arrange their living quarters and daily routines to minimize unnecessary use of energy and unnecessary stress on joints.

4. Maintain strength and range of motion. The patient is encouraged to maintain at least minimal involvement in the majority of self-care tasks to preserve active range of motion. Daily activities may be supplemented with active range of motion exercises targeted for specific joints.

5. Avoid positions of deformity. Positions or motions that stress the joints toward positions of deformity are to be avoided or eliminated. Ulnar stresses, twisting motions, and lateral pinch forces are to be avoided.

6. Use stronger muscles and larger joints. The patient is taught adaptive techniques in which less stress is placed on the smaller joints and weaker muscles of the hand. Items should be carried close to the body or cradled in the entire arm to distribute loads rather than relying on the smaller muscles and joints of the hand to bear the entire load.

7. Use adaptive equipment and splints. The patient is provided with information on specific adaptive devices that are helpful in reducing or eliminating positions of deformity or unnecessary stress on smaller joints. Splints are fabricated as indicated to preserve joint integrity and avoid positions of deformity.

8. Avoid activities that cannot be interrupted or stopped: Strenuous activities that may cause severe pain or joint stress should be avoided. Activities such as lifting a small child or carrying a hot pan should be discouraged since the patient not only risks danger of joint stress, but also risks injury to others or further injury to himself if the hand cannot withstand the joint forces.

9. Avoid sustained positions. Sustained gripping should be eliminated. The patient is encouraged to use frequent rests or adaptive equipment to avoid static positions that facilitate joint stress and muscle fatigue.

Splinting regimens are commonly used in treatment of the arthritic hand. The type of splint fabricated is based on the desired therapeutic goal and the patient's level of cognition and compliance. For the arthritic hand, splints are used to rest inflamed joints, maintain proper joint alignment, improve functional control, and support weak structures. The most commonly used splints include the resting hand splint, ulnar deviation splint, tripoint proximal interphalangeal joint splint, and thumb spica splint. Each splint should be fabricated to minimize interference with uninvolved joint function and maximize independence in activities of daily living. As with any splinting regimen, the patient is provided with instructions on the splint wear times, splint care procedures, donning and doffing procedures, and skin precautions.

Moist heat modalities such as warm water soaks or paraffin baths are used in the treatment of the nonacute arthritic hand. Contraindications for using heat on an arthritic hand include acute exacerbation of joint inflammation, peripheral neuropathies or other sensory disturbances, skin irritations, and open wounds.[56] Gentle range-of-motion exercises of all digits are to be performed following the application of moist heat. Exercises should include active, active assistive, or passive exercises in all anatomic planes of motion. The number and frequency of exercises varies from patient to patient, but five to ten repetitions of each motion two to three times daily is considered a safe starting point.[56]

Patient information pamphlets are available from many of the local community chapters of the Arthritis Foundation. These pamphlets provide patient information ranging from a description of the etiology and clinical manifestations of arthritis to specific exercises and ADL self-help techniques.

The evaluation of rheumatoid arthritis or osteoarthritis of the hand should assess:

1. Joint pathologies and joint stability
2. Joint pain and inflammation
3. Limitations in active and passive range of motion
4. Grip and pinch strength deficits
5. Limitations in hand dexterity
6. Degree of ADL independence

The treatment for rheumatoid arthritis or osteoarthritis often includes:

1. Rest of the involved joints
2. Modifications of activities that stress joints
3. Joint protection/work simplification instruction
4. Splinting regimens
5. Heat modalities followed by gentle active range-of-motion exercises
6. Resistive exercises and functional activities

Digital arthroplasty is frequently performed on the arthritic hand to eliminate pain, improve joint stability, and increase joint mobility.[49] The combination of these improvements is aimed at improving the overall functional ability of the hand. In order for functional improvement to occur, the surgical repair must be followed by a consistent and carefully monitored rehabilitation regimen.[63] Preoperative counseling is an integral part of the rehabilitation regimen. The patient is informed of the rehabilitation process, expectations, and goals. An explanation of the specific splints to be used is also emphasized. The postoperative rehabilitation program consists of an exercise regimen and either a dynamic or static splinting program. The selection of a particular rehabilitation program is based on the surgeon's discretion and directly related to the specific joint(s) being reconstructed and the surgical procedure used. If early controlled motion in a dynamic splint is initiated, rehabilitation is aimed at restoring maximal range of motion, reducing edema, monitoring splint fit, and preserving joint mobility. If static splinting or cast immobilization is used, therapy is directed towards maintaining range of motion in the uninvolved digits, reducing edema, and monitoring splint fit. Strengthening exercises are initiated only with the approval of the surgeon and should be graded based on the patient's level of function and

cooperation. In both rehabilitation regimens, the therapist must always annotate the patient's compliance and response to treatment. This information should be reviewed regularly with the patient's surgeon and the rehabilitation regimen adjusted accordingly.

Hand Weakness

Another common problem associated with the elderly population is hand weakness. Hand weakness can be attributed to single or multiple system failures to include degenerative joint disease, cervical radiculopathy, peripheral vascular disease, neurological impairments, trauma, or connective tissue disorders. Hand weakness, however, is associated most commonly with muscular dysfunction secondary to a disruption in the nerve innervation. Of the many possible nerve entrapments, carpal tunnel syndrome, compression of the median nerve in the carpal, is most prevalent. Carpal tunnel syndrome can be caused by an increased volume with the carpal canal as well as an inflammation of the median nerve itself. In the elderly, bony spurs in the carpal canal secondary to rheumatoid arthritis, osteoarthritis, or old wrist trauma may exacerbate symptoms of carpal tunnel syndrome.[69] In carpal tunnel syndrome, the patient complains of numbness, tingling, and aching of the hand, particularly in the median nerve distribution. Subjective complaints of painful dysesthesia in the hand that radiates to the shoulder are also common. These symptoms are often reported to be more intense at night and typically disrupt sleep. The patient may also complain of a general weakness and clumsiness, which results in a loss of fine motor control.[30, 53]

Physical examination may also reveal a positive Tinel's sign, a positive Phalen's test, diminished two-point discrimination in the median innervated digits and intrinsic atrophy or loss of strength of the thenar muscles.[53] Electromyographic (EMG) and nerve conduction velocity (NCV) studies also provide information regarding the extent of nerve compression. It is important to note that a negative physical examination does not negate the possibility of a compressive median neuropathy. The patient's subjective reports are a key factor in the diagnosis of carpal tunnel syndrome. Evaluation of sensory and motor function, however, may not only support the patient's subjective complaints but may provide a good baseline of the effectiveness of therapeutic interventions.

The nonoperative management of carpal tunnel

syndrome includes a static splinting program and patient instruction on ergonomically efficient body mechanics. A variety of prefabricated splints and patterns for custom-fitted thermoplastic splints is available. There are no studies that support the benefits of using a custom-made splint rather than a prefabricated splint. The choice of splint is based on availability, patient activity patterns, and patient comfort. Whether worn volarly or dorsally, the splint maintains the wrist in 15 to 30 degrees of extension and allows uninterrupted function of all digits (Fig 15–4). The splint is worn during sleep and also when the patient is engaged in activities requiring repetitive or forceful use of the hand. Restricting the active motion of the wrist may decrease the amount of compromise in the carpal canal and help to control the irritation and swelling in this area.

Instruction in joint protection and work simplification is advantageous. The patient's daily activity patterns are to be assessed and suggestions are made regarding the most ergonomically efficient method of performing specific daily activities.

If the symptoms of carpal tunnel syndrome persist despite conservative management or when there is noted muscle atrophy or sensory loss, a carpal tunnel release is performed. The wrist is immobilized for 2 to 4 weeks to allow for adequate healing of the transverse carpal ligament. During the period of wrist immobilization, patients are given a specific home exercise program to maintain joint mobility of the digits and prevent disuse atrophy of the intrinsic musculature. Gentle active range-of-motion wrist ex-

ercises are initiated following the immobilization. Graded resistive exercises can be initiated 4 weeks postsurgically. In some instances, a volar wrist splint is worn during daily activities for several more weeks to prevent reinjury to the transverse carpal ligament. In addition to range-of-motion exercises, the patient is instructed on scar massage to soften and desensitize the scar formation at the incision site. The range-of-motion and strengthening exercises, scar massage, and resumption of activity level must be carefully graded so as not to reinstate an inflammatory process that would once again compromise the median nerve in the carpal tunnel.

Ulnar nerve entrapments are also common in the elderly. Entrapments at Guyon's canal at the wrist occur secondary to prolonged inappropriate grasping of walking canes. Cubital tunnel syndrome at the elbow is typically seen in patients who are confined to a wheelchair or spend much of the day in an armchair or bed.[23, 27] These entrapments are treated conservatively using splinting regimens, exercise programs, and instruction in work simplification and joint protection techniques.

Phases of Rehabilitation

Many of the hand problems associated with aging, including joint deterioration, muscle weakness, nerve compression, and hand trauma, result in stiffness and loss of hand function. Prevention of the stiff hand is of paramount importance in the overall rehabilitation of the elderly person. Controlled-mo-

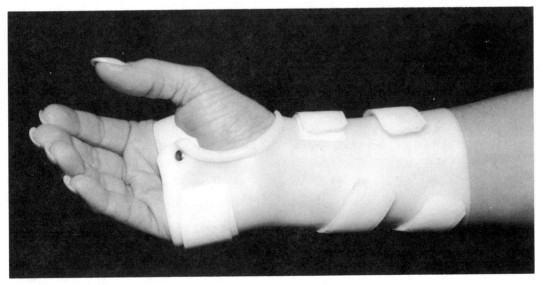

FIG 15–4.
Custom-fabricated wrist orthosis; allows for maximum digit motion and wrist stability in the management of carpal tunnel syndrome.

tion regimens are to be initiated as soon as possible.

The amount of motion or extent of passive stretch is determined based on the normal phases of wound healing. Following trauma to the hand, the wound progresses through three general phases of healing: the inflammatory phase, the proliferative phase, and the remodeling phase. Three distinct phases of rehabilitation coincide with these major phases of wound healing. These are the immobilization phase, the controlled motion phase, and the functional training phase.

The immobilization phase of rehabilitation corresponds with the inflammatory phase of wound healing. During this phase, which begins at the time of injury and subsides within several days, the injured hand or digit should be managed conservatively with rest or immobilization. Static splints or bulky compressive dressings are used most often during this phase. Edema control is the main therapeutic goal. Once the inflammation subsides, a program of controlled motion is initiated.

The controlled motion phase of rehabilitation corresponds with the proliferative phase of wound healing, which begins several days following injury and continues for 2 to 4 weeks. This phase of wound healing is characterized by a rapid and random formation of collagen fibers, which are primarily responsible for scar formation and increased tensile strength. Since collagen forms in a random formation and at a rapid rate, it is essential that the rehabilitation regimen incorporate a graded program of controlled motion through passive, active assistive, and active range of motion. A supplemental program of splinting for protection, passive stretch, and/or exercise may be initiated as indicated by the biologic state of the wound. The primary objective during the controlled motion phase of rehabilitation is to decrease adhesion formation, increase tendon gliding and tensile strength, decrease edema, and maintain joint mobility. Active, active assistive, and passive range of motion exercises of the uninvolved digits are also initiated during this phase to maintain joint mobility and decrease edema.

The functional training phase of rehabilitation corresponds with the remodeling phase of wound healing. During this phase of healing, there is an increase in the metabolic activity of the wound, which may last upwards to a year following the initial injury. The rate of metabolic activity of the remodeling scar in the elderly is slower, therefore, the length of rehabilitation necessary to restore function may be longer than the rehabilitation required for a younger person with a comparable injury. The ultimate reha-

bilitation goal during this phase of wound healing is to restore maximal independence in functional activity. Depending on the injury, the functional training phase of rehabilitation may include graded resistive activity, functional splinting, pressure garments or dressings, sensory reeducation, desensitization, and/or work hardening. Adaptive devices may be indicated during this stage of rehabilitation to maximize functional independence if an injury resulted in a permanent disability.

Communications between the therapist, surgeon, and patient are of utmost importance during each phase of rehabilitation. Patient education regarding the rehabilitation process improves the patient-therapist rapport and may increase the patient's overall cooperation in the treatment process. Progress towards the rehabilitation goals must be assessed during each treatment session. Changes in patient progress should be discussed with the surgeon and the patient. A more conservative treatment approach may be indicated for patients who are not cooperative or who have demonstrated poor cognitive understanding of the treatment regimen.

Early Controlled Motion Following Tendon Injuries

Early controlled motion regimens following flexor and extensor tendon injuries of the hand have been described in the literature.[16–19, 21, 43] With few exceptions, most treatment regimens include a period of dynamic splinting supplemented by a program of carefully controlled active and passive range-of-motion exercises. Following the repair of hand flexor tendons, the wrist and the metacarpophalangeal joint(s) of the involved digit(s) are splinted in a protective flexed position according to the surgeon's specifications and the surgical zone of injury. A dynamic traction apparatus, which substitutes for the repaired flexor tendon, is attached to the involved digit(s). The dynamic component of the splint provides the desired degree of passive flexion and is adjusted to allow for active extension of the involved digit(s) within the limits of the static component of the splint. In the elderly population there is an increased risk of joint stiffness if the joints are maintained in prolonged maximal flexion. The palmar pulley apparatus as described in the literature[17, 19] therefore is not recommended for use with this population (Fig 15–5). The splint is worn continuously for 4 weeks. Two to three days following the repair, a program of controlled active extension and passive flexion is initiated. The patient is in-

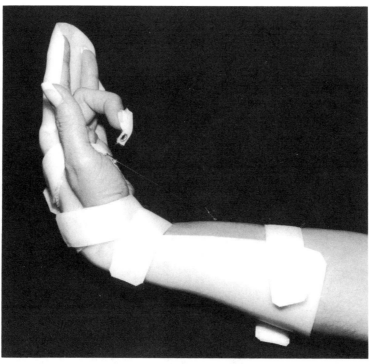

FIG 15–5.
Dynamic flexion–assist orthosis positions the wrist and metacarpophalangeal joints in flexion. The traction device provides passive flexion to the finger's joints and allows for the desired degree of active extension.

structed to actively extend the digit(s) against the rubber band traction ten times every waking hour. During the initial 2 to 3 weeks of rehabilitation, therapist-assisted passive motion of the interphalangeal joints are necessary to maintain joint mobility and prevent adhesions (Fig 15–6). When the patient demonstrates full active extension of the interphalangeal joints within the limits of the splint, the passive range-of-motion exercises are discontinued. Active extension exercises are continued. On the 28th postoperative day (or when ordered by the surgeon), active flexion exercises are initiated within the confines of the splint. Splint wear is discontinued at the end of the sixth postoperative week. Any residual stiffness is managed using gentle passive range-of-motion exercises and dynamic splinting.[17, 19]

Extensor tendon injuries distal to the proximal interphalangeal joint (mallet finger deformities) require 6 to 8 weeks of immobilization prior to the initiation of any type of exercise regimen. Rehabilitation following hand extensor tendon repairs proximal to the proximal interphalangeal joint, however, incorporate an early controlled-motion regimen. A dynamic splint and active and passive range-of-motion exercises are used to maximize ten-

don glide, maintain joint mobility, and prevent contractures. The splint is designed to maintain the wrist in 45 degrees of extension and to maintain all joints proximal to the injury in complete extension. A dynamic traction apparatus, which substitutes for the repaired extensor tendon, is attached to the involved digit(s). The dynamic component of the splint maintains the involved digit(s) in extension while at rest (Fig 15–7). The traction device is adjusted to allow for graded active flexion of the involved digit(s) within the limits of the static component of the splint. Two to three days following the repair, a program of controlled active flexion is initiated. During the first postoperative week, the patient actively flexes the metacarpophalangeal joint of the involved digit(s) 15 to 30 degrees against the rubber band traction, ten times every waking hour. Active flexion of the metacarpophalangeal joint(s) is increased weekly as follows: 30 to 45 degrees, postoperative week 2; 45 to 60 degrees, postoperative week 3; 60 degrees to full flexion, postoperative week 4. At the end of the fourth postoperative week, the patient is allowed to make a full fist and active extension is initiated. The splint is worn for protection until the completion of the fifth postoperative week. Any residual stiffness is managed using

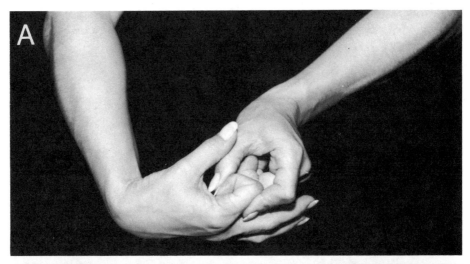

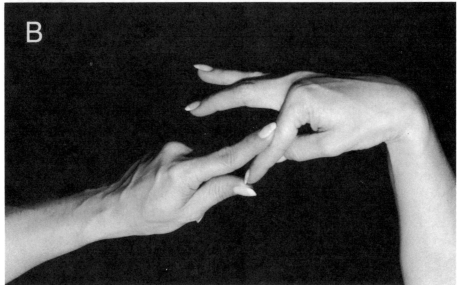

FIG 15–6.
A, passive interphalangeal joint flexion exercises. **B,** passive interphalangeal joint extension exercises to prevent joint flexion contractures following flexor tendon repair.

gentle passive range-of-motion exercises and dynamic splinting.[16, 18]

Firm scar massage using lanolin, cocoa butter, or vitamin E is initiated 2 to 3 weeks postinjury to soften and desensitize the scar. The patient is instructed to perform scar massage for a minimum of 10 to 15 minutes, three times daily. Vigorous scar massage is followed by the appropriate exercise regimen. An ice pack may be applied to the injured area if edema is noted following the scar massage or exercise regimen. The application of ice is contraindicated, however, if there is a neurologic or vascular compromise of the involved hand.

The Stiff Hand

Physiologic and psychological factors affecting the elderly such as degenerative joint disease, pain, paresis, peripheral neuropathies, vascular compromise, noncompliance, and cognitive dysfunction may complicate the rehabilitation process. Every effort must be made to design a rehabilitation program that minimizes potential complications in patients with complex medical problems. A common challenge in hand rehabilitation of the elderly is prevention of joint stiffness, persistent edema, and chronic pain syndromes. Active, active assistive, and pas-

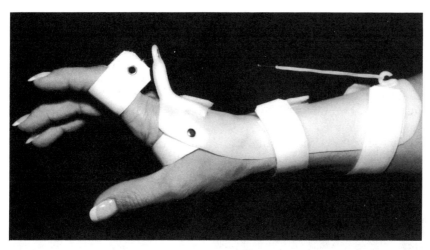

FIG 15–7.
Dynamic extension–assist orthosis positions the wrist and metacarpophalangeal joints in extension. The traction device provides passive extension to the metacarpophalan- geal joints and allows for the desired degree of active meta- carpophalangeal joint flexion.

sive range-of-motion exercises, dynamic and static splinting, therapeutic modalities, and functional activities must be systematically incorporated into the rehabilitation regimen to minimize these potential complications.

Prevention of a stiff hand begins with patient education, edema control, and therapeutic exercise during the acute phase of injury. It is important for the therapist to educate the patient regarding the nature and extent of injury, as well as the rehabilitation expectations and goals. This helps to alleviate the patient's anxiety related to the injury and encourages the patient to progress towards the restoration of function.

Acute inflammation and edema are an essential part of the healing process. Excessive and persistent edema, however, results in decreased mobility and increased joint stiffness. Ice, elevation, active range of motion, compression, and retrograde massage are the most effective ways to reduce edema in the acutely and chronically stiff hand.[6, 13, 32, 40, 41, 47]

Therapeutic cold takes the form of direct ice pack application or cold whirlpool bath. Both of these cold modalities result in a local vasoconstriction and therefore temporarily reduce inflammation and edema. Previously stated contraindications for cold application should be considered prior to using this modality.

Elevation of the injured hand above the level of the heart and active range-of-motion exercises will allow gravity to assist in venous drainage. Active range-of-motion exercises of the digits, alternating from flexion to extension, produce a pumping effect that forces the fluids from the edematous region and prevents stasis.

Intermittent compression pumps, compression wraps, air splinting, and pressure gradient garments also assist in edema reduction. The selection of a specific compression modality is dependent on the particular stage of healing, extent of edema, and patient comfort and cooperation. A combination of compression techniques may be used as deemed effective via the patient's response to treatment. Caution must be taken to ensure that the compressive forces do not cause an ischemic response. Compression must be adjusted or the compression modality changed if constriction or ischemia occurs.

Retrograde massage assists in venous and lymph flow. The massage is performed in a distal-to-proximal direction with the hand elevated. This form of edema reduction is most effective if performed several times daily. The patient or a family member should be instructed in the massage technique so that this modality can be performed at home.

Dynamic splinting is effective in regaining range of motion of the stiff hand. Factors contributing to the loss of motion include scarring, adhesions, muscle contracture, capsular tightness, and tendon and ligament shortening. The dynamic splint provides gentle, graded, and prolonged tension to the involved joint(s), which is more effective in elongating soft tissue than passive range of motion. The type of dynamic splint and the degree of force application depends on the joint(s) and soft tissues affected.[9] Several of the more commonly used dynamic splints and their functions are described in Figure 15–8.

Passive exercises are performed by the therapist in a gentle, slow, and deliberate fashion to increase range of motion. The goal of passive exercise is to move the involved joint(s) to the point of maximal stretch. The amount of passive stretch must be carefully monitored. Excessive stretching that results in persistent pain after completion of the exercise is contraindicated. The use of excessive force may damage soft tissues and reinstate an inflammatory process, resulting in increased edema and decreased joint mobility. Passive range-of-motion exercises are most effective if performed for frequent, short intervals each day. Patients may be instructed to perform passive range-of-motion exercises as part of their home program. The patient must have a thorough understanding of the exercise goals, degree of maximal tension, and potential complications of passive range of motion. The direction of motion, number of repetitions, and duration of passive exercise must be well understood by the patient prior to initiating any home program.[40] The use of continuous passive mo-

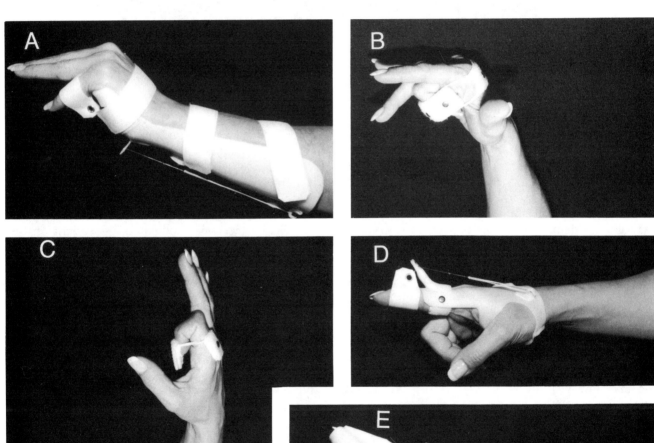

FIG 15–8.
A, dynamic metacarpophalangeal joint flexion–assist orthosis. Note the incorporation of the thumb to prevent the distal migration of the orthosis during use. **B,** dynamic proximal interphalangeal joint flexion–assist orthosis. **C,** dynamic finger flexion–assist loop; provides composite interphalangeal joint flexion. **D,** dynamic proximal interphalangeal joint extension assist orthosis; note the use of the strapping to prevent metacarpophalangeal joint hyperextension and maximize the effectiveness of the traction tension. **E,** dynamic extension–assist orthosis to provide composite extension. Used to manage stiffness resulting from extrinsic causes.

tion may be used to supplement manual passive range-of-motion exercises. The decision to use continuous passive motion must be made in coordination with the therapist, referring physician, and patient. Continuous passive motion or passive range-of-motion exercises should supplement and not replace active range-of-motion exercises.

Active range of motion is of paramount importance in restoration of function. Active range-of-motion exercises are performed on all joints of the involved extremity to maintain joint mobility, control edema, increase circulation, and prevent disuse atrophy. These exercises are initiated as early as possible in the rehabilitation process. They are performed several times each day until maximal functional use of the extremity is achieved. As with passive range-of-motion exercises, a home program is initiated only after the patient competently demonstrates the exercise program.

Resistive activities are designed to strengthen the involved extremity for maximal return of function. The activity selected and the amount of resistance applied depends on the patient's response to treatment, the type of injury, and the corresponding stage of wound healing. The resistance applied is carefully graded. Typical devices used for resistive exercises include weights, hand grippers, graded elastic tubing, therapy putty, and clothespins. A variety of work simulators and work samples are commercially available. This type of therapeutic equipment can be used for both upper extremity strengthening and ADL/work evaluation.

Functional activities are encouraged throughout the entire treatment process. New activities commence once the patient demonstrates the required skills to successfully complete a particular task. Functional activities require a combination of dexterity, coordination, range of motion, and strength. Use of functional activities as a therapeutic modality allows the therapist to realistically assess hand function.

Activities requiring simple grasp, release, and pinch prehensions should be incorporated in the treatment regimen as early as possible. This provides the patient with feedback regarding the extent of the injury and the effect of rehabilitation on functional performance. As the patient begins to use the hand for normal activities, functional limitations are identified. Therapeutic activities can be designed or modified to overcome these limitations and provide the patient with an opportunity to practice specific activities in a protected and supervised environment.

The evaluation of the stiff hand should assess:

1. Degree of swelling
2. Limitations in active and passive range of motion
3. Grip and pinch strength deficits
4. Patient's perception of pain limitations
5. Limitations in hand dexterity
6. Degree of ADL independence

The treatment of the stiff hand often includes:

1. Edema control techniques
2. Splinting regimens
3. Active, active assistive, and passive range-of-motion exercises
4. Resistive exercises and functional activities

Management of Chronic Pain Syndromes

Chronic pain is characterized by persistent pain lasting longer than 6 months. The initial onset of pain may be secondary to acute trauma (e.g., Colles' fracture, amputation, crush injury, surgery) or a specific disease process (e.g., arthritis, carpal tunnel syndrome, diabetes). Typically, pain is accompanied by diffuse swelling, stiffness, and/or sudomotor and vasomotor changes. If left untreated, secondary complications include osteoporosis, fibrosis, disuse atrophy, ischemia, and dysfunction.[51, 52] Chronic pain is accompanied by a strong psychological component owing to the stresses produced by long-term pain and the inability to perform normal ADL.[51]

There is much in the literature devoted to the clinical management of chronic pain syndromes. Although there is no one recommended treatment approach, the primary treatment goals are consistent and include symptom reduction and restoration of functional mobility. This is achieved through a combination of medical and therapeutic modalities.

Medical intervention is aimed at reducing pain using pharmaceutical and surgical measures.[52] This may include oral nonsteroid anti-inflammatory drugs (NSAIDs), corticosteroids, percutaneous injections for local anesthesia, and chemical sympathetic nerve blocks. The medication selected is based on the physician's discretion depending on the extent and duration of pain and the patient's response to previous treatment modalities. Surgical sympathectomy is performed in extreme cases where repeated chemical blocks are necessary for long-term pain relief.[52]

The most commonly used therapeutic modality for pain management is transcutaneous electrical nerve stimulation (TENS). The frequency and pulse-width application of the TENS is dependent upon the stage of the pain syndrome[28] and the patient's individual tolerance level.[52] TENS is effective in reducing pain so that other therapeutic modalities aimed at restoring function can be tolerated.[28, 51] TENS electrode placement varies depending on the degree and location of the pain. Electrodes may be placed over the involved peripheral nerve proximal to the painful area, at the perimeter, or directly over the painful area.[28] Other modalities that can be useful in pain management include massage, ice pack application, compression splinting, paraffin bath, ultrasound, muscle stimulation, and vibration.[52] Graded upper extremity weight-bearing activities that increase proprioceptive input are also effective in pain management.[52]

Once pain reduction or relief is achieved, therapeutic activities similar to those used in the management of the stiff hand must be incorporated into the treatment regimen. Passive range of motion should be used cautiously and judiciously and all other activities must be performed within the patient's pain tolerance so as not to increase the sympathetic pain response. The patient's participation in functional activities aids in reducing the psychological stresses associated with chronic pain. Each new accomplishment can be viewed as a step towards recovery and reintegration into normal activity patterns.

The evaluation of chronic pain in the hand should assess:

1. Degree of swelling
2. Limitations in active or passive range of motion
3. Vasomotor changes
4. Grip and pinch strength deficits
5. Level of muscle atrophy
6. Limitations in hand dexterity
7. Level of ADL independence

Treatment for chronic pain in the hand often includes:

1. Clinical modalities useful in pain management
2. Edema control techniques
3. Splinting regimens
4. Active, active assistive, and passive range-of-motion exercises
5. Resistive exercises and functional activities

With age, prolonged use, and continuous demands, the normal functions of the hand become disrupted. The muscles lose strength, the bones become brittle, the joints become worn and narrowed, ligaments become less elastic, and nerves may become less tactilely discriminate.

Treatment of the hand begins with a thorough evaluation. The evaluation should include information to understand the past demands placed on the hand, the level of present hand function, and the patient's perception of the problem as well as the baseline data of active and passive range of motion, sensation, strength, and dexterity. The overall effectiveness of the treatment will be dependent on the therapist's understanding of the hand's anatomy, familiarity with the pathologies associated with the geriatric patient, and appreciation of the impact of wound healing stages in the rehabilitation program.

REFERENCES

1. American Medical Association: *Guide to the Evaluation of Permanent Impairment*, ed 2. Chicago, American Medical Association, 1984.
2. American Society for Surgery of the Hand: *The Hand: Examination and Diagnosis*, ed 2. New York, Churchill Livingstone, 1983.
3. Aulicino PI, DuPuy TE: Clinical examination of the hand, in Hunter JM, Schneider LH, Mackin EJ, et al (eds): *Rehabilitation of the Hand*, ed 2. St Louis, Mosby-Year Book, 1984, pp 261–271.
4. Baxter PL, Ballard MS: Evaluation of the hand by functional tests, in Hunter JM, Schneider LH, Mackin EJ, et al (eds): *Rehabilitation of the Hand*, ed 2. St Louis, Mosby-Year Book, 1984, pp 91–100.
5. Bear-Lehman J, Colin-Abreu B: Evaluating the hand: Issues in reliability and validity. *Phys Ther* 1989;69:1025–1032.
6. Beasley RV: Principles of managing acute hand injuries, in Converse J, McCarthy J, Littler JW, et al (eds): *Reconstructive Plastic Surgery*, ed 2. Philadelphia, W.B. Saunders, 1977, pp 3000.
7. Bennett GK: *Hand Tool Dexterity Test* ed 2. New York, The Psychological Corp, 1981.
8. Brand PW: The mind and spirit in hand therapy. *J Hand Ther* 1988; 1:145–147.
9. Brand PW: The forces of dynamic splinting: Ten questions before applying a dynamic splint to the hand, in Hunter JM, Schneider LH, Mackin EJ, et al (eds): *Rehabilitation of the Hand*, ed 2. St Louis, Mosby-Year Book, 1984, pp 847–852.
10. Callahan AD: Sensibility testing: Clinical methods, in Hunter JM, Schneider LH, Mackin EJ, et al (eds): *Rehabilitation of the Hand*, ed 2. St Louis, Mosby-Year Book, 1984, pp 407–431.
11. Cambridge CA: Range of motion measurements in the hand, in Hunter JM, Schneider LH, Mackin EJ, et al (eds): *Rehabilitation of the Hand*, ed 2. St Louis, Mosby-Year Book, 1984, pp 79–90.
12. *Crawford Small Parts Dexterity Test Manual*. New York, The Psychological Corp, 1956.

13. Curtis RM: Management of the stiff hand, in Hunter JM, Schneider LH, Mackin EJ, et al (eds): *Rehabilitation of the Hand*, ed 2. St Louis, Mosby-Year Book, 1984, pp 209–215.
14. Dellon AL: Touch sensibility in the hand. *J Hand Surg (Br)* 1984; 9:11–13.
15. Dellon AL, Mackinnon SE, Crosby PM: Reliability of two-point discrimination measurement. *J Hand Surg (Am)* 1987; 12:693–696.
16. Dovelle S, Heeter PK: Early controlled mobilization following extensor tendon repair in zone V and VI of the hand. *Contemp Orthop* 1985; 11:41–44.
17. Dovelle S, Heeter PK: Early controlled motion following flexor tendon grafting. *Am J Occup Ther* 1988; 42:457–463.
18. Dovelle S, Heeter PK: Rehabilitation following extensor tendon repair using early controlled motion. *Am J Occup Ther* 1988; 43:115–119.
19. Dovelle S, Heeter PK: The Washington regimen: Rehabilitation of the hand following flexor tendon injuries. *Phys Ther* 1989; 69:1034–1040.
20. Doyle JR: Anatomy of the finger flexor tendon sheath and pulley system. *J Hand Surg (Am)* 1988; 13:473–484.
21. Duran RJ, Houser RG, Coleman CR, et al: Management of flexor tendon lacerations in zone 2 using controlled passive motion postoperatively, in Hunter JM, Schneider LH, Mackiin EJ, et al (eds): *Rehabilitation of the Hand*, ed 2. St Louis, Mosby-Year Book, 1984, pp 273–276.
22. Eaton RG, Littler WJ: A study of the basal joint of the thumb, *J Bone Joint Surg (Am)* 1969; 51:661–668.
23. Ebeling P, Gilliett RW, Thomas PK: A clinical and electrical study of ulnar nerve lesions of the hand. *J Neurol Neurosurg Psychiatr* 1960; 23:1–11.
24. Fess EE: Documentation: Essential elements of an upper extremity assessment battery, in Hunter JM, et al (eds): *Rehabilitation of the Hand*, ed 2. St Louis, Mosby-Year Book, 1984, pp 49–78.
25. Fess EE: The need for reliability and validity in hand assessment instruments. *J Hand Surg (Am)* 1986; 11:621–623.
26. Fess EE: Using research terminology correctly: Validity. *J Hand Ther* 1988; 1:148.
27. Gay JR, Love JG: Diagnosis and treatment of tardy paralysis of ulnar nerve based on a study of 100 cases. *J Bone Joint Surg (Am)* 1947; 29:1087.
28. Goldner JL, Nashold BS, Hendrix PC: Peripheral nerve electrical stimulation. *Clin Orthop* 1982; 163:33–41.
29. Hamilton GF, Lachenbruch PA: Reliability of goniometers in assessing finger joint angle. *Phys Ther* 1969; 49:465–469.
30. Harrell LE, Massey EW: Hand weakness in the elderly. *J Am Geriatr Soc* 1983; 31:223–227.
31. Hunter JM: Anatomy of flexor tendons, pulley, vincular, synovia and vascular systems, in Spinner M (ed): *Kaplan's Functional and Surgical Anatomy of the Hand*, ed 3. Philadelphia, J. B. Lippincott, 1984, pp 65–92.
32. Hunter JM, Mackin EJ: Edema and bandaging, in Hunter JM, Schneider LH, Mackin EJ, et al (eds): *Rehabilitation of the Hand*, ed 2. St Louis, Mosby-Year Book, 1984, pp 146–153.
33. Jaeger SH, Mackin EJ: Primary care of flexor tendon injuries in Hunter JM, Schneider LH, Mackin EJ, et al (eds): *Rehabilitation of the Hand*, ed 2. St Louis, Mosby-Year Book, 1984, pp 261–271.
34. Jebsen RH, Taylor N, Triegchmann R, et al: An objective and standardized test of hand function. *Arch Phys Med Rehabil* 1969; 50:311–319.
35. Kaplan EB, Hunter JM: Extrinsic muscles of the fingers, in Spinner M (ed): *Kaplan's Functional and Surgical Anatomy of the Hand*, ed 3. Philadelphia, J.B. Lippincott, 1984, pp 93–112.
36. Kaplan EB, Hunter JM: The muscles and the tendon systems of the fingers, in Spinner M (ed): *Kaplan's Functional and Surgical Anatomy of the Hand*, ed 3. Philadelphia, J.B. Lippincott, 1984, pp 53–64.
37. Kaplan EB, Riordan DC: The thumb, in Spinner M (ed): *Kaplan's Functional and Surgical Anatomy of the Hand*. ed 3. Philadelphia, J.B. Lippincott 1984, pp 113–142.
38. Kasch MC: Acute hand injuries, in Pedretti LW, Zolton B (eds): *Occupational Therapy: Practice Skills for Physical Dysfunction*, ed 3. St Louis, Mosby-Year Book, 1990, pp 477–506.
39. Labi ML, Greshman GE, Ruthey UK: Hand function in osteoarthritis. *Arch Phys Med Rehabil* 1982; 63:438–440.
40. Laseter GF: Management of the stiff hand: A practical approach. *Orthop Clin North Am* 1983; 14:749–765.
41. Laseter GF: Postoperative management of capsulotomies, in Hunter JM, et al (eds): *Rehabilitation of the Hand*, ed 2. St Louis, Mosby-Year Book, 1984, pp 246–252.
42. Levin S, Pearsall G, Ruderman RJ: Von Frey's method of measuring pressure sensibility in the hand: An engineering analysis of the Weinstein-Semmes pressure aesthesiometer. *J Hand Surg (Am)* 1978; 3:211–216.
43. Lister GD, Kleinert HE, Kutz JE, et al: Primary flexor tendon repair followed by immediate controlled mobilization. *J Hand Surg (Am)* 1977; 2:441–451.
44. Mathiowitz V, Kashman N, Volland G, et al: Grip and pinch strength: Normative data for adults. *Arch Phys Med Rehabil* 1985; 66:69–74.
45. Mathiowitz V, Rennels C, Donahue L: Effect of elbow position on grip and key pinch strength. *J Hand Surg (Am)* 1985; 10:694–697.
46. Mathiowitz V, Weber K, Volland G, et al: Reliability and validity of grip and pinch strength evaluations. *J Hand Surg (Am)* 1984; 9:222–226.
47. McEntee PM: Therapist's management of the stiff hand, in Hunter JM, et al (eds): *Rehabilitation of the Hand*, ed 2. St Louis, Mosby-Year Book, 1984, pp 216–230.
48. McKenna F, Wright V: Clinical manifestations, in Utsinger PD, et al (eds): *Rheumatoid Arthritis: Etiology, Diagnosis, Management*. Philadelphia, J. B. Lippincott, 1985, pp 283–307.
49. Millender LH, Nalebuff EA, Amadio P, et al: Interpositional arthroplasty for rheumatoid carpometacarpal joint disease. *J Hand Surg (Am)* 1978; 3:533–541.
50. *Minnesota Rate of Manipulation Test Examiner's Manual.* Circle Pines, Minn, American Guidance Services, 1969.

51. Mullins PT: Management of common chronic pain problems in the hand. *Phys Ther* 1989; 69:1050–1058.

52. Omer GE: Management of pain syndromes in the upper extremity, in Hunter JM, et al (eds): *Rehabilitation of the Hand*, ed 2. St Louis, Mosby-Year Book, 1984, pp 503–507.

53. Phalen GS: The carpal tunnel syndrome. *Clin Orthop* 1972; 83:211–228.

54. Phillips CA: Rehabilitation of the patient with rheumatoid hand involvement. *Phys Ther* 1989; 69:1091–1098.

55. Posner MA, Kaplan EB: The fingers: Osseous and ligamentous structures, in Spinner M (ed): *Kaplan's Functional and Surgical Anatomy of the Hand*, ed 3. Philadelphia, J. B. Lippincott, 1984, pp 23–50.

56. Quinet RJ: Osteoarthritis: Increasing mobility and reducing mobility. *Geriatrics* 1986; 41:36–50.

57. Schmidt RT, Towes J: Grip strength as measured by the Jamar dynamometer. *Arch Phys Med Rehabil* 1970;5:321–327.

58. Schultz RJ, Kaplan EB: Nerve supply to the muscles and skin of the hand, in Spinner M (ed): *Kaplan's Functional and Surgical Anatomy of the Hand*, ed 3. Philadelphia, J. B. Lippincott, 1984, pp 222–243.

59. Sorenson MK: The edematous hand. *Phys Ther* 1989; 69:1059–1064.

60. Stokes HM: The seriously injured hand—weakness of grip. *J Occup Med* 1983; 25:683–685.

61. Strickland JW: Anatomy and kinesiology of the hand, in Fess EE, Phillips CA (eds): *Hand Splinting: Principles and Methods*, ed 2. St Louis, Mosby-Year Book, 1987, pp 3–41.

62. Swanson AB: Pathogenesis of arthritic lesions, in Hunter JM, Schneider LH, Mackin EJ, et al (eds): *Rehabilitation of the Hand*, ed 2. St Louis, Mosby-Year Book, 1984, pp 631–637.

63. Swanson AB, deGroot-Swanson G, Leonard J: Postoperative rehabilitation programs in flexible implant arthroplasty of the digits, in Hunter JM, Schneider LH, Mackin EJ, et al (eds): *Rehabilitation of the Hand*, ed 2. St Louis, Mosby-Year Book, 1984, pp 665–680.

64. Swanson AB, Goran-Hagert C, deGroot-Swanson G: Evaluation of impairment of hand function in Hunter JM, Schneider LH, Mackin EJ, et al (eds): *Rehabilitation of the Hand*, ed 2. St Louis, Mosby-Year Book, 1984, pp 101–132.

65. Teraoka T: Studies in the perculiarity of grip strength in relation to body positions and aging. *Kobe J Med Sci* 1979; 25:1–17.

66. Tiffin J: *Purdue Pegboard Examiner's Manual*. Lafayette, Ill, Lafayette Instrument Co, 1988.

67. Werner JL, Omer GE: Evaluating cutaneous pressure sensation in the hand. *Am J Occup Ther* 1970; 24:347–356.

68. Wilgis EFS, Kaplan EB: The blood supply of the hand, in Spinner M (ed): *Kaplan's Functional and Surgical Anatomy of the Hand*, ed 3. Philadelphia, JB Lippincott, 1984, pp 203–221.

Chapter 16

Hip Injuries: An Orthopedic Perspective

Ari Ben-Yishay, M.D.
Joseph D. Zuckerman, M.D.

Hip injuries in the geriatric patient population present major challenges to the health care system. The impact of these injuries extends far beyond the obvious orthopedic injury into the domains of medicine, rehabilitation, psychiatry, social work, and medical economics. A hip fracture remains one of the most potentially devastating injuries in the elderly. It evokes great fear because its occurrence is often considered the start of a steady decline resulting in loss of independence, increasing debilitation, and possibly death. In this chapter we will discuss the spectrum of common hip disorders from degenerative and inflammatory arthritis to hip fractures and pelvic fractures. An overview of the etiology, evaluation, management and anticipated outcomes of these disorders and injuries will be presented.

NORMAL CHANGES WITH AGE

Bone Quality

Osteoporosis is the most common age-related pathologic condition of bone. Osteoporosis can be defined as an absolute decrease in bone density to the point at which fractures begin to occur.[105] The bone that remains is normal. Osteoporosis results from an identifiable underlying disease process in approximately 20% of cases (endocrine disorders, drug effect, neoplasm, collagen disorders[106]). In 80% of cases, the condition is considered involutional and a product of normal aging.[106]

Two types of osteoporosis have been identified, each with different biochemical and clinical characteristics.[105] Type 1 osteoporosis is postmenopausal osteoporosis. It occurs primarily in women within 15 to 20 years of menopause and is related to accelerated bone loss. Trabecular bone is primarily affected, resulting most commonly in fractures of the distal radius and vertebral compression fractures. These areas are composed primarily of trabecular bone. Type 2 or age-related osteoporosis is characterized by a slower rate of bone loss, which begins around age 50 and continues throughout life.[93, 105] Trabecular and cortical bone are both affected. Hip fractures occur much more commonly in patients with type 2 osteoporosis.

The factors associated with type 1 osteoporosis are primarily hormonal. The loss of estrogen production associated with menopause results in accelerated bone loss that is most rapid within the first 3 years.[1] Although the etiology of the accelerated bone loss is unclear, different theories have been proposed, including the inability to utilize dietary calcium and a decrease in calcitonin levels resulting in unopposed vitamin D and parathormone activity.[93, 122] This is characterized at the cellular level by increased osteoclastic activity, with each osteoclast creating a wider area of resorption.[51]

The etiology of type 2 osteoporosis is multifactorial. Factors that have been implicated include decreased calcium intake,[92] decreased calcium resorption,[3, 30] decreased vitamin D synthesis,[23, 62] decreased levels of physical activity,[103] and increased urinary excretion of calcium.[93]

Other factors associated with osteoporosis may contribute to the incidence of hip fractures. These factors include low percentage of body fat, low calcium intake, alcohol ingestion, smoking, and inactivity.

Articular Cartilage

The function of all synovial joints, including the hip joint, is highly dependent on articular cartilage. Articular cartilage, because of its unique structure, distributes loads and minimizes the peak stresses on subchondral bone. The aging process affects both the cellular and matrix components of articular cartilage. With increasing age, the cellularity of the articular cartilage, particularly of the superficial layers, decreases.[102] Biochemical changes noted with increasing age include a decrease in proteoglycan content, specifically chondroitin sulfate, as well as decreasing hyaluronic acid chain size.[29] These age-related changes in the extracellular matrix may be the result of alterations in chondrocyte synthetic function or degradation of proteoglycans within the matrix, or both.

Microscopically, fibrillation of the superficial layer may be seen by age 30 years.[69] This may be followed by the development of small areas of ulceration.[117] As these degenerative changes progress, osteoarthritis may result. It is, however, unclear at which point the changes associated with the normal aging of articular cartilage become those of osteoarthritis. Although age, sex, and mechanical factors have been implicated in the development of osteoarthritis, a causal relationship between mechanical overuse and osteoarthritis has not been convincingly established.[102]

OSTEOARTHRITIS

Osteoarthritis may be divided into primary and secondary forms. Primary osteoarthritis develops in the absence of any predisposing diseases and most typically affects women in their fifth and sixth decades. Usually there is a gradual onset of symptoms, with the hips less frequently involved than the knees and the hands. Occasionally the process may mimic acute inflammatory arthritis with a sudden onset of symptoms and a rapidly deteriorating course.

Secondary osteoarthritis is characterized by an underlying hip abnormality (trauma, osteonecrosis, congenital hip deformity, Perthes' disease, slipped capital femoral epiphysis), which leads to mechanical incongruity and progressive hip deterioration. Osteoarthritis is characterized by a brief period of morning stiffness, which is frequently attenuated by normal activity during the day but may reappear after periods of inactivity and may be aggravated by excessive activity. Patients frequently present with buttock, medial thigh, or greater trochanteric pain from weight bearing. The pain may radiate to the anterior thigh as far down as the knee and may be present at night, occasionally disturbing sleep.

The radiographic findings for osteoarthritis of the hip include loss of the superior and lateral joint space, superior migration of the femoral head, osteophytes, sclerosis, and the presence of subchondral cysts. Laboratory examinations are unremarkable except when there is an underlying etiology such as previous infection or endstage rheumatoid disease.

The mainstays of treatment of osteoarthritis of the hip include use of salicylates and nonsteroid anti-inflammatory drugs (NSAIDs) as well as resting the joint by using ambulatory aids such as a cane, crutches, or walker to unload the hip. If the condition is debilitating and is no longer responsive to these measures, artificial joint replacement may be necessary (Fig 6–1).

Other disorders that may lead to degenerative hip disease in the elderly include inflammatory arthritis of infectious and noninfectious etiologies. Inflammatory, noninfectious arthritis can be further characterized into seropositive arthritis such as rheumatoid arthritis, seronegative arthritis such as psoriatic arthritis, and crystal-induced arthritis such as pseudogout. An in-depth discussion of these disorders is beyond the scope of this chapter. Diagnosis of these disorders is usually established by appropriate history and physical examination, including a recognized pattern of other joint involvement. Laboratory examination, including white blood cell count, sedimentation rate, rheumatoid factor and antinuclear antigen as well as HLA tissue typing will often lead to the appropriate diagnosis. The mainstays of treatment of the inflammatory, noninfectious arthropathies include salicylates, NSAIDs, and immunosuppressive treatment for severe and resistive cases. Total hip replacement is performed for advanced inflammatory arthritis with excellent or good results in over 90% of cases.

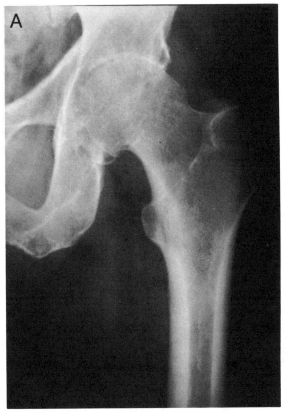

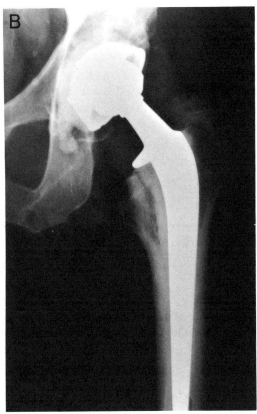

FIG 16–1.
A, 76-year-old man with advanced osteoarthritis of the left hip. There is complete loss of the joint space superiorly with sclerotic changes of the acetabulum and femoral head. The superior portion of the femoral head is mildly flattened. In addition, there is a medial osteophyte, which results in some lateral subluxation of the femoral head. **B,** a cemented total hip replacement was performed with excellent relief of pain and improvement of overall function.

BURSITIS

Bursitis is frequently overlooked as a cause of hip pain in the elderly because the peak incidence occurs between the fourth and sixth decades. Three syndromes of bursitis about the hip have been characterized based on the presence of three anatomically distinct bursae. These include the trochanteric, ischiogluteal, and iliopsoas bursae.

Trochanteric bursitis is the most common bursitis about the hip joint. It usually presents with a deep, dull, aching pain that may sometimes cause a burning and tingling sensation in the lateral aspect of the upper thigh. The pain may radiate along the L2 dermatome or down the thigh to the knee. The condition is exacerbated by activity, especially with the affected leg crossed. It may be intermittent or chronic and may disturb sleep owing to local pain from pressure over the greater trochanter.

Physical examination reveals pain over the bony prominence of the greater trochanter. Rarely is there a decreased range of motion, although the patient may have pain with extremes of external rotation. There is often pain with active hip abduction against resistance. X-ray evaluation may show irregularity of the greater trochanter, and/or supratrochanteric calcification if calcific tendinitis is also present.

Ischial bursitis is characterized predominantly by the presence of buttock pain, which may occasionally radiate down the leg, mimicking sciatica. The pain is worse in the sitting position and is relieved when the affected side is held off the seat. The pain may be exacerbated by bending forward and during long strides during gait. On physical examination there is tenderness over the ischial tuberosity, which is palpated best when the hip is in a flexed position.

Iliopsoas bursitis may present with gradually increasing groin pain that may radiate down the anterior and medial aspect of the thigh to the knee. On physical examination there is usually local tenderness over the medial and proximal thigh. The pain is exacerbated by extension of the hip joint and may radiate down the thigh. This pattern of findings can simulate femoral nerve compression.

All three syndromes of bursitis may be relieved by avoiding offending positions and activities. Application of ice or heat may provide some pain relief as well. NSAIDs are usually helpful. If these measures are unsuccessful, relief can be obtained by injection of the bursa with lidocaine and steroids.

HIP FRACTURES: OVERVIEW

Epidemiology

It is currently estimated that more than 270,000 hip fractures occur each year in the United States,[59] most of them in patients over 65 years of age. Since the majority of these fractures are treated surgically, hip fracture surgery represents one of the most common orthopedic procedures performed in the elderly population. It is estimated that by the year 2040 the number of hip fractures occurring annually will double, making hip fracture surgery even more significant in the future.[27]

Numerous studies have been devoted to the problem of hip fractures in the elderly, particularly with respect to risk factors and mortality. Age remains an important risk factor. The incidence of hip fractures increases with advancing age beyond age 50, possibly even doubling with each additional decade.[44] Hip fractures occur more commonly in women by a ratio of at least 2:1.[40] Elderly white women are at the greatest risk while black men are at the lowest risk.[21] Institutionalized patients also have a higher incidence of hip fracture.[64, 74] This is most likely related to dementia, other comorbid conditions, and the use of psychotropic medications.

The mortality rate following hip fracture in the elderly remains significant. Recent studies focusing on elderly hip fracture patients treated operatively in the 1980s found a 1-year mortality rate of approximately 25%.[121, 139] This is significantly greater than the anticipated mortality for an age- and sex-matched population who have not sustained hip fractures.[78] The highest risk for mortality occurs within the first 6 months following fracture. After 1 year, mortality rates approach those for an age- and sex-matched non–hip fracture population. Factors that increase mortality risk include age,[78, 139] signifi-

cant comorbid medical conditions,[60] male sex,[65] underlying cognitive disorders,[91,123] institutional prefracture living environment,[44] poor prefracture mobility,[15, 38] and the presence of postoperative complications.[2, 42] Factors not necessarily associated with increased mortality include fracture type,[46, 71] and timing of surgical treatment.[20, 59, 78] Frequently, more than one risk factor is present, making it difficult to pinpoint the contribution of any one factor to mortality risk. This remains an important area to be studied because identification of risk factors may lead to more effective treatment approaches.

Fracture Types

Fractures of the proximal femur are generally classified according to their anatomic location and include femoral neck, intertrochanteric, and subtrochanteric fractures. Based upon our experience with over 600 hip fractures in patients over age 65 at the Hospital for Joint Diseases, more than 95% are femoral neck or intertrochanteric fractures. These fractures occur with an approximately equal frequency.[61] The remaining 5% are subtrochanteric fractures. These fractures occur more commonly in younger patients, usually as a result of high-energy injuries.

FEMORAL NECK FRACTURES

Fractures of the femoral neck occur in the proximal femur in an area beginning just inferior to the articular surface of the femoral head and ending just superior to the intertrochanteric region. The intracapsular location of femoral neck fractures has important implications on fracture healing and the development of femoral head osteonecrosis. The primary blood supply for the femoral head arises from the medial and lateral femoral circumflex arteries, which enter the posterior and anterior portions of the femoral neck (Fig 16–2). They form an extracapsular arterial ring at the base of the femoral neck, which in turn gives rise to ascending cervical arteries. These traverse the neck proximally and form an intracapsular ring at the junction of the femoral head and neck. This blood supply is distally based. Displaced femoral neck fractures may therefore result in disruption of the blood supply, resulting in significant risk of osteonecrosis and fracture nonunion. These are two complications that have resulted in

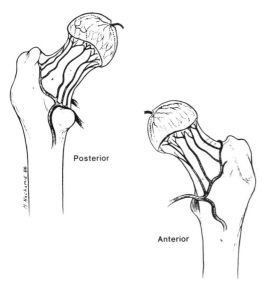

FIG 16–2.
The blood supply to the femoral head (see text). It is important to note that the blood supply to the femoral head traverses the femoral neck in a distal-to-proximal direction. Therefore, femoral neck fractures that disrupt the ascending cervical arteries deprive the femoral head of its blood supply. (From Zuckerman JD (ed): *Comprehensive Care of Orthopaedic Injuries in the Elderly.* Baltimore, Williams & Wilkins, 1990. Used by permission.)

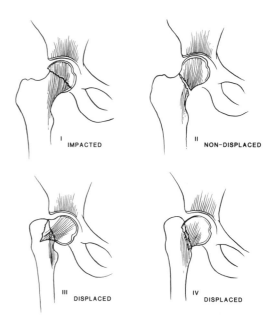

FIG 16–3.
Garden classification of femoral neck fractures (see text). It is important to recognize that type I (impacted) and type II are nondisplaced fractures while type III and type IV are displaced fractures. It is usually difficult to differentiate type III and type IV fractures. (From Zuckerman JD (ed): *Comprehensive Care of Orthopaedic Injuries in the Elderly.* Baltimore, Williams & Wilkins, 1990. Used by permission)

displaced femoral neck fractures being referred to as the "unsolved fracture."

The majority of femoral neck fractures occur as a result of a simple fall. These are low-energy injuries that result in a fracture owing to the inability of the osteoporotic bone of the proximal femur to withstand the relatively low stresses involved.

A number of different classification systems have been used for femoral neck fractures,[47, 63, 101] the most popular of which is the Garden classification system (Fig 16–3). This divides femoral neck fractures into four types and is based upon the degree of displacement. Type I is an incomplete, impacted fracture in which the bony trabeculae of the inferior portion of the femoral neck remain intact (Fig 16–4, A). This category includes valgus impaction fractures. Type II is a complete fracture without displacement of the fracture fragments (Fig 16–4, B). Type III is a complete fracture with partial displacement (Fig 16–4, C). Type IV is a complete fracture with total displacement of the fragments (Fig 16–4, D). It is often difficult to differentiate the four types radiographically. Therefore, a simpler system has evolved in which types 1 and 2 are considered nondisplaced fractures and types III and IV are displaced fractures.[142] The degree of displacement has

very important implications on the development of healing complications.

Clinical Evaluation

The clinical presentation of femoral neck fractures is dependent primarily on the type of fracture. Patients with nondisplaced or impacted fractures may have only minimal pain at the extremes of motion and may remain ambulatory with mild discomfort. More often, however, there may be significant symptoms that preclude ambulation. Displaced fractures are generally more symptomatic at presentation. Patients are unable to stand or ambulate and the affected lower extremity may be externally rotated and shortened. Any motion of the hip will be painful. Standard radiographic examination of the hip includes an anteroposterior (AP) view of the pelvis and a cross-table lateral view. The AP view of the pelvis allows a comparison with the uninvolved hip, which may be helpful in identifying nondisplaced or impacted fractures. Displaced fractures are easily identified with the standard radiographic evaluation. An internal rotation view of the hip may also be helpful in identifying nondisplaced or impacted

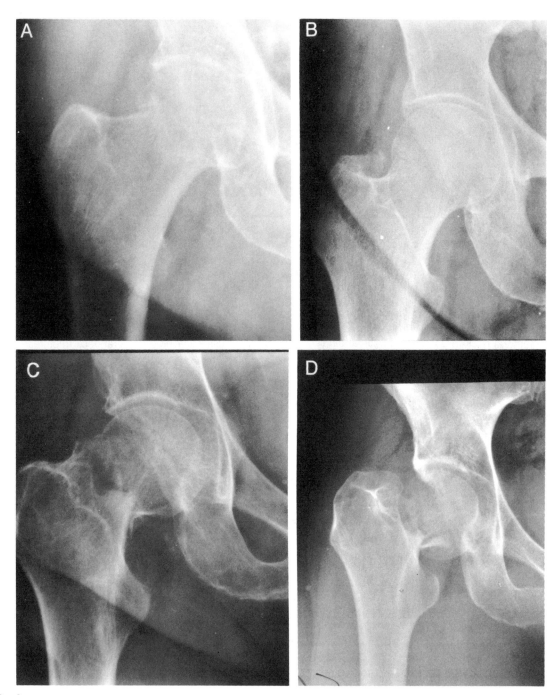

FIG 16–4.
Four types of femoral neck fractures based upon the Garden classification. **A,** type I. **B,** type II **C,** type III. **D,** type IV. (From Zuckerman JD (ed): *Comprehensive Care of Ortho-* *paedic Injuries in the Elderly.* Baltimore, Williams & Wilkins, 1990. Used by permission)

fractures. This view is taken with the lower extremity internally rotated approximately 15 degrees, permitting visualization of the entire femoral neck. When a femoral neck fracture is suspected but is not apparent on standard radiographs, a technetium bone scan is often helpful in establishing the diagno- sis. This is a sensitive indicator of an unrecognized femoral neck fracture.[57] The importance of maintaining a very high index of suspicion for femoral neck fractures in all elderly patients with hip pain cannot be overemphasized.

Treatment

All patients with femoral neck fractures should be admitted to an acute care facility and maintained on a regimen of strict bed rest. Whereas light skin traction has been utilized in the past, we prefer to maintain the leg in a position of comfort, which is usually slight hip flexion and external rotation supported by pillows. All patients should undergo prompt medical evaluation and preparation for surgical management of the fracture.

There is general agreement among orthopedic surgeons that surgical management is the treatment of choice for almost all femoral neck fractures. There are, however, some exceptions to this general rule. Patients with severe medical problems and significant risk of perioperative mortality can be considered for nonoperative management; however, prolonged bed rest and traction also pose a significant medical risk to these patients. Nonoperative treatment should consist of early mobilization with acceptance of the resultant malunion or nonunion. Demented, nonambulatory patients may also be considered for nonoperative management.[140] The goal in these patients, as in all hip fracture patients, is return to their prefracture level of function. These patients may be surprisingly comfortable following a few days of restricted activity followed by bed-to-chair transfers.

The type of surgical procedure chosen depends on many factors and will vary from surgeon to surgeon. These factors can be divided into two categories: patient factors and fracture factors. Patient factors include the patient's age, ambulatory ability, functional status, mental status, associated medical problems, and the ability to participate in a rehabilitation program. Fracture factors include the degree of displacement, osteoporosis, comminution, and the age of the fracture. While all of these factors are important, the most important differences in treatment approach are determined by fracture displacement. Nondisplaced and displaced femoral neck fractures will be considered separately.

Nondisplaced fractures include Garden type 1 and 2 fractures. Type 1, impacted fractures, are inherently stable owing to the impaction at the fracture site. While there has been some support for nonoperative management of these fractures in the past, problems with late displacement and healing complications[16, 17, 68] have led to support for operative management. Type 2, nondisplaced fractures are not impacted and do not have the inherent stability of impacted fractures. They carry a very high

risk for further displacement. Therefore, internal fixation is the treatment of choice.

Impacted and nondisplaced femoral neck fractures should undergo in situ internal fixation using multiple pins or screws (Figs 16–5 and 16–6). Use of cannulated screws or 6.5-mm cancellous screws[37, 127, 132] is preferable because of the improved lag effect provided by the outside thread diameter and the relatively short length of threads. The optimal number of screws or pins to be used has not been determined.[131] Use of three screws placed in parallel on both the AP and lateral views of the proximal femur is preferred by these authors. The screws should be inserted under fluoroscopic control. Permanent AP and lateral radiographs are essential at the completion of surgery.

Postoperative management of these patients is directed at early mobilization to prevent the complications of prolonged recumbency. The patient should be out of bed on the first postoperative day and begin ambulation on the second postoperative day. Weight bearing is allowed as tolerated with assistive devices as needed. There does not appear to be any advantage to restricted weight bearing following internal fixation of these fractures.[5] Limiting weight bearing in these patients is often disadvantageous owing to the difficulty elderly patients have in ambulating with restricted weight bearing.

Whereas virtually all younger patients with displaced femoral neck fractures should be treated with internal fixation, such is not the case for displaced femoral neck fractures in the elderly. A relatively high risk of nonunion and osteonecrosis has led to the development and popularity of primary prosthetic replacement as a treatment option. Since both symptomatic nonunion and osteonecrosis following internal fixation are treated by prosthetic replacement, primary prosthetic replacement has been advocated for these high-risk fractures as a means of decreasing the need for reoperation. In reality, the choice of internal fixation vs. prosthetic replacement may be difficult. It should be based upon careful consideration of the patient's age, fracture, comminution, bone quality, age of the fracture, and associated medical conditions. The treatment approach favored by the authors is based upon these factors.

For displaced fractures in active, healthy patients under the age of 70 years, the authors feel that treatment by anatomic reduction and internal fixation is preferred over primary prosthetic replacement (Fig 16–7). This approach should be considered for patients between the ages of 70 and 75 years if good bone quality is present and an acceptable re-

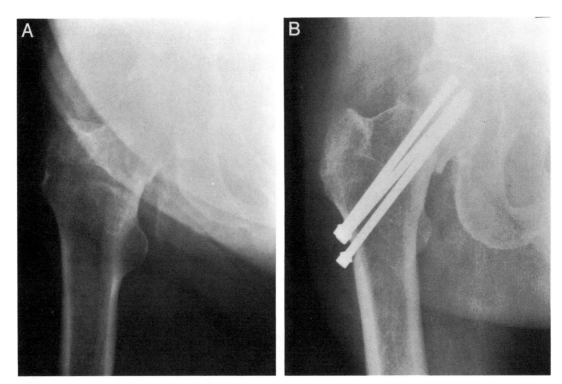

FIG 16–5.
An 80-year-old woman with impacted valgus femoral neck fracture **(A)** treated by internal fixation with three cannulated screws **(B)**.

duction with secure fixation can be obtained. Ideally, the fracture is treated urgently, with rapid medical stabilization and surgical treatment whenever possible within 24 hours of admission. Treatment consists of a closed reduction of the fracture under fluoroscopic control. This is the most important and frequently the most difficult step. Closed reduction should be attempted by flexing the hip to 45 degrees and externally rotating the femur to disengage the fracture fragments. Traction is then applied as the

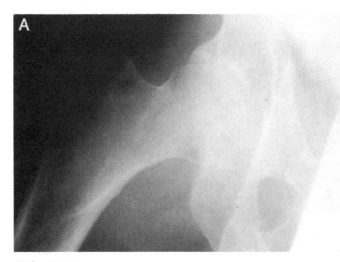
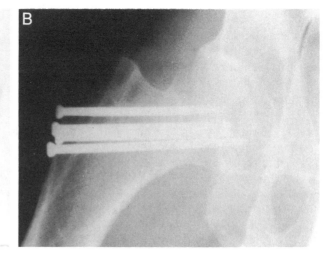

FIG 16–6.
Nondisplaced femoral neck fracture **(A)** in a 62-year-old woman treated by internal fixation with 6.5 mm AOI cancellous screws **(B)**. (From Zuckerman JD (ed): *Comprehensive Care of Orthopaedic Injuries in the Elderly.* Baltimore, Williams & Wilkins, 1990: Used by permission.)

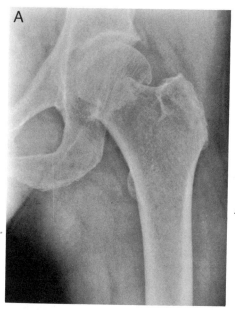

FIG 16–7.

A, a 63-year-old woman sustained a displaced femoral neck fracture as a result of a fall at work. Two attempts at closed reduction were unsuccessful. An open reduction was performed using an anterolateral approach. **B** and **C,** postreduction radiographs showed acceptable alignment without evidence of significant posterior comminution. **D** and **E,** internal fixation was performed using cannulated screw. (From Zuckerman JD (d): *Comprehensive Care of Orthopaedic Injuries in the Elderly.* Baltimore, Williams & Wilkins, 1990. Used by permission.)

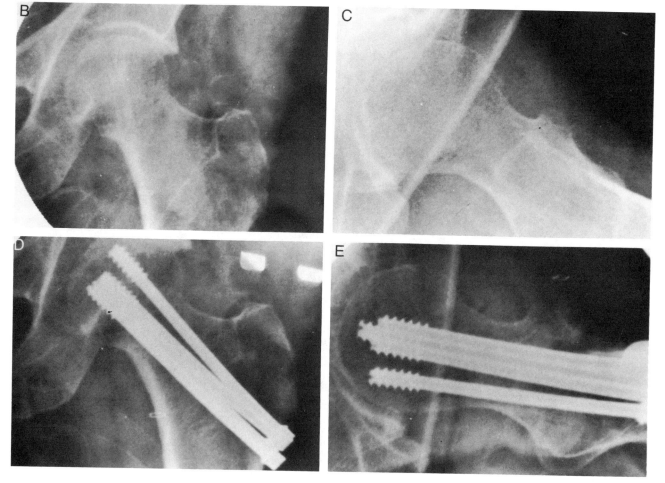

leg is internally rotated and brought to full extension. Traction is maintained by placing the extremity in the foot holder of the fracture table. Careful evaluation of AP and lateral views is essential in determining the next step in treatment. If an obvious malreduction is present, the reduction maneuver should be repeated. A gentle closed reduction should be attempted up to three times before reevaluating the treatment options. If significant posterior comminution of the femoral neck is present that would ultimately compromise internal fixation, a primary prosthetic replacement should be performed. If the reduction is acceptable and posterior comminution is not significant, then internal fixation should be performed using multiple screws or pins as described previously. The inability to obtain an adequate closed reduction, the presence of significant posterior comminution, and/or poor bone qual-

ity are all factors favoring primary prosthetic replacement (Fig 16–8).

Postoperative management of these patients has been a source of controversy. While some have recommended restricted weight bearing until the fracture is healed,[47, 73, 99] the authors encourage weight bearing as tolerated for virtually all femoral neck fractures. An adequate reduction and secure internal fixation are the mainstays of treatment and guarded weight bearing postoperatively will have little effect on the ultimate outcome of treatment.

Special Situations

There are special situations that may modify the approach to patients with femoral neck fractures. Patients with Parkinson's disease who sustain femoral neck fractures have higher morbidity and mortal-

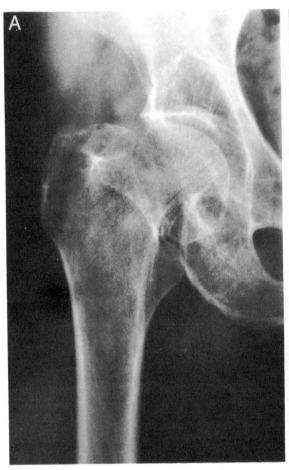
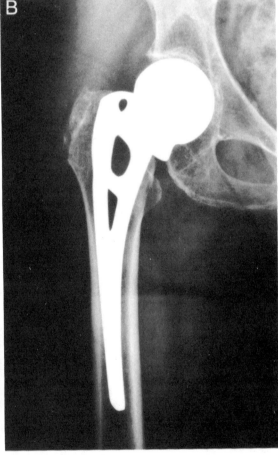

FIG 16–8.
A, an 84-year-old woman sustained a displaced femoral neck fracture when she fell in the bathroom in her home. **B,** an uncemented Austin-Moore hemiarthroplasty was performed. Two years earlier she had sustained a similar frac-ture of the left hip treated with a hemiarthroplasty. (From Zuckerman JD (ed): *Comprehensive Care of Orthopaedic Injuries in the Elderly*. Baltimore, Williams & Wilkins, 1990. Used by permission.)

ity rates than hip fracture patients without Parkinson's disease.[39, 47, 55] In deciding upon an appropriate treatment plan, it is essential to consider the status of the disease. Parkinson's disease is a movement disorder with clinical manifestations that range from mild tremors without significant functional limitations to complete incapacitation with severe contractures. The following guidelines are preferred by the authors. Patients with nondisplaced or impacted fractures should be treated with multiple screw fixation and early mobilization regardless of age. Patients with displaced femoral neck fractures who are relatively young and active and whose disease is well controlled should be treated with anatomic reduction and internal fixation using the approach previously described. Older patients with displaced fractures and those patients with poorly controlled disease and significant loss of function can be treated by primary prosthetic replacement.

Elderly patients with Paget's disease present with two types of femoral neck fractures: incomplete or fissure fractures and complete fractures. Different reports have documented the increased incidence of healing complications following internal fixation of femoral neck fractures in Paget's disease.[49, 90, 98] Reports of treatment with prosthetic replacement reported both satisfactory[49] and unsatisfactory results.[14] Primary prosthetic replacement is the treatment of choice for complete femoral neck fractures in patients with Paget's disease. The question to be answered is whether an endoprosthesis or total hip replacement is preferred. In answering this question, it is important to determine the presence and severity of prefracture hip symptoms as well as the extent of pagetoid involvement in the acetabulum. If there is no history of preexisting symptoms and acetabular disease is minimal, then a hemiarthroplasty should be performed. When significant prefracture symptoms are present or acetabular involvement is extensive with secondary degenerative changes, total hip replacement is the preferred treatment.

Complications

The age and medical fragility of the elderly patient population sustaining femoral neck fractures increases the risk of postoperative complications. Cardiopulmonary complications such as pneumonia, congestive heart failure, myocardial infarction, and arrhythmias, as well as urinary tract infections and thromboembolism, occur with significant frequency. The incidence of clinically significant thrombophlebi-

tis has been reported as 15% to 20%, while the incidence of radiographically documented thrombophlebitis has been reported to be as high as 50%.[43, 66, 94] Fatal pulmonary embolism occurred in 4% to 7% of patients who did not receive thromboembolic prophylaxis.[52] Prophylactic anticoagulation using a variety of regimens has been effective in decreasing the incidence of thromboembolic complications. Urinary tract infection and decubitus ulcers have been reported in up to 30% of cases.[72, 96] Many of these complications can be prevented by aggressive respiratory therapy and early surgery followed by rapid mobilization, judicious management of fluid and electrolyte replacement, and meticulous nursing care.

Complications following internal fixation of femoral neck fractures include loss of fixation, nonunion, osteonecrosis, and infection. Early fixation failure within 3 months after surgery occurs in 12% to 24% of displaced femoral neck fractures.[12, 28, 68] Factors associated with early loss of fixation include age, initial fracture type/displacement, presence of posterior comminution of the neck, and delay of surgery for more than 7 days after injury.[11, 12, 86, 116]

Infections following internal fixation of femoral neck fractures have become uncommon. Superficial as well as deep infection has been reported in up to 5% of cases.[35, 107, 124, 125] Perioperative antibiotic prophylaxis has now become standard in the management of elderly hip fracture patients and is responsible in part for the low rates of infection.[76]

Nonunion of femoral neck fractures is related to fracture type.[37, 127] Nonunion occurs in 0% to 5% of nondisplaced fractures[12, 37]; However, for displaced fractures, the incidence of nonunion has been reported from 9% to 35%.[10, 31, 37, 124, 125] Nonunions are more common following inadequate reduction and in the presence of posterior comminution[5, 11, 12] (Fig 16–9).

The development of osteonecrosis following femoral neck fracture reflects the vulnerability of the femoral head circulation to disruption. The incidence of osteonecrosis following nondisplaced femoral neck fractures has been reported to be as high as 15% but in general is approximately 5% to 8%.[10, 17, 118] The incidence of osteonecrosis following displaced femoral neck fractures has been reported as 9% to 35%, with most series reporting 20% to 35%.[10, 12, 35, 37, 87, 130] Factors associated with an increased incidence of osteonecrosis include inadequate reduction, delay of reduction and fixation, and the use of sliding hip screws or nail-plate devices. In general, approximately one third of patients devel-

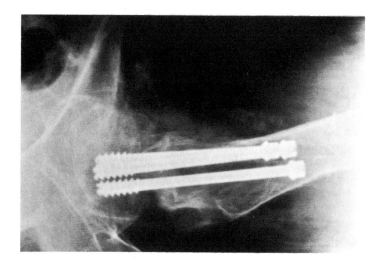

FIG 16-9.
Femoral neck nonunion is evident in 64-year-old woman 7 months following internal fixation of a displaced femoral neck fracture. (From Zuckerman JD (ed): *Comprehensive* *Care of Orthopaedic Injuries in the Elderly*. Baltimore, Williams & Wilkins, 1990. Used by permission.)

oping osteonecrosis require reoperation from disabling symptoms. The remainder are either asymptomatic or have symptoms that are not disabling.[12]

Complications following primary prosthetic replacement for acute femoral neck fractures include infection, dislocation, and pain associated with acetabular erosion and/or prosthetic loosening. A recent series using mostly bipolar endoprostheses reported infection rates of 2% to 8%.[26, 32, 107, 136] The incidence of dislocations following prosthetic replacement has varied from 1% to 10% with the posterior surgical approach associated with a higher dislocation rate as compared with the anterior approach.[19, 33, 45, 75, 134]

INTERTROCHANTERIC FRACTURES

Intertrochanteric hip fractures occur in the anatomic region between the greater and lesser trochanters. They are purely extracapsular fractures, indicating that the fracture line is distal to the anatomic limits of the capsule of the hip joint. The metaphyseal cancellous bone in this area is well vascularized. Consequently, the problems of nonunion and osteonecrosis encountered with intracapsular femoral neck fractures are rarely a problem with intertrochanteric fractures.

These fractures are usually a result of direct or indirect forces that are transmitted to the intertro-

chanteric area. This may result from a direct blow to the area of the greater trochanter or from indirect forces transmitted along the axis of the femur. Both of these mechanisms come into play in association with falls. This was confirmed with recent reports in which 77% to 81% of patients reported a fall from a standing height associated with a fracture.[86]

Many classifications systems have been proposed for intertrochanteric hip fractures.[8, 24, 53, 135] The most important aspect of any classification system is determining the stability of the fracture pattern and the ability to achieve a stable reduction. The key to a stable reduction in intertrochanteric fractures rests in the ability to restore posteromedial cortical continuity. In stable fracture patterns, the posteromedial cortex remains intact and a stable reduction can be obtained. Unstable fracture patterns are characterized by comminution of the posteromedial cortex. These fractures, therefore, are inherently unstable but can be converted to a stable configuration if medial cortical apposition is obtained.

Intertrochanteric fractures may be classified into stable and unstable fracture patterns. Therefore, the first step in the evaluation of these fractures is to differentiate the stable from the unstable fracture patterns. Fractures with associated posteromedial comminution, intertrochanteric fractures with subtrochanteric extension, and reverse obliquity fractures all represent unstable fracture patterns (Fig 16-10). The treatment protocol that follows is based on the fracture pattern present.

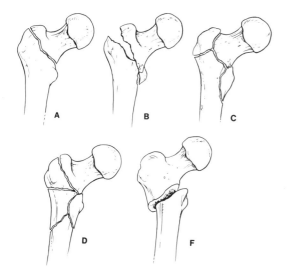

FIG 16–10.
Classification of intertrochanteric fractures. **A,** a two-part fracture that is stable. **B,** also a stable pattern because the medial fragment is small and does not significantly compromise the posteromedial buttress. **C,** unstable fracture because of the large posteromedial fragment. **D,** unstable intertrochanteric fracture with subtrochanteric extension. **E,** reverse obliquity pattern, which is also unstable because of the tendency for the shaft to displace medially. This classification is a combination of those described by Evans[54] and Kyle et al.[81] (From Zuckerman JD (ed): *Comprehensive Care of Orthopaedic Injuries in the Elderly.* Baltimore, Williams & Wilkins, 1990. Used by permission.)

Clinical Evaluation

Patients who sustain intertrochanteric hip fractures are rarely able to stand or ambulate following the injury. The clinical deformity present on examination is dependent upon the degree of displacement and comminution of the fracture. Nondisplaced fractures may present with virtually no clinical deformity. Displaced intertrochanteric fractures classically present with a shortened, externally rotated extremity. On examination there is usually tenderness in the area of the greater trochanter and groin. Range of motion of the hip is extremely painful and should be avoided. Following thorough medical evaluation and admission to the hospital, 5 pounds of light skin traction to the involved extremity should be used to provide patient comfort and to prevent additional injury.

Standard radiographic examination of intertrochanteric fractures includes an AP and cross-table lateral view of the hip. It may be difficult to obtain a lateral radiograph owing to patient discomfort; however, it is very important to have a complete radiographic evaluation prior to surgery. When a fracture is suspected but not identified on standard radiographs, a technetium bone scan will often aid in identification of the fracture.[56]

General Treatment

The primary goal of treatment of intertrochanteric fractures, as in all fractures of the elderly, is prompt restoration to their preinjury level of function. The method of obtaining this goal has changed dramatically over the past 50 years. Treatment was originally nonoperative, consisting of prolonged bed rest in traction until fracture healing occurred. This was then followed by a lengthy program of ambulation training. This prolonged period of recumbency was associated with a very high complication rate including decubitus ulcers, pneumonia, thromboembolic complications, urinary tract infections, and joint contractures.[54, 77, 81] Healing generally occurred with significant malunion and shortening at the fracture site secondary to strong deforming muscular forces that were unrelieved by traction. It soon became apparent that early mobilization of the patient was necessary to avoid the problems of prolonged recumbency. To achieve this, operative management consisting of reduction and stabilization of the fracture was necessary. Techniques of internal fixation that have developed over the last 30 years have overcome the earlier problems encountered. Operative management has become the treatment of choice for intertrochanteric fractures because it allows early mobilization of the patient, thereby avoiding many of the associated complications of prolonged bed rest.

Patients with intertrochanteric fractures require prompt evaluation and treatment. In most cases, surgery can be performed within the first 24 to 48 hours following admission. If the patient is unstable medically, it is essential to delay surgery until he or she is stabilized. The primary goal of operative management is achieving a stable fracture reduction maintained with internal fixation allowing early ambulation and mobilization of the patient. For stable fracture patterns, achievment of this goal is usually straightforward. However, for unstable fracture patterns, it is much more difficult.

The choice of the internal fixation device is important. At present, the sliding hip screw is the most commonly utilized device (Fig 16–11). This device allows for controlled impaction at the fracture site, thereby decreasing the stress on the implant, which further decreases the incidence of implant failure. Although these devices are "forgiving" by al-

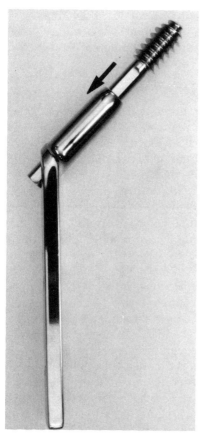

FIG 16–11.
The sliding hip screw allows controlled impaction to occur at the fracture site. Screw sliding within the barrel of the plate *(arrow)* effectively shortens the bending movement and reduces the risk of loss of fixation and implant failure. (From Zuckerman JD (ed): *Comprehensive Care of Orthopaedic Injuries in the Elderly.* Baltimore, Williams & Wilkins, 1990. Used by permission.)

lowing impaction at the fracture site, they must be inserted properly for this to occur. In addition, a stable reduction must be obtained at the time of surgery. Sliding hip screws are available in plate angles varying from 125 to 155 degrees, of which 135 degrees is the plate angle most commonly used. While some authors have recommended the use of the 150-degree sliding hip screw, comparative studies have failed to show a significant advantage over the 135-degree device.[95, 141]

Other devices have been used for the internal fixation of intertrochanteric fractures, of which flexible intramedullary (Ender) nails have the largest experience. Ender nails are inserted through portals in the distal femur just proximal to the femoral condyles in a retrograde manner under fluoroscopic guidance. Proposed advantages of this procedure include decreased blood loss, decreased anesthetic and operative time, and reduced mortality.[22, 79, 109] Although excellent results with this device have been reported,[138] the majority of studies have shown a significant incidence of complications associated with their use, including rotational malalignment, supracondylar femur fractures, proximal migration of the nails through the femoral head, and backing out of the nails from the proximal portals, causing knee pain and stiffness.[34, 50, 67, 70, 80, 120] At the present time, flexible intramedullary nails are best utilized by surgeons with significant experience in their use.

Some authors have reported satisfactory results using prosthetic replacement for comminuted intertrochanteric fractures in osteoporotic bone[108, 128, 129]; however, this option has been used to only a limited extent, and thus far the specific indications for its use have been difficult to define. Our indications for primary prosthetic replacement are an elderly patient with a comminuted, unstable intertrochanteric fracture in whom a stable reduction and secure internal fixation cannot be achieved. Although prosthetic replacement results in prolonged operative and anesthetic time and increased blood loss, it is certainly preferred to accepting a poor reduction and inadequate stabilization leading to early loss of fixation.

Treatment

Stable Fractures
Stable intertrochanteric fractures are those in which the posteromedial cortical buttress is intact and medial cortical opposition can be reestablished. These fractures may be nondisplaced or displaced. Nondisplaced fractures do not require reduction. Displaced fractures require reduction, which can usually be performed by closed manipulation (Fig 16–12). If this is unsuccessful, open reduction is necessary. The fracture table and image intensifier should be used for internal fixation of all intertrochanteric fractures. The feet and ankles of both lower extremities must be protected with soft padding when placed in the foot holders to prevent skin problems from excessive pressure. Closed reduction is performed by gentle traction and either abduction or adduction, depending upon the position of the fragments. The reduction should be evaluated using the image intensifier on both the AP and lateral views. At this point, surgery is performed through a direct lateral approach. The 135-degree sliding hip screw may be utilized for virtually all intertrochan-

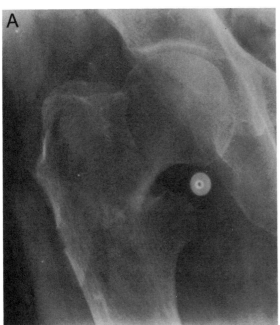

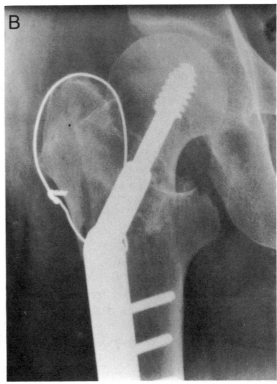

FIG 16–12.
A, stable intertrochanteric fracture with comminution of the greater trochanter. **B,** a cerclage wire is placed under the abductor tendon and around the plate barrel to act as a tension band for fixation of the greater trochanter. (From Zuck-erman JD (ed): *Comprehensive Care of Orthopaedic Injuries in the Elderly.* Baltimore, Williams & Wilkins, 1990. Used by permission.)

teric fractures. A few technical points should be emphasized. First, the guide wire placed within the femoral neck and head should be in a central position. A superior and anterior position should be avoided owing to the increased risk for "cutting out" through this weakened area of bone. Second, the compression screw should be located approximately 0.5 to 1 cm from the articular surface into the subchondral bone for best fixation. Third, the fracture should be impacted prior to fixation of the plate to the shaft of the femur. This impaction maneuver is necessary to enhance the stability of the reduction and to avoid excessive impaction postoperatively that may exceed the sliding capacity of the nail. Permanent AP and lateral radiographs should be obtained at the end of the procedure for accurate evaluation of the reduction and placement of the device. Postoperatively, patients are out of bed to a chair on the first postoperative day. This is followed by weight bearing as tolerated with assistive devices as needed beginning on the second postoperative day. This postoperative regimen is most compatible with optimal recovery.

Unstable Fractures

Unstable intertrochanteric fractures are characterized by loss of the posteromedial buttress. This comminution can extend to the subtrochanteric area, thereby increasing the degree of instability. In general, the goal in treatment of unstable intertrochanteric fractures is to convert the fracture to a stable configuration and obtain secure internal fixation.

The general approach for unstable intertrochanteric fractures is as described for stable fracture patterns. However, a stable reduction may be difficult to obtain by closed manipulation and open reduction is often necessary. Different reduction techniques have been developed over the years because of the high failure rate associated with the use of fixed-angle nail plate devices. In general, these techniques have resulted in a significantly lower complication rate when fixed-angle nail plates were used. Examples of these reduction techniques include the Dimon and Hughston medial displacement osteotomy, the Sarmiento valgus osteotomy and the Wayne County lateral displacement.[48, 77, 112, 114]

In our opinion, the importance of these reduction techniques has been significantly diminished with the development of the sliding hip screw. The authors prefer anatomic alignment with the sliding hip screw for the treatment of unstable intertrochanteric fractures. If a large posteromedial fragment is present, an attempt should be made to internally fix the fragment in a near anatomic position. This aids in restoring the posteromedial cortical support. Fixation of this fragment may be difficult, particularly if comminution is present. It is important to recognize that an anatomic reduction of this fragment is not required. The fragment should be brought back to the area of the posteromedial defect and secured in that position to provide an effective buttress to prevent varus displacement. One or two cerclage wires may be used for the fixation of this fragment. After the posteromedial fragment is reduced and an acceptable reduction is obtained, the sliding hip screw should be inserted in the usual manner (Fig 16–13). It is important to note that the unstable nature of this fracture often makes it necessary to manually hold the reduction during insertion of the internal fixation device. Again, it is important to be certain that an adequate amount of sliding capacity remains following insertion of the device. If this is not present, then a plate with a short barrel should be used to increase the sliding capacity. In comminuted fractures, a longer plate is often necessary. The plate should be securely fixed to the femoral shaft with eight to ten cortices of fixation in the distal fragment.

Postoperatively, management follows the same guidelines as described for stable fractures. Patients are mobilized out of bed to chair on the first postoperative day and begin ambulation with weight bearing as tolerated on the second postoperative day.

Complications

Elderly patients with intertrochanteric fractures are subjected to the same medical complications as patients with femoral neck fractures. Urinary tract infections, decubitus ulcers, cardiopulmonary problems, and deep venous thrombosis occur with equal frequency among the two groups. In addition, mortality following intertrochanteric fractures does not differ significantly from that associated with femoral neck fractures.[4, 46, 139] The use of prophylactic antibiotics has significantly decreased the incidence of wound infection, with a recent reported incidence of less than 3%.[100] The risk factors for wound infection include a urinary tract infection, decubitus ulcers, prolonged operative time, disorientation that inter-

feres with proper wound care, and proximity of the incision to the perineum.[13]

The complications most frequently encountered with the sliding hip screw include varus displacement of the proximal fragment, malrotation, and nonunion. Osteonecrosis, failure of the fixation device, and migration of the screw into the acetabulum are extremely uncommon occurrences.[83, 84] Varus displacement of intertrochanteric fractures following internal fixation is associated with unstable fractures with a lack of posteromedial support. Varus displacement may be severe enough to result in a screw "cutting out" through the anterosuperior portion of the femoral head. Factors contributing to this complication include placement of the screw into the anterosuperior aspect of the femoral head, improper reaming, inability to obtain a stable reduction, excessive collapse of the fracture that exceeds the sliding capacity of the device, and severe osteoporosis, which limits secure fixation. It should be emphasized that the best way to prevent postoperative loss of fixation and varus displacement is by achieving a stable reduction intraoperatively with proper technical insertion of the sliding hip screw.

Rotational deformities at the fracture site usually result from internal rotation of the distal fragment at the time of internal fixation of unstable fractures. This technical error can be prevented by careful attention to the position of the extremity during the device insertion. Nonunion of intertrochanteric fractures occurs in less than 2% of cases.[85] For most elderly patients, conversion to a calcar replacement endoprosthesis is the treatment of choice.

SUBTROCHANTERIC FRACTURES

Subtrochanteric fractures occur much less frequently in the elderly than femoral neck or intertrochanteric fractures. At the Hospital for Joint Diseases, they account for approximately 5% of hip fractures in patients over 60 years of age. When these fractures occur in the elderly, they are usually the result of a simple fall, while in younger patients they are often the result of high-energy trauma.[18] The subtrochanteric area is also a frequent site for pathologic fractures from neoplastic disease.[111]

Subtrochanteric fractures start at or below the lesser trochanter and involve the proximal portion of the femoral shaft. This area of the proximal femur is the site of very high biomechanical stresses with

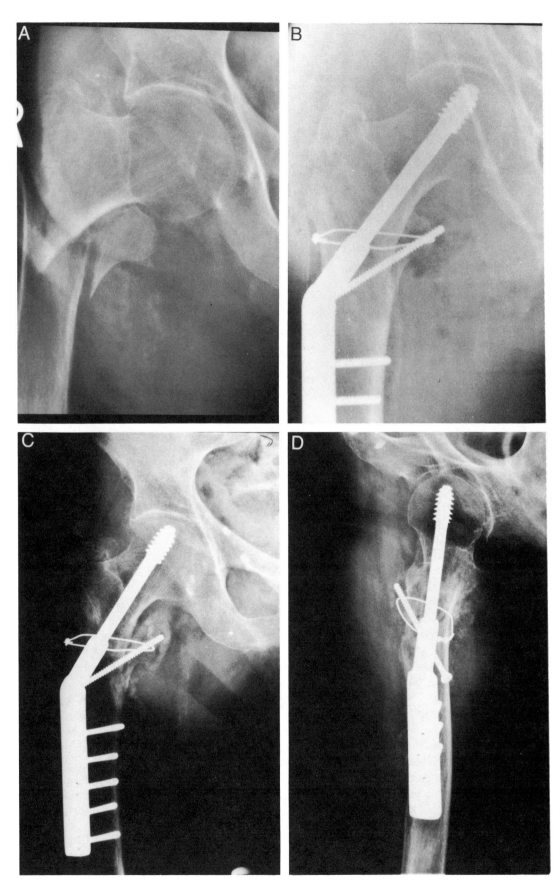

FIG 16–13.
A, unstable intertrochanteric fracture in an 82-year-old woman. **B,** the large posteromedial fragment was reduced to a "near-anatomic" position and fixed with a crew and cerclage wire. **C** and **D,** 6 weeks later, the position of the frag-

ment and fixation is unchanged and the fracture has healed. (From Zuckerman JD (ed): *Comprehensive Care of Orthopaedic Injuries in the Elderly.* Baltimore, Williams & Wilkins, 1990. Used by permission.)

high compressive forces medially and posteromedially and high tensile forces over the lateral cortex.[115] This asymmetric loading pattern is an important consideration in the selection of internal fixation devices and in understanding the causes of fixation failure and healing disturbances in the subtrochanteric area.[115] In addition, the decreased vascularity of the cortical bone in the subtrochanteric region compared with the vascular cancellous bone of the intertrochanteric region further exacerbates the potential for healing disturbances.

Different classification systems have been proposed by Fielding and Magliato,[58] Mueller et al,[97] Waddell et al,[137] and Seinsheimer.[119] We have modified Seinsheimer's system into stable and unstable fracture types to specifically address this important aspect of fracture classification (Fig 16–14). The key determinant of fracture stability is an intact or reconstructible posteromedial cortical buttress. If posteromedial cortical continuity can be reestablished, internal fixation devices will act as tension bands and compression forces will be transmitted along the medial cortex.

Clinical Evaluation

Elderly patients usually report a history of a fall or high-energy trauma. If the mechanism of injury is the latter, a comprehensive evaluation is indicated to identify associated chest, abdominal, or musculoskeletal injuries. Patients complain of hip and thigh pain and are unable to ambulate. Displaced fractures usually result in a shortened and externally rotated lower extremity. Thigh swelling may be significant since this fracture results in more bleeding than intertrochanteric fractures. A neurovascular examination of the involved extremity should be performed in all patients.

Radiographic evaluation includes AP and lateral views of the femur, including the hip and knee. The radiographs should be carefully evaluated to determine the location of the fracture, extent of comminution and the degree of osteoporosis. The proximal fragment is often flexed and abducted by the pull of the iliopsoas and abductors, respectively. The distal femoral shaft fragment is often displaced medially by the adductor muscles and may result in considerable shortening of the involved extremity.

Treatment

The initial management of patients with subtrochanteric fractures parallels that of patients with

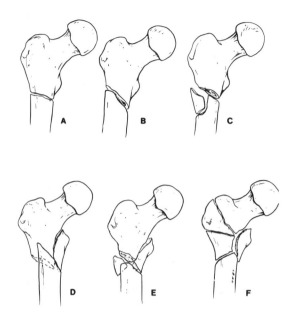

FIG 16–14.
Classification of subtrochanteric fractures. **A–C,** stable fracture patterns are characterized by an intact posteromedial cortical buttress. **D–F,** unstable fracture patterns are characterized by loss of the posteromedial cortical buttress. (From Zuckerman JD (ed): *Comprehensive Care of Orthopaedic Injuries in the Elderly.* Baltimore, Williams & Wilkins, 1990. Used by permission.)

intertrochanteric fractures. Patients require careful initial medical evaluation and stabilization. The increased blood loss associated with these fractures requires close monitoring of the patient's hematocrit with blood replacement if necessary. If surgery is anticipated within 48 hours of admission, 5 pounds of Buck's skin traction will be adequate. If a longer delay is anticipated, patients should be placed in skeletal traction with a proximal tibial pin to maintain alignment and length and prevent additional soft-tissue injury.

Both nonoperative and operative management approaches have been described. Nonoperative management generally consists of skeletal traction followed by spica casting or cast bracing. This method is poorly tolerated in elderly people because of the need for prolonged bed rest and the possibility of skin problems associated with spica casting. The results of nonoperative management generally reported increased morbidity and mortality as well as nonunion, delayed union, and malunion.[36, 113, 133] Nonoperative management should be reserved for those elderly patients who are such poor operative risks that surgery cannot be undertaken. In these cases, nonambulators may be amenable to nonoperative management consisting of early bed-to-chair mobilization. However, whenever possible, operative management is favored and non-operative management is reserved for carefully selected patients who are not candidates for surgery.

Operative management is the treatment of choice to achieve the goals of early rehabilitation and optimal functional recovery. Restoration of postero-medial cortical continuity is the most important aspect in obtaining a successful result. Different devices have been used to treat subtrochanteric fractures. These include fixed angle nail plates, intramedullary devices, and plate-screw assemblies. The implant of choice depends on numerous factors including the location of the fracture, the fracture pattern, the degree of osteoporosis, the patient's functional limitations and ability to participate in the postoperative rehabilitation program, and the experience of the surgeon.

Based upon a review of the many available fixation devices, a general approach can be formulated. The fracture pattern is very important. Stable fractures in which the medial cortex is intact should be treated by intramedullary fixation by closed technique whenever possible (Fig 16–15). This minimizes the surgical procedure and decreases anesthesia time and blood loss. Our preference has been the Zickel nail or a locked intramedullary rod, depending on the location of the fracture. The treatment of unstable fractures depends on the location of the fracture and the quality of the bone. Proximal subtrochanteric fractures or subtrochanteric-intertrochanteric fractures can be treated with a sliding hip screw because the location of the fracture allows impaction to occur by the sliding mechanism. Again, any posteromedial fragment or subtrochanteric extension should be stabilized with cerclage wires to enhance the stability of the implant-fracture construct. More distal unstable fractures cannot be treated with the sliding hip screw. Intramedullary devices can be used for these fractures when combined with supplemental fixation to improve stability. Both the Zickel nail and locked intramedullary nails can be used for unstable fractures if the other criteria are met. Extensively comminuted subtrochanteric fractures are the most difficult to treat. Cancellous bone grafting or methyl methacrylate may be necessary for augmentation with care taken to avoid intrusion of cement into the fracture site.

Postoperative management is directed at early mobilization of the patient with close monitoring for medical complications. Weight-bearing status must be individualized based upon the fracture type, fixation device, and security of the fixation. Whenever possible, early weight bearing is preferred in elderly patients; however, this may not be advisable for certain fractures and fixation devices. In these situations, restricted weight bearing will be necessary, although probably difficult, until signs of healing are evident.

Complications

Complications of fixation (nonunion, malunion, and implant failure) have been reported to be more common following subtrochanteric fractures than for intertrochanteric or femoral neck fractures.[6, 7, 9, 25, 115] It is important to remember that fractures with loss of the posteromedial cortical buttress, especially those in which it cannot be restored, are at greatest risk for healing complications. Symptomatic nonunion with or without implant failure generally requires reoperation. Treatment usually consists of removal of the implant, exposure and curettage of the nonunion site, bone grafting, and internal fixation using an intramedullary device if possible. Prosthetic replacement is not an option because of the location of the fracture.

PELVIC AND ACETABULAR INJURIES

Pelvic fractures comprise a spectrum of injuries ranging from stress or insufficiency fractures in osteoporotic bone to life-threatening disruptions of the pelvic ring. An in-depth discussion of the classifications, evaluation, and management of these injuries is well beyond the scope of this chapter. This section is meant to provide an overview of those injuries most commonly encountered in the elderly patient population.

Stress Fractures

Fractures seen more commonly in the elderly are insufficiency fractures of the pelvis. These fractures are usually seen in patients with marked osteoporosis. Supraacetabular fractures can be seen on routine radiographs as hazy bands of sclerosis located immediately above and parallel to the acetabular roof. These fractures may be an unsuspected cause of hip pain, especially in older women. A significant number of these fractures are not evident on routine radiographs and require a bone scan to establish the diagnosis. Bed rest may be required initially, but early mobilization is recommended.

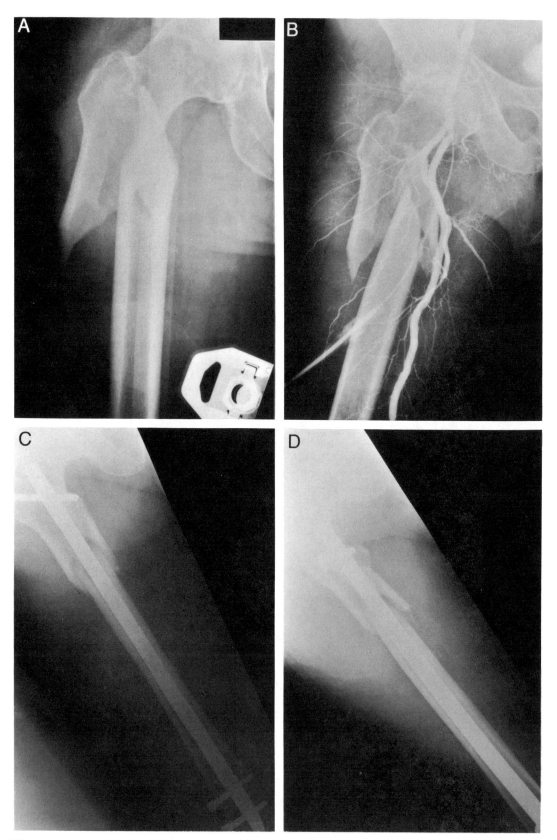

FIG 16–15.
A, 75-year-old man sustained a comminuted subtrochanteric fracture when he was struck by an automobile. **B,** angiogram obtained because of a diminished distal pulse was negative. **C** and **D,** immediate interlocking closed femoral nailing was performed. (From Zuckerman JD (ed): *Comprehensive Care of Orthopaedic Injuries in the Elderly.* Baltimore, Williams & Wilkins, 1990. Used by permission.)

Fractures of a Single Ramus of the Pubis or Ischium

The single ramus fracture is the most common pelvic fracture in the elderly. In one large series of pelvic fractures, 69% of all fractures involved the pubic bone, with 28% involving the ischium.[104] Emergency room views of the hip may not allow adequate visualization of the pelvic bones. Four standard radiographic views are recommended for evaluation of pelvic and acetabular fractures.[82] These include a standard AP view of the entire pelvis, a standard AP view centered on the affected hip, and two oblique views taken accurately at 45 degrees (Judet views). Additional views such as the inlet and outlet views may be necessary to complete the evaluation of pelvic ring fractures.

Isolated ramus fractures are intrinsically stable fractures that are extremely unlikely to displace with continued normal activities. Analgesia and relief from full weight bearing by the use of crutches or a walker may allow an early return to normal activities and avoid prolonged bedrest.

Sacral Fractures

Sacral and coccygeal fractures are often caused by a fall onto the buttocks. The fracture pattern is usually transverse, may traverse a sacral foramen, and may be angulated. Forward angulation may be best appreciated on lateral sacral views of the pelvis. Bimanual examination, with one finger in the rectum, may reveal mobility of the distal segment or the presence of angulation.

A short period of bed rest is usually sufficient to alleviate most symptoms. Sitting on an inflatable rubber or foam ring as well as in a semireclining position is useful. Rarely is resection of the coccyx necessary. If a painful nonunion occurs, coccygeal resection should be considered.

Acetabular Fractures

The diagnosis and correct analysis of acetabular fractures is important. The ultimate fate of the hip joint may rest on the recognition and appropriate management of these intra-articular fractures. Undisplaced fractures may be treated with bed rest and light longitudinal traction for 1 to 2 weeks. Gradual touch-down weight-bearing mobilization has been encouraged and is continued for 8 to 12 weeks. This may be followed by progressive weight bearing. Early use of continuous passive motion is probably beneficial to the healing of articular cartilage[110] and

should be used. Posttraumatic arthritis may develop, even after undisplaced acetabular fractures. Total hip replacement is the treatment of choice for elderly patients suffering this complication.[41]

Displaced acetabular fractures may be treated either nonoperatively or operatively. The basic principle of nonoperative treatment is skeletal traction applied to the lower extremity, usually by a distal femoral pin. A recent review of 25 patients older than 65 years of age with unilateral acetabular fractures managed nonoperatively showed that 30% of the patients had an unacceptable functional result. Poor results were associated with displaced posterior column fractures, osteoporosis, femoral head fractures, delayed diagnosis, inappropriate traction, and early weight bearing.[126]

The long-term prognosis of an acetabular fracture is directly related to the degree of articular congruency. If the congruency is perfectly restored, the prognosis is good, whatever the type of treatment. The greater the amount of residual incongruence, the more likely and more quickly that degenerative arthritis will occur. Displaced acetabular fractures may be treated nonoperatively if there is an adequate acetabular dome, as determined by roof-arc measurements.[88, 89]

Surgical treatment of displaced fractures allows visual control of the reduction of the fracture line and is the only procedure that consistently allows restoration of articular congruency. Surgery is also the only way to maintain a perfect reduction by means of plates and screws, allowing early passive and active motion. The joint should be explored and thoroughly irrigated. Loose bony fragments may be responsible for early deterioration and debilitating arthritis. Surgery allows early mobilization in the elderly which may reduce the morbidity of prolonged bedrest. The protocol for progressive weight-bearing ambulation is essentially the same as that for a nondisplaced acetabular fracture.

Although the patient's age is an important factor in making management decisions, advancing age is not a contraindication to operative management of displaced acetabular fractures. There has been a trend to treat displaced acetabular fractures nonoperatively in the elderly in anticipation of simply performing a total hip replacement once the fractures have united. Unfortunately, complications such as malunion, nonunion, and acetabular bone deficiency may compromise the outcome following total hip replacement.

The choice of the appropriate surgical approach and methods of internal fixation are beyond the scope of this discussion. However, it is important to note that the treatment of displaced acetabular fractures needs to be individualized with careful consideration given to the fracture configuration, the patient's physiologic age as well as bone quality, and the expertise of the treating surgeon.

CONCLUSION

Hip disorders in the elderly continue to challenge the resources and expertise of health care professionals. As a growing number of Americans enter the latter decades of life, we will be faced with an increasing number of hip fractures and related disorders. Research oriented towards the prevention of osteoporosis, improvement of treatment regimens, and the establishment of comprehensive geriatric hip fracture programs may prove to be very beneficial in reducing the impact these injuries have on our patients as well as the health care system.

REFERENCES

1. Abraham GE, Lobotsky J, Lloyd CW: Metabolism in normal and ovariectomized women. *J Clin Invest* 1969; 48:696–703.
2. Agarwal N, Reyes JD, Westerman DA, Cayten CG: Factors influencing DRG 210 (hip fracture) reimbursement. *J Trauma* 1986; 26:426–431.
3. Alevizaki CC, Ikkos DG, Singhelakis P: Progressive decrease in intestinal calcium absorption with age in normal man. *J Nucl Med* 1973; 14:760–762.
4. Alffram PA: An epidemiological study of cervical and trochanteric fractures of the femur in an urban population. *Acta Orthop Scand (Suppl)* 1964; 65:1–109.
5. Arnold WD: The effect of early weight-bearing on the stability of femoral neck fractures treated with Knowles pins. *J Bone Joint Surg (Am)* 1984; 66A:847–852.
6. Aronoff PM, David PM, Wickstrom JK: Intramedullary nail fixation as treatment of subtrochanteric fractures of the femur. *J Trauma* 1971; 11:637–650.
7. Aronoff PM, Davis PM, Wickstrom JK: Subtrochanteric fractures of the femur treated by intramedullary nail fixation. *South Med J* 1972; 65:147–153.
8. Astrom J, Ahngvist S, Beertema J, et al: Physical activity in women sustaining fracture of the neck of the femur. *J Bone Joint Surg (Br)* 1987; 69B:381–383.
9. Baker HR: Ununited intertrochanteric fractures of the femur. *Clin Orthop* 1960; 18:209–220.
10. Banks HH: Factors influencing the result in fractures of the femoral neck. *J Bone Joint Surg (Am)* 1962; 44A:931–964.
11. Banks HH: Nonunion in fractures of the femoral neck. *Orthop Clin North Am* 1974; 5:865–885.
12. Barnes R, Brown JT, Garden RS, et al: Subcapital fractures of the femur. *J Bone Joint Surg (Br)* 1976; 58B:2–24.
13. Barr JS: Diagnosis and treatment of infections following internal fixation of hip fractures. *Orthop Clin North Am* 1974; 5:847–864.
14. Barry HC: Fractures of the femur in Paget's disease of bone in Australia. *J Bone Joint Surg (Am)* 1967; 49A:1359–1370.
15. Beals RK: Survival following hip fracture. Long follow-up of 607 patients. *J Chronic Dis* 1972; 25:235–244.
16. Bentley G: Impacted fractures of the neck of the femur. *J Bone Joint Surg (Br)* 1968; 50B:551–561.
17. Bentley G: Treatment of nondisplaced fractures of the femoral neck. *Clin Orthop* 1980; 152:93–101.
18. Bergman G, Winquist R, Mayo K, et al: Subtrochanteric fracture of the femur: Fixation using the Zickel nail. *J Bone Joint Surg (Am)* 1987; 69A:1032–1040.
19. Bochner RM, Pellicci PM, Lyden JP: Bipolar hemiarthroplasty for fracture of the femoral neck. Clinical review with special emphasis on prosthetic motion. *J Bone Joint Surg (Am)* 1988; 70A:1001–1010.
20. Bogoch ER, Ovellette G, Hastings DE: Failure of internal fixation of femoral neck fractures in rheumatoid arthritis patients, paper #228, Presented at *annual meeting of the American Academy of Orthopaedic Surgeons*, Las Vegas, February 11, 1989.
21. Bollett AJ, Engh G, Parson W: Epidemiology of osteoporosis. *Arch Intern Med* 1965; 16:191–194.
22. Bos CFA, Vanderlist W: Ender nailing of trochanteric and subtrochanteric fractures in 146 patients. *Acta Orthop Belg* 1982; 48:811–822.
23. Bouillon RA, Auwerx JH, Lessens WD, et al: Vitamin D status in the elderly: Seasonal substrate deficiency causes 1,25-dihydroxycholecalciferol deficiency. *Am J Clin Nutr* 1987; 45:755–763.
24. Boyd HB, Griffin LL: Classification and treatment of trochanteric fractures. *Arch Surg* 1949; 58:853–866.
25. Boyd HB, Lipinski SW: Nonunion of trochanteric and subtrochanteric fractures. *Surg Gynecol Obstet* 1957; 104:463–470.
26. Bray TJ, Smith-Hoefer E, Hooper A, et al: The displaced femoral neck fracture: Internal fixation versus bipolar endoprothesis results of a prospective, randomized comparison. *Clin Orthop* 1988; 230:127–140.
27. Brody JA: Commentary: Prospects for an ageing population. *Nature* 1985; 315:463–466.
28. Brown T, Court-Brown C: Failure of sliding nail-plate fixation in subcapital fractures of the femoral neck. *J Bone Joint Surg (Br)* 1979; 61B:342–346.
29. Buckwalter JA, Kuettner KE, Thonar EJ: Age-related changes in articular cartilage proteoglycans: Electron microscopic studies. *J Orthop Res* 1985 3:251–257.
30. Bullamore JR, Gallagher JC, Wilkinson R, et al: Effect of age on calcium absorption. *Lancet* 1970; 2:535–537.
31. Calandruccio RA, Anderson WE: Post-fracture avascular necrosis of the femoral head: Correlation of experimental and clinical studies. *Clin Orthop* 1980; 152:49–84.
32. Cassebaum WH, Nugent G: The predictability of bony union in displaced intracapsular fractures of the hip. *J Trauma* 1963; 3:421–424.

33. Chan RN, Hoskinson J: Thompson prosthesis for fractured neck of the femur. *J Bone Joint Surg (Br)* 1975; 57B:437–443.

34. Chapman MW, Bowman WE, Csongradi JJ, et al: The use of Enders pins in extracapsular fractures of the hip. *J Bone Joint Surg (Am)* 1981; 63A:14–28.

35. Christie J, Howie C, Armoir P: Fixation of displaced femoral neck fractures: Compression screw fixation versus double divergent pins. *J Bone Joint Surg (Br)* 1988; 70B:199–201.

36. Cleveland M, Bosworth DM, Thompson FR: Intertrochanteric fractures of the femur. *J Bone Joint Surg* 1947; 29:1049–1067.

37. Cobb AG, Gibson PH: Screw fixation of subcapital fractures of the femur—a better method of treatment. *Injury* 1986; 17:259–264.

38. Cobey JC, Cobey JH, Conant L, et al: Indications of recovery from fractures of the hip. *Clin Orthop* 1976; 117:258–262.

39. Coughlin L, Templeton J: Hip fractures in patients with Parkinson's disease. *Clin Orthop* 1980; 148:192–195.

40. Coventry MB: An evaluation of the femoral head prosthesis after ten years of experience. *Surg Gynecol Obstet* 1959; 109:243–244.

41. Coventry MB: The treatment of fracture-dislocation of the hip by total hp arthroplasty. *J Bone Joint Surg (Am)* 1974; 56A:1128–1134.

42. Craxford AO, Stevens J: Proximal femoral fractures in psychiatric patients. *Injury* 1979; 11:19.

43. Culver D, Crawford JS, Gardiner JH, et al: Venous thrombosis after fracture of the upper end of the femur: A study of incidence and site. *J Bone Joint Surg (Br)* 1970; 52B:61–69.

44. Cummings SR, Kelsey JL, Nevitt MC, et al: Epidemiology of osteoporosis and osteoporotic fractures. *Epidemiol Rev* 1985; 7:178–208.

45. D'Arcy J, Devas M: Treatment of fractures of the femoral neck by replacement with the Thompson prosthesis. *J Bone Joint Surg (Br)* 1976; 58B:279–286.

46. Dahl E: Mortality and life expectancy after hip fractures. *Acta Orthop Scand* 1980; 51:163–170.

47. DeLee JC: in Rockwood CA, Green DP (eds): *Fractures in Adults*, ed 2, vol 2. Philadelphia, JB Lippincott, 1984, pp 1211–1357.

48. Dimon JH, Hughston JC: Unstable intertrochanteric fractures of the hip. *J Bone Joint Surg (Am)* 1967; 49A:440–450.

49. Dove J: Complete fractures of the femur in Paget's disease of bone. *J Bone Joint Surg (Br)* 1980; 62B:12–17.

50. Elabdien BS, Olerud S, Karlstrom G: Ender nailing of pertrochanteric fractures: Complications related to technical failures and bone quality. *Acta Orthop Scand* 1985; 56:138–144.

51. Eriksen EF, Mosekilde L, Melsen F: Trabecular bone resorption depth increases with age: Differences between normal males and females. *Bone* 1985; 6:141–146.

52. Eskeland C, Solheinik H, Skjorten F: Anticoagulant prophylaxis, thromboembolism and mortality in elderly patients with hip fractures. A controlled clinical trial. *Acta Chir Scand* 1966; 131:16–29.

53. Evans EM: The treatment of trochanteric fractures of the femur. *J Bone Joint Surg (Br)* 1949; 31B:190–203.

54. Evans EM: Trochanteric fractures. *J Bone Joint Surg (Br)* 1951; 33B:192–204.

55. Eventor I, Moreno M, Geller E, et al: Hip fractures in patients with Parkinson's syndrome. *J Trauma* 1983; 23:98–101.

56. Eversmann WW: Entrapment and compression neuropathies, in Green DP (ed): *Operative Hand Surgery* ed 2. New York, Churchill Livingstone, 1988, pp 1430–1440.

57. Fairclough J, Colhoun E, Johnson D, et al: Bone scanning for suspected hip fractures. *J Bone Joint Surg (Br)* 1987; 69B:251–253.

58. Fielding JW, Magliato HJ: Subtrochanteric fractures, *Surg Gynecol Obstet* 1966; 122:555–560.

59. Galasko CSB: Skeletal metastases. *Clin Orthop* 1986; 210:18–30.

60. Galasko CS, Rushton S, Sylvester BS, et al: The significance of peak expiratory flow rate in assessing prognosis of elderly patients undergoing operations on the hip. *Injury* 1985; 16:398–401.

61. Gallagher JC, Melton LJ, Riggs BL, et al: Epidemiology of fractures of the proximal femur in Rochester Minnesota. *Clin Orthop* 1980; 150:163–167.

62. Gallagher JC, Riggs BL, Eisman J, et al: Intestinal calcium absorption and serum Vitamin D metabolites in normal subjects and osteoporotic patients. *J Clin Invest* 1979; 64:729–736.

63. Garden RS: Low angle fixation in fractures of the femoral neck. *J Bone Joint Surg (Br)* 1961; 43B:647–663.

64. Gates B, Fairbaum A, Craxford AD: Broken necks of the femur in a psychogeriatric hospital. *Injury* 1986; 17:383–386.

65. Gordon PC: The probability of death following fracture of the hip. *Can Med Assoc J* 1971; 105:47–62.

66. Hamilton HW, Crawford JS, Gardiner JH, et al: Venous thrombosis in patients with fractures of the upper end of the femur: A phlebographic study of the effect of prophylactic anticoagulation. *J Bone Joint Surg (Br)* 1970; 52B:268–289.

67. Harper MC, Walsh T: Ender nailing for pantrochanteric fractures of the femur: An analysis of indications, factors related to mechanical failure and postoperative results. *J Bone Joint Surg (Am)* 1985; 67A:79–88.

68. Holmberg S, Kalen R, Thorngren KG: Treatment and outcome of femoral neck fractures. *Clin Orthop* 1987; 218:42–52.

69. Jee WSS: The skeletal tissues, in Weiss L (ed): *Histology and Tissue Biology*, New York, Elsevier, 1983.

70. Jensen JS, Sonne-Holm S, Tondevold E: Unstable interbiochanteric fractures: A comparative analysis of four methods of internal fixation. *Acta Orthop Scand* 1980; 51:949–962.

71. Jensen JS, Tondevold E: Mortality after hip fractures. *Acta Orthop Scand* 1979; 50:161–167.

72. Jensen TT, Juncker V: Pressure sores common after hip operations. *Acta Orthop Scand* 1987; 58:209–211.

73. Jewett EL: One piece angle nail for trochanteric fractures. *J Bone Joint Surg* 1941; 23:803–810.

74. Johnell O, Sernbo I: Health and social status in patients with hip fractures and controls. *Age Ageing* 1986; 15:285–291.

75. Johnston CE, Ripley LP, Bray CB: Primary endoprosthetic replacement for acute femoral neck fractures. *Clin Orthop* 1982; 167:123–130.

76. Jones S, DiPito JT, Nix DE, et al: Cephelosporins for prophylaxis in operative repair of femoral fractures: Levels in serum, muscle and hematoma. *J Bone Joint Surg (Am)* 1985; 67A:921–924.

77. Kaufer H, Matthews LS, Sonstegard D: Stable fixation of intertrochanteric fractures. *J Bone Joint Surg* 1974; 56A:899–907.

78. Kenzora JE, McCarthy RE, Lowell JD, et al: Hip fracture mortality. *Clin Orthop* 1984; 186:45–56.

79. Kuderna H, Bohler N, Collon DJ: Treatment of intertrochanteric and subtrochanteric fractures of the hip by the Ender method. *J Bone Joint Surg (Am)* 1976; 58A:604–611.

80. Kuokkanen H, Korkala O, Lauttamus L: Ender nailing of trochanteric fractures: A review of 73 cases. *Arch Orthop Trauma Surg* 1986; 105:46–48.

81. Kyle RF, Gustilo RB, Premer RF: Analysis of 622 intertrochanteric hip fractures: A retrospective study, *J Bone Joint Surg (Am)* 1979; 61A:216–221.

82. Letournel E, Judet R: in Elson RA, (trans and ed): *Fractures of the Acetabulum*. New York, Springer-Verlag, 1981, pp 29–31.

83. Lichtblau S: A pitfall in the insertion of a sliding screw. *Bull Hosp Joint Dis* 1986; 46:60–62.

84. Manoli A: Malassembly of the sliding screw-plate device. *J Trauma* 1986; 26:916–922.

85. Mariani EM, Rand JA: Nonunion of intertrochanteric fractures of the femur following open reduction and internal fixation. *Clin Orthop* 1987; 218:81–89.

86. Martens M, Van Audelercke R, Mulier JC, et al: Clinical study on internal fixation of femoral neck fractures. *Clin Orthop* 1979; 141:199–202.

87. Massie WK: Treatment of femoral neck fractures emphasizing long term follow-up observations on aseptic necrosis. *Clin Orthop* 1973; 92:16–62.

88. Matta JM, Anderson LM, Epstein H, et al: Fractures of the acetabulum. A retrospective analysis. *Clin Orthop* 1986; 205:230–240.

89. Matta JM, Mehne DK, Roffi R: Fractures of the acetabulum. Early results of a prospective study. *Clin Orthop* 1986; 205:241–250.

90. Milgram JW: Orthopaedic management of Paget's disease of bone. *Clin Orthop* 1977; 127:63–69.

91. Miller CW: Survival and ambulation following hip fracture. *J Bone Joint Surg (Am)* 1978; 60A:930–934.

92. Morley JE: Nutritional status of the elderly. *Am J Med* 1986; 81:679–695.

93. Morley JE, Gorbien MJ, Mooradian AD, et al: UCLA geriatric grand rounds: Osteoporosis. *J Am Geriatr Soc* 1988; 36:845–859.

94. Moskovitz PA, Ellenberg SS, Feffer HL, et al: Low dose heparin for prevention of venous thromboembolismin total hip arthroplasty and surgical repair of hip fractures, *J Bone Joint Surg (Am)* 1978; 60A:1065–1070.

95. Mulholland RC, Gunn DR: Sliding screw plate fixation of intertrochanteric femoral fractures. *J Trauma* 1972; 12:581–591.

96. Mullen JO: Relationship of admission mental status, hospital confusion, and mortality in hip fractures: A prospective study. Presented at *52nd annual meeting, American Academy of Orthopaedic Surgeons*, Las Vegas, Jan 24, 1985.

97. Muller ME, Allgower M, Willeneger H: *Manual of Internal Fixation*. New York, Springer-Verlag, 1970.

98. Nicholas JA, Killoran P: Fracture of the femur in patients with Paget's disease. *J Bone Joint Surg (Am)* 1965; 47A:450–461.

99. Nieminen S: Early weight-bearing after classical internal fixation of medial fractures of the femoral neck. *Acta Orthop Scand* 1975; 46:782–794.

100. Norden CW: A critical review of antibiotic prophylaxis in orthopedic surgery. *Rev Infect Dis* 1983; 5:928–932.

101. Pauwels F: *Der Schenkelhalsbruch, ein Mechanisches Problem: Grundlagen des Heilungsvorganges, Prognose und Kausale Therapie*. Stuttgart, Ferdinand Enke Verlag, 1935.

102. Peyron JG: Osteoarthritis: The epidemiologic viewpoint. *Clin Orthop* 1986; 213:13–19.

103. Pocock NA, Eisman JA, Yeates MG, et al: Physical fitness is a major determinant of femoral neck and lumbar spine bone mineral density. *J Clin Invest* 1986; 78:618–621.

104. Rankin LM: Fractures of the pelvis. *Ann Surg* 1937; 106:266–277.

105. Riggs BL: Pathogenesis of osteoporosis. *Am J Obstet Gynecol* 1987; 156:1342–1346.

106. Riggs BL, Melton LJ: Involutional osteoporosis. *N Engl J Med* 1986; 314:1676–1686.

107. Rodriguez J, Herrara A, Canales V, et al: Epidemiologic factors, morbidity and mortality after femoral neck fracture in the elderly. *Acta Orthop Belg* 1987; 53:472–479.

108. Rosenfeld RT, Schwartz DR, Alter AH: Prosthetic replacement for trochanteric fractures of the femur. *J Bone Joint Surg (Am)* 1973; 55A:420.

109. Russin LA, Sonni A: Treatment of intertrochanteric and subtrochanteric fractures with Ender's intramedullary rods. *Clin Orthop* 1980; 148:203–212.

110. Salter RB, Minster RR, Clements N, et al: Continuous passive motion and the repair of full thickness articular cartilage defects: A one year follow-up. *Orthop Trans* 1982; 6:266–267.

111. Sangeorzan BJ, Ryan JR, Salciccroli GG: Prophylactic femoral stabilization with the Zickel nail by closed technique. *J Bone Joint Surg (Am)* 1986; 68A:991–999.

112. Sarmiento A: Intertrochanteric fractures of the femur: 150-degree-angle nail-plate fixation and early rehabilitation: A preliminary report of 100 cases. *J Bone Joint Surg (Am)* 1963; 45A:706–722.

113. Sarmiento A: Unstable intertrochanteric fractures of the femur. *Clin Orthop* 1973; 92:77–85.

114. Sarmiento A, Williams EM: The unstable intertrochanteric fracture: Treatment with a valgus osteotomy and I-Beam nail-plate. *J Bone Joint Surg* 1970; 52A:1309–1318.

115. Schatzker J, Waddell JP: Subtrochanteric fractures of the femur. *Orthop Clin North Am* 1980; 11:539–554.

116. Scheck M: The significance of posterior comminution in femoral neck fractures. *Clin Orthop* 1980; 152:138–142.

117. Scileppi KP: Aging of the musculoskeletal system, in

Sculco TP (ed): *Orthopaedic Care of the Geriatric Patient.* St Louis, Mosby-Year Book, 1985, pp 3–11.

118. Scott WA, Allum RL, Wright K: Implant induced trabecular damage in cadaveric femoral necks. *Acta Orthop Scand* 1985; 56:145–146.

119. Seinsheimer F: Subtrochanteric fractures of the femur. *J Bone Joint Surg (Am)* 1978; 60A:300–306.

120. Sernbo I, Johnell O, Gentz G, et al: Unstable intertrochanteric fractures of the hip: Treatment with Ender pins compared with compression hip screw. *J Bone Joint Surg (Am)* 1988; 70A:1297–1303.

121. Sexson SB, Lehner JT: Factors affecting hip fracture mortality. *J Orthop Trauma* 1988; 1:298–305.

122. Siverberg SJ, Lindsay R: Postmenopausal osteoporosis, *Med Clin North Am* 1987; 71:41–57.

123. Sisk TD: Fractures, in Edmonson AS, Crenshaw AH (eds): *Campbell's Operative Orthopaedics.* St Louis, Mosby-Year Book, 1980, pp 1719–1720.

124. Skinner PW, Powles D: Compression screw fixation for displaced subcapital fracture of the femur: Success or failure? *J Bone Joint Surg (Br)* 1986; 68B:78–82.

125. Soreide O, Mölster A, Raugstad TS: Internal fixation versus primary prosthetic replacement in acute femoral neck fractures: A prospective, randomized clinical study. *Br J Surg* 1979; 66:56–60.

126. Spencer RF: Acetabular fractures in older patients. *J Bone Joint Surg (Br)* 1989 71B:774–776.

127. Stappaerts KH, Broos PL: Internal fixation of femoral neck fractures: A follow-up study of 118 cases. *Acta Chir Belg* 1987; 87:247–251.

128. Stern MB, Angerman A: Comminuted intertrochanteric fractures treated with Leinbach prosthesis. *Clin Orthop* 1987; 218:75–80.

129. Stern MB, Goldstein TB: The use of the Leinbach prosthesis in intertrochanteric fracture of the hip. *Clin Orthop* 1977; 128:325–331.

130. Stromquist B, Hansson L, Nilsson L, et al: Hook pin fixation in femoral neck fractures: A two year follow-up study of 300 cases. *Clin Orthop* 1987; 218:58–62.

131. Swiontkowski MF, Harrington RM, Keller TS, et al: Torsion and bending analysis of internal fixation techniques for femoral neck fractures: The role of implant design and bone density. *J Orthop Res* 1987; 5:433–444.

132. Swiontkowski MF, Winquist RA, Hansen ST: Femoral neck fractures in patients aged 12–49. *J Bone Joint Surg (Am)* 1984; 66A:837–846.

133. Taylor GM, Neufield AJ, Nickel VL: Complications and failures in the operative treatment of intertrochanteric fractures of the femur. *J Bone Joint Surg (Am)* 1955; 37A:306–316.

134. Testa NN, Mazur K: Heterotopic ossification after direct lateral approach and transtrochanteric approach to the hip. *Orthop Rev* 1988; 18:965–971.

135. Tronzo RG: Special considerations in management. *Orthop Clin North Am* 1974; 5:571–583.

136. Waddell JP: Femoral head preservation following subcapital fracture of the femur. *Instr Course Lect* 1984; 33:179–190.

137. Waddell JP: Subtrochanteric fractures of the femur: A review of 130 patients. *J Trauma* 1979; 19:583–592.

138. Waddell J, Czitrom A, Simmons EH: Ender nailing in fractures of the proximal femur. *J Trauma* 1987; 27:911–916.

139. White BL, Fisher WD, Laurin CA: Rate of mortality for elderly patients after fracture of the hip in the 1980s. *J Bone Joint Surg (Am)* 1987; 69A:1335–1340.

140. Winter WG: Non-operative treatment of proximal femoral fractures in the demented, non-ambulatory patient. *Clin Orthop* 1987; 218:97–103.

141. Wolfgang GL, Bryant MH, O'Neill JP: Treatment of intertrochanteric fracture of the femur using sliding screw plate fixation. *Clin Orthop* 1982; 163:148–158.

Hip Injuries: A Rehabilitation Perspective

Kathy Kampa, M.S., P.T.

The hip joint is a common site of dysfunction in the geriatric population. Not only can localized and referred pain to the hip region create discomfort, but it can also interfere with an individual's mobility and independence. Hip dysfunction can limit a person's ability to live alone, walk alone, and most importantly, to enjoy his or her surroundings.

This chapter will first present an overview of the anatomy, physiology, and biomechanics of the hip joint. Normal aging and commonly seen pathologic changes occurring within the aging hip joint will be discussed. Expected changes during objective evaluation of the geriatric hip will be presented. The chapter will also include guidelines for the physical therapist treating a patient with either a nonoperative or operative hip dysfunction. The chapter will present views regarding the prognosis and follow-up of hip injuries and concepts in the prevention of these injuries in the geriatric population.

ANATOMY

The hip joint is a synovial ball-and-socket joint located just inferior to the midline of the inguinal ligament.[26] The hip joint consists of the bony articulation between the proximal portion of the femur and the acetabulum, which is formed by the ilium, ischium, and pubic bones. The head of the femur is shaped in such a way to enable a great deal of motion within this acetabular cup (Fig 17–1).

The femoral head is covered by articular carti-

lage, except for a central area where the ligamentum teres connects the femur with a rich vascular supply from the acetabulum. The ligamentum teres, unlike the strong capsular ligaments at the hip, does not restrict hip motion.

A thickening in the articular cartilage of the superior acetabulum called the *labrum* increases the socket depth, encapsulating more of the femoral head. The acetabular labrum is much like the glenoid labrum in the shoulder, which serves to deepen and cushion the articulating surface within the joint. The acetabular labrum allows increased yet stable hip motion.

The head of the femur is held in the acetabulum by a strong joint capsule. The attachment of the joint capsule defines areas of the proximal femur as being intracapsular or extracapsular. The fibrous capsule is strong and dense. It extends from the surface above the acetabulum across the actual hip joint to the trochanteric line of the femoral neck. The capsule is thicker at the proximal portion of the joint, where it sustains greater forces.[26]

The joint capsule has thickenings or ligaments that strengthen the integrity of the capsule when in a stretched position (Fig 17–2). Anteriorly, the iliofemoral ligament or ligament of Bigelow is described as an inverted Y, which extends from the anterior inferior iliac spine to the region of the trochanteric line. This ligament resists excessive hip extension and internal rotation. Posteriorly, the pubofemoral and ischiofemoral ligaments reinforce the joint capsule. The pubofemoral ligament, running from the pubis to an area anterior to the lesser trochanter, resists excessive lower extremity abduction

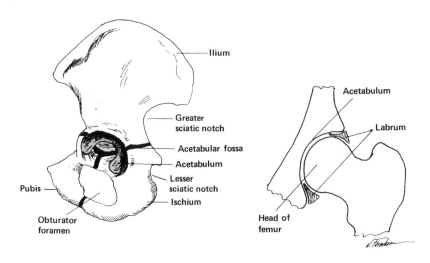

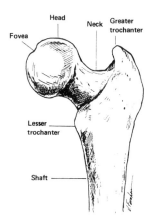

FIG 17–1.
The hip joint. Articulating surfaces on the pelvis. *Top left,* the drawing of a left hip bone shows the acetabulum located on the lateral aspect. *Top right,* lateral view of the hip joint shows the acetabulum labrum grasping the head of the femur. *Bottom,* an anterior view of the proximal portion of the left femur shows the normal relationship between the head, neck, and femoral shaft. (From Norkin C, Levangie P: *Joint Structure and Function.* Philadelphia, FA Davis, 1983, pp 259–260. Used with permission.)

and internal rotation. The ischiofemoral ligament, rising from the ischium to the superior posterior femoral neck, resists hip extension and internal rotation.

These ligaments blend in a twisting fashion into the joint capsule so that there needs to be an added unwinding to stretch the ligament. Both amputees and paraplegics with weak hip extensors are taught to use the inherent stability in the ligaments to maintain an upright position. This is referred to by some as "hanging on the Y ligaments," and can be done by moving the body's center of gravity posterior to the hip joint axis producing an extension moment at the hip.

The closed, packed position of the hip joint is extension, abduction, and external rotation.[26] This is why the surgeon operating on the hip will flex, ad-

duct, and internally rotate the hip to more easily gain access to the hip joint capsule.

Muscles of the Hip Joint

Six major hip motions are produced by the muscles surrounding the hip joint. The hip joint muscles are usually discussed in terms of the motions for which they are most responsible. A few, however, are able to produce motions different from those with which they are commonly associated, depending on the amount of hip flexion present. For example, a prime hip adductor may be a secondary hip flexor when the hip is flexed.

The muscles producing hip flexion are the psoas major and iliacus. Secondary hip flexors include the pectineus, rectus femoris, sartorius, adductor lon-

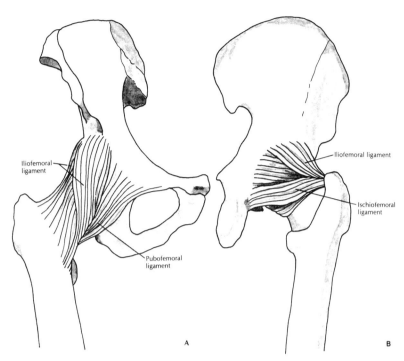

FIG 17–2.
Ligaments of the hip joint. **A,** anterior. **B,** posterior. (From Hertling D, Kessler R: Management of common musculoskeletal disorders, in Hertling D, Kessler R (eds): *Physical* *Therapy Principles and Methods,* ed 2. Philadelphia, JB Lippincott, 1990, p 277. Used with permission.)

gus, brevis, and magnus (oblique fibers), and tensor fasciae latae.

Muscles responsible for hip extension are the gluteus maximus, semitendinosus, semimembranosus, and biceps femoris (long head).

Hip abduction is primarily achieved by the gluteus medius and gluteus minimus. Secondary hip abductors include the tensor fascia latae and gluteus maximus (upper fibers).

Primary hip adduction is achieved by contraction of the adductor longus, adductor brevis, and adductor magnus. The pectineus and gracilis are secondary hip adductors.

Hip internal rotation is obtained by tensor fasciae latae, the anterior portion of gluteus minimus, gluteus medius, semitendinosus, and semimembranosus.

External rotation is primarily achieved by the obturator muscles, the gemelli, and quadratus femoris. Secondary external rotators are the piriformis, gluteus maximus, sartorius, and biceps femoris (long head).[6, 26]

Bursae

Bursae decrease friction between muscles and the bony prominences they traverse. The bursae are named according to their anatomic relationships: i.e., bony landmarks or muscles. The four bursae located in close proximity to the hip joint include the superficial and deep trochanteric, the iliopectineal, and the ischiogluteal. The superficial trochanteric bursa is found just below the skin over the greater trochanter and separates the gluteus maximus and medius muscles from the greater trochanter of the femur. The deep trochanteric bursa is found directly posterior to the greater trochanter near to the insertion of the gluteus maximus. The iliopectineal bursa lies on the anterior hip joint capsule, providing a smooth surface over which the iliopsoas muscle glides. The ischiogluteal bursa covers the ischial tuberosity, lessening the friction between the gluteus maximus and the tuberosity during contraction of the gluteus maximus.

Innervation

Innervation of the hip joint comes from lumbar segments L2-S1.[6, 10, 26] Anteriorly the hip joint is supplied by the femoral and posterior division of the obturator nerves. Posteriorly the hip is supplied by the nerve to quadratus femoris and the superior gluteal nerve.

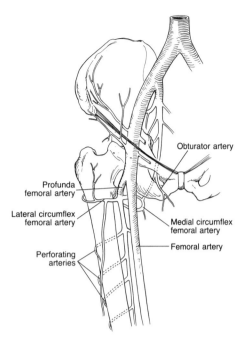
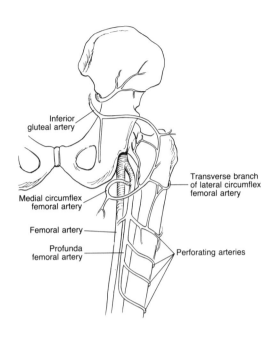
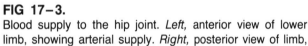

FIG 17–3.
Blood supply to the hip joint. *Left,* anterior view of lower limb, showing arterial supply. *Right,* posterior view of limb, showing arterial supply. (Adapted from Moore K: *Clinically Oriented Anatomy.* Baltimore, Williams & Wilkins, 1980.)

Blood Supply

Blood supply to the hip joint capsule is plentiful, while the head of the femur has only single blood supply. The anterior capsule and joint are supplied by the lateral femoral circumflex artery, the posterior portion by the medial circumflex artery, the most superior portion of the joint capsule by the inferior gluteal artery, and the head of the femur is supplied by a branch of the obturator artery[26] (Fig 17–3). Because there is no secondary circulation to the head of the femur, it is important that the integrity of its blood supply be confirmed after an injury to the area.

BIOMECHANICS

The bony framework and designs of each individual femur create different hip joint configurations. These variations alter the entire lower extremity's biomechanics. An alteration of the biomechanics of an extremity, especially a weight-bearing extremity, is thus capable of changing the energy consumption during different activities of daily living (ADL).

The femur itself is the longest bone in the hu-

man body.[26] It articulates proximally with the acetabulum and distally with the tibia. The diaphysis of the femur ends superiorly in the region of the greater trochanter, where the femur angulates superomedially. This section of the femur is called the femoral neck. The angle created between the diaphysis and the neck is called the angle of inclination. A normal angle of inclination is approximately 125 degrees. A larger angle between the femoral neck and shaft is termed coxa valga; a smaller angle is called coxa vara. The femoral neck then connects to the femoral head, creating a mechanism for the stance leg to receive the weight of the upper body and trunk.

The femur also exhibits antetorsion. Antetorsion describes the position of the femoral head anterior to the sagittal plane of the femur. Normal antetorsion is an angle of approximately 15 degrees. The degree of antetorsion determines the amount of femoral head surface area that articulates with the acetabulum. Normally, in upright stance, weight bearing is limited to a small section of the posterior superior femoral head.

Retroversion, an antetorsion angle of less than 15 degrees, limits internal rotation of the hip and often creates a toe-out gait. Anteversion, an angle of more than 15 degree, limits hip external rotation and is characterized by a toe-in gait pattern. Biomechanically, increased anteversion will increase the moment arm of the gluteus maximus and is therefore important to consider during a total hip replacement procedure. If the moment arm of the gluteus maximus is increased the patient does not need to contract the gluteus maximus to the same degree as when the moment arm was shorter. The surgeon can thus artificially create an anteverted femoral head to ensure that the surgically disrupted hip extensor does not need to contract with preoperative force.

The degree of antetorsion, therefore, can also be another factor in the progressive wear of the hip joint surfaces. Decreased muscular efficiency from lack of exercise or decreased antetorsion tends to promote degenerative joint changes.

Trabecular Patterns

The femoral neck is able to withstand incumbent weight owing to bony architecture and muscular support. Within the neck and greater trochanter areas of the femur a model of bone organization works to absorb compressive, loading, and shear-bending forces directed through the femoral neck. This bony framework is the setup of trabeculae in three organized systems (Fig 17–4). The arcuate trabeculae bundle, which traverses from the greater trochanter superiomedially towards the femoral head, resists shearing forces directed through the femoral head. The vertical trabeculae bundle running from the medial femoral shaft superiorly to the superior femoral head resists downward compression forces through the femoral head and neck. The trochanteric trabeculae bundle running laterally from the medial base of the femoral neck to the greater trochanter resists the tensile forces of contracting muscles that are attached to the greater trochanter. In the region where these trabecular bundles cross, there is an increase in bone strength. Where there is no bundle, or where there are one or two bundles only, there is an inherent weakness in the bone, limiting the amount of compressive, tensile or shear forces that can be absorbed. Trabecular patterns are important in the study of hip fractures, where there is often a change in both bone stock and density.

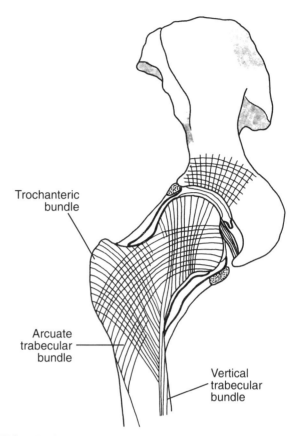

FIG 17–4.
Trabecular patterns of the upper femur. (From Hertling, Kessler: Management of Common Musculoskeletal Disorders, in: *Physical Therapy Principles and Methods*, ed 2. Philadelphia, JB Lippincott, 1990. p 276. Used with permission.)

EVALUATION OF THE HIP JOINT

Evaluation of the hip joint entails not only a thorough understanding of hip anatomy and pathology, but knowledge also of the pelvis, lumbar spine, and knee. Not only must the hip joint be clearly suspected as the originating site of the symptoms, but a thorough hip evaluation should eliminate the presence of a pelvic, spine, or knee dysfunction that may be the actual source of symptoms at the hip.

On the basis of subjective and objective information, the physical therapist must first determine if the dysfunction is taking place in contractile or noncontractile tissue. (The work of Cyriax is recommended for review.[4, 5]) Once the location of the dysfunction is determined, a more defined physical therapy diagnosis is needed. In order for appropriate treatment to begin, the physical therapy evaluation must begin with the patient's subjective report or the history of the present problem. Patient questioning should include:

1. When did the pain or problem originate?
2. Was there any previous trauma to the hip, pelvis, or lower extremity?

3. Is there a family history of hip dysfunction?
4. Is there a contributory medical history?
5. What medications are taken and have there been any injections, such as cortisone injections, into the hip joint?
6. How far can the patient walk before having to stop and relieve weight from the involved hip?
7. Is it possible to cut the toenails on the involved side in a tailor's position? Is hip range of motion limited?
8. Is there any pain? If so, where? Does it spread?
9. What makes the pain better?
10. What makes the pain worse?
11. Is there any night pain?
12. Has there been any recent weight loss or gain?
13. Is any numbness or parasthesia present?
14. Are there any other specific activities that may be limited owing to hip pain?

A differential physical therapy diagnosis can be set up after listening to the patient's report of symptom onset, symptom progression, and ADL limitations. With the addition of an account of the patient's past medical history and a thorough clinical examination, a more accurate physical therapy diagnosis can be formed.

The objective part of the examination should begin with gait analysis as the patient enters the clinic. Notations of assistance needed, devices used, and gait deviations present must be made (Table 17–1). While taking the patient's history, the clinician should note if the patient is able to sit comfortably or if he or she must stand. Sitting is generally more comfortable for patients with osteoarthritis of the hip because weight has been removed from the involved leg. Patients with spinal stenosis will also get relief upon sitting, whereas patients with lumbar disc disease or herniation are often more comfortable standing or while walking than sitting.

Inspection of sitting and standing posture, if it is possible for the patient, is next performed. Degree of symmetry between right and left anatomic landmarks can indicate the presence of spinal rotations, deformities, and muscular atrophy. Accurate bony palpation will aid in postural analysis (Fig 17–5). Posture should be assessed from the front, side, and behind the patient. This is a convenient time during the evaluation to scan the body for other deformities and past surgical incisions, as well as varicosities, hair growth, and trophic nail changes.

TABLE 17–1.

Common Gait Deviations and Possible Causes[10, 21]

Deviation	Possible Causes
1. Lurch toward weight-bearing limb	1. Weak hip abductor on stance side
	2. Pain in stance hip
	3. Coxa vara of stance hip
	4. Hip dislocation on stance side
	5. Shorter leg on stance side
2. Lurch posteriorly on weight bearing	1. Weak hip extensor on stance side
	2. Weak hip flexor on swing side
3. Anterior trunk bend	1. Weak quadriceps during stance
	2. Weak gluteus maximus during stance
4. Increased lumbar lordosis when weight bearing	1. Poor flexibility and strength in stance hip flexors
	2. Generalized hip weakness
5. Dropping of pelvis on stance side	1. Abductor weakness on stance side
6. Vaulting	1. Shorter leg on stance side
	2. Extension ankylosis of swing hip
7. Increased base of support	1. Hip abductor contracture, either hip
	2. Joint instability, either hip
	3. Pain, either hip
	4. Leg length discrepancy, either leg

The evaluation can then continue with the patient in a short sitting position with assessment of sensation, deep tendon reflexes and proprioception. Gross muscle testing can be done with the patient in a sitting position, with more precise testing performed in the supine or side-lying position as needed.

With the patient supine, palpation of anterior and lateral hip surfaces is possible. Soft-tissue palpation locates tenderness and the presence of muscle spasm. Masses may also be detected with accurate soft tissue inspection. Masses must be described precisely in terms of location, size, consistency, and tenderness, and reported to the referring physician immediately. Any areas of suspected swelling or atrophy must be objectively measured bilaterally for present and future comparison.

Range of motion can be evaluated by allowing the patient while supine to flex, rotate, abduct, and adduct the hip. Hip extension is most easily evaluated with the patient in a prone or side-lying position. Alternatively, internal and external rotation can be assessed with the patient in short sitting, and hip

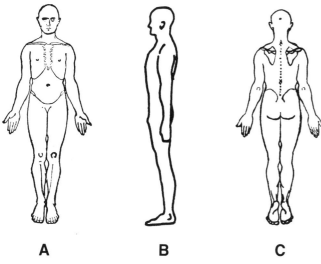

A   **B**   **C**

FIG 17–5.
Posture evaluation: bony landmarks. **A,** anterior view: head position, shoulder levels, midline sternum orientation, lower extremity rotation, iliac crests, anterior superior iliac spine, medial malleoli, navicular tubercle, first metatarsal head. **B,** lateral view: head position, shoulder position, thoracic kyphosis, lumbar lordosis, hip flexion contracture, knee flexion contracture, genu recurvatum. **C,** posterior view: head position, shoulder levels, scapular position and height, posterior superior iliac spine, gluteal folds, greater trochanters, popliteal folds, fibular heads, alignment of hindfoot.

TABLE 17–2.
Hip Range of Motion*

Type of Motion	Range (Degrees)
Flexion	125
Extension	15
Abduction	45
Adduction	45
Internal Rotation	45
External Rotation	45

*Data from Daniels and Worthingham.[6]

extension can as well be measured in the standing position.

Assessment of passive range of motion would not be complete without note given to the quality of the motion. Notation of crepitus, clicking, snapping, or pain during the motion, as well as the quality of motion end feel, is important. Crepitus elicited during passive range-of-motion testing may denote arthritic changes of the joint surfaces being examined, while clicking may be indicative of a loose joint body or of a nearby tendon catching on a bony prominence. Snapping also may represent a tendon moving across a bony landmark. Pain often designates underlying dysfunction and should be further assessed as well as reproduced during evaluation. Severity, location and reproducibility of patient-reported pain is important. The ability to clearly reproduce the patient's stated pain complaints may help in determining the mechanism of injury and the treatment of such an injury.[4]

Normal ranges of hip motion can be found in Table 17–2. It is important to note that while range of motion values are expected to decrease with aging, there are few research studies examining age or sex differentials in range-of-motion values. James

and Parker reported in 1989 that hip abduction declined most among those aged 70 to 92 years who participated in a lower limb mobility study. Hip abduction was found consistently among elderly subjects to be the only hip motion to show a significant and consistent decline with increasing age. These researchers also found limitations in hip internal and external rotation among their subjects, although to a lesser degree than the abduction limitation. The study results also describe a general increased joint mobility found among the female compared with the male population aged 70 to 92 years.[13]

Special Tests

The Thomas Test.—This test can be used to detect a shortened iliopsoas muscle. Tightness in this muscle will be revealed by increased lumbar lordosis when the patient is placed supine with the hip at 0 degrees flexion and knee at 90 degrees flexion (Fig 17–6, A–C).

Ely's Test.—Performed with the patient in the prone position, Ely's test will rule out a tight iliopsoas in the presence of a tight rectus femoris. Knee flexion in the prone position that produces hip flexion points to a tight iliopsoas. Production of increased lumbar lordosis will detect a tight rectus femoris.

Ober's Test.—When performed with the patient in the side-lying position, Ober's test will detect a tightness in the tensor fasciae latae. The top leg is extended and adducted to observe for tightness in the ipsilateral tenso. A positive Ober's sign may also indicate bursitis or tendinitis at the ipsilateral greater trochanter (Fig 17–6, D and E).

Fabere or Patrick Test.—This test will aid the clinician in reproducing symptoms from a painful hip

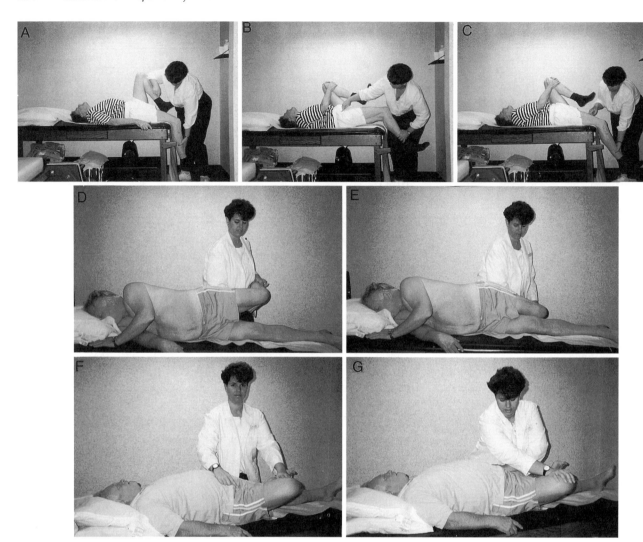

FIG 17–6.
A, negative Thomas test. **B,** positive Thomas test for hip flexor tightness. **C,** positive Thomas test for (rectus femoris) quadriceps tightness. **D,** positive Ober's test. **E,** negative or sacroiliac joint. The leg to be examined is ab-

Ober's test. Fabere or Patrick test: **G,** hip joint dysfunction; **F,** sacroiliac dysfunction.

ducted, flexed, and externally rotated. The lateral malleolus of the involved leg rests on the uninvolved side's knee. If pain is produced in the ipsilateral anterior groin, hip pathology can be suspected (Fig 17–6,F). Symptoms of sacroiliac involvement are reproduced when pressure is applied to the ipsilateral knee and contralateral anterior ilium concurrently (Fig 17–6, G).

Compression.—Compression of the hip joint during internal and external rotation of the flexed hip will detect specific areas of the hip joint that may have articular or osseous changes.

Distraction.—In a painful hip with severe osteoarthritic changes, distraction may decrease pain.

Leg Length.—Leg length measurements are of value in detecting causes for gait deviations and secondary osteoarthritis. Many surgeons wish leg length measurements to be done 8 to 12 weeks after hip surgery, to allow shortened joint capsules and muscles to lengthen before addressing the leg length discrepancy with a heel or shoe lift. It is important to reassure the patient who feels a difference in leg length that although there may in fact be a difference, time must be allowed for stretching previously tightened structures.

CHANGES WITHIN THE HIP WITH AGE

There are many normal "expected" changes that take place within each individual human with aging. Some of these alterations begin earlier than was perhaps first realized. In simpler terms, the body is always changing and completing an aging process from the time each of us is born. Some may argue as well that we are aging from the moment of conception. In some instances these modifications are adaptations that assist the organism to continue to live. In other instances the adaptation conflicts with the organism's ease of living. Disease processes may initiate, cultivate, or redirect the natural aging process of either the entire system or a separate portion, such as the hip joint.

The effects of a more forwardly directed head and shoulders and an increase in thoracic kyphosis can promote a hip flexion posture. Lack of stretching tight hip flexor musculature can also promote anterior trunk flexion, protracted shoulders, and increased thoracic kyphosis. More often than not, hip flexors become tight with age. Joint flexibility diminishes with time as the elastic fibers of the capsule, ligaments, and tendons become less pliable.[12, 16] These less elastic structures will then limit hip motion. Limitations in hip motion then affect the positions and activities of the hip joint. With normal aging the extent to which the hip musculature can contract is limited, as well as the amount of force attained via muscle contraction. Muscles that are either tight or stretched are limited in their ability to generate force. Owing to the length-tension association of muscle fiber components, a lengthened muscle has less mechanical advantage to create filament binding and subsequent muscle shortening. A shortened and contracted muscle cannot generate force by shortening further.[24]

The formation of osteophytes along the brim of the acetabular cup is a common change with aging. Progressive impact loading from the head of the femur to the acetabulum gradually thins and even erodes the articular cartilage lining of both surfaces. As articular cartilage does not regenerate, continued wear and tear may create bony changes called osteophytes, which are created by the subchondral bone in response to a force. A common area of such osteophyte proliferation is at the superolateral acetabular rim and superolateral femoral head. Osteophytes can produce pain and a subsequent antalgic gait pattern. Primary hip osteoarthritis is this naturally occurring osteophyte formation and resultant joint space narrowing. Primary hip osteoarthritis is differentiated from secondary hip osteoarthritis in that there is no history of damage to the hip joint.

There are often few telltale signs of osteoarthritis before joint destruction has begun, as articular cartilage is aneural. The synovial joint lining is also aneural, but the fibrous joint capsule is highly innervated.[9] The first observation is often an antalgic gait pattern with a shift in the body's center of gravity over the deteriorated hip, so as to decrease further joint reaction forces and limit the production of pain.

During the degenerative process chondrocyte production halts, with resultant production of proteolytic enzymes that produce synovial capsule inflammation. Capsule fibrosis soon follows the joint capsule inflammation, creating a less resilient cartilaginous surface. Further stress, shear, and impact loading of the hip joint will then produce fibrillation of the superior layers of cartilage. In time and with progressive wear and destruction of the joint's articular cartilage, forces are transposed to the articulating bony surfaces. Subchondral bone responds accordingly to Wolff's law by the further laying down of bone to respond to the increased stress, which only promotes the hip deterioration and dysfunction.[26]

COMMON DISEASE PROCESSES AFFECTING THE HIP JOINT

Hip Fracture

In the United States, there were 197,000 hip fractures in 1970; 267,000 in 1980; and an expected 500,000 or more per year by the year 2000. The incidence of hip fracture has been reported to double every 5 years after the age of 50. One of every 20 women after age 65 is expected to suffer at least one hip fracture in her remaining years. Presently one out of five women aged 80 years or more has sustained or will sustain a hip fracture. When considering the many cases of hip fractures among elderly, as well as the increasing number of aged people the management of elderly patients with a hip fracture must become an area of special consideration to all physical therapists in both acute care and community settings.[1, 14–17]

Hip fractures are categorized into two major categories. Intracapsular hip fractures are fractures occurring within the borders of the hip capsule. Examples of these are femoral neck fractures (supcapital, transcervical, and basicervical). Extracapsular fractures occur outside the hip joint capsule. Examples of extracapsular hip fractures are intertrochanteric and subtrochanteric fractures. Both intracapsular and extracapsular hip fractures can be described as either nondisplaced or displaced, comminuted or noncomminuted.

Secondary Osteoarthritis

Secondary hip osteoarthritis, or degenerative joint disease, is of presumedly known etiology. Secondary osteoarthritis of the hip is an advanced and progressive degeneration of articular surfaces. The onset or predisposing factor to secondary osteoarthritis may be any previous osseous damage in either lower extremity, which then would alter the normal and smooth hip joint arthrokinematics. The result of such joint surface erosion may be a change in the shape of and painful function of the femoral head within the acetabulum.

Osteoporosis

Osteoporosis is often referred to as the reason that all older women have "brittle bones." Osteoporosis is a process in which the bone stock is broken down, but this does not occur to every aging woman. Bone health and growth depends on many factors. Osteoporosis may be the result of many factors. Some of these factors are gravity's weight-bearing effect through the bone; nutrition; vitamin D and calcitonin levels; testosterone and estrogen production; and proper functioning of the thyroid gland.[20]

Two types of osteoporosis have been identified. The first, more commonly seen in postmenopausal women, affects trabecular bone content. Decreased bone calcification is cited as the primary reason for this type of osteoporosis. Resorption of cortical and trabecular bone, the second type of osteoporosis, affects males and females equally. This second type of osteoporosis is associated more with increased age and is the only type of osteoporosis to be influenced by dietary calcium intake.[20]

Rheumatoid Arthritis

Rheumatoid arthritis is observed in females more than males and is much less common than os-

teoarthritis. Rheumatoid arthritis usually manifests itself earlier in the lifespan than osteoarthritis. Synovial inflammation of the hip joint decreases available pain-free hip range of motion. When the inflammation process lingers, as in the case of a rheumatoid arthritis flare-up, decreased joint mobility fostered by stiffness and pain encourage decreased mobilization. The cycle of decreased motion–increased pain with range of motion–decreased mobilization owing to painful range of motion–decreased motion, is then enabled. During examination of a hip joint with rheumatoid arthritis, the duration of morning stiffness and the quality and velocity of gait should be documented.

Avascular Necrosis

Avascular necrosis of the femoral head may have several causes. The primary etiology is often disruption of the blood supply to the head of the femur. This may occur when a fracture of the pelvis or femur results in perforation of the arteries that supply the femoral head. Avascular necrosis may also occur secondary to other conditions that disrupt femoral head blood supply. Some examples include long-term steroid use or multiple steroid injection history. Alcohol abuse, gout, and failure of an internal fixation of a intracapsular hip fracture may also be possible causes of avascular necrosis of the hip.

Osteopenia

The term osteopenia describes an evenly systemic decrease in bone density below an expected level. Therefore, femoral osteopenia is not unilateral or limited to the femur. This systemic condition, when present, is radiologically detectable in other regions of the body. The result of femoral osteopenia is a decrease in bone density, which may precede fracture. Rehabilitation after a hip fracture resulting from an osteopenic bone condition is very arduous for adults with biliary tract or intestinal disease.[23]

Osteomalacia

Osteomalacia is a softening of bone owing to poor mineralization. Pain, tenderness, and weakness are often symptoms, as is concurrent weight loss. Vitamin D and calcium deficiencies are usually present. Osteomalacia most often presents in patients with biliary tract or intestinal disease, in whom vitamin D absorption is decreased.

Osteitis Deformans

Osteitis deformans or *Paget's disease* refers to a bone disease where there are continuous resorption and repair cycles. The resultant bone appears deformed and larger on radiologic examination. When the disease is present in the femur, bowing, usually anterolateral, takes place. Often fractures occur in the areas of marked resorption. Fixation of these fractures is often not sufficient to progress to full weight-bearing ambulation postoperatively. In such a case fracture bracing may be used to limit forces through and around the fracture site.

SOFT-TISSUE INJURIES OF THE HIP JOINT

Bursitis

Bursitis at the hip joint is most common to the trochanteric bursa. Symptoms include localized and at times locally referred pain, and tenderness on palpation. A painful isometric contraction of the overlying muscle usually confirms inflammation of a bursa. Treatment in the geriatric population is typical and no different from treatment of any other age group. Rest, ice, and anti-inflammatory medication should be the first course of treatment. Cross-friction massage, ultrasound, stretching, and strengthening of the involved area should follow when tolerated. Finding the cause of the inflammation process, however, should be a priority.

Tendinitis

Tendinitis is treated likewise without respect to the age of the patient. Care, however, should be given during any muscle stretching. A decrease in pliability of the muscle's elastic fibers, due to injury or to the aging process, permits less stretching of the musculotendinous junctions.

Synovitis

Synovitis, an inflammation of the hip joint synovium, is characterized by painful joint range of motion and swelling. Treatment is no different in the geriatric population than in others, and should include rest, anti-inflammatory medication, and range-of-motion exercises.

Capsular Tightening

Capsular tightening without a concurrent disease process should be addressed and treated promptly. The common capsular pattern for the hip joint is internal rotation and abduction greater than flexion and extension, which is more limited than external rotation.[5] When a hip joint is found to be restricted an underlying disease process should be suspected even if the patient is symptom free. Modalities that can increase the capsule's extensibility and surrounding soft tissue flexibility should be used. In coordination with these modalities, stretching and mobilization of the hip joint aids in regaining hip joint motion.

After trial of modalities, mobilization, and soft-tissue techniques to promote healing of a hip dysfunction, further nonoperative treatment may include the use of a cane for ambulation activities. In active cases of bursitis or tendinitis a cane may as well be of value to the patient who has a severe antalgic gait pattern, in order to decrease the forces across the painful hip (Fig 17–7).

As depicted in Figure 17–7, a small force through a cane in the hand opposite the painful hip will reduce the force needed to be generated across the painful hip. These forces across the painful hip are determined by the length of the moment arms over which the forces (muscles) act.[2, 22, 24]

PRESURGICAL CONSIDERATIONS

If the patient is to undergo elective surgery there is opportunity in some instances to evaluate the patient preoperatively, noting range of motion and muscular strength. Most important is the ability to note muscular imbalances and gait deviations present preoperatively. If given enough time prior to surgery, therapeutic exercise and gait training can begin, to aid the patient's full recovery. It is usually easier for a patient familiar with physical therapy and therapy goals to proceed with postoperative rehabilitation.

If the surgery is emergency surgery, rehabilitation goals should be considered immediately by the examining medical team. In most cases of injury to the hip joint where trauma such as fracture occurs, significant internal bleeding and damage may have occurred. Owing to the proximity of major neurovascular structures, major medical emergencies are possible.

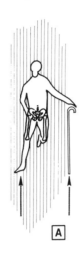
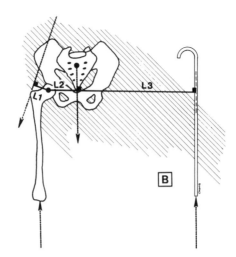

FIG 17–7.
A, vectors of forces must be equal to maintain balance situation. **B,** this illustration breaks down vectors on left into abductor muscle force and body weight. Vector on right: cane force. Vectors on left multiplied by cane moment arms must equal cane force multiplied by cane moment arm. Thus, with W = abductor force:

$$W \times L_1 = W \times L_2 - \text{cane force} \times (L_2 + L_3)$$

Because the cane moment arm is larger than the body weight moment arm, small cane forces can balance the equation. (From Pugh J: Biomechanics of the hip. *Orthopedic Surgery Update Series*, part 1, vol 2, lesson 7. Princeton, NJ, Continuing Professional Education Center, 1982. Used with permission.)

Where there has been injury solely to the hip joint, it is necessary to medically clear the patient and operate as soon as possible. During this time, the nursing and emergency room team need to gather as much information as possible regarding the cause of injury and the patient's ambulatory and activity levels prior to injury. It is also important to determine mental orientation, living arrangements, and available family and social network before corrective surgery is contemplated. It is necessary for the orthopedist to repair a hip fracture as quickly as possible for the medical well-being of the patient. It is of next priority for the surgeon to repair the hip in view of the patient's usual activities. Preinjury activity level can vary from bedbound to fully independent in ambulation and ADL without an assistive device. A bedbound patient does not need a fixation that will help him or her to ambulate more easily. This patient would, however, benefit from a fixation allowing access to the perineum for hygiene care. The avid walker who is independent or a member of the work force would benefit from a fixation or replacement which allows a quick and successful return to the prior functional level.

It is important to assess mental activity before injury, where possible, in order to determine the effects of shock and anesthesia on the patient's mental awareness. In addition, the surgeon needs to know whether a patient can be expected to follow instructions postoperatively. For those patients who could not follow instructions easily before injury, the fixation should allow full weight bearing. Where there is any question of the patient's ability to alter weight bearing, a joint replacement or a fixation allowing full weight bearing should be considered. If the patient is noncomplaint, this issue must be addressed.

As discussed in the previous chapter, the orthopedic surgeon's choice of fixation or joint replacement is decided after consideration of the type and location of fracture, the patient's age, medical condition, preinjury activity level, and preinjury mental orientation. Most importantly, the fracture site and type must be identified.

In a fracture situation where blood supply to the femoral head is interrupted, a replacement of the proximal femur may be necessary to avoid future avascular necrosis of the femoral head. In an instance of a severely comminuted fracture where solid fixation may be difficult, joint replacement may then eliminate the future need for revision of an internal fixation failure. In cases where the fracture is simple and through good bone stock it may be possible to fix the fracture with pins or plates and screws.

Age is important in choosing a type of joint replacement. While a noncemented prosthesis will last longer than the 10-year average for cemented total hip replacements, postoperative rehabilitation is more energy consuming and inappropriate for many geriatric patients. More demanding postoperative rehabilitation may be unwarranted for a patient with a life expectancy of less than 10 years, or in the case of a patient with complex medical problems. The energy required for more difficult ambulation procedures such as non–weight-bearing ambulation may prove too taxing to a system where available energy levels are already depleted.

The patient's medical condition requires particular consideration. There may be internal organ damage if the patient has been involved in a motor vehicle (or high-velocity impact) accident, or there may be more nutrition-related problems to cope with in an elderly hip fracture patient. Many times in instances of hip fracture occurring at home, the victim is found many hours after the time of the accident. Most commonly there are complications of internal damage with accompanying blood loss, dehydration, and malnutrition. Cardiac status must be checked and closely monitored in all patients.

Often times the anesthesiologist recommends use of general anesthesia for the healthy patient and a spinal epidural local anesthetic for the "at-risk" patient who may not tolerate general anesthesia well. An epidural block, while reducing anesthesia risks, increases surgical site bleeding. In the hip, where surgery is often bloody, increased bleeding owing to epidural anesthetic brings added risk to the patient.

GOALS OF PREOPERATIVE AND POSTOPERATIVE REHABILITATION

The management of any postoperative hip surgery patient should first be approached in a generic way where overall goals are much the same. Bed mobility and progressive out-of-bed activities and exercises are the rule to start. As standing and ambulation activities begin, goals for each patient become more select depending on the individual patient and operative procedure.

It is the goal of the entire rehabilitation team from the orthopedic surgeon down the line to the nursing aide to get the postoperative patient out of bed and ambulatory as quickly as possible. Each day the postoperative patient spends in bed allows fears and anxieties to increase. This produces more obstacles to conquer during the patient's return toward

preinjury status. The patient who is ambulatory within 2 days of surgery has not been given the time to become too fearful of walking and the automatic response to walk may take over. Assurance that the fracture is fixed and that the leg will not give out is usually all that is needed to win a patient's trust. While the fear of falling may be present, patients who ambulate within 2 days of surgery, in most cases progress much more easily.

POSTOPERATIVE PHYSICAL THERAPY EVALUATION

Physical therapy evaluation of a postoperative hip surgery patient includes a thorough review of the patient's chart. The events necessitating the hip surgery, be it a traumatic fracture, progressive osteoarthritis, or a pathologic fracture, are important in planning the physical therapy program. If surgery is necessitated by traumatic fracture, were any other body parts injured? More importantly, what was the cause of the fall or trauma? If hip surgery was done because of advanced osteoarthritis, was the patient accustomed to ambulating long distances with a cane or walker? If the hip dysfunction was the result of a pathologic fracture it is important to know what the underlying disease process was and if it has spread to other areas of the body. Metastatic disease found in the opposite lower extremity or one of either arms may decrease the amount of weight bearing possible through these extremities. With these examples in mind, the evaluation can continue. It is necessary that each patient, fracture, and fixation be considered unique. This will ensure that each patient's rehabilitation is directed in view of his or her own set of circumstances.

Alertness, orientation, and memory are important to assess on initial postoperative evaluation so as to determine whether or not the patient will follow and remember instructions. It is within reason to expect a patient recovering from general anesthesia to be confused and forgetful. It is also within reason that a patient with Alzheimer's disease will act in much the same way. The patient suffering from anesthesia-induced confusion should be expected within a day or two to become more lucid. It is important to identify the patients who do not, so as to present physical therapy treatment in a different manner. Patients with Alzheimer's or Parkinson's disease often show exaggerated behaviors after major surgery. It is the physical therapist who most often first realizes that the patient will need more assistance postoperatively owing to a disease progression that was not identified prior to surgery. In some cases the first signs of Alzheimer's and Parkinson's diseases are first identified by a therapist working with a postoperative patient.

Sensation, circulation, and edema next need to be evaluated. Examination of the surgical dressing is important to monitor bloody or serous drainage. Normally no drainage is expected to occur through the surgical bandage. When drainage is present, the surgeon or nurse often outlines the area in ink and record the time of day the drainage was measured. Any additional drainage that seems significant in view of the recorded measurement should be brought to the primary nurse's attention before further exercise or ambulation is attempted. When the dressing is removed the incisional site should be examined daily for any signs of infection. Any wound seepage should be documented, as well as the presence of foul smell if noted. During examination of the wound site, the buttocks and legs can be inspected for early signs of skin breakdown. Daily skin breakdown checks can potentially be life saving.

Postoperative Day 1

On postoperative day 1 (POD 1), informal physical therapy should begin at the bedside with the evaluation described above. It is important that the orthopedic surgeon or orthopedic surgical resident be directly consulted as to the proper weight-bearing status if ambulation orders are received via an intermediary. For the total hip–replacement patient, precautions and contraindicated motions can be clarified with the surgeon. Any increased hip pain or difficulty with ambulation activities should be brought to the attending surgeon's attention.

Those patients who have undergone total hip replacement should be first instructed in proper precautions, which are determined by the surgical approach to the hip joint (anterior or posterior). Most common is a lateral incision with a posterior approach to the hip joint. In these instances combined motions of hip flexion, adduction, and internal rotation are allowable to a degree, but generally avoided so as to eliminate confusion. It is important that the patient not only be aware of the motions to be avoided, but to be cognizant of the daily activities that may place the operated hip in jeopardy of dislocation.

If medically stable on POD 1, a bed-to-chair transfer with nursing help is appropriate. It is important for the therapist and patient to establish a rapport as well as set goals and ground rules. When a postoperative patient is doing well medically on POD 1, it is important that he or she begin getting out of bed. While assisting the patient with verbal cues, the therapist should offer as little physical assistance as is necessary. In this manner the patient does not become overly dependent nor reliant on some one else to move. Allowing the patient to get out of bed as he or she did prior to surgery, with cues as necessary, initiates the patient's regaining independence. This practice will only be successful when the entire nursing staff replicates transfers in much the same manner.

Once in a seated position, even if only with legs dangling over the side of the bed, balance, range of motion, and muscular strength can be assessed. Time out of bed on POD 1 is determined according to the patient's tolerance. Signs of orthostatic hypotension and fatigue dictate the patient's ability to remain out of bed. Vital signs should be monitored throughout each treatment session. The mere experience of getting out of bed on POD 1 usually enables easier transfers on POD 2. Either in the sitting or in the supine position, traditional exercises such as quadricep and gluteal setting, ankle pumping, and active knee flexion and extension can begin. Swelling in the affected lower extremity can be controlled to some degree by elevation of the extremity when supine with concomitant ankle pumping and quadricep setting exercise.

Postoperative Day 2

On POD 2, or on POD 1 where possible, sit-to-stand transfers and ambulation must begin. Coordination and balance in standing are then assessed. The patient should be instructed in proper weight bearing and weight shifting within the walker (or parallel bars when necessary). It should be the goal of every orthopedic surgeon to fix a hip fracture in an elderly individual so that "full weight bearing as tolerated" ambulation is possible on POD 1. Gradually orders such as non–weight bearing and toe-touch weight bearing for open reduction of hip fractures are disappearing. Surgeons, with the help of physical therapists, are seeing better results postoperatively in those patients who are allowed earlier mobilization and progressive weight bearing through the affected limb. In fact, many activities, such as lifting the buttocks to use a bedpan, straight leg raising, and non–weight-bearing ambulation, place more stress across the hip joint than partial or full weight bearing. This same concept explains why placing the whole foot on the floor, partial weight bearing, is more comfortable than toes-only weight bearing. The surgically interrupted gluteus muscle group needs to actively contract to keep the affected lower extremity off the ground for non–weight-bearing ambulation. During partial weight bearing and full weight bearing the gluteus muscles do not have to contract to elevate the leg, resulting in less surgical site pain during ambulation.

When weight shifting and appropriate weight bearing are possible, ambulation using a three-point gait pattern for unilateral hip surgery and a four-point gait pattern for bilateral hip surgery can begin. A reciprocal walker should be used to allow a comfortable four-point gait pattern for bilateral total hip replacement patients.

It is important when first beginning ambulation training to set distance goals with the patient. The first goal might be to walk the distance needed to reach the bathroom to prepare the patient for bathroom privileges. It is always important for the patient to be instructed in the reasons behind physical therapy activities to increase motivation and to promote the attainment of more difficult goals.

Exercises, while important, should be secondary to ambulation during initial physical therapy sessions. Survival time is reported by Crane and Kernek, as cited by Barnes and Dunovan, to be correlated with a hip fracture patient's ability to walk preoperatively and postoperatively.[1] When the patient has ambulated the maximum distances (at least two walks per therapy session), exercises can be done to improve breathing patterns, active range of motion, strength, and endurance. It is very easy for

patients to convince therapists that exercises have worn them out for the day and that ambulation would be much too taxing.

Postoperative Day 3

From POD 3 on there should be progressive increases in distances ambulated with weight bearing as directed by the orthopedic surgeon. The goal of each therapy session should be to increase distances ambulated. If a patient should reach a plateau and either be unable to increase walking distance or find that it is no easier to walk each day consistently for 3 days or more, the medical team needs to determine possible reasons for this lack of goal attainment. Often a change in diet or roommate or increased psychological support will be all that is needed to return the patient to progressive ambulation training.

Progression from a walker to crutches (most often Lofstrand crutches) to a cane should take place as tolerated and agreed upon by the attending orthopedist. Stair training and ADL instruction should begin as soon as possible to enable the patient's return toward maximum independence. For patient's who have undergone total hip replacement, it is necessary that further precaution instruction be given. Often patients do not carry over precaution guidelines to daily activities.

Appendix 17–1 is a sample of a total hip replacement protocol used at Vanderbilt University Medical Center in Nashville, Tennessee. The protocol for both clinician and patient use is quite complete in terms of rehabilitation expectations and time frames postoperatively. Table 17–3 is an example of a summary of hip precautions and instructions to be given

---

TABLE 17–3.

Hip Precaution Guidelines for Patients After Total Hip Replacement

To permit your hip to fully heal, and to ensure its stability, the following guidelines should be
  observed unless altered by your orthopedic surgeon.
When lying in bed
  • Lie on your back; do not turn on your side
  • Both legs should be separated 6 to 8 in. at the knees
When sitting
  • Your legs should not be crossed
  • The level of your knees should be lower than the level of your hips
  • Don't reach for objects on the floor by bending your trunk
  • Do not tie your shoes by bending over in the chair
Walking
  • Continue to use your walker, crutches, or cane until your surgeon or physical therapist tells you
    otherwise
  • Be sure not to pivot on your operated leg; pick up each foot and take small steps when turning
Walking on steps
  • Up: unoperated leg first, then operated leg, then assistive device
  • Down: assistive device first, then operated leg, then unoperated leg

to patients on discharge from the hospital. Postoperative therapy, however, should not end on discharge from the hospital. Home care services are essential for the most optimally safe return home.

HOME CARE

Physical therapists who work with postoperative hip fracture and hip replacement patients after hospital discharge learn quickly during evaluations that the most important points to ascertain are the patient's functional ability and support network. The patient's ability to readapt to his or her surroundings must be assessed as well. It is not uncommon to find that an elderly patient returning home is apprehensive. The hip injury may have occurred in the home, with which fears will be associated. In addition, all postsurgical patients have had 1 to 3 weeks to ponder their return home. This time has enabled the patient to magnify potential difficulties and problems.

The home care therapist can most easily confirm that a patient can assimilate back into his or her surroundings. Safety checkouts in bed mobility, bathroom or commode use, and opening the main entrance door are most important. Any difficulties in these basic areas need to be brought to the attention of the physician, home care nurse, and family. Additional services may be indicated and available to aid the patient in these areas.

Therapy goals can then advance to progressive ambulation and strengthening activities. When indicated, the patient's ability to leave the home independently should be assessed. When cleared by the orthopedic surgeon, activities such as sit or stand to floor and back transfers are important, especially for the patient living alone. This activity gives patients the confidence that getting off the ground is possible if they should fall. Many patients at first may associate the floor with a previous fall and become even more frightened of the floor.

Home care discharge goals vary from patient to patient. When the patient who lives alone is able to leave home for continued outpatient therapy, formal home care physical therapy services are often discontinued. For the patient who has reached a plateau and who lives with a spouse, family member, or companion, home care physical therapy can be discontinued when the caregiver is able to safely transfer, exercise, and ambulate the patient, as directed. In few instances maintenance-type home care physical therapy is warranted.

FALL PREVENTION

Accident Facts reported that in 1987 74% of deaths resulting from falls occurred in the population aged 65 years and older. Of these deaths, 82% were among persons 75 years and older.[18] Fall prevention is an area that is often neglected during inpatient, outpatient, and home care physical therapy sessions. Prevention of the many falls among the elderly population undoubtedly decreases the number of geriatric hip fractures. In turn, the number of elderly who die after hip fracture may also be decreased.

Physical therapists have already cited the growing need for tracking and organizing information regarding falls among the elderly. It has been noted that many of the falls among elderly people were falls from a chair or toilet or occurred during out-of-bed transfer or during ambulation activities. Using this information, preventive programs can be designed to concentrate on problem areas.

Combining a structured exercise and activity session to encompass daily transfer and ambulation skills may help to make elderly people more aware of the dangers of falls and of methods to prevent falls. The addition of an educational session during which common causes of accidents could be reviewed with specific prevention examples may help patients to recognize potential problems in their own homes or communities.

CONCLUSION

In order to assist in an efficient evaluation and treatment of the geriatric client with hip pain, hip injury, or recent hip surgery, the following "quick tips" lists have been formulated. These lists are not intended to be "quicky" evaluation/treatment solutions, but rather to aid in the direction of patient care.

Patient With Hip Pain:

1. Is pain reproducible on examination?
2. Correlate patient history with clinical examination; in conjunction with physician rule out serious pathology when it is suspected.
3. Use analgesic modalities, exercises, and assistive devices to decrease pain.
4. Maintain or regain passive range of motion.
5. Strengthen hip muscles as well as providing total conditioning to joints below the hip, i.e., knee and ankle, and joints above, i.e., spine, in both static and dynamic activities.
6. Use coordination and balance activities for motor reeducation to incorporate increased strength into functional activities.

Patient Who Has Undergone Hip Surgery:

1. Establish range-of-motion and activity precautions and weight-bearing guidelines with surgeon.
2. Begin formal physical therapy as soon as possible via deep breathing exercises, active range-of-motion and isometric exercises, and patient education at bedside.
3. Initiate bed mobility, as well as transfers and ambulation when medically cleared.
4. Increase time out of bed and ambulation distance/endurance with appropriate assistive device. Progress weight bearing as per surgeon's instructions and patient's tolerance.
5. Restore hip active range of motion as tolerated by patient within guidelines of surgeon.
6. Strengthen LE muscles with isometric and isotonic exercises per guidelines of surgeon.
7. Incorporate activities of daily living and stair climbing into physical therapy session as patient's endurance increases.
8. Total hip replacement positioning precautions should be phased out by orthopedist only.

Acknowledgment

This chapter is dedicated to the many elderly patients with whom I have worked. At times they intended not to return home from the hospital, but to die following hip surgery. Many of their injuries would have been catastrophic for any aged person to cope with. When these injuries were coupled with poor medical status and poor social networks from which to gain support and encouragement, many of these patients felt that death was the easier solution. I promised each that if for no other reason than to teach me something about hip injury prevention or treatment their injury and successful return home would benefit someone else. I thank each one for the many helpful experiences that help me to convey principles of the evaluation and treatment of geriatric hip dysfunction.

REFERENCES

1. Barnes B, Dunovan K: Functional outcomes after hip fracture. *Phys Ther* 1989; 67:1675–1679.
2. Brand R, Crowninshield R: The effect of cane use on hip contact force. *Clin Orthop* 1980; 147:181–84.
3. Ceder L, Thorngren K-G, Wallden B: Prognostic indicators and early home rehabilitation in elderly patients with hip fractures. *Clin Orthop* 1980; 152:173–184.
4. Cyriax J: *Textbook of Orthopaedic Medicine,* vol 1. *Diagnosis of Soft Tissue Lesions.* Baltimore, Williams & Wilkins, 1975.
5. Cyriax J: *Illustrated Manual of Orthopaedic Medicine.* London, Butterworths, 1983.
6. Daniels L, Worthingham C: *Muscle Testing,* ed 4. Philadelphia, W.B. Saunders, 1980.
7. *Dorland's Illustrated Medical Dictionary,* ed 25. Philadelphia, W.B. Saunders, 1981.
8. Echternach J (ed): *Clinics in Physical Therapy of the Hip.* New York, Churchill Livingstone, 1990.
9. Gould J, Davies G (eds): *Orthopaedic and Sports Physical Therapy.* St Louis, Mosby–Year Book, 1985.
10. Hertling D, Kessler R: *Management of Common Musculoskeletal Disorders,* ed 2. Philadelphia, J.B. Lippincott, 1990.
11. Hoppenfeld S: *Physical Examination of the Spine and Extremities.* Norwalk, Conn, Appleton-Century-Crofts, 1976.
12. Jackson O: *Physical Therapy of the Geriatric Patient.* New York, Churchill Livingstone, 1983.
13. James B, Parker AW: Active and passive mobility of lower limb joints in elderly men and women. *Am J Phys Med Rehabil* 1989; 68:162–167.
14. Jette SM, Harris BA, Cleary PD, et al: Functional recovery after hip fracture. *Arc Phys Med Rehabil* 1987; 68:735–740.
15. Kampa K: Mortality of hip fracture patients within one year of fracture. . . . an overview. *Geritopics* 1991; 14:10–11.
16. Lavine L, Doppelt S: Rehabilitation management of the patient with hip fracture and other orthopaedic problems. *Surg Rounds Orthop,* Sept 1990; pp 29–36.
17. Lewinnek G, Kelsey J, White A, et al: The significance and a comparative analysis of the epidemiology of hip fractures. *Clin Orthop* 1980; 152:35–43.
18. National Safety Council: *Accident Facts.* Chicago, National Safety Council, 1988.

19. Norkin C, Levangie P: *Joint Structure and Function.* Philadelphia, F.A. Davis, 1983.
20. Parfitt AM: Definition of osteoporosis: Age related loss of bone and its relationship to increased fracture risk. *National Institutes of Health Consensus Development Conference Statement,* 1984; pp 15–19.
21. Prosthetics and Orthotics New York University Postgraduate Medical School: *Lower-Limb Orthotics: NYUPMS,* New York, 1981.
22. Pugh J: Biomechanics of the Hip. *Orthopaedic Surgery Update Series,* part 1, vol 2, lesson 7, Princeton, Continuing Professional Education Center, 1982.
23. Rodman G, Schumacher H (ed): *Primer on the Rheumatic Diseases,* ed 8. Atlanta, Arthritis Foundation, 1983.
24. Soderberg G: *Kinesiology—Application to Pathological Motion.* Baltimore, Williams & Wilkins, 1986.
25. Somjen G: *Neurophysiology—the Essentials.* Baltimore, Williams & Wilkins, 1983.
26. Williams P, Warwick R (Eds): *Gray's Anatomy,* ed 36. Philadelphia, W.B. Saunders, 1980.

APPENDIX 17–1

Vanderbilt University Medical Center Department of Physical Therapy: Physical Therapy Treatment Protocol for Total Hip Arthroplasty

Preoperative—1 Month Prior to Hospitalization:

1. Attend total joint class on hip arthroplasty. Material covered in the class includes discussions on anatomy of normal and abnormal hip joint, components and types of hip prosthesis, admission procedures for VUH, inpatient preoperative care, intraoperative sequence of events, identification of postoperative complications and preventative measures, inpatient/home rehabilitation via physical therapy, and occupational therapy and postdischarge needs. Class personnel include nursing, PT, OT, and SW.

Preoperative—Day of Admission:

1. Preoperative evaluation of range of motion, strength, limb length discrepancy, pain, gait, etc.
2. Review basic precautions and instruct in immediate postoperative exercises.
3. Fit walker/crutches and instruct in appropriate gait pattern—three-point gait if one extremity is involved, four-point gait if both lower extremities are involved; WBAT if ce-

mented prosthesis is to be used, TDWB if noncemented prosthesis is used.

Postoperative Day 1:

1. Begin lower extremity isometrics and ankle pumping exercises.
2. Initiate bilateral upper extremity and contralateral limb strengthening exercises.
3. Begin bed-to-chair transfers with assistance to a chair of appropriate height. Patients are not required to "slouch" sit and may sit in an upright position if comfortable.

Postoperative Day 2:

1. Review lower extremity isometrics and ankle pumping exercises.
2. Begin active-assisted lower extremity range of motion exercises to the operative extremity in bed. Operative limb motions should be to the patients tolerance and the limb should be kept in a single plane of motion.
3. Begin assisted walker/crutch ambulation with weight-bearing status dependent upon prosthesis design and implantation.

Postoperative Days 3–5:

1. Continue supine exercises.
2. Instruct patient in sitting exercises.
3. Instruct in bathroom transfers—patients are to use an over-the-commode chair, which the nursing staff will secure for their use while hospitalized.
4. Continue gait training on level surfaces.

Postoperative Days 6–Discharge:

1. Review and reinforce supine and sitting exercises.
2. Reinforce postoperative precautions.
3. Further gait refinement to achieve maximum, safe, energy-efficient gait pattern with appropriate weight bearing status.
4. Instruct in stair climbing.
5. Begin and complete discharge plans and arrangements for follow-up home/outpatient physical therapy (follow-up physical therapy services arranged for 6 weeks with three sessions per week).
6. Review home instructions and exercise program with patient and family members.

After Discharge:

First clinic follow-up visit—approximately 2–3 weeks from hospital discharge; seen in orthopedic clinic with surgeon.

1. Review home instructions and exercise program.
2. Instruct in hip abduction exercises—standing only, and instruct in supine IT band stretches.
3. Continue walker/crutch ambulation with appropriate weight-bearing status.

Second Clinic Follow-up Visit—Approximately 6 Weeks Postoperative

1. Review complete exercise program.
2. Instruct in hip abduction exercises—side-lying and instruct in supine IT band stretches.
3. Instruct in increased activity schedule.
4. If *cemented* prosthesis, begin cane ambulation. Continue to use the cane until patient is able to ambulate without a Trendelenburg limp.
5. If *noncemented* prosthesis, begin on progressive weight-bearing program using walker/crutches.

Third Clinic Follow-up Visit—Approximately 12 Weeks Postoperative

1. Review complete exercise and activity program.
2. *Noncemented* prosthesis, begin cane ambulation. Continue to use cane until patient able to ambulate without a Trendelenburg limp.

All Other Clinic Follow-up Visits

1. Continue to review and reinforce exercises and activity regimens.

APPENDIX 17–2

Vanderbilt University Hospital Physical Therapy Department

Hip Arthroplasty General Instructions

1. The exercise program should be carried out 2 to 3 times per day building up to 20 repetitions of each exercise.

2. You may sit for up to 30 minutes at one time, as often as desired, as long as you walk or lie flat on your back or stomach for a few minutes between sitting periods.
3. It is very common to note swelling of the lower leg when first home; do not be concerned as long as the swelling is down in the morning.
4. Do not sleep on your operative side until approved by your surgeon.
5. Sexual activity may be resumed when comfortable.
6. Try to keep your operative leg positioned in bed so that the toes and kneecap point upwards toward the ceiling when your are backlying.
7. When advised by your surgeon, you may take a shower (tub baths are not advised). You may wish to put a chair in your shower to sit in while bathing (mesh lawn chairs work very well).
8. Low, soft contour-type chairs should be avoided.
9. Dining out: Do not sit in booths or low chairs.
10. Walk in short sessions as tolerated to gradually improve your physical endurance. You may walk out of doors when stamina and strength are adequate.
11. You may return to work at the discretion of your surgeon.
12. *Walking:*
    a. Keep erect posture at all times with buttocks tucked under shoulders.
    b. Look straight ahead.
    c. Walk in a heel-to-toe sequence, with toes pointed straight ahead.
    d. Tighten your buttocks and the knee of the supporting leg until the heel of the moving leg hits the ground.
    e. Never lean on your crutches. Distribute your weight on the hand grips.
13. *Stairs:*
    Up: Step up with your _____ leg first. Lean slightly forward and push down on your crutches. Raise your other leg. After both feet are firmly on the stair above, raise your crutches.
    Down: Come to the edge; lower your crutches to the stair below as you bend your knees. Lower your _____ leg, then lower your other leg.

Additional Comments:

APPENDIX 17–3

Vanderbilt University Hospital Physical Therapy Department: Hip Arthroplasty Home Exercise Program

Starting Position: Lying on Your Back, Legs Straight.

1. *Quad Sets:* Tighten the muscles on the front of the thighs. Hold for a count of 5. Relax. Repeat 10 times.
2. *Gluteal Sets:* Tighten the buttocks. Hold for a count of 5. Relax. Repeat 10 times.
3. *Ankle Pumps:* Pump feet up and down. This may be done as often as you can, but at least 3–4 times a day.
4. *Hip Rotation:* Keeping legs flat on the bed and slightly apart, roll both knees inward towards each other and then out away from each other. Hold. Relax. Repeat 10 times.
5. *Hip Abduction/Adduction:* Start with legs slightly apart, keeping knees and toes pointed upward. Slide your _____ leg out to the side, with heel turned out slightly. Return to starting position. Relax. Repeat 10 times.
6. *Hip Flexion/Extension:* Keeping the knee straight and the toes pointed upwards, bend your _____ knee up towards your chest; then return your leg to the starting position on the bed. Relax. Repeat 10 times.

Starting Position: Lying on Your Side.

1. *Side-lying Leg Lifts:* Lie on your _____ side with the lower hip and knee bent. Your top leg should be in a straight line with your body. Raise and lower the top leg (towards the ceiling) keeping the knee straight. Do not roll forward or backward. Relax. Repeat _____ times.

Starting Position: Sitting

1. Feet flat on the floor, rock the weight of the legs up on the toes and back on the heels. Repeat several times.
2. *Knee Extensions:* Straighten one knee by raising the foot out in front of you. Do not lean backwards. Return to the starting position. Repeat with the opposite leg. Repeat 10 times.
3. *Hip Flexion:* Raise your knees upwards alternately as if marching. Repeat 10 times.
4. *Hip Abduction/Adduction Isometrics:* Start with two fists between your knees. Bring your feet together while trying to push your knees towards one another, keeping feet flat on the floor. Relax. Repeat 10 times. Then, place your fists outside your knees and try to push your knees outward away from one another, keeping feet flat on the floor. Relax. Repeat 10 times.

Starting Position: Standing (Using Your Crutches For Supports)

1. *Hip Abduction Isometrics:* Stand facing forwards with your _____ leg approximately 4 inches from the wall. Using your crutches for support and keeping the knee straight, push outwards with the _____ leg as if you were trying to push the wall over. Hold for a count of 5. Relax. Repeat _____ times.
2. *Hip Abduction:* Using your crutches for support, and keeping your body straight (facing forwards), raise your _____ leg sideways in the air. Do not raise your pelvis. Hold for a count of 3. Return to the starting position. Relax. Repeat _____ times.

Additional Comments or Suggestions:

Chapter 18

Knee Injuries: An Orthopedic Perspective

Stephen Smith, M.D.

Casual observation would lead one to think that the knee joint is a simple hinge; however, it is not. Both anatomically and biomechanically, the knee joint is quite complex. Being a weight-bearing joint, and by virtue of its interposition between the two other major weight-bearing joints of the body, the hip and the ankle, it is subject to enormous stresses and strains, which ultimately over a period of many years in some people give rise to painful and disabling conditions. Being a very large joint with a rich blood supply it is also subject to other painful and disabling conditions of nontraumatic etiology.

It is of interest to note that many of the anatomic features of the human knee share quite distinct characteristics with knee joints found in ancient fossilized animal forms thought to be more than 300 million years old. In an excellent article by Dye, entitled "An Evolutionary Perspective of the Knee,"[17] it is shown that the chicken's knee, well hidden under the wing in most birds, shares many anatomic features of the human knee, including a bicondylar cam-shaped distal femur, nearly flat tibial plateaus, a patella, intra-articular cruciate ligaments, menisci, a broad, flat medial collateral ligament, and a more cylindrical lateral collateral ligament (Fig 18–1). In this elegant study of the comparative anatomy of the human with other life forms, the author demonstrates that the tetrapod knee can be divided into three broad categories based on the weight-bearing form of the foot. There are the unguligrades, including pigs, horses, and sheep; the digitigrades, including carnivores such as cats and dogs, and plantigrades, including *Homo sapiens*. In the unguiligrade knee full extension is lacking and the knee is permanently loaded in flexion. In the digitigrade knee, the knee can be extended fully but functionally it is loaded in at least slight flexion. In the plantigrade knee at least part of the gait cycle involves full extension of the knee.

The importance of the functional integrity of the knee joint can hardly be overstated. One of the most important factors determining independence in elderly persons is the ability to rise unaided from the seated position. Implicit in this important and deceptively simple act is a smoothly functioning knee joint as well as a strong extensor mechanism. Four major factors giving rise to potential or actual disability at the level of the knee joint are pain, weakness, stiffness, and deformity. Frequently a combination of these exists in any one individual. Shephard, in reviewing the Canada Health Survey published in 1982, stated that death is usually preceded by 8 to 10 years of some disability and about a year of total dependency.[63] Not infrequently the knee can be implicated in progressive disability in the elderly.

CLINICAL EXAMINATION OF THE KNEE

The examination of the knee joint is a demanding and time-consuming process. The importance of a concise and accurate history cannot be overstated. Not only is a correct diagnosis predicated on an accurate history, but increasingly, important medicolegal issues hinge on the facts as stated in the initial evaluation and subsequent progress notes. The commonplace nature of litigation and insurance company peer review makes it essential that the perti-

Gallus domesticus

Homo sapiens

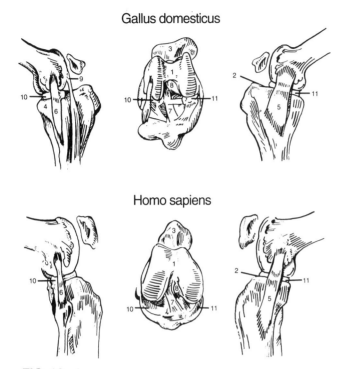

FIG 18–1.
Comparative morphology of the knee in *Gallus domesticus* and *H. sapiens*. 1 = bicondylar cam-shaped distal part of the femur; 2 = flat tibial plateaus; 3 = osseous patella; 4 = fibular articulation with lateral femoral condyle (in *G. domesticus* only); 5 = flat medial collateral ligament with distal tibial insertion; 6 = cord-shaped lateral ligament; 7 = anterior cruciate ligament; 8 = posterior cruciate ligament; 9 = origin of extensor digitorum longus on lateral femoral condyle (in *G. domesticus* only); 10 = lateral meniscus; and 11 = medial meniscus. (From Dye SF: *J Bone Joint Surg (Am)* 1987; 69A:977, 980. Used by permission.)

nent facts surrounding the onset of symptoms be stated accurately and rechecked if possible on subsequent visits.

When the onset of pain or disability is related to trauma most often the patient can state precisely when, where, and how the symptoms began. Often, however, the onset of symptoms is insidious and the patient has only a vague idea of when and how the symptoms began. It is worthwhile to be as thorough as time will permit in trying to obtain how and when the symptoms began, as well as a detailed history of the progression, or in some cases, the stable nature of the symptoms. It is important to realize that not all knee pain has its origin in the knee and it is wise to inquire as to the possible coexistence of other symptoms, such as low back, buttock, thigh, calf, or foot pain. It has been the experience of this author to have patients scheduled for knee proce-

dures when in fact they are suffering from lumbar spine pathology and its consequent sciatic pain. It has also been the author's experience to see patients with distal thigh and knee pain have significant osteoarthritis of the hip uncovered in the course of the examination. While this pitfall is most notorious in cases of slipped capital femoral epiphysis of late childhood and early adolescence, it is by no means unheard of in elderly people with afflictions of the spine, pelvis, and hip.

The following is a list of of questions that may be appropriate when obtaining a preliminary history from a patient with knee pain. Once the history helps clarify the category of pathology—acute vs. chronic, traumatic vs. degenerative, etc., one might appropriately ask less general question in order to work down the history taking algorithm. The following are examples of questions the examiner might consider:

1. Did the pain start with an injury?
2. Did the pain start suddenly or gradually?
3. Is the pain an aching, burning, sharp, or dull pain?
4. Is the pain intensified with weight bearing?
5. Is the pain diminished or absent at rest?
6. Do the symptoms awaken the patient from sleep or prevent him or her from falling asleep?
7. Does the pain radiate proximally or distally?
8. Are the symptoms aggravated by ascending or descending stairs, driving a car, getting up from the seated position?
9. Are the symptoms relieved by resting the knee in the extended position?
10. Is there associated swelling? Has the knee been previously aspirated of fluid by a physician?
11. Is there associated swelling in any other joints?
12. Has the patient been experiencing any fever, sweats, chills, or weight loss?
13. Is there associated clicking, popping, or grinding?
14. Is there associated locking or catching within the knee?
15. Does the knee give way or feel as if it might give way and is this associated with other symptoms of pain or catching within the joint?

Examination of the patient's knee is as important as but no more important than the history taking. It is advisable to observe and record the following characteristics of the knee joint in the course of evaluating a patient with knee complaints:

1. Gait characteristics including stride length, cadence, weight-bearing time.
2. Additional gait characteristics, including presence of external rotation of the foot as well as extension of the knee. Does the knee fully extend in the stance phase or is it held in the flexed position? Does the patient require walking aids such as cane, crutches, or walker?
3. Does the knee joint appear stable or is there abnormal motion in the joint in weight bearing?

With the patient seated on the examination table so that active flexion and extension is unimpeded, observe the following:

1. Can the patient fully extend the knee against gravity?
2. Can the knee be fully extended with gravity eliminated by providing a base of support for the heel?
3. Does the patella appear to be in the midline, tilted, riding abnormally high?
4. Is the quadriceps muscle group atrophied?
5. Does the knee appear swollen, tense, red?
6. Is the knee warm to the touch compared with the opposite knee?
7. Is there a palpable defect above the patella in the area of the quadriceps tendon or below the patella in the area of the patellar ligament?
8. Is there tenderness over the tibial tubercle?
9. Is there a palpable, well-localized lump or bulge? If there is, is it movable?

In measuring the knee with a goniometer, it should be accepted that there is an inherent probability of error of ± 5 to 10 degrees, especially in patients with knee problems. This might be explained to patients when in the course of rehabilitation the level of desired flexion or extension is slightly less or more then it might have been measured on a prior visit in order to modify unwarranted pessimism or optimism.

Next with the patient in the reclining position the clinician uses the following examination sequence:

1. Observe the ability of the patient to fully extend the knee.
2. Observe the degree of flexion obtainable both actively and passively both on the symptomatic and the contralateral side.
3. Observe once again the position of the kneecap.
4. Observe the relative valgus or varus position of the knee both on the symptomatic and contralateral side.
5. Test for instability with a gentle valgus and then varus stress both in full extension and in 30 degrees of flexion.
6. Perform a Lachman's test by asking the patient to completely relax and then by proceeding to pull and push the tibia forward and back on the femur passively while stabilizing the distal femur with the opposite hand. This is performed with the knee in slight flexion.
7. Palpate for an effusion in the knee joint.
8. Palpate for tenderness at the level of the joint line, beneath the patella, over various tendinous insertions and very gently over any spot which the patient might indicate as painful or tender.
9. Observe the patient's ability to perform a straight leg raising maneuver with the knee extended.

This section was intended as a general introduction to the clinical examination of the knee. Remember that even in asymptomatic people there may be performance differences between the right and left knees. The results of these tests must, therefore, be considered in the context of the patient's symptoms.

ANATOMY

Functionally, the knee can be considered to be tricompartmental. The femorotibial joint consists of both a medial and a lateral compartment. Each femoral condyle articulates with expanded and flattened portions of the proximal tibia known as the tibial plateaus. Interposed between the femoral condyles and the tibial plateaus are the medial and the lateral menisci. Both the patella, a sesamoid bone, and the quadriceps tendon articulate with the distal femur between the femoral condyles in the groove known as the patellar groove.

The patellofemoral joint may be subject to a host of conditions giving rise to pain, disability, and deformity completely independent from the femorotibial joint, or it may be subject to the same degenerative or inflammatory processes involving the femorotibial articulation.

The femoral condyles form the expanded distal portion of the femur. They are covered with hyaline cartilage and articulate with both the patella and the tibial plateaus. Viewed from the lateral aspect, both the anterior and posterior aspects of the femoral condyles approximate a portion of a circle. The lateral femoral condyle is slightly shorter in its anterior-posterior dimension as well as being somewhat flatter on its articular surface in comparison to the medial femoral condyle. The thickness of the articular cartilage of the femoral condyles was measured by Hall and Wysak[22] using data from 430 arthrograms. For males the average thickness of the cartilage on the medial femoral condyle was 4.3 mm and on the lateral femoral condyle 3.9 mm. Among females, the medial femoral condyle had an average articular cartilage thickness of 3.6 mm with 3.3 mm as the average for lateral femoral condyles. Thickness of the articular cartilage is related to the stress borne by the articular cartilage. The thickness of the cartilage gradually diminishes towards the periphery of the joint surface where the weightbearing stress is diminished.

The tibial plateaus have a slight backward slope relative to the axis of the tibia. The medial tibial plateau has a shallow concavity, whereas the lateral tibial plateau is actually slightly convex. Separating the medial and lateral tibial plateaus is the intercondylar eminence with its medial and lateral intercondylar tubercles. The areas directly anterior and posterior to the intercondylar eminence are the site of attachment for both the cruciate ligaments and the menisci. The lateral tibial plateau has a rounded-off contour posteriorly, which permits the lateral meniscus to slide posteriorly in flexion of the knee.

The patella, a sesamoid bone embedded in the distal quadriceps tendon, when viewed from the front is roughly pentagonal in shape. Its articular surface has a longitudinal vertical ridge separating a smaller medial and a somewhat larger lateral facet. The tendinous expansion covering the anterior surface of the patella is thought to originate entirely from the tendon of the rectus femoris muscle. The cartilage on the articular surface of the patella is the thickest in the human body. In full extension the patella rides superior to the articular margin of the femoral groove and in most cases the lateral facet is

in contact with the lateral femoral condyle. The medial patellar facet articulates with the medial femoral condyle to a very minimal extent until nearly complete flexion is achieved. The total vertical excursion of the patella from full extension to full flexion is approximately 8 cm. In a study by Boone and Azen,[10] range of motion was measured in the knees of 109 male subjects. The range of motion averaged 142.5 degrees. Subjects under 19 years had a slightly higher range of motion, measuring 143.8 degrees ± 5.1 degrees. Subjects older than 19 years had an average range of motion of 141.2 degrees ± 5.3 degrees.

The principal extra-articular tendinous structures that cross the knee joint giving it the power to flex and extend, as well as providing dynamic stabilization, are the quadriceps muscles, hamstrings, gastrocnemius muscles, and the popliteus muscle and tendon. The quadriceps muscle group is described as a trilaminar structure inserting onto and around the patella. In addition to the rectus femoris, vastus medialis, intermedius, and vastus lateralis, there are additional small but functionally important muscles known as the vastus medialis obliquus inserting onto the superomedial border of the patella and the vastus lateralis obliqus inserting into the superolateral border of the patella. These small but significant musculotendinous units have been studied intensively in regard to their role in normal and pathologic patellar alignment. The patellar tendon originates from the distal pole of the patella and inserts into the bony prominence on the anterior crest of the proximal tibia known as the tibial tubercle. The patellar tendon length closely approximates patellar height. An abnormally long patellar tendon as measured in a lateral radiograph indicates a condition known as patella alta, thought to be one of the conditions responsible for chronic patellar pain.

Three of the four medial hamstrings, the sartorious, gracilis, and semitendinosus, insert on the anteromedial aspect of the proximal tibia. This collective insertion is known as the *pes anserinus,* which translated from Latin is *goose foot.* This important group flexes the knee and provides internal rotation. The significant lateral hamstring muscle is the biceps femoris, which inserts collectively into the fibular head, lateral aspect of the tibia, and the posterolateral capsule of the knee. It, too, flexes the knee and in addition provides an external rotatory force. The broad, thick tendinous structure spanning the lateral and distal thigh is known as the iliotibial band. Its posterior third is the iliotibial tract, which inserts into the lateral epicondyle of the femur as well as into the bony prominence on the anterolateral aspect of the proximal tibia known as Gerdy's tubercle.

The popliteus muscle originates from the lateral femoral condyle, from the fibula, and occasionally from the posterior portion of the lateral meniscus. The arcuate ligament is formed by the confluence of the femoral and fibular origins where they are joined by the capsule and occasionally the meniscus. It was once thought that the popliteus tendon had a consistent attachment to the lateral meniscus, drawing it down and backwards in flexion; however, in a study by Tria et al,[77] in 82.5% of the knees dissected the popliteus tendon had no major attachment to the lateral meniscus. The popliteus muscle is a medial rotator of the tibia as flexion begins.

The semimembranosus muscle, the additional member of the medial hamstring group, is an important posterior and posteromedial stabilizer. It has five distal tendinous expansions acting to support various portions of the posterior and posteromedial portion of the knee. The direct head of the semimembranosus attaches to the posterior aspect of the medial tibia below the joint line.

The important extra-articular ligamentous structures will be briefly summarized. These are the static stabilizers of the knee, in contrast to the previously described musculotendinous units, which are the dynamic stabilizers. The capsule of the knee joint is a dense fibrous structure surrounding the joint. It is more well-developed medially then laterally. The capsule becomes thinner anteriorly with reinforcement provided by the medial and lateral retinacular expansions. The medial capsule may be divided into three anatomically distinct areas: the anteromedial, midmedial, and posterior medial capsules. Reinforcing the midmedial portion of the capsule is the medial collateral ligament also known as the tibial collateral ligament. It originates from the femoral condyle and epicondyle and inserts onto the tibia below the joint line. The medial meniscus is attached to the inner portion of the ligament dividing it into meniscofemoral and meniscotibial portion. The meniscofemoral portion is anatomically longer and stronger. The medial collateral ligament is the primary static restraint to valgus stress on the knee joint.

The central portion of the posterior medial capsule runs distally and posteriorly in an oblique direction from the adductor tubercle of the femur into the proximal tibia posteriorly near the insertion of the direct head of the semimembranosus tendon. This structure contributes significantly to the stability of the knee posteromedially.

The most important intra-articular structures of the knee joint are the medial and lateral menisci as well as the anterior and posterior cruciate ligaments. The menisci, which were once thought to be vestigial structures, have been shown in fact to have very important anatomic and biomechanical functions. In an article by Beaupré et al,[7] the menisci of the human knee were shown to be essential in transmission of load, stability, and lubrication. Sections made vertically through the midsections of the menisci demonstrated two well-defined regions. The inner or medial two thirds and an outer third were identified, each having a different orientation of the collagen bundles. The menisci are roughly C-shaped structures with firm peripheral capsular attachments. In cross section they are V-shaped with a sharp inner margin. As demonstrated by Beaupré, the inner two thirds of the meniscus is formed by radially oriented collagen bundles, with the peripheral third comprising large collagen bundles oriented horizontally and running circumferentially parallel to the tibial surface. The inner two thirds with its radial orientation of fibers is biomechanically best suited for the compressive forces generated by axial loading of the femur on the tibia, whereas the circumferential fibers in the peripheral portion are best suited to resist the tension and stress from the axial forces, which tend to dislocate the menisci laterally. This explains why bucket-handle tears of the meniscus typically occur at the junction of the inner and outer portions of the meniscus, a potentially weaker zone owing to the change in orientation of the collagen fibers.

The anterior cruciate ligament, which has demanded increasing attention over the past two decades, is described, along with the posterior cruciate ligament, as being intraarticular but extrasynovial. This is to say that the cruciate ligaments, while lying near the center of the joint, are not in contact with the synovial fluid secreted by the inner layer of the synovial membrane, which otherwise bathes, nourishes, and lubricates the articular surfaces of the joint as well as the menisci. The anterior cruciate ligament has two major portions, a small anteromedial portion and a larger, stronger posterolateral contribution. The anterior cruciate arises on the posterior aspect of the medial surface of the lateral femoral condyle. The ligament passes distally and obliquely anteriorly to insert broadly anterolateral to the anterior tibial eminence. The tibial attachment is triangular, with the apex directed posteriorly. The anatomy of the anterior cruciate ligament is complex, with three functional bundles described as anteromedial, intermediate, and posterolateral. Each of these bundles has a relatively discrete origin and insertion. It should be noted that none of the bundles attaches directly to the tubercles or spines of the intercondylar eminence. Apparently straight anterior instability of the knee can be increased by severing the intermediate bundle of the anterior cruciate ligament and anterolateral rotary instability is enhanced by dividing the anteromedial bundle of the anterior cruciate ligament. The anterior cruciate ligament has approximately the same tensile strength as the tibial collateral ligament and is approximately half as strong as the posterior cruciate ligament. In knee flexion, the so-called anteromedial band of the anterior cruciate ligament is taut, whereas the bulky posterolateral portion of the anterior cruciate ligament is in extension.

Johansson et al[34] showed that the cruciate ligaments are richly innervated. Nerve tissue contributed 1.0% to 2.5% of the total volume of the anterior cruciate ligament. The cruciate ligaments are innervated by the posterior articular nerve. This study noted that four types of discrete nerve endings are found in the cruciate ligaments, including Ruffini endings, pacinian corpuscles, Golgi tendon organlike structures, and free nerve endings. The pacinian corpuscles are dynamic mechanoreceptors; the Golgi tendon organlike endings measure the tension in the ligament at the extremes of movement. The free nerve endings giving rise to painful stimuli are activated when subjected to abnormal mechanical deformation or chemical agents. Because deafferentation affects the normal sensory feedback during knee movement, on theoretical grounds primary anterior cruciate ligament repair should be attempted in order to preserve the important sensory function of the anterior cruciate ligament as well as its important role as a static stabilizer.

The posterior cruciate ligament, larger and two times stronger than the anterior cruciate ligament, arises from the posterior portion of the lateral surface of the medial femoral condyle and inserts onto the posterior tibia near the midline below the articular surface. The posterior cruciate ligament is oriented more vertically than the anterior cruciate ligament. It serves as the axis for internal and external rotation of the tibia on the femur. The posterior cruciate ligament has a larger anterior component and a smaller, less strong posterior component. Its role as a stabilizer will be discussed under the section on the biomechanics of the knee.

The blood supply of the knee joint is derived from five major arteries, which form a rich anasto-

mosis.[65] The arteries are the superior medial and superior lateral genicular arteries, the middle or posterior geniculate artery and the inferior medial and lateral geniculate arteries. The descending genicular arteries also form an anastomosis with the anterior tibial recurrent artery. The peripheral attachment and the outer one third or one half of the menisci is richly vascularized. Additionally, there are anastomoses between the cruciate ligaments and the menisci. The middle peripheral portion of the medial meniscus has significant vascular anastomoses with the vessels supplying the medial collateral ligament.

BIOMECHANICS OF THE KNEE

It is tempting to picture the knee as a simple hinge. Closer analysis of the complex biomechanics of the knee joint, however, reveals that the knee is anything but a simple hinge. The knee joint is described as having six degrees of freedom, three transitional and three rotational (Fig 18–2). Pennock and Clark[56] in a review of the literature, noted that the knee can be described kinematically as a three-cylindric open chain. A cylindric joint is a two degree of freedom joint that permits translation along and a rotation about a common axis. In the knee joint, the three rotation axes are skewed and do not intersect. The three axes along which the translations occur are not coordinate with the three axes about which the rotations occur. Pennock and Clark go on to describe the knee joint as a general geometry six-link open chain connected by three prismatic and three revolute joints.[56] In an article by O'Connor[54] the description of the cruciate ligaments with the tibia and femur as constituting a four-bar kinematic linkage was attributed to Strasser (Fig 18–3). The cruciates are considered the main ligamentous elements in the sagittal plane linkage of the knee. According to O'Connor, an important property of the cruciate linkage, on which much geometric and mechanical theory depends, is that the point where the ligaments cross is the instant center of the joint.[52] The full title of this phenomenon is the "instant center of zero velocity of the femur relative to the tibia," which is equivalent to the flexion axis. In this system the femur slides forward while rolling backwards on the tibia during flexion and must slide backwards while rolling forwards during extension. This occurs because contact between the bones lies distal to the flexion axis. It makes necessary a more extensive ar-

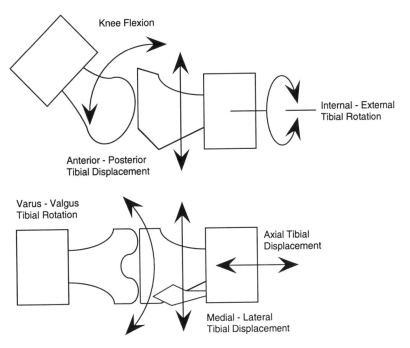

FIG 18–2.
Schematic representation of the six degrees of freedom of the knee on tibiofemoral joint—three rotational, three trans- lational. (From Sullivan D. et al: *J Bone Joint Surg* (Am) 1984; 66A:932. Used by permission.)

ticular surface on the femur than on the tibia. The distance between successive contact points on the femur is three to four times greater than the corre- sponding points on the tibia.

O'Connor further notes that the polycentric and polyradial nature of the knee was described by Strasser and that all the published data show that the flexion axis of the human knee penetrates both the cruciates and the medial collateral ligament, the anterior fibers of which stretch and the posterior fi- bers of which slacken during passive flexion.[54] The axis of flexion passes anterior to the lateral collateral ligament, all the fibers of which slacken during pas- sive flexion. The internal rotation axis of the knee is said to be fixed in and move with the tibia. The com- pression distraction axis is defined as perpendicular to the tibial plateau and located through the mid- point of the medial spine of the tibial eminence. As previously noted, the knee has a differentially greater rollback of the lateral femoral condyle on the lateral tibial plateau. The radii of curvature of the tibial plateaus and femoral condyles also are differ- ent. During flexion, the weight-bearing surfaces in the knee were found to move backward on the tibial

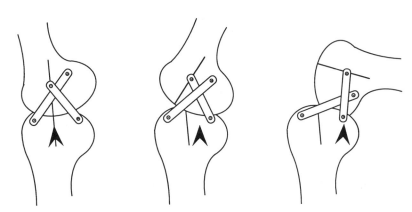

FIG 18–3.
Schematic representation of the knee as a four-bar linkage system demonstrating posterior displacement of the point of femorotibial contact with flexion. (From Dye SF: *J Bone Joint Surg (Am)* 1987; 69A:977, 980. Used by permission.)

plateaus and become progressively smaller. This was demonstrated in an article by Maquet et al.[47] Total weight-bearing surface in the human knee was noted to be between 18.22 cm^2 to 21.95 cm^2 in full extension diminishing to 11.6 cm^2 between 90 and 100 degrees of flexion. The area of weight-bearing surface with the menisci intact is much greater than after total meniscectomy. The menisci represent a large part of the weight-bearing surface in any position of knee flexion.

In further consideration of the biomechanical role of the menisci, Shoemaker and Markolf[66] demonstrated that the anteroposterior (AP) displacement of the knees at full extension in the absence of a compressive load was increased by 43% after meniscectomy. Under compressive load there was a 24% increase in anterior-posterior motion after medial and lateral meniscectomy. Therefore, it is clearly demonstrated that the menisci aid in passive stability of the knee. It is now well accepted that the menisci act as weight-bearing structures to distribute compressive forces across the knee joint during axial loading. Shoemaker and Markolf further noted that in 20 degrees of flexion there was no significant increase on laxity either loading the knee or in the unloaded model. Furthermore, it was demonstrated that the compressed menisci, under physiologic joint loading, do resist anterior subluxation in the absence of the anterior cruciate ligament.

Radin et al[58] demonstrated that the proportion of load borne by the meniscus is dependent on the degree of flexion. He stated that the menisci transmit approximately 50% of the load during walking and that this load was approximately equal to five to six times body weight.

Of course, any discussion of the biomechanics of the knee separate from the consideration of the mechanics of gait has limited clinical relevance. Apkarian et al[2] described a three dimensional kinematic and dynamic model of the lower limb. They stated that at heel contract there is a flexor moment as the knee actively flexes to absorb the impact force. They further noted that from flat foot to midstance there is an increasing extensor moment as the knee extensors control knee flexion and then actively extend the knee at midstance. At heel lift-off the knee flexor moment increases as active knee flexion begins. At toe-off there is a short extensor moment to slow down knee flexion. In late swing a flexor moment acts to decelerate the rotation of the shank in preparation for heel contact. In the frontal plane a valgus moment stabilizes the knee as the external force vector lies medial to the knee joint and places a varus

stress upon it. In the transverse plane, variable rotational moments are seen. The pattern of internal rotation moment followed by an external rotation moment appears necessary to stabilize the knee against an opposing moment at the hip.

There is some controversy as to the exact proportion of compressive load in the medial vs. the lateral compartments. One study suggests that under physiologic loading during gait, the weight borne by each tibial plateau is approximately equal. In an article by Hsu et al[27] it was demonstrated that the medial tibial plateau force equaled approximately 72.8% of body weight in standing and the shear forces change from 1.9% body weight in males and 0.35% in females age 25 to 40 years, to 1.6% body weight in males and 0.5% body weight in females ages 41 to 60 years (Table 18–1). Hattin et al[25] described a 50% increase in AP sheer forces and 28% increase in compressive forces between fast and slow cadences. They further noted that fatigue had a significant effect on the magnitude of the articular force components. In studying deep knee bends with heavy loads, Hattin and coinvestigators found that training elicited improvements exhibited not only by increased muscle forces, but also by biomechanical patterns that resulted in increased compressive forces and reduced shear forces across the knee joint.[25] This is to say that anteroposteriorly directed shear forces exhibit a greater increase as a result of fatigue than the compressive forces. The mediolateral shear forces in the knee are mainly assumed by the conformity of the intercondylar eminences in the intercondylar notch of the femur. The work of Hattin and co-workers, therefore, demonstrated that load, cadence, and fatigue all had important effects on the articular force components at the tibiofemoral joint. They further noted that maximum anterior-posterior sheer and compressive forces consistently occurred during knee bends at the lowest position of weight, i.e., when the posterior thighs were parallel to the ground.

In a study of the kinematics of the sit-to-stand maneuver, Jeng et al[32] noted that maximum knee flexion in this maneuver measured 85 degrees ± 6 degrees. In an interesting discussion of the relationship between the moments at the L5-S1 level to hip and knee joint when lifting, Schipplein et al[61] reviewed the inverse correlation between the compressive forces at the L5-S1 level and the knee joint. They showed that as the back forces increase, the knee forces decrease. They further noted that the muscle cross-sectional area of the erector spinae muscles in the back is larger than that of the quadri-

TABLE 18–1.

Knee Joint Contact Pressure Distribution in a Population Divided According to Gender and Age (Assuming Normal Cartilage and Upper-Body Gravity Location, IR = 0.8)*

Joint Alignment Parameters	Men		Women		Overall (n = 120)
	25–40 Years (n = 30)	41–60 Years (n = 30)	25–40 Years (n = 30)	41–60 Years (n = 30)	
Normal force at knee joint, % BW	95.3 ± 5.9	93.6 ± 3.6	94.1 ± 5.1	94.3 ± 6.8	94.3 ± 5.4
Shear force at knee joint, % BW	−1.9 ± 2.5	−1.6 ± 2.6	0.3 ± 3.5	0.5 ± 2.1	−0.9 ± 2.9
Joint peak pressure, % BW/mm	3.6 ± 1.0	3.3 ± 0.9	4.3 ± 1.1	3.8 ± 1.4	3.8 ± 1.2†
Med. plateau force, % knee force	77.7 ± 10.6	72.8 ± 12.7	76.5 ± 11.4	72.8 ± 12.6	75.0 ± 12.0
Med. plateau contact area, % joint area	60.0 ± 8.8	58.6 ± 5.8	61.2 ± 10.4	59.2 ± 4.9	60.0 ± 7.8
LCLF, % BW	3.5 ± 5.9	1.6 ± 3.6	2.1 ± 5.2	2.5 ± 5.7	2.4 ± 5.2

*From Hsu, RWN, et al: *Clin Orthop* 1990; 255:222. Used by permission.
†Significantly different between men and women for both age groups at $p < .05$.
BW = body weight; LCLF = lateral collateral ligament force.

ceps muscles. They felt that this explains why a subject changes from a flexed leg to a straight leg method of lifting heavier objects. They stated that the knee moment restricts the flexed leg method. This is the rationale for the strengthening of the quadriceps in the rehabilitation of back patients. This, of course, would be especially true in patients who need to lift relatively heavy objects on a daily basis.

In an important study by Markolf et al[48] in vivo knee stability testing revealed an average of 3.7 mm of AP laxity in full extension. There was a 5.5 mm AP laxity in 20 degrees of flexion and 4.8 mm of laxity in 90 degrees of flexion. Mean valgus-varus laxity was 6.7 degrees in full extension. Individual right and left differences averaged 26% to 35%, but ranged from 35% to 50% for laxity and from 19% to 24% for stiffness. When requested to tense the "knee muscles," subjects were able to increase the knee stiffness an average of two to four times while knee laxity was diminished 25% to 50% of the normal value. They went on to state that even though the clinical varus-valgus test is performed at 20 degrees of flexion based on prior ligament sectioning studies, the extended position was felt to be the ideal position for measurement of ligament disruption.

Watkins et al[82] described the effect of patellectomy on the function of the quadriceps and hamstrings. All patients studied achieved full active extension against gravity but demonstrated significant limitations in functional activities. When compared to the untreated side, peak torque values after patellectomy were diminished by 54% using the Cybex isokenetic test speed of 30 degrees/sec and 49% at 180 degrees/sec. A residual deficit in quadriceps function was also demonstrated by the significant delay in the time of onset of the quadriceps torque curve during alternating reciprocal contractions. In addition to altering the length of the lever arm, patellectomy also changes the angle of the pull of the quadriceps, increasing the joint compression force and diminishing the rotatory force, particularly with the knee in the flexed position.

Huberti and Hayes,[28] in a discussion of patellofemoral contact pressures noted that the patellar contact area shifted from the distal margin of the patellar cartilage at 20 degrees of flexion to the most proximal margin at 120 degrees of flexion (Fig 18–4). The maximum contact of the articular surface of the patella was achieved at 120 degrees of flexion. This included the entire proximal third of the vertical crest. Patellofemoral contact pressures were highest at 60 to 90 degrees of flexion and not 120 degrees of flexion. Peak pressures were not found on the vertical crest where the highest incidence of chondromalacia has been found. A uniform pressure was found on the articular patellar surface on all knees and was not related to the Wiberg classification of patellar shape. Maximum contact force at 90 degrees of flexion on the patellar surface was estimated to be 6.5 times body weight. In trained male athletes, the contact pressure could in fact achieve 12 times body weight. During weight lifting a maximum force of 25 times body weight could occur at 90 degrees of flexion. Twenty times body weight has been estimated

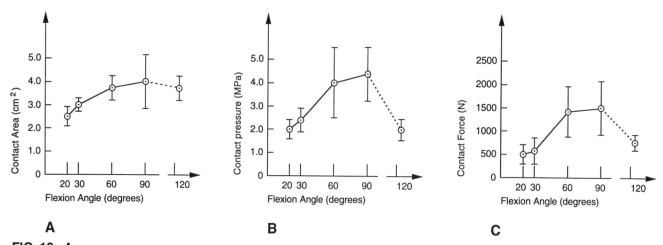

A   **B**   **C**

FIG 18–4.
Graphs showing relationship between flexion angle of the knee and patello-femoral contact area *(A)*, contact pressure *(B)*, and contact force *(C)* (From Huberti II, Hayes WC: *J Bone Joint Surg (Am)* 1984; 66A:717. Used by permission.)

in jumping maneuvers. Contact between the quadriceps tendon and the femoral groove may play a significant role in reducing patellofemoral pressure at high angles of flexion. Tendofemoral contact seems to be important biomechanically. This may explain the increased incidence of chondromalacia in patients with patella alta. Findings also suggest that both increased and decreased Q angles may be pathologic and may lead to chondromalacia.[21]

In a discussion of the biomechanics of the knee extension exercise Grood et al[22] noted that the effective moment arm of the extensor mechanism of the knee was maximal at 20 degrees of flexion and rapidly diminished as full extension was reached. Furthermore, it was noted that the quadriceps force increased rapidly as terminal extension was reached. It was also noted in this empirical study that the addition of 7 pounds at the foot doubled the quadriceps force required to extend the leg.

Biomechanical walking patterns in fit and healthy subjects were studied by Winter et al.[84] They noted that the initiation of gait is an unstabilizing event, with the body's center of gravity falling forward beyond the stance foot. By the time cadence is selected and achieved, the only stabilizing period is double support stance. Even during the two 10% double-support stance periods, the feet are not flat on the ground. During the first half of stance, the hip extensor intervenes to control diminished inertial load, joining with the knee muscles, in what was described as a "tight coupling." The tight coupling of these two motor patterns has been described as "an index of dynamic balance."[84] This study went on to note that the natural cadence of fit and healthy elderly people was no different than that of young

adults except for a significantly shorter stride length and increased stance time. Additionally it was noted that the "vigor of push-off" in the elderly person was markedly diminished, which resulted in a shorter step length and increased double-stance time. Furthermore, flatfooted landing during gait in the elderly was noted.

During monarticular quasistatic extension of the knee, a cocontraction of the hamstrings with quadriceps has been described.[16] With hamstring exercises done prone rather than seated, there is an absence of coactivation of the quadriceps with the hamstrings. In the seated position the anterior cruciate ligament is stressed with quasistatic extension of the knee, whereas in the prone position it is not tensed.

Hsieh and Walker[26] in studying the stabilizing mechanisms of the loaded and unloaded knee joint noted that the geometric conformity of the condyle is the most important factor for diminished laxity under load-bearing conditions. They noted that on the medial side the tibial plateau is doubly concave giving reasonably good conformity with the femoral condyle, but that the lateral plateau, being convex in the average knee, gave less geometric conformity. They noted that the menisci increased the conformity both medially and laterally. They describe the "uphill effect": it is seen that in order to perform anterior-posterior, rotary, or mediolateral movements, the femur must ride upward or "uphill" on the convexity of the tibial plateaus, particularly with intact menisci. They pointed out that one notable exception when rotary stability would not be operative under a compression load is in the presence of a valgus or varus force sufficient to reduce the compressive force in one compartment or the other to zero.

They further pointed out that intrinsic factors such as the major ligaments, capsule, and menisci provide stability of the joint under non–load-bearing conditions and that the cruciates were most important in anterior and posterior movement, with the medial collateral being most important in rotation. They further noted that given the laxity of the joint, under certain conditions of compression certain extrinsic factors, including muscle force and gravity, were sufficient to prevent dislocation of the knee after all the intrinsic structures had been removed.

In a discussion of the influence of design on the transmission of torque across a knee prosthesis, Werner et al[83] noted that torque in the knee joint in normal subjects during level walking averaged 100 in.-lb (11.3 Newton-meters [Nm]). Tibial fracture occurs at an average of 417 in.-lb (47.1 Nm). In full extension rotation increases resistance to torque so that by 6 degrees of internal-external rotation, torque is increased to approximately 50 in.-lb (5.5 Nm). Maximal torque normally occurs at between 70% and 80% of stance phase and at this point there is near–full-knee extension.

It is easily seen from the above discussion that the biomechanics of the knee joint is a complex and intriguing topic. It will be difficult for the reader to integrate all the facts presented above into a simple scheme of knee function; nevertheless, it is hoped that a rough approximation of the biomechanics of the human knee joint is better appreciated.

KNEE PAIN

A separate discussion of the incidence and etiology of knee pain is worthwhile in order to set the stage for the forthcoming discussion of the various entities affecting the knee joint, including those of degenerative, traumatic, and inflammatory origin. A discussion by Brandt[12] concerning pain, synovitis, and changes in the articular cartilage found in osteoarthritis reviews the various origins of pain in the osteoarthritic knee joint. These included inflamed synovium, stretching of nerve endings in the periosteum in the region of osteophytes, microfractures of subchondral trabecular bone, venous hypertension, distention of the joint capsule by accumulation of joint fluid, and muscle spasm. These causes of pain, of course, are not limited to osteoarthritis alone and may occur singly or in combination as the cause of pain in numerous other conditions. In the case of acute trauma with an intra-articular fracture, the free nerve endings in the torn periosteum and the tense hemarthrosis distending the joint capsule, as well as the direct ligamentous and capsular damage may give rise to intense pain, some of which may be alleviated with splinting and immobilization. Intense pain of joint distention can be relieved only with aspiration of the joint. In the case of an acutely septic joint with a pyarthrosis, inflammatory exudates give rise to the same intense pain as is experienced with cellulitis or abscess formation in parts of the body remote from a joint, in addition to the pain from the mechanical distention arising from the septic effusion.

Bergenudd et al[8] in a study of knee pain in middle age and its relationship to occupational work load and psychosocial factors noted that in 55-year-old residents of Malmö, Sweden, there was a 10% prevalence of knee pain. In men, the knee pain was related to more strenuous work and interestingly was also related to decreased job satisfaction. There was no statistical correlation to the type of work or level of job satisfaction with knee pain in women in this study.

In a quantitative analysis of walking patterns in patients with osteoarthritis, Blin et al[9] noted several different compensatory mechanisms, including a decrease in support phase duration during gait and diminished amplitude of knee movement. External rotation of the hip on the affected side was observed in some patients. Additionally, decreased ground support accompanied by damping of foot contact leading to a shuffling gait was observed. In this case, the foot remains close to the ground and step length is diminished on the affected side leading to a decrease in forward and backward velocity. In the case of stiffness of the knee limping, owing to functional inequality of leg length, may occur.

It is sometimes useful to point out to patients during the course of treatment the importance of the ability of the knee to generate painful stimuli as a protective mechanism. It was the privilege of this author to observe an entire family with a type of congenital insensitivity to pain known as acrodystrophic neuropathy.[5] Among the numerous acquired deformities exhibited by all the members of this family were deformed joints. The role of deafferentation of a joint as an etiologic factor in the development of degenerative changes has been controversial. Brandt noted that deafferentation alone did not result in arthropathy.[12] Degenerative changes occurred rapidly if the anterior cruciate ligament was transected in addition to deafferentation.

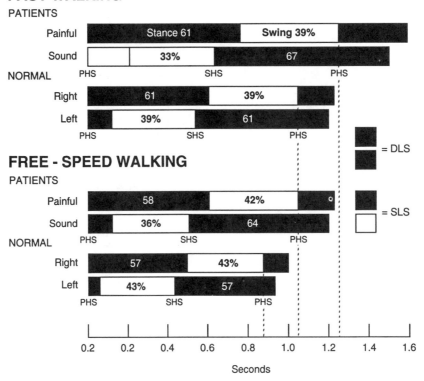

FIG 18-5.

Average stance and swing durations (expressed in percent of the walking cycle duration) during free-speed and fast walking for the painful and sound limbs of 35 men with unilateral knee pain and for both limbs of 60 normal men. The instants of heel strike are indicated for the painful (PHS) and sound (SHS) limbs of patients and for the right (RHS) and left (LHS) limbs of the normal men. (From Murray MP, et al: *Clin Orthop* 1985; 199:195. Used by permission.)

Antalgic maneuvers during walking in men with unilateral knee disability were studied by Murray et al.[53] In a study of 35 males with a major complaint of unilateral knee pain, of which 26 cases were secondary to osteoarthritis and 9 to internal derangement of the knee, various patterns of limping were observed. Out-toeing of the foot on the painful side was noted to be a pain-avoidance maneuver in most of the cases. Increased lateral lurching was thought to increase the lateral dimension of the base of support while walking, giving an increased sense of security. Additionally, diminished hip flexion with increased anterior tilting of the pelvis and ankle dorsiflexion was noted. Diminished walking speed, diminished motion of the painful joint, and diminished time in single-limb support with rapid forward movement of the body during the painful single-limb–support phase was appreciated Fig 18–5. The effect was to produce uneven successive step lengths. Some of these abnormalities were mirrored on the normal side in an attempt to minimize so-called "dysrhythmic gait."[53]

STIFFNESS AND CONTRACTURE

In a review of the origins of stiffness of joints, Siegler and Beck[68] noted that the patients may describe a variety of symptoms as stiffness. These include pain, restriction of motion, fatigue, soreness, or nonspecific joint discomfort. It was noted that stiffness may arise in the central nervous system (CNS) or peripherally in the muscle itself or from changes within the joint proper. Proximal stiffness suggests a rheumatologic syndrome or early Parkinson's disease. Unilateral stiffness might be an indication of stroke-induced spasticity but could also be related to early Parkinson's disease. Stiffness occurring on both flexion and extension occurs with so-called extrapyramidal syndromes and gegenhalten but generally is limited to either flexion or extension with other more classic patterns of spasticity. Furthermore, it was noted that only joint contractures per se prevent full passive manipulation of a joint. Stiffness resulting from spasticity or gegenhalten is velocity dependent. Stiffness secondary to arthridities, myotonia, or polymyalgia rheumatica tends to be related to periods of inactivity and improves after light exercise.

The stiffness associated with rheumatoid arthritis is believed to result from a combination of accumulation of fluid within the joint, thickening of the joint capsule, and synovial congestion. Joint contractures per se develop as a result of restricted or prolonged immobilization from splinting, casting, or from the limited range of motion resulting from rheumatologic disease. Changes in an immobilized joint can occur in a matter of weeks. These changes included invasion of the joint by fibrofatty connective tissue adherent to the articular cartilage. Cartilage atrophy with tearing of the surface following joint manipulation has been noted. Additionally, adhesions between synovial folds and random orientation of ligamentous (collagen) fibers and their insertion during the healing phase of injury can be a source of disabling stiffness. Biochemical as well as mechanical changes also occur in an immobilized joint. Increased collagen synthesis and degradation with a net collagen loss and an increase in collagen cross-linking has been demonstrated. Glycosominoglycans as a group are said to be reduced.[68]

Spasticity, of course, presents an entirely different problem in regard to joint contractures as the limited range of motion may be purely the result of increased rigidity of the muscle in the absence of permanent changes in the so-called static restraints within the joint itself. Remember that the stiffness of spasticity is to a large extent velocity dependent and that a "clasp-knife" effect may be seen in which the stiffness suddenly releases during passive range of motion. Another interesting and relatively common form of relative joint rigidity is termed gegenhalten, also known as oppositional rigidity or paratonia. It is frequently associated with organic brain syndrome causing dementia, and degenerative CNS conditions.[68] Its pathophysiology is not clear. The rigidity in paratonia may vary from very slight to quite severe, causing the patient to become bedridden.

Parkinson's disease causes a type of rigidity that is classed neurologically as extrapyramidal. Extrapyramidal rigidity may also result from certain encephalopathies, heavy metal toxicities, and adverse reactions to the class of drugs known as neuroleptics.[68] In some cases the rigidity resulting from an adverse reaction to a neuroleptic agent is permanent.

Primary muscle diseases resulting in contractures are for the most part genetic and the diagnosis is frequently made before adulthood. In some forms, as in Duchenne's muscular dystrophy, the patient does not live into middle life, but there are other forms that can affect patients into their middle years and beyond. It should be realized that muscle requires energy in the form of adenosine triphosphate (ATP), not merely for contraction but for relaxation as well. Myotonia, a nonspecific term denoting a delay in relaxation of a muscle following a forceful contraction, is secondary to an energy-requiring active contraction. Of the three broad groups in which muscle contractures are observed, congenital deficiency of glycolytic enzymes, malignant hyperthermia, and rigor mortis, only the first is of clinical significance to the therapist.[68]

Keenan et al[37] in a discussion of hamstring releases for knee flexion contractures in spastic adults noted an approximate 50% correction of knee flexion deformity could be achieved at the time of surgery by simple release of the medial and lateral hamstrings. They noted that further correction was limited by tethering of the neurovascular structures. The majority of patients in this study had spasticity resulting from closed head injury or stroke. Ten percent were ambulatory preoperatively vs. 43% postoperatively. The number of patients able to transfer independently went from 3% to 17%. Overall, 83% of the patients in this study had good to excellent results. It was further noted that intra-articular surgery in limbs that lack motor control generally resulted in unwanted joint stiffness.

In summary, then, contractures of the knee joint can involve and generally do involve multiple tissues, including the skin, subcutaneous tissue, muscle, tendon, ligament, joint capsule, vessels, and nerves. The more common reasons for the development of knee flexion contractures include prolonged immobilization or long-term stress deprivation of soft tissues. Botte et al[11] in a discussion of the physiologic aspects of the formation of spasticity and contracture noted the following nine general areas or conditions leading to contracture:

1. Casting
2. Splinting
3. Severe or neglected spasticity
4. Paralysis
5. Sepsis
6. Inflammatory or degenerative arthritis
7. Congenital disorders
8. Prolonged bedrest associated with chronic illness
9. Mechanical incongruity of joint surfaces

Joint contracture results in secondary biomechanical and biochemical changes within the joint. Biomechanically there is an increase in joint stiffness, which is the equivalent of increased torque required to extend or flex the joint. Biochemically there may be a decreased water content in the soft tissues of the joint with concomitant loss of joint space and diminished lubrication. In the discussion of physiologic aspects of contracture formation, Botte et al[11] noted that in a stiff joint there was an associated increased rate of turnover of collagen with degradation being greater than synthesis equaling a net loss in collagen mass averaging 10%. A 5% loss at 9 weeks was noted, whereas there was an observed 25% loss of collagen mass by 12 weeks of immobilization. Also noted was a qualitative change in the matrix of the cartilage with an increase in the reducible collagen cross-linking and a decrease in glycosominoglycans by 20%.

Review of the literature has revealed several other systemic illnesses resulting in knee flexion contractures. Kapoor and Sibitt[36] noted that the syndrome of limited joint mobility associated with diabetes mellitus occurs in 30% to 40% of type 1 diabetics and in some type 2 as well. They suggested that this condition should be suspected in all patients with diabetes mellitus who complain of stiffness or loss of strength in their extremities. The joint contractures are most commonly seen in the joints of the fingers, but in severe and long-standing cases it was noted that the joint contractures could extend to include the elbows, shoulders, knees, and the axial skeleton as well. An additional condition described by Harper et al[24] was that of flexion contractures secondary to adrenocortical insufficiency. They noted that adrenocortical insufficiency had a predilection for the lower extremities and that the contractures were often severe and progressive being entirely resistant to splinting or physical therapy. They failed to speculate on this unusual phenomenon, but stated that it was unlikely to be related to structural, capsular, or ligamentous changes. Furthermore, in the case described in their report, there was dramatic and rapid improvement with the appropriate glucocorticoid replacement. They further noted that a low serum sodium level may be the key to the diagnosis of adrenocortical insufficiency.

OSTEOARTHRITIS

It is estimated that somewhere in the neighborhood of 18 million to 20 million North Americans are suffering from symptoms secondary to osteoarthritis of the knee. Patients with varus deformity associated with osteoarthritis, by far the most common pattern seen, complain primarily of pain, whereas with valgus deformity or patellofemoral arthritis the primary complaints are related to weakness, instability, or the deformity per se. Because pain, of course, is the most common reason for seeking medical attention, patients with the varus deformity pattern of idiopathic osteoarthritis of the knee may be seen earlier. The research done by Barrett and co-workers shows a relationship between the prevalence, age, and pattern of deformity seen in osteoarthritis of the knee (Table 18–2).[6] Odenbring[54] and his fellow researchers found the incidence of medial osteoarthritis of the knee negligible below age 50 to a 3% incidence at 75 years in women. Their study was aimed primarily at determining the prognosis for patients with medial arthritis producing a varus type defor-

TABLE 18–2.
Prevalence and Bilaterality of Roentgenographic Patterns of Deformity in Symptomatic Idiopathic Osteoarthritis of the Knee*

Deformity Pattern†	Total No. of Knees	% of Total Knees	Average Age (yr)	Distribution (F/M)	Patients With Bilateral Deformity
DJD varus	1383	63.0%	72	Equal	17%
DJD valgus	349	16.0%	79	2:1	9%
Primary PFA	84	3.8%	84	7:1	79%
DJD varus PFA	157	7.0%	74	Equal	15%
DJD valgus PFA	143	6.5%	81	2.5:1	9%
Nonproliferative DJD varus	81	3.7%	73	Equal	11%

*From Barrett JP, et al: *Clin Orthop* 1990; 253:182. Used by permission.
†DJD = degenerative joint disease; PFA = patellofemoral arthritis

mity. Of those patients studied long term, only 9 of 31 patients treated nonsurgically were considered to have a satisfactory knee. Lindberg and Montgomery,[46] in a study relating heavy manual labor to the occurrence of osteoarthritis of the knee, noted that approximately 4% of men engaged in 30 years or more of heavy labor had radiologic evidence of osteoarthritis, which was double that of the two control groups.

Osteoarthritis is generally considered to be a roentgenographic diagnosis; that is to say, the definitive means of arriving at a diagnosis in this particular condition is not by physical examination nor by examination of joint fluid or blood chemistries, but by skillful interpretation of radiographs of the patient's knee joint. Perhaps the single most useful view of the knee joint is that which is sometimes referred to as the 6-foot anterior-posterior standing view, or modifications of this view (Fig 18–6 A,B). In the absence of weight bearing, significant changes in the alignment of the knee, of paramount importance in making the diagnosis, are missed. In standing, particularly with most of the weight borne on the knee being studied, significant narrowing of the arthritic compartment, which might otherwise be missed, is clearly seen. The classic hallmarks of osteoarthritis as seen roentgenographically are joint space narrowing, subchondral sclerosis, peripheral osteophyte formation, flattening, or irregularity of the joint surface, subchondral cyst formation, and abnormal valgus or varus alignment secondary to unequal joint space narrowing (Fig 18–7).

There is undoubtedly an underlying genetic component in osteoarthritis. It is not uncommon for patients to describe a pattern of deformity as well as age of onset similar to their own in describing one or both of their parents. The prospective study of the natural history of osteoarthritis in human beings is difficult and time consuming, to say the least. The disease process spans at least 30 years. The earliest recognizable pathologic changes seen histologically, i.e., on a cellular basis, may of course not be appreciated clinically in terms of pain, deformity, or joint effusion. It may take years for a patient to experience symptoms severe enough to warrant medical attention from what were probably the earliest detectable cellular abnormalities of the joint cartilage in idiopathic osteoarthritis. The situation is somewhat different, however, in the type of osteoarthritis that develops secondary to severe joint injury, including intra-articular fractures. This condition is termed posttraumatic osteoarthritis and while it generally shares many if not most of the histologic features of idiopathic osteoarthritis—radiologic features may occasionally be characteristic—articular fractures or deformity secondary to fractures are causative.

In a study by Kettlekamp and co-workers,[40] in a discussion of degenerative arthritis of the knee secondary to fracture malunion, 15 knees in 14 patients were followed up for an average of 31.7 years. Osteoarthritis, which was primarily unicompartmental in either medial or lateral compartments of the knee, was associated with significant residual angular deformities of the bone after fractures of the shafts of the tibia or femur. In this series it was noted that the knee was better able to tolerate increased valgus (knock-knee) then increased varus (bowleg) deformity. These researchers noted that in standing, the medial and lateral tibial plateaus have approximately equal forced distribution, whereas with walking, the

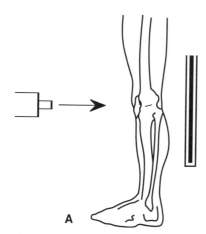 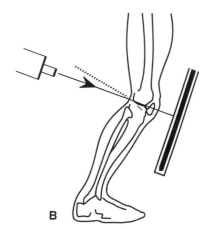

FIG 18–6.
Anteroposterior weight-bearing radiographs. **A,** full extension; **B,** 30 degree flexion standing tunnel view. (From Messieh SS, et al: *J Bone Joint Surg [Br]* 1990; 72B:639. Used by permission.)

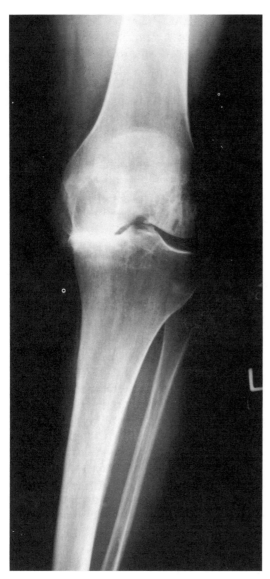

FIG 18–7.
Radiograph taken in the erect weight-bearing position showing closure of medial joint space, varus deformity, and sclerotic reaction of subchondral bone.

medial plateau has a much greater force than the lateral. They further noted that articular cartilage was very tolerant to prolonged excessive loading. Articular cartilage is in fact extremely resistant to compressive loads but less so to sheer forces.

In addition to the disability consequent to the pain and stiffness inherent in advanced degenerative arthritis of the knee, Waters et al[81] demonstrated that patients with osteoarthritis of the knee had a 19% increase in oxygen consumption with walking. These patients averaged 59.7 years in age. The question is often asked as to whether running has a direct effect on the pathogenesis of the osteo-

arthritis of the hips or knees. This is of course a particular concern to the older population who feel they are at much higher risk and for whom physical fitness can be a preoccupation, albeit a healthy one. In a study by Sohn and Micheli[71] there was no association between running at moderate levels of approximately 25 miles per week and the development of osteoarthritis. It was further stated that heavy mileage, in the range of 50 to 140 miles per week, was probably not associated with osteoarthritis of the knee. Furthermore, they noted no correlation between the number of years running and the development of osteoarthritis of the knee. This and other similar studies should be of great reassurance to those young and old alike who find running important in their lives (Tables 18–3 and 18–4).

Early and moderate osteoarthritis presents a definite therapeutic challenge. It may be years before the clinical and radiographic findings are severe enough to warrant either high tibial osteotomy for realignment of the knee or, in more severe cases, total knee replacement arthroplasty. Both of these procedures entail definite risks, and results occasionally fail to meet patient expectations. Treating the patient with mild to moderate osteoarthritis of the knee must be individualized by the physician. Some patients are obese and simply refuse to lose weight, whereas other patients are very cooperative in this regard. Furthermore, some patients, even though elderly, are quite resistant to the helpful regimen of using a cane. Others, even middle-aged and

TABLE 18–3.

Average Miles Run per Week During Running Career*

Age (yr)	Reporting Pain	No Pain
70+	18.8	18.75
60–69	17.9	16.3
50–59	30	24.87
40–49	33.4	27.9
0–40	58.5	54.0

*From Sohn RS, Micheli LJ: *Clin Orthop* 1985; 198:108. Used by permission.

TABLE 18–4.

Average Number of Years Running*

Age (yr)	Reporting Pain	No Pain
70+	8.5	8.47
60–69	9.5	9.8
50–59	12.1	12.4
40–49	14.8	13.5
0–40	10.5	13.1

*From Sohn RS, Micheli LJ: *Clin Orthop* 1985; 198:108. Used by permission.

younger patients, quickly adapt to the use of a cane and therefore accrue the benefits of this simple but effective means of lessening the load in the affected joint. Response to nonsteroidal anti-inflammatory agents is unpredictable. It has been this author's experience that some patients will obtain excellent long-term relief from one or even many different classes of this medication, whereas, there are other patients who obtain almost no relief despite trials of a wide variety of these agents.

The use of intra-articular corticosteroids in osteoarthritis remains somewhat controversial. In a study by Gray and Gottlieb[20] it was noted that despite what they described as "extensive favorable anecdotal evidence" there was limited carefully controlled studies to suggest any long-term benefit to be accrued from intra-articular corticosteroids in cases of osteoarthritis of the knee. Nevertheless, they went on to state that despite popular belief to the contrary, there was little evidence to suggest a deleterious effect of intra-articular steroid preparations. It has been this author's experience that, once again, the effect of intra-articular corticosteroids is unpredictable. Some patients experience almost complete relief of symptoms for many months after a single injection, whereas other patients return to state that they received only a few hours or at best a few days of relief from the injection administered into their osteoarthritic knee joint. However, once a full-blown bone-on-bone situation is seen radiographically, the chance of an intra-articular corticosteroid injection giving significant relief of more than a few days is unusual. Frequently neglected by orthopedic surgeons, but less so by rheumatologists, is the addition of a muscle-strengthening regimen for the patient with osteoarthritis of the knee. As the joint space diminishes with the progressive loss of height of the articular cartilage, the spacer, or shim effect of the cartilage in providing stability to the knee is diminished, thereby allowing greater shear forces to develop, which in themselves may be harmful to the joint. On theoretical grounds, strengthening the dynamic stabilizers, i.e., the musculotendinous units crossing the knee joint, is worthwhile. This will be discussed in a later chapter.

RHEUMATOID ARTHRITIS

While there are many systemic inflammatory conditions producing arthritic manifestations, space permits discussion of only a few of the more common and important types. Perhaps the most important in terms of prevalence and destructive potential is rheumatoid arthritis. Rheumatoid arthritis has a prevalence approaching 1% in the adult Western population. Approximately two thirds of patients with rheumatoid arthritis are female. Onset is usually around age 50 years. Approximately 80% of the population with rheumatoid arthritis can be classified as having the disease in functional class 1 or 2, which allows them to function reasonably well for activities of daily living (ADL) despite their disease. Rheumatoid arthritis may involve muscles either directly or indirectly, resulting in the vicious cycle of joint damage, muscle wasting, muscle weakness, and therefore enhanced joint damage. In addition to a primary myopathy in rheumatoid arthritis, rheumatoid neuropathy has also been described. In mild rheumatoid arthritis there appears to be a preferential atrophy of type 2, or fast-twitch type muscle fibers.[62] In rheumatoid arthritis, low muscle ATP content in addition to diminished muscle blood flow has been demonstrated. Electromyographic (EMG) changes are said to be similar to primary muscle disease. Additionally, certain pharmaceutical agents used to treat rheumatoid arthritis such as cortisone and chloroquine may induce myopathy.

Semble et al[62] in a discussion of therapeutic exercise for rheumatoid arthritis and osteoarthritis noted that diminished muscle strength might result from several factors including a primary myositis, inactivity, corticosteroids, and the inhibition of muscle contractions secondary to a joint effusion. It has been demonstrated that there is a spinal reflex arc inhibiting quadriceps power with joint distention. In rheumatoid arthritis, the joint becomes stiff with diminished range of motion for several reasons, including voluntary limitation of motion as a result of pain consequent to the inflammation. As with any inflammatory process, pain, swelling, redness, and increased warmth may accompany an acute rheumatoid flare. Semble et al[62] further noted that the maximum isometric muscle strength of knee flexion and extension was approximately two-thirds lower on average in rheumatoid patients then in control subjects. They noted that well-supervised exercise programs helped maintain range of motion, strength in muscles, increased endurance, and increased bone density. Further noted was a 40% to 60% decrease in functional ability in patients with rheumatoid arthritis class 2 or 3 in carrying out such simple tasks as walking on level ground, ascending stairs, or stepping up onto a foot stool. Maximum aerobic capacity was diminished in this study by 25%. Statistically significant functional improvement was noted in those patients who participated in an aerobic and a standard physical rehabilitation program including weight training and flexibility exercises, compared with those who participated in what was described as "standard physical therapy and rehabilitation alone."[62] Mean joint counts, for example, pain and swelling, were diminished in the aerobic exercise group.

In a rheumatoid patient, practically speaking, isometric and isotonic muscle training should be and in fact can be performed only during periods of low disease activity. Compliance with an exercise program is only about 50%. Range-of-motion exercises, however, are useful in rheumatoid arthritis. The above authors stated that an acutely inflamed joint should be put through passive or gentle active-assisted range of motion at least once daily.[62] The range-of-motion program should be administered when the patient is feeling his or her best; for example, after a warm shower. They suggest starting with two to three repetitions and gradually increasing the number up to ten daily according to patient tolerance. Isometric exercise is appropriate for restoring or maintaining strength in rheumatoid patients because there is minimal associated joint motion. A maximum of six 6-second contractions should be done with a 20-second rest period between contractions. Isometric exercises are also helpful in improving gait in rheumatoid arthritic patients by increasing the strength of the quadriceps and the hip muscle groups as well. Isometric exercises using low resistance and few repetitions may be performed in rheumatoid arthritis after the pain or the joint inflammation has been controlled.

With active disease, or rheumatoid flare, patients improve most with rest; however, with less active disease more improvement is noted with physical activity. Rest should be limited according to Semble and co-authors[62] to periods of active joint disease. These authors further noted that patients with severe disease had preferentially type 1 muscle fiber atrophy but those with less severe disease had type 2 muscle fiber atrophy. The general goal in the therapeutic exercises administered for rheumatoid arthritis is to minimize the biomechanical forces acting on the joint in order to diminish the risk of joint damage. Even in ADL, the forces acting on weight-bearing joints are high and in excess of what may be experienced during training exercises.

While there is little scientific documentation of long-term benefits of intra-articular administration of corticosteroids in patients with osteoarthritis, the benefits of using intra-articular corticosteroids in rheumatoid arthritis patients, given appropriate circumstances, has been well established.

Patients with rheumatoid arthritis who have severe polyarticular disease are among the most disabled of patients. They live not only with stiffness and weakness but frequently in unremitting pain. They are among the most stoic of patients. They bravely accept their limitations and are grateful for even small gains in function and for brief remissions from their chronic pain. Their expectations generally are not great and their level of cooperation is usually quite high. Rheumatoid arthritis has been described as an autoimmune-type disease in which some foreign agent may trigger a response causing immune complexes to form. The exuberant proliferation of the synovium within the joints affected by the disease process, i.e., synovitis, destroys the articular surface of the joints by growing onto the cartilage in a richly vascularized membrane termed pannus. Pannus, characteristic of rheumatoid arthritis, has a remarkable erosive effect on the hyaline cartilage of joint surfaces. Additionally, rheumatoid synovitis can erode tendinous structures, most notably the extensor tendons of the hands, causing sudden but potentially catastrophic rupture of the tendons. The rheumatoid inflammatory cell mass, or pannus, is not the only source of damage in rheumatoid arthritis. Rheumatoid synovial fluid also contains enzymes derived from white blood cells which have a degradative action on the articular cartilage of the joint. Furthermore, the deleterious biomechanical effect of a chronic joint effusion should not be overlooked. It is of interest to note that histologic examination of hypertrophic and inflamed synovium from certain patients with osteoarthritis is indistinguishable from that removed from patients with rheumatoid arthritis.

The American Rheumatism Association's criteria for the diagnosis of rheumatoid arthritis includes morning stiffness, pain of motion or tenderness in at least one joint, swelling in at least one joint continuously for more than 6 weeks, swelling of at least one other joint occurring within 3 months of a prior joint flare, symmetrical joint swelling with simultaneous involvement of the same joint on both sides of the body, subcutaneous nodules over bony prominences on extensor surfaces or in juxta-articular regions, radiologic changes typical of rheumatoid arthritis including osteoporosis localized to or around involved joints, positive tests for rheumatoid factor, poor mucin precipitate from synovial fluid, characteristic histologic changes in the synovial membrane, and characteristic histologic changes in nodules. Definite diagnosis of rheumatoid arthritis requires at least five of the above criteria with a total duration of joint symptoms of at least 6 weeks. Probable rheumatoid arthritis rests upon the appearance of at least three of the above criteria and a total duration of joint symptoms of at least 4 weeks.

Further consideration of the destructive processes at work in rheumatoid arthritis reveals that in contrast to the proteoglycans of the articular cartilage, the collagen in the joint surfaces is eroded only where pannus is present. The knee is the most common single joint initially involved in rheumatoid arthritis. One unusual and characteristic complication of rheumatoid arthritis is rupture of a large popliteal or Baker's cysts. These cysts are contiguous with the joint, contain joint fluid, and occasionally extend deep into the calf musculature. The joint fluid pressure is increased significantly with flexion of the knee and occasionally cyst rupture occurs causing a clinical picture practically indistinguishable from acute thrombophlebitis of the calf.

GOUTY ARTHRITIS

Space permits the discussion of only two types of crystal-induced disease of the knee joint. The first, which has been recognized from antiquity, is gout. Clinically gout is characterized by recurrent episodes of acute arthritis. It is the result of a crystal-induced synovitis. In gout, the offending agent is microcrystalline monosodium urate. The most important factor accounting for urate deposition and the clinical presentation of the gouty state is hyperuricemia or elevated levels of plasma uric acid. The concentration of uric acid in human beings is closely regulated and the normal range in men is between 3 and 7 mg/dL. In women it is 2 to 6 mg/dL. In patients manifesting levels above 10 mg/dL, the chances for an acute gout attack are greater than 90%. Hyperuricemia, and therefore gout itself, is multifactorial. The primary metabolic form of gout, has several known causes, as does the renal form, most of which are related to diminished renal function on an acute or chronic toxic basis. Both share the common result of hyperuricemia.

An acute attack of gouty arthritis affecting the knee presents more of a diagnostic than a therapeutic challenge. Because an acute attack presents with rapid onset of pain, tenderness, swelling, redness, and joint stiffness, it may be difficult to distinguish from an infected or septic joint. The diagnosis is usually made on microscopic examination of aspirate removed from the knee by and arthrocentesis performed under aseptic conditions. The joint fluid, under these circumstances, might also be subjected to gram stain in order to detect bacteria. In the case of gout, the negatively birefringent needlelike crystals of monosodium urate will be seen with the aid of polarizing light microscopy.

Gout is more common in males than in females and is more common in middle age and in the elderly. In women, it is most likely to occur after menopause. Gout that begins in young adulthood may have a worse prognosis than that of the elderly.

Approximately 50% of all the initial attacks of gout involve the first metatarsophalangeal joint, which is at the base of the big toe. Gout attacks involve not only joints but may also involve bursae and tendon sheaths as well. Most commonly the olecranon and prepatellar bursae are involved. Sometimes more than one joint is initially involved; when this happens, it is usually joints of the lower extremity that exhibit the acute disease process. It may be many years between the initial acute attack of gout and the appearance of chronic gouty arthritis, manifested by progressive and irreversible changes of the articular surfaces of a given joint such as the first metatarsophalangeal joint, the knee, or the finger joints. Certain patients have only a few acute attacks and are spared the sequelae of chronic arthritis; however, after 10 to 20 years most patients present with the findings of chronic gouty arthritis. These findings include chalky-appearing urate deposits covering the surface of the articular cartilage as well as urate deposits embedded in the synovium and perhaps the surrounding periarticular soft tissues such as the tendon and ligaments as well. Radiographically, the destructive lesions which include a cellular response to the focal deposit of monosodium urate crystals, produce erosions of the articular cartilage and bone. Histologically the findings of gout and rheumatoid arthritis share many similar characteristics, including an infiltrate in the synovium that closely resembles pannus.

A variety of pharmaceutical agents are used both in the prevention of recurrent attacks and in attacks of gout in order to hasten the resolution of these attacks once they occur. Gout attacks themselves are self-limited, usually subsiding within a few days to a few weeks even in the absence of medical treatment. Several factors may precipitate gout attacks, including local trauma, overindulgence in certain foods, and consumption of alcohol, particularly if the intake is excessive.

In an acute gouty attack involving the knee it is necessary first to make a definite diagnosis. As noted above, this is done by examination of the synovial fluid under the microscope to observe the presence or absence of the monosodium urate crystals. Usually these are seen within the white blood cells present in the synovial fluid, but not necessarily so. Once the diagnosis is established, treatment may involve the oral administration of either colchicine or anti-inflammatory agents. Intra-articular cortisone injections may also provide rapid relief of symptoms; however, if there is any possibility of joint sepsis, the intra-articular administration of glucocorticoid preparation can be catastrophic. Additionally, as comfort measures, until the acute attack subsides the patient is advised to rest with the affected extremity elevated and when ambulating to use crutches with as little weight bearing on the affected joint as possible.

PSEUDOGOUT

Masuda and Ishikawa[49] described the clinical features of pseudogout attack. They noted in their report that calcium pyrophosphate dihydrate crystals were first described as a cause of an acute crystal induced synovitis in 1961. Pseudogout, or calcium pyrophosphate dihydrate deposition disease, is common in the elderly. Like gout, it may be difficult to distinguish from septic arthritis of the knee. The knee is the site most frequently affected by pseudogout. It is somewhat paradoxical that intra-articular glucocorticoid injection, which may be necessary for early successful treatment, may actually precipitate an attack of pseudogout. Characteristic of pseudogout is a condition termed chondrocalcinosis, which is a radiographic finding denoting the calcification of the cartilage within the joint. In long-standing pseudogout the menisci become densely calcified as seen on radiographs.

Diagnosis, as in gout, rests primarily on the microscopic examination of synovial fluid using polarized light microscopy. In the case of pseudogout, intracellular or extracellular rhomboid crystals with positive birifringence are noted. Unlike gout, pseudogout frequently involves more than one joint. Fever and mental confusion have been noted in pseudo-

gout attacks. Patients with calcium pyrophosphate deposition arthropathy have normal plasma levels of inorganic pyrophosphate but increased concentrations of inorganic pyrophosphate in the synovial fluid. The prevalence of calcium pyrophosphate deposition disease increases with age and is associated with certain diseases such as hyperparathyroidism and hemochromatosis. Furthermore, deposition of crystalline calcium pyrophosphate dihydrate is seen in patients with hypothyroidism, as well as those who have gout.

Pseudogout, technically speaking, signifies the acute attacks of arthritis associated with the intracellular and extracellular presence of the calcium pyrophosphate dihydrate crystals. Joints involved in prior attacks tend to be the site of subsequent attacks. Unlike the case with gout, involvement of the first metatarsophalangeal joint is rare. Crystal deposition with calcification can also occur in the synovium, tendons, bursae, and joint capsules as well. Within the knee joint, crystal deposition usually involves the inner two thirds of the meniscus and assumes either a striped or spotted pattern. It is curious to note that the deposition of calcium pyrophosphate dihydrate may be asymptomatic and may be noted only incidentally on radiographic examination of the knee joint. In other cases, chronic symptoms affecting several joints and giving rise to a clinical picture not unlike rheumatoid arthritis may occur. In these patients various symptoms, including muscle aching, fatigue, and characteristic morning stiffness, may occur. In other patients a clinical and radiographic picture resembling osteoarthritis may occur, with joint narrowing secondary to erosion of the articular cartilage and peripheral osteophyte formation. This may represent one of many potential osteoarthritic responses to joint injury. Instead of the macrotrauma causing posttraumatic osteoarthritis or possibly giving rise to the so-called idiopathic osteoarthritis, this may represent a case of chemical trauma. Krane[41] noted that a valuable diagnostic clue to the osteoarthritic response to calcium pyrophosphate deposition was the presence of osteophytes in the knee joint and contractures in other joints that were not normally affected by osteoarthritis. He further notes that patients with the osteoarthritic form of calcium pyrophosphate dihydrate crystals deposition disease may have superimposed episodes of pseudogout. Further, joint destruction may be so severe and advanced that it appears to be neuropathic Charcot's arthritis. (The absence of pain or normal sensation leads to a destructive arthritis, described in the 19th century by the eminent French physician Charcot. This term originally referred to joints rendered insensate by syphilis.)

SEPTIC ARTHRITIS

The knee is the most common site of septic arthritis in adults. Gonococcal *(Neisseria gonorrhoeae)* infection is the most common form of septic arthritis of the knee in the adult population. Over 80% of nongonococcal joint infections are due to gram-positive cocci. *Staphylococcus aureus* is the most common gram-positive bacterium, with *Streptococcus pneumoniae* and other streptococcal species accounting for the bulk of the other gram-positive infections. Gram-negative bacilli are responsible for approximately 10% to 12% of the nongonococcal arthridies, with *Salmonella* accounting for 10% to 20% of these.[73]

The acute destructive potential of septic arthritis cannot be overemphasized; this is indeed one of the more urgent conditions confronting the orthopedic surgeon. Once again the treating physician is confronted first with the challenge of differentiating the presenting complaint from other acute inflammatory conditions such as gout or pseudogout. Additionally, the organism responsible for the infection must if possible be identified, first via Gram stain and then culture techniques, in order to provide optimal antibiotic therapy.

It is not always possible to determine how the joint became infected. Most commonly the route is hematogenous, that is, through the bloodstream. There may be remote infections responsible for the septic joint, such as a urinary tract infection, respiratory tract infection, or an infected wound elsewhere. Initially the infection involves the synovium of the joint; however, the septic synovitis rapidly becomes a septic arthritis affecting the joint fluid and the entire joint space as well. Usually a tense and painful effusion forms quickly, causing a distended, tender, and exceedingly uncomfortable joint. Destruction of the joint occurs by several mechanisms, including the degradative enzymes present and the pressure from the joint effusion itself. Articular cartilage is rapidly destroyed. The joint capsule may also be infected and weakened. Subchondral bone may be damaged by the infection.

The second task presented to the physician when confronted with a septic joint is treatment.

Rest and elevation, as a therapeutic and comfort measure, are necessary initially. Once the infection is under control, gentle active and active assisted range of motion will help prevent joint stiffness. Ivey and Clark,[31] in a study defining the efficacy of arthroscopic debridement of the knee in septic arthritis, noted that the goals of therapy in septic arthritis were decompression, joint sterilization, and full functional rehabilitation. They stated that loss of ground substance and collagen matrix of articular cartilage as a result of the activity of lysosomal enzymes could occur in the absence of viable bacteria within the joint. They felt that inadequately drained joint fluid would continue to destroy the articular cartilage by enzymatic means and advocated arthroscopy rather than aspiration as a more effective approach to treatment. Loculated deposits of inflammatory exudate were said to be better drained with arthroscopy than with repeated aspiration using a hypodermic needle and syringe. In a study of septic arthritis and treatment considerations, Lane et al[43] noted that certain organisms seem to necessitate open drainage procedures rather than aspiration. Particularly they noted that only 3 of 14 patients with *S. aureus* responded favorably to repeated aspirations whereas 6 of 6 responded favorably to open surgical drainage. They further noted that patients with gram-negative infections were not managed well with repeated aspiration alone. Only 22% of the knees under treatment responded successfully to aspiration in the face of gram-negative infection. They further noted that the length of time between the onset of symptoms and initiation of treatment was statistically significant. If the symptoms were present for more than 3 days before treatment was initiated, 89% of the patients failed management by repeated aspiration. Furthermore, patients with compromised host resistance or limited immune response showed poor response to repeated aspirations and intravenous antibiotics alone. Only 32% of patients with underlying disease states responded to this manner of treatment. Occasionally in the face of clinically resistant infections, which result in repeated joint effusions despite repeated aspiration and/or arthroscopic drainage along with intravenous antibiotic therapy, arthrotomy and synovectomy may be necessary. This presents the additional challenge of avoiding permanent joint stiffness after the infection itself has been eradicated. Osteomyelitis of the bones contiguous to the joint must not be overlooked and if found mandates a more prolonged course of antibiotic therapy.

KNEE SPRAINS AND DISLOCATIONS

Broadly speaking, traumatic conditions involving the knee joint include sprains, which may be defined as partial ligament injuries, ligament ruptures, and fractures. While the era of sports medicine has certainly advanced the knowledge of ligamentous injuries to the knee, focus has centered primarily on the young athlete and the treatment generally recommended reflects the goals of active participation in sports, not necessarily reflecting the desires or physiology of the more elderly population. Nevertheless, research into the area of the pathomechanics and pathophysiology of knee injuries in younger athletes has contributed to a better understanding of certain acute posttraumatic conditions affecting the older patient as well.

In addition to sprains, ligamentous ruptures and fractures, there is also the problem of the dislocated knee joint. To the lay person, the expression "dislocated knee" most often refers to a laterally dislocated patella. To the orthopedist or trauma surgeon, however, dislocation of the knee means something far more serious. This type of traumatic rearrangement of the anatomy of the tibiofemoral joint carries with it a high incidence of permanent and catastrophic consequences, not the least of which may be amputation of the leg at or above the level of the knee. In a study by Sisto and Warren[70] the incidence of popliteal artery rupture with complete knee dislocation was 33%, with a range of 16% to 64% in various other studies. Anterior dislocation of the knee tended to cause traction injuries to the poplpiteal artery and posterior dislocation tended to cause more complete tears. Anterior dislocation has been reported to have a higher incidence of popliteal artery injury overall. The incidence of peroneal nerve injury was also to be high, ranging from 14% to 35%. In the author's opinion, and in the opinion of others, both cruciate ligaments must tear in order for dislocation of the knee to occur.[70] Further, unlike isolated cruciate ligament tears, in the case of complex dislocation, the ruptures tended to occur as avulsions at the origin or insertion rather than in the mid substance. The authors, in a study of complex knee dislocation as a follow-up to operative treatment, recommended that anterior dislocation should be immobilized following reduction in flexion to prevent redislocation and should be maintained in extension in cases of posterior dislocation. They further recommended operative approach in young,

active patients. Frassica et al,[18] in a study of the treatment for complete dislocation of the knee, noted that vascular injuries were seen in 10 of 11 patients initially. Of 30 patients, 13 had early operative repair of the major knee ligaments and capsular structures. In all 13, both the anterior cruciate and posterior cruciate ligaments were torn. All surgical repairs were done within 5 days of injury. The knee was immobilized postoperatively in 30 degrees of flexion in these cases. Twelve patients were seen in follow-up, of whom five had excellent results and six were said to have good or fair results.

By virtue of the commonly associated significant vascular injuries, knee dislocations are considered to be true orthopedic emergencies. Extensive ligamentous damage to the joint is a necessary consequence of the dislocation. Knee dislocations can usually be reduced by closed methods and in the author's experience, intravenous sedation is usually adequate anesthesia. Circulation needs to be assessed constantly for at least 1 week following closed reduction. Occasionally, particularly in cases of posterolateral dislocation, closed reduction may be difficult or impossible.

Rupture of the extensor mechanism of the knee joint may involve either the quadriceps tendon or the patellar tendon. In the elderly, quadriceps rupture generally occurs during stair climbing. The site of rupture is said to be close to the patella. In patients younger than 50, quadriceps ruptures occur generally as a result of a fall on stairs or a direct blow, or secondary to other systemic disease processes and occasionally following corticosteroid injections.[45] Underlying disease processes that may predispose to rupture of the patellar tendon include rheumatoid arthritis, chronic renal failure with hypoparathyroidism, or systemic lupus erythematosis. In many cases, the patients have been receiving systemic steroid therapy.[64] It is a well-established principal in orthopedics that tendon rupture does not occur in the midsubstance of the tendon unless the tendon is affected by a degenerative process because of the enormous mechanical strength of the substance. In the absence of predisposing degenerative process of the tendon, rupture will generally occur as an avulsion at the site of insertion into the bone, as a fracture of the bone where the tendon inserts, or as a tear of the muscle or the musculotendinous junction. Failure of the extensor mechanism usually involves the patellar tendon (frequently referred to as the patellar ligament) in patients 40 and younger and more frequently involves the quadriceps tendon in the older age group (Fig 18–8). It is distressing to

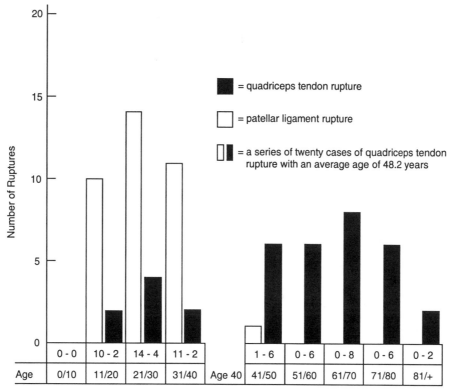

FIG 18–8.
Distribution of quadriceps tendon and patellar ligament ruptures according to age group. (From Siwek CW, Rao JP: J Bone Joint Surg [Am] 1981; 63A:936. Used by permission.)

note how frequently the diagnosis of rupture of the extensor mechanism, either quadriceps or patellar tendon, is initially missed. The consequences of missing this diagnosis can be catastrophic, as late repair is difficult. Results of early repair, particularly of the quadriceps tendons, are quite good. The results of repair of ruptures of the patellar tendon are less satisfactory. Following repair of complete ruptures of either the patellar tendon or the quadriceps tendon, 6 weeks of immobilization is necessary with extremely protected weight bearing strictly enforced. Following the period of immobilization, the process of repairing full flexion is a slow and frequently difficult process, taxing the patient, the physician, and the therapist administrating the rehabilitation program.

First-, second-, and third-degree medial collateral ligament sprains are occasionally seen in the elderly as isolated injuries.[21] In a discussion of the ligamentous and capsular restraints preventing straight medial and lateral laxity in intact human cadaver knees, it was noted that the long parallel fibers of the superficial portion of the medial collateral ligament were the primary restraining mechanism limit-

ing medial opening. A small increase in laxity (5 to 8 mm) indicated significant tearing of the primary restraint (medial collateral ligament). The midmedial and midlateral capsular structures provide important attachments for the menisci but do not have important primary roles in limiting straight medial and lateral laxity. The lateral collateral ligament is the primary restraint limiting lateral joint opening. The lateral collateral ligament provides greater restraining moment than that exerted by the entire lateral half of the capsule plus the iliotibial tract, popliteus tendon, and cruciate ligaments combined. It was further noted by the above authors that the insertion of the biceps femoris into the lateral collateral ligament may enable this muscle to tighten the lateral collateral ligament.

Nonoperative treatment of complete tears of the medial collateral ligament of the knee was described by Indelicato[29] in 1984. Nonsurgically managed patients were treated with a cast brace. Both groups, surgically repaired and those treated with a cast brace, showed a clinically insignificant jog of laxity on valgus stressing at 30 degrees of flexion. The residual laxity had no apparent functional significance.

It is now accepted that the medial collateral ligament and the medial collateral ligament complex are capable of normal or near-normal functional recovery, even with a complete tear. Indelicato[29] stated that the key to success with nonoperative treatment was to establish that the medial collateral ligament injury was an isolated one and not associated with other significant ligamentous ruptures, particularly that of the anterior cruciate ligament or significant meniscal tears. Other studies have challenged the concept that medial collateral ligament injuries associated with anterior cruciate ligament injuries are best treated surgically. In a study by Jokl[34] discussing nonoperative treatment for severe injuries to the medial and anterior cruciate ligaments of the knees, Hastings was credited with the finding that medial instability of more than 11 mm with a valgus stress was diagnostic of a concomitant anterior cruciate tear.

Tension studies of human knee ligaments performed by Kennedy et al[39] noted several clinically important features of knee ligament injuries. Human ligaments are viscoelastic, absorbing more energy and requiring more force to rupture as the loading rate is increased. At faster loading rates, failure tends to be more intraligamentous. Ligaments may be stressed to ultimate failure in the absence of macroscopic disruption. These researchers further noted that the tibial collateral ligament is the most frequently disrupted, followed by the anterior and then posterior cruciate ligaments. They further noted that the anterior cruciate ligament was approximately equal to the tibial collateral ligament in strength in the course of in vitro testing, whereas the posterior cruciate ligament was twice as strong. Pope et al,[57] in a discussion of the role of the musculature in injuries to the medial collateral ligament, felt that the quadriceps mechanism was generally regarded as the most important muscle group for protection against valgus force. Through contraction of the quadriceps retinaculum, the muscle fibers cause the anteromedial and anterolateral parts of the joint capsule to become tense.

Jonsson et al,[35] in an article on kinematics of active knee extension after tear of the anterior cruciate ligament noted that in normal knee motion, passive flexion to 30 degrees is usually coupled with an internal rotation that is decreased in the anterior cruciate ligament–absent knee. They further noted that pushing the flexed tibia backwards passively might further reduce the internal rotation or even cause an external rotation in the absence of the anterior cruciate ligament. When the tibia is displaced anteriorly, as in the pivot-shift test, the internal rotatory laxity increases. Furthermore, these authors noted that increased varus laxity has been observed in anterior cruciate ligament–deficient knees.

The natural history of the posterior cruciate–deficient knee was studied by Torg et al.[78] Those patients with unidirectional posterior instability did not require repair or reconstruction, whereas there was a much poorer prognosis with multidirectional instability. In those patients with multidirectional instability, there were diminished functional results and an increased incidence of degenerative changes seen radiographically. Additionally, there was an increased incidence of patellofemoral dysfunction. Therefore the authors recommended surgical repair in cases of multidirectional instability. They further stated that the prognosis might be dependent on good quadriceps tone.

Templeman and Marder[75] studied the association of knee ligament injuries and tibial shaft fractures. They noted that 22% of patients with tibial shaft fractures had an associated second- or third-degree ligamentous disruption of the knee. They noted further in cases of femoral shaft fracture there was a 25% to 35% incidence of knee ligament injury. These potentially problematic injuries are not infrequently overlooked, as the attention of the treating physician is diverted to the painful and unstable long bone fracture. It is difficult to test the human knee joint in a normal fashion in the presence of a femoral or tibial shaft fracture. Nevertheless, an attempt to test for knee ligament injuries in the case of long bone fractures of the lower extremity is prudent. Dalamarter et al,[15] in discussing knee ligament injuries associated with tibial plateau fractures, found that ligament injuries occurred in 20% to 25% of patients with this injury, the most common being the medial collateral ligament. The usual types of tibial plateau fractures associated with ligamentous injuries were the so-called local compression and split compression types. It was noted that patients in whom the injury caused greater than 10 degrees of instability had generally poor results. Cruciate injury associated with tibial plateau fractures also had a poor prognosis for functional outcome.

It is sometimes difficult in the middle-aged and elderly population to determine whether meniscal tears noted on imaging studies, particularly magnetic resonance imaging (MRI) films, are clinically significant. Certainly most of these do not appear to be of major clinical significance. Therefore, the mere presence of a degenerative-type horizontal cleavage tear of the meniscus is not an indication for surgical intervention. Traumatic tears of the menisci, however, which may be of clinical significance, can occur in middle-aged and older patients. The standard arthroscopic approach to these tears may give quite satisfactory results, although in many cases there is associated pathology of the articular cartilage indicative of early to moderate osteoarthritis. In these cases, the arthroscopic procedure per se may have limited therapeutic benefit and the generally progressive nature of osteoarthritis should be explained to the patient. Terry et al[76] discussed an interesting pathologic entity giving rise to symptoms that may be clinically confused with a meniscal tear. They studied isolated chondral fractures of the articular surface of the knee. They stated that the patient's physical examination was highly suggestive of a meniscal injury. What they described as "an incomplete lesion" was detected only by probing the articular cartilage during arthroscopy, revealing the partial separation of the articular cartilage from the underlying subchondral bone. These authors felt that torsion of a flexed knee as well as impaction might cause the chondral fractures. They noted that impaction injuries to hyaline cartilage, when produced experimentally either from a single event or from repetitive loading, could cause permanent damage once the critical threshold was reached. They noted that even in the absence of gross fracture, these lesions could progress rapidly to osteoarthritis.

OSTEONECROSIS OF THE KNEE

Ahuja and Bullough[1] credited Alback with the first description of subchondral segmental idiopathic avascular necrosis of the femoral condyle in 1968. Alback and associates described radiolucent lesions of the medial femoral condyle in 39 patients all over the age of 60 years. This condition is now generally referred to by the simplified term osteonecrosis of the knee. Osteonecrosis of the nonidiopathic type may be associated with osteoarthritis. Association with rheumatoid arthritis is rare and usually involves the lateral femoral condyle rather than the medial femoral condyle. Bone scans will reveal the lesion well in advance of the typical changes seen on plain film radiographs. The successive stages in the development of the osteonecrotic lesion are first, fracture of necrotic bone; second, fragmentation and collapse of the articular cartilage followed by breakdown of the necrotic segment. This in turn is followed by fibrillation of the articular cartilage, subchondral osteosclerosis and lastly secondary osteoarthritis.[1]

Rozing et al[58] in studying spontaneous osteonecrosis of the knee noted that clinically the condition presents with sudden onset of pain, usually on the medial side of the knee. The condition is acutely painful causing swelling and tenderness over the medial femoral condyle with loss of motion in both flexion and extension. They noted that the technetium 99m bone scan showed intense uptake in the area of the lesion within a few days of the onset of symptoms. The lesion rarely occurs on the medial tibial plateau. Symptoms subsided within 6 months with limited weight bearing and use of anti-inflammatory agents and analgesics combined with straight leg–raising exercises in two thirds of patients. It was noted, however, that mild pain might persist permanently. One third of the patients were noted to have persistent and disabling symptoms for more than 6 months. These patients were felt to be possible surgical candidates.

Motohashi et al,[50] studying the clinical course and roentgenographic changes of osteonecrosis in the femoral condyle treated conservatively, noted in their series that the average age at diagnosis was 62.8 years. In lesions measured radiographically as less than 3.5 cm in diameter, conservative treatment was successful unless there was associated severe pain or varus deformity. In lesions noted to have a maximum width of not greater than 1 cm, there appeared to be no significant progression in the size of the lesion nor deformity of the limb.

REFLEX SYMPATHETIC DYSTROPHY AND REGIONAL MIGRATORY OSTEOPOROSIS

Several conditions giving rise to knee pain should be mentioned before moving to other traumatic conditions affecting the knee joint. In recent years, reflex sympathetic dystrophy of the knee has been recognized with increasing frequency as a source of severe and disabling pain. In an article by

Tietjen[77] it was stated that a suspicion of reflex sympathetic dystrophy should be raised when a patient presents with pain out of proportion to the original injury or out of proportion to the usual course of events postoperatively. Tietjen described the pain as possibly burning in nature, persistent or intermittent, and usually worsening with ambulation or weight bearing. A common presenting complaint in addition to pain is that of stiffness of the joint, although most patients will have an entirely normal range of motion when examined gently or under anesthesia. Additionally, the confusing presence of mechanical complaints such as locking or buckling may also occur. Diffuse swelling is a common complaint that may not be actually observed clinically by the examiner. Tietjen stated that the initial radiographs may be entirely negative but within 2 to 4 weeks radiographic changes are frequently noted. There include regional osteoporosis involving the patellofemoral joint and most commonly involving the medial femoral condyle and the medial tibial plateau. It was felt that the skyline view of the patella is helpful because the patella is uniformly involved. Bone scans were noted to be positive two thirds of the time in this particular study. Passive range of motion was said to increase the pain and active assisted range of motion apparently was the treatment of choice.

Regional migratory osteoporosis was described by Banas et al.[4] They attributed the first description to Duncan in 1967. It is said to be an uncommon entity most frequently seen in middle-aged women and characterized by arthralgias in the lower-limb weight-bearing joints. Severe focal osteoporosis develops with symptoms persisting for 6 to 9 months. The pain is increased markedly with weight bearing and apparently peaks in intensity somewhere between the second and third months in the course of the disease. The patient presents with a warm, swollen joint. Limited range of motion is noted. The patient also demonstrates an antalgic gait and muscle atrophy. In this condition, radiographic findings lag behind the onset of symptoms for 4 to 6 weeks. Once again, the bone scan is generally positive with focal intense uptake prior to appearance of typical radiographic changes. Additionally, the bone scan may reveal changes in other joints before the symptoms actually appear. The knee is the most commonly involved joint, followed by ankle, foot and then less commonly, the hip. Remineralization of the lesion radiographically may be delayed for up to 2 years.[68]

FRACTURES

Fractures of the tibial plateau most commonly occur in patients in later middle age and older. Lansinger et al[44] in reviewing tibial plateau fractures reviewed 260 patients with these fractures. The mean age was 55 years with peak incidence of tibial condylar fractures occurring between 50 and 59 years. They noted the common feature in the pattern of injury is that the lateral condyle was involved first; therefore, the main damage to the joint surface is generally found in the area of the lateral tibial plateau. The surface of the medial condyle was seldom disrupted and medial compression was rare. These authors state that the decision for surgical treatment should not be based on the radiographic appearance but on the presence or absence of instability. The indication for surgical intervention would therefore be medial or lateral instability, unacceptable deformity, or any combination of these. The knee should be tested in extension to determine the presence or absence of instability with tibial plateau fractures. More than 10 degrees of increase in medial or lateral deviation with testing is considered a possible indication for operative treatment. The notable exception in this case is the pattern of bicondylar fractures (Fig 18–9) in which stability is either difficult or impossible to assess. If there is a central compression greater than 10 mm in depth the lesion should be reduced, possibly with bone grafting, and fixed by some type of internal fixation. Lansinger[44] recommended nonoperative treatment of tibial plateau fractures by the use of a plaster cast for 2 weeks followed by flexion and extension exercises without weight bearing for an additional 4 weeks. Weight bearing following 6 weeks was resumed.

Fractures of the patella are quite common in elderly people and may occur either from a direct blow, such as in contact with the dashboard in a motor vehicle accident, or in an avulsion fracture such as might occur in a misstep off of a curb or loss of balance while descending stairs (Fig 18–10). When examining the patient with a patellar fracture, it is useful to determine whether or not straight leg raising is possible with the patient in the supine position. With a displaced transverse fracture through the patella, if straight leg raising is not possible, it is assumed there is an associated rupture or tearing of both the medial and lateral quadriceps expansions. In addition to open reduction and internal fixation of

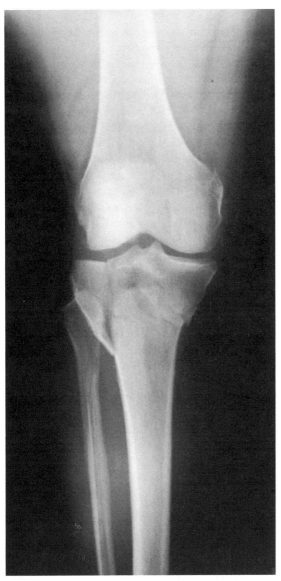

FIG 18–9.
Radiograph showing a comminuted fracture of the proximal tibia including the lateral tibial plateau. A good result was obtained in this case using open reduction and internal fixation.

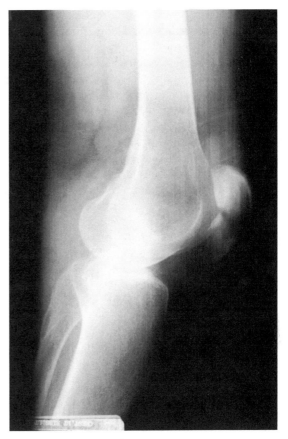

FIG 18–10.
Lateral radiograph of the knee showing a separation of the fragments of a transverse fracture of the patella. Open reduction and internal fixation produced an excellent result in this case.

the fracture, repair of the torn medial and lateral retinacula should also be performed. Even in nondisplaced fractures of the patella as observed roentgenographically the patient should be asked during the course of the examination to maintain the extended position of the knee when performing a straight leg–raising maneuver. If there is minimal separation of the patellar fragments and the patient can perform a straight leg–raising maneuver without assistance, then treatment in a knee immobilizer or cylinder cast generally will provide satisfactory results after 4 to 6 weeks of immobilization.

Various types of repair have been advocated for fractured patellae including excision of small inferior fragments with repairs of the tendinous portions. Patellectomy may be advisable in the case of highly comminuted fractures. It has been this author's experience, however, that even highly comminuted patellar fractures with some degree of separation of the fragments may do remarkably well in well-motivated patients given vigorous physical therapy after sufficient healing has occurred.

HIGH TIBIAL OSTEOTOMY

In an attempt to lessen the symptoms experienced by patients with unicompartmental osteoarthritis, particularly in the medial compartment with a varus deformity, high tibial osteotomy, either by wedge resection, dome osteotomy, or drill osteoclasis, has proven to be a reliable and effective procedure. The procedure is particularly applicable for patients for whom, because of their relative youth, total knee replacement arthroplasty seems ill-advised. The principle of high tibial osteotomy for medial compartment osteoarthritis of the knee is to realign the weight-bearing axes so that the pressure borne within the joint is shifted laterally into the area of the intercondylar eminence and tibial spines rather than concentrated in the medial compartment. Proximal tibial varus osteotomy for osteoarthritis of the lateral compartment of the knee is performed less often, as lateral compartment osteoarthritis is much less common and the results, owing to the different biomechanics of valgus deformity, are less predictable. In a study on gait analysis in patients with gonarthrosis of the knee treated with high tibial osteotomy, Iversson and Larsson[30] noticed that following high tibial osteotomy for medial compartment osteoarthritis, pain was consistently and significantly reduced, but there was not a significant improvement in terms of gait velocity. They called gait velocity a "central parameter in gait analysis." Patients with rheumatoid arthritis ambulate with 36% of normal velocity on average, whereas patients with osteoarthritis in the knee walk with an average of 55% of normal. These authors cited Murray and co-workers as reporting the walking velocity among men with unilateral knee disability to be 62% of that of normal individuals. In this study, the preoperative velocity was and remained 61% of normal for somewhat younger adults.

In a report by Keene et al[38] the results of high tibial osteotomy were found to deteriorate over time. In their study only 47% of 51 knees had good or excellent results in a 5-year follow-up, whereas 78% of these patients had good to excellent results at 2 years. After a minimum follow-up of 5 years the 38 knees with minimal lateral compartment arthritis had the same clinical result as the 13 knees with moderate to marked lateral compartment degenerative arthritis. It is somewhat surprising to note that the patients did as well with radiographic evidence of more severe arthritis in the lateral compartment following valgus high tibial osteotomy as those patients with much less severe disease in the lateral compartment, considering that the operative procedure shifts the weight-bearing axis laterally. The same author noted gradual postoperative loss of correction and in particular recurrent varus deformity.

This has frequently been implicated as a cause of deteriorating clinical results. They further noted, as a result of their study, the degree of valgus alignment achieved at surgery was not always successful in preventing recurrence of varus deformity. They described a low adduction moment across the knee as being a clinically good predicator, whereas patients with high adduction moment had significantly poorer results (Fig 18–11). In fact, 100% of the patients with low adduction moments had excellent to good results, whereas only 50% of patients with high adduction moments had good results. The patient with high adduction moments at the knee had recurrent varus angulation and those with low adduction moments did not experience a deterioration in surgical correction.[38]

In a similar study by Rudan and Simurda[59] 80% of patients followed for 9 years maintained good to excellent results following valgus high tibial osteotomy for medial compartment arthritis; 70% had good to excellent results after 10 years. The revision rate for surgery was 10.9%. They further noted there was no difference in the results in patients who were younger than 60 or in patients who were older than 60 at the time of the surgical procedure. These authors cited conflicting reports regarding the effect

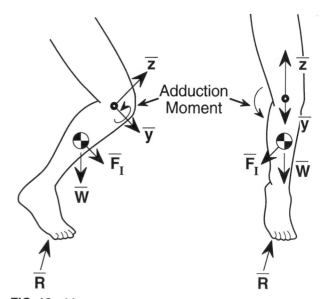

FIG 18–11.
The adduction moment is resolved about an axis ($\bar{y}$) that moves with the tibia in the sagittal plane. The longitudinal axis of the tibia ($\bar{z}$) is perpendicular to the $\bar{y}$ axis and is also in the sagittal plane. The moment is calculated from the ground-reaction force ($\bar{R}$) the limb-segment inertia ($\bar{F}_1$), and the limb-segment weight ($\bar{W}$). (From Wang et al: *J Bone Joint Surg [Am]* 1990; 72A:906. Used by permission.)

of high tibial osteotomy on the outcome of subsequent total knee replacement arthroplasty. Coventry[13] at the Mayo Clinic, who is credited with popularizing the high tibial osteotomy procedure, published the results of proximal tibial varus osteotomy for osteoarthritis of the lateral compartment of the knee. He noted that while load will be transferred to the lateral compartment after a valgus osteotomy performed for the valgus deformity of the medial compartment arthritis, a comparable load cannot be transferred to the medial compartment by a varus osteotomy because of the inherent anatomic valgus alignment of the femur on the tibia. He further noted that weight was shifted medially but also to the lateral portion of the intercondylar area in a varus osteotomy for lateral compartment arthritis.

High tibial osteotomy is a reliable and time-proven method of providing significant relief for the patient under 60 years of age with predominantly medial compartment osteoarthritis and varus deformity. Patients with high adductor moments statistically do not do as well as those with low adductor moments. This is not easily predictable preoperatively. Furthermore, the operative procedure is technically demanding requiring skillful osteotomy at precisely the right level. No more and no less than the correct amount of bone may be removed when the wedge osteotomy method is used. Intraoperative roentgenograms are essential during the procedure to check the placement of the guide pins prior to osteotomy. Postoperatively, immobilization must be maintained until solid union is achieved. Overzealous physical therapy performed too early can contribute to delayed or nonunion. Overcorrection can result in cosmetically unacceptable and functionally inferior results. Recurrent deformity over time will occur in a certain percentage of patients, ultimately necessitating either a repeated high tibial osteotomy or total knee replacement arthroplasty. There is no question in this author's mind that total knee replacement arthroplasty is technically more difficult in patients who have had prior high tibial osteotomy, although whether or not the ultimate functional result is compromised remains somewhat controversial. Obesity appears to be a relative contraindication for a high tibial osteotomy.

The high tibial osteotomy procedure is performed by making, in the case of the wedge resection, two transverse cuts across the flare of the tibial metaphysis several centimeters below the joint line (Fig 18–12). The more proximal cut, closest to the joint itself, is made parallel to the joint surface, whereas the lower cut is made at an angle. Cuts are made so that the wedge removed is based laterally. The osteotomy should leave some medial cortex intact to function as a hinge. At the end of the procedure, the assistant surgeon applies a strong valgus force to close the osteotomy, at which point the sur-

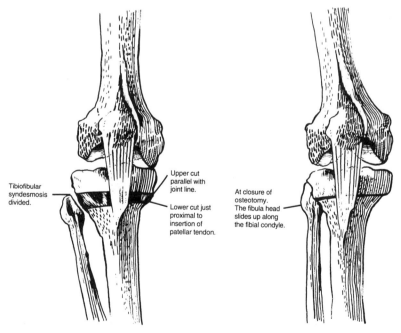

FIG 18–12.
Lateral closing wedge valgus high tibial osteotomy performed for medial compartment osteoarthritis and osteone-crosis of the medial femoral condyle. (From Insall JN, et al: *J Bone Joint Surg [Am]* 1984; 66A:1042.

geon will usually drive a staple or use some other fixation device to hold the osteotomy closed. The functional effect is to move the foot laterally so the weight-bearing axis is shifted laterally. In addition to delayed union or nonunion, peroneal nerve palsy is a potentially serious complication, although in many cases gradual resolution of the foot drop will resolve if the nerve itself has suffered only a stretch or contusion and has not been severed.

TOTAL KNEE REPLACEMENT ARTHROPLASTY

While there is no question that enormous advancements have been made in the art and science of prosthetic arthroplasty for the knee joint, this should still be undertaken with a great degree of circumspection and restraint. Salvage in the case of failed total knee replacement arthroplasty is not simple and the results are occasionally less than desired by both the patient and the operating surgeon. An indication for total knee replacement arthroplasty is chronically disabling pain in a knee joint affected by an arthritic process. It is not indicated in severely demented or bedridden patients. Absolute contraindications include an infection within the joint or an acute infection elsewhere in the body. A high rate of postoperative sepsis has been noted in patients with prior osteomyelitis in the bones adjacent to the knee joint. Charcot arthropathy or absence of sensation in the joint is a contraindication inviting failure. Spasticity, particularly if severe and associated with contractures, should also be considered a contraindication. The author has experienced disappointing results when attempting to address the painful arthritic deformities sometimes encountered in spastic patients.

The design of the various knee prosthesis have gradually merged so that there are relatively minor differences between most of various types now available on the market.

Prosthetic designs are classified as constrained, semiconstrained, or minimally constrained. Fully constrained prostheses are actually hinges. Because the knee joint does not function as a simple hinge, as discussed earlier in this chapter, these prostheses have a high failure rate. There are, in fact, few indications for the use of the hinge-type prosthesis today. The semiconstrained prothesis is used when the posterior cruciate ligament is either absent or

sacrificed, and may be necessary in cases of revision of previous total replacement arthroplasty. It is designed to prevent subluxation or dislocation of the tibiofemoral joint resulting from the absence of static restraints, i.e., important ligamentous structures. The minimally constrained prosthesis, the type most frequently used, reproduces the anatomic contours of the knee joint to a large extent. The normal anatomy and contour of the distal femur are reproduced in the highly polished metallic surface applied to the distal femur. The tibial portion, however, has a concavity machined into the high-molecular-weight polyethylene both on the medial and lateral compartment. In most modern prostheses this is inserted on a metal tray, which is itself affixed to the proximal tibia after the required amount of bone has been osteotomized from the tibia. The patellar components vary somewhat in size and shape. Over the past several years, the use of metal-backed patellar components has been discontinued as polyethylene wear leading to exposure of the metal backing has caused scoring of the femoral component.

The goal in total knee replacement arthroplasty is to provide the patient with a stable, pain-free knee joint with a functional range of motion. Modern surgical techniques include a number of intraoperative jigs and cutting guides to assist the surgeon in the osteotomies necessary for precise fit of the prosthetic components and the alignment necessary to ensure good long-term results. Varus malalignment following total knee replacement arthroplasty is not well tolerated and the chance for ultimate failure via loosening is definitely increased.

One of the major postoperative problems, well known to therapists, is that of knee stiffness. While this is to some degree unpredictable, many reports have cited the preoperative degree of flexion as being an important predictor in the postoperative outcome. A study by Shoji et al[67] relating to factors affecting postoperative flexion following total knee arthroplasty noted that 90 degrees of flexion was considered a minimum requirement for ADL. They noted that more flexion is necessary in at least one knee so that the sit-to-stand maneuver is possible. In a retrospective study[67] it was discovered that range of motion did not change significantly after 1 year from the time of surgery. These authors further noted that in total knee replacement arthroplasty, the four-bar linkage system described under the section of biomechanics is of necessity disrupted. A tight extensor mechanism such as that resulting from quadriceps adhesions or dense adhesions within the suprapatellar pouch will naturally limit flexion. Results of this particular study showed good preoperative flexion, intense physical therapy, and avoidance of increasing patellar thickness intraoperatively are important factors in maintaining good flexion. Furthermore, postoperative manipulation did not produce excellent results but did prevent the compromised results that might have otherwise occurred if limited flexion had been allowed to persist untreated. In this published series,[74] poor preoperative flexion did, in fact, improve following total knee replacement arthroplasty but not to the point of producing excellent flexion. It was stated that in cases where preoperative flexion is good, pain may be a limiting factor in achieving satisfactory range of motion following surgery. Thereafter the rate of improvement diminished (Fig 18–13), and at 6 months further improvement was noted to be minimal. Of all the parameters that correlated best with the overall knee rating velocity was noted to be the most significant.[72] Three months postoperatively the mean knee score was increased an average of 21 and this was primarily in the category of diminished knee

pain. The correlated with the ± 3% increase in walking velocity secondary to longer stride. At 6 months, the mean knee score had increased only another 8%. After 6 months, walking velocity and knee ratings changed very little. These authors[72] felt that arthritis related abnormalities of the opposite limb may have been the most significant single factor in causing measurable gait abnormalities beyond 6 months from surgery. Simon et al,[69] in discussing quantitative gait analysis after total knee arthroplasty for monarticular degenerative arthritis, stated that of the multiple types of measurement only four parameters show statistically significant differences between the patient undergoing total knee arthroplasty and controls. These were percent of weight acceptance time, knee flexion and stance phase, external moments of the knee joint, and cadence (Table 18–5).

Kroll et al[42] studied the relationship of stride characteristics to pain before and after total knee replacement arthroplasty (Table 18–6). They noted that a marked early reduction in pain postopera-

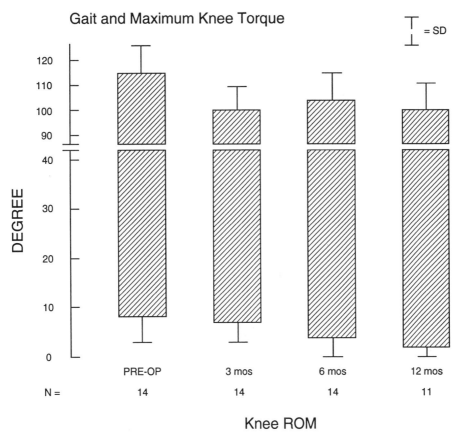

FIG 18–13.
Gait and maximum knee torque following arthroplasty (From Steinen ME, et al: *Clin Orthop* 1989; 238:177. Used by permission.)

TABLE 18-5.

Gait Analysis: Patients*

Case No.	Velocity (m/sec)	Cadence (Steps/min)	Ratio of Step Length to Lower-Limb Length	Ratio of Step Length of Involved to Uninvolved Limb	Step Width (cm)	Ratio of Swing Time to Stance Time		Weight Acceptance (% of Cycle Time)	
						Involved	Uninvolved	Involved	Uninvolved
1	0.92	102	1.16	1.01	16.7	0.42	0.39	20.7	22.4
2	0.97	103	1.21	1.13	13.3	0.46	0.50	17.5	17.5
3	0.89	100	1.17	0.91	14.5	0.44	0.44	18.6	20.3
4	0.91	94	1.23	0.98	12.8	0.57	0.53	14.3	15.8
5	1.50	115	1.62	1.01	15.8	0.55	0.55	15.7	13.7
6	0.99	100	1.32	1.18	11.6	0.51	0.55	15.2	15.2
7	0.92	102	1.19	1.67	12.5	0.57	0.50	15.5	17.2
8	1.15	107	1.21	0.96	9.8	0.46	0.50	18.2	18.2
9	1.15	98	1.31	1.07	9.8	0.54	0.58	16.3	18.3
10	0.93	92	1.34	0.96	5.0	0.40	0.42	20.3	21.9
11	1.06	97	1.29	1.26	10.0	0.53	0.52	16.4	19.7
12	1.17	96	1.42	1.00	12.5	0.75	0.80	9.8	13.1
Mean	1.05	100.6	1.29	1.09	12	0.52	0.54	16.5	17.8
Standard deviation	0.17	5.8	0.13	0.19	3.3	0.09	0.09	2.8	2.9

*From Simon SR et al: *J Bone Joint Surg (Am)* 1983; 65A:608. Used by permission.

tively correlated well to increased velocity and stride length within 5 months of surgery. There was a significant increase in five of eight stride characteristics over the short term, which was felt to be independent of changes in pain. In the period from 5 to 13 months preoperatively, there were also significant increases of four of eight stride characteristics, which were not related to diminished pain. There was felt to be no change in active range of motion from preoperatively to 5 months, but significant increase in the period from 5 to 13 months. Normal gait velocity in the older man was said to average 75 m/min.

Arafiles and Gustilo[3] discussed joint replacement arthroplasty in nonambulatory patients. They noted that involvement of the upper extremities prolonged the time needed for rehabilitation but did not actually appear to affect the ultimate functional results. They further noted that preoperative rehabilitation programs functioned best to determine the level of motivation and did not appear to be a worthwhile means of increasing the strength of the muscles preoperatively. In none of the patients studied was the rehabilitation program preoperatively instrumental in improving the objective muscle rating. In one published study discussing the range of mo-

TABLE 18-6.

Mean and SD of the Stride Characteristics, Range of Motion, and Pain Scores for the 3 Test Days*

Stride Characteristics†	Preoperative		Postoperative			
			5 mo		13 mo	
	M	SD	M	SD	M	SD
VELFR (m/min)	50.4	12	59.0	9	64.1	5.7
CADFR (steps/min)	92.3	10.9	103.4	12.1	109.7	10.7
SLFR (m)	1.04	0.21	1.15	0.14	1.18	0.13
SSTFR (% normal)	77.3	18.3	85.5	11.5	88.2	9.3
VELFS (m/min)	67.2	19.8	80.2	13.4	86.3	12.4
CADFS (steps/min)	115.6	16.4	126.9	18.4	132.5	16.5
SLFS (m)	1.15	0.27	1.27	0.18	1.30	0.20
SSTFS (% normal)	79.3	18.7	85.3	13.6	91.2	10.9
Pain (cm)	7.2	1.8	1.3	1.1	0.9	0.8
ROM (degree)	101	17	98	13	107	9

*From Kroll MA, et al: *Clin Orthop* 1989; 239:192. Used by permission.
†FR = free speed; FS = fast speed; velocity = VELFR, VELFS; cadence = CADFR, CADFS; stride length = SLFR, SLFS; single-limb support time = SSTFR, SSTFS; M = mean; SD = standard deviation.

tion following total knee replacement in ankylosed joints, a vigorous postoperative physical therapy program produced results matching those in knees with excellent preoperative flexion.[52] Following a vigorous range of motion protocol in thirteen joints having range of motion between 16 and 48 degrees, the knees achieved a significant increase in postoperative range of motion actually matching that achieved by a comparable group of patients with greater than 90 degrees of preoperative flexion.

Moreland[50] noted eight primary mechanisms of failure in total knee replacement arthroplasty. First was postoperative instability, either anterior or posterior, valgus or varus and patellofemoral. Knees are usually stable on extension but there is inherently less stability in flexion. Additionally, he noted malalignment of the knee following surgery, and poor range of motion particularly less than 90 degrees flexion as contributing to unsatisfactory results. Additional modes of failure included postoperative sepsis, loosening, loss of extensor power, fractures, and failure of the prosthetic components themselves (Fig 18–14). Instability in the joint, if mild, can be tolerated if the knee joint is well aligned. If there is malalignment created at the time of surgery even minor degrees of tibiofemoral instability are not well tolerated. In full extension there should be virtually no valgus-varus instability of the knee following surgery. It is of course difficult to evaluate valgus/varus instability with the knee in flexion because of the associated hip rotation. Antero-posterior stability at the time of surgery should be achieved in both flexion and extension. AP instability in extension is unusual because the interface between the prosthetic surfaces provides mechanical stability.

Patellar instability may vary from frank patellar dislocation to painful or annoying snapping or recurrent clicking. Patellar instability may result from various factors including excessive valgus reconstruction of the knee, malpositioning of the tibial component, or malrotation of the femoral component. Grace and Rand[19] noted that the etiology of patellar instability following total knee arthroplasty can be separated into three categories: errors in surgical technique, quadriceps imbalance, and postoperative trauma. They felt that the need for surgical revision resulting from patellar instability was uncommon and necessary only in 0.4% of the cases. They noted that incorrect placement of the tibial component in an internally rotated position caused lateral displacement of the tibial tubercle. In one study cited by the above authors[19] investigating causes for patellar instability, tibial component mal-

alignment was found to be the source of patellar instability in 25% of the cases.

Supracondylar fractures of the femur following prosthetic knee arthroplasty occurred in one study with a reported incidence of 0.6% to 2.5%.[14] This disastrous complication was usually associated with either notching of the anterior femoral cortex when performing the anterior osteotomy necessary for fitting the femoral component, or with preexisting neurologic disease. It was felt that unrecognized excessive osteoporosis was also a possible etiology. Following supracondylar fracture, the treatment that was shown to preserve the best quality of function was open reduction-internal fixation combined with early postoperative motion. It is said that notching the anterior femoral cortex by only 3 mm reduces torsional strength by 30%.[14]

Wasilewski and Frankel[80] discussed the utility of arthroscopy in diagnosing painful dysfunctional total knee replacement. They noted increasing concern regarding failure of metal backed patellar components. Arthroscopy was believed to provide a less invasive surgical means for early diagnosis of this problem, permitting early patellar revision, perhaps eliminating the need for revising the femoral component or complete revision if significant scoring of the femoral component had not yet occurred. These authors felt that the indications for arthroscopy after total knee replacement included lateral release for subluxing patella, lysis of dense adhesions, removal of loose bodies of methyl methacrylate, and for diagnosis of suspected fracture or wear of the polyethylene component of the patella or tibial plateau. It was felt that arthroscopic lysis of adhesions in patients with total knee replacement arthroplasty contributed significantly to diminished pain and increased function.

There is no question that prosthetic design and surgical technique play significant roles in the ultimate results following total knee replacement. Nevertheless, there are certain less tangible factors that also seem to play a major role in functional outcome. Following surgery, the first priority is to allow wound healing. While continuous passive motion has not in most studies been shown to inhibit or interfere with wound healing, the author prefers to maintain the knee immobilized in extension with a knee immobilizer for the first 5 postoperative days. After 5 days, the wound is inspected and if it appears to be healing well, gentle active and active assisted range of motion is commenced. Skin staples remain in place for approximately 2 weeks. They may be left in place longer if there is no apparent ir-

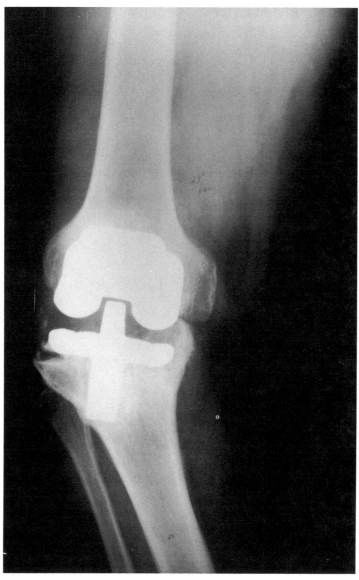

FIG 18–14.
AP radiograph of the knee depicting a loose semicon-strained total knee prosthesis in a markedly obese middle-aged male. The prosthesis appears to have implanted in ex-cessive varus alignment, predisposing to failure.

ritation from the staples. Frequently, however, pa-tients feel a noticeable difference once the staples are removed and feel their ability to flex the knee is en-hanced.

There are multiple means of regaining knee flex-ion postoperatively, such as wall slides, weight-as-sisted gravity flexion in a seated position, skate-board devices, pure passive flexion, and squatting maneuvers. A postoperative total knee rehabilitation program must of course be individualized based on the patient's age, strength, understanding, motiva-tion, and not least important, pain tolerance. It has been the author's experience that patients who claim

to be highly motivated may sometimes be manifest-ing marked anxiety and in the long run are among the most difficult patients to rehabilitate in terms of regaining good flexion. Generally speaking, the happy, relaxed and good-natured patient manifest-ing little in the way of worry or anxiety tends to re-gain flexion easily, and therefore good postoperative function returns almost effortlessly. Levels of pain tolerance certainly vary and those experiencing higher levels of postoperative pain will usually re-quire a much longer time to gain full benefit from their therapy program and frequently will not have the good functional outcome of the patient with the higher pain threshold. While total knee replacement arthroplasty is and will remain an important means of treating end stage knee arthritis, we must continue to strive to preserve function by nonoperative means if possible. The simple use of a cane used on the side opposite that of the painful knee can, in many cases, prolong the interval from the onset of symptoms to the time when surgery may ultimately be necessary.

Prevention is the goal of every conscientious physician. This applies as well to orthopedic care of the knee. The patient should be made to understand the importance of maintaining strong dynamic stabilizers of the knee joint. The consequences of ignoring options to preserve function including therapeutic exercises, limiting certain activities and in some circumstances protected weightbearing may be significant. Some of the treatments described in this chapter are in reality salvage procedures, requiring lengthy rehabilitation. Aggressive attempts to improve function and decrease pain by nonsurgical means first may be wise.

REFERENCES

1. Ahuja SC, Bullough PG: Osteonecrosis of the knee. *J Bone Joint Surg (Am)* 1978; 60A:191–196.
2. Apkarian J, Naumann S, Cairns B: A 3-dimensional kinematic and dynamic model of the lower limb. *J Biomech* 1989; 22:143–155.
3. Arafiles RP, Gustilo RB: Joint replacement in nonambulatory patients. *J Bone Joint Surg (Am)* 1979; 61A:892–897.
4. Banas MP, Kaplan FS, Fallon MD, et al: Regional migratory osteoporosis. *Clin Orthop* 1990; 250:303–309.
5. Banna M, Foster JB: Roentgenologic features of acrodystrophic neuropathy *Clin Orthop* 1972; 115:186–190.
6. Barrett JP Jr, Rasleoff E, Sirna E, et al: Correlation of roentgenographic patterns and clinical manifestations of symptomatic idiopathic osteoarthritis of the knee. *Clin Orthop* 1990; 253:179–183.
7. Beaupré A, Choulsroun R, Guidouin R, et al: Knee menisci: Correlation between microstructure and biomechanics. *Clin Orthop* 1986; 208:72–75.
8. Bergenudd H, Nilsson B, Lindgarde F: Knee pain in middle age and its relationship to occupational work load and psychosocial factors. *Clin Orthop* 1989; 255:210–215.
9. Blin O, Pailhouse J, Tafforgue P, et al: Quantitative analysis of walking in patients with knee osteoarthritis: A method of assessing the effectiveness of nonsteroidal anti-inflammatory treatment. *Ann Rheum Dis* 1990; 49:990–993.
10. Boone DC, Azen SP: Normal range of motion of joints in male subjects. *J Bone Joint Surg (Am)* 1980; 61A:408–413.
11. Botte MJ, Mickel UL, Abeson WH, et al: Spasticity and contracture; Physiologic aspects of formation. *Clin Orthop* 1988; 233:7–18.
12. Brandt KD: Pain, synovitis and articular cartilage changes in osteoarthritis. *Semin Arthritis Rheum* 1989; 18:77–80.
13. Coventry MB: Proximal tibia varus osteotomy for osteoarthritis of the lateral compartment of the knee. *J Bone Joint Surg (Am)* 1987; 69A:32–38.
14. Culp RW, Schmidt RG, Hanks G, et al: Supracondylar fracture of the femur following prosthetic knee arthroplasty *Clin Orthop* 1987; 222:212–222.
15. Delamarter RB, Hohl M, Happ E Jr: Ligament injuries associated with tibial plateau fractures. *Clin Orthop* 1990; 250:226–233.
16. Draganich LF, Jaeger RJ, Kralj AR: Coactivation of the hamstrings and quadriceps during extension of the knee. *J Bone Joint Surg (Am)* 1989; 71A:1075–1081.
17. Dye SF: An evolutionary perspective of the knee. *J Bone Joint Surg (Am)* 1987; 69A:976–983.
18. Frasica FJ, Sim AH, Staeheli JW, et al: Dislocation of the knee, *Clin Ortho* 1991; 213:150–153.
19. Grace JN, Rand JA: Patellar instability after total knee arthroscopy. *Clin Orthop,* Dec 1988, pp 184–189.
20. Gray RG, Gottlieb NL: Intra-articular corticosteroids, *Clin Orthop* 1983; 177:235–263.
21. Grood ES, Noyes FR, Butler DL, et al: Ligamentous and capsular restraints preventing straight medial and lateral laxity in intact human cadaver knees. *J Bone Joint Surg (Am)* 1981; 63A:1257–1269.
22. Grood ES, Suntay WJ, Noyes FR, et al: Biomechanics of the knee-extension exercise. *J Bone Joint Surg (Am)* 1984; 66A:725–734.
23. Hall FM, Wyshak G: Thickness of articular cartilage in the normal knee. *J Bone Joint Surg (Am)* 1980; 62A:408–413.
24. Harper WM, Wray CC, Burden AC, et al: An unusual cause of flexion deformity of the hips and knees. *J Bone Joint Surg (Am)* 1989:71A:1418.
25. Hattin HC, Pierrynowski MR, Ball K: The effect of load, cadence and fatigue on the tibiofemoral joint force during a half squat. *Med Sci Sports Exerc* 1989; 21:613–618.
26. Hsieh HH, Walker PS: Stabilizing mechanisms of the loaded and unloaded knee joint. *J Bone Joint Surg (Am)* 1976; 58A:87–93.
27. Hsu RWW, Himeno S, Coventry MB, et al: Normal axial alignment of the lower extremity and load bearing distribution of the knee. *Clin Orthop* 1990; 255:215–227.
28. Huberti HH, Hayes WC: Patellofemoral contact pressures. *J Bone Joint Surg (Am)* 1984; 66A:715–724.
29. Indelicato PA: Non-operative treatment of complete tears of the medial collateral ligament of the knee. *J Bone Joint Surg (Am)* 1984; 66A:741–744.
30. Iversson I, Larsson LE: Gait analysis in patients with gonarthrosis treated by high tibial osteotomy. *Clin Orthop* 1989; 239:185–190.
31. Ivey M, Clark R: Arthroscopic debridement of the knee for septic arthritis. *Clin Orthop* 1985; 199:201–206.
32. Jeng SF, Scheulsman M, O'Riley P, et al: Reliability of a clinical kinematic assessment of the sit-to-stand movement. *Phys Ther* 1990; 70:511–520.

33. Johansson H, Sjolander P, Sojka P: A sensory role for the cruciate ligaments. *Clin Orthop* 1991; 268:161–178.

34. Jokl P, Kaplan N, Stowell P,et al: Non-operative treatment of severe injuries to the medial and anterior cruciate ligaments of the knee. *J Bone Joint Surg (Am)* 1984; 66A:741–744.

35. Jonsson H, Karrholm J, Elmqvist LG: Kinematics of active knee extension after tear of the anterior cruciate ligament. *Am J Sports Med* 1989; 17:796–802.

36. Kapoor A, Sibitt WL Jr: Contractures in diabetes mellitus: The syndrome of limited joint mobility. *Semin Arthritis Rheum* 1989; 18:168–180.

37. Keenan MA E, We K, Smith CW, et al: Hamstring release for knee flexion contracture in spastic adults. *Clin Orthop* 1988; 236:221–226.

38. Keene JS, Mouson DK, Roberts M, et al: Evaluation of patients for high tibial osteotomy. *Clin Orthop* 1989; 268:157–160.

39. Kennedy JC, Hawkins RJ, Willis RB, et al: Tension studies of human knee ligaments. *J Bone Joint Surg (Am)* 1976; 58A:350–355.

40. Kettlekamp DB, Hillberry BM, Murrish DE, et al: Degenerative arthritis of the knee secondary to fracture malunion. *Clin Orthop* 1988; 234:159–169.

41. Krane SM: Crystal induced joint diseases. *Sci Am Med* 1984; 2:1–15.

42. Kroll MA, Otis JC, Seuko JP, et al: The relationship of stride characteristics to pain before and after total knee arthroplasty. *Clin Orthop* 1989; 239:191–195.

43. Lane JG, Falahee MH, Waztys E, et al: Pyarthrosis of the knee: Treatment considerations. *Clin Orthop* 1990; 252:198–204.

44. Lansinger O, Bergman B, Korner F, et al: Tibial condylar fractures, *J Bone Joint Surg (Am)* 1986; 68A:13–19.

45. Larsen E, Lund PM: Ruptures of the extensor mechanism of the knee joint. *Clin Orthop* 1986; 213:150–153.

46. Lindberg H, Montgomery F: Heavy labor and the occurrance of gonarthrosis. *Clin Orthop* 1987; 214:235–236.

47. Maquet P, VanDeBerg A, Simonet J: Femorotibial weightbearing areas. *J Bone Joint Surg (Am)* 1975; 57A:766–771.

48. Markolf KL, Graff-Radford A, Amstutz HC: In vivo knee stability. *J Bone Joint Surg (Am)* 1978; 60A:664–674.

49. Masuda I, Ishikawa K: Clinical features of pseudogout attack. *Clin Orthop* 1988; 229:173–181.

50. Moreland JR: Mechanisms of failure in total knee arthroplasty. *Clin Orthop* 1983; 226:49–64.

51. Motohashi M, Morii T, Koshino T: Clinical course and roentgenographic changes of osteonecrosis in the femoral condyle under conservative treatment. *Clin Orthop* 1991; 266:156–161.

52. Mullen JO: Range of motion following total knee arthroplasty in ankylosed joints. *Clin Orthop* 1983; 179:200–203.

53. Murray MP, Gore DR, Sepic SB, et al: Antalgic maneuvers during walking in men with unilateral knee disability. *Clin Orthop* 1985; 199:192–200.

54. O'Connor JJ, Shercliff TL, Bider E, et al: The geometry of the knee in the sagittal plane. *Proc Inst Mech Eng* 1989; 203:223–233.

55. Odenbring S, Lindstrand D, Egund N, et al: Prognosis for patients with medial gonarthrosis, *Clin Orthop* 1991; 266:152–155.

56. Pennock GR, Clark KJ: An anatomy based coordinate system for the description of the kinematic displacements of the human knee. *J Biomech* 1990; 23:1209–1218.

57. Pope MH, Johnson RJ, Brown DW, et al: The role of the musculature in injuries to the medial collateral ligament. *J Bone Joint Surg (Am)* 1979; 61A:398–402.

58. Radin EL, DeLaMotte F, Maquet P: Role of the menisci in the distribution of stress in the knee, *Clin Orthop* 1984; 185:290–294.

59. Rozing PM, Insall J, Bohne WH: Spontaneous osteonecrosis of the knee. *J Bone Joint Surg (Am)* 1980; 62A:2–7.

60. Rudan JF, Simurda MA: Valgus high tibial osteotomy. *Clin Orthop* 1991; 268:157–160.

61. Schipplein OD, et al: Relationship between moments at the L5/S1 lever, hip and knee joint when lifting. *Biomechanics* 1990; 23:907–912.

62. Semble EL, Loeser RF, Wise CM: Therapeutic exercise for rheumatoid arthritis and osteoarthritis. *Semin Arthritis Rheum* 1990; 20:32–40.

63. Shepard RJ: The scientific basis of exercise prescribing for the very old. *J Am Geriatr Soc* 1990; 38:60–70.

64. Sherlock DA, Hughes A: Bilateral spontaneous concurrent rupture of the patellar tendon in the absence of associated local or systemic disease. *Clin Orthop* 1988; 237:179–183.

65. Shim SS, Leung G: Blood supply of the knee joint. *Clin Orthop* 1986; 208:119–125.

66. Shoemaker S, Markolf K: The role of the meniscus in the anterior-posterior stability of the loaded anterior cruciate deficient knee. *J Bone Joint Surg (Am)* 1986; 68A:71–79.

67. Shoji H, Solomonow M,Yoshino S, et al: Factors affecting postoperative flexion in total knee arthroplasty. *Orthopaedics* 1990; 13:643–649.

68. Siegler EL, Beck LH: Stiffness: A pathophysiologic approach to diagnosis and treatment. *J Gen Intern Med* 1989; 4:533–540.

69. Simon SR, Frieslunana HW, Burdett RG, et al: Quantitative gait analysis after total knee arthroplasty for monarticular degenerative arthritis. *J Bone Joint Surg (Am)* 1983; 65A:605–613.

70. Sisto D, Warren R: Complete knee dislocation: A follow-up study of operative treatment. *Clin Orthop* 1985; 198:94–101.

71. Sohn RS, Micheli LJ: The effect of running on the pathogenesis of osteoarthritis of the hips and knees. *Clin Orthop* 1985; 198:106–109.

72. Steiner ME, Simon SR, Pisciotta JC: Early changes in gait and maximum knee torque following knee arthroplasty. *Clin Orthop* 1989; 238:174–182.

73. Swartz MN, Calin A: Infectious arthritis. *Sci Am Med* 1979; 8:1–9.

74. Tanser M, Miller J: The natural history of flexion contracture in total knee arthroplasty. *Clin Orthop* 1989; 248:129–134.

75. Templeman DC, Marder RA: Injuries of the knee associated with fractures of the tibial shaft. *J Bone Joint Surg (Am)* 1989; 71A:1392–1395.

76. Terry GC, Flandry F, Vorwood TA, et al: Isolated chondral fracture of the knee. *Clin Orthop* 1990; 234:226–233.

77. Tietjen R: Reflex sympathetic dystrophy of the knee, *Clin Orthop* 1986; 209:234–243.

78. Torg JS, Barton TM, Pavlov H, et al: Natural history of the posterior cruciate ligament-deficient knee. *Clin Orthop* 1989; 246:208–216.

79. Tria AJ Jr, Johnson CD, Zawadsky JP: The popliteus tendon. *J Bone Joint Surg (Am)* 1989; 71A:714–716.

80. Wasilewski SA, Frankel A: Arthroscopy of the painful dysfunctional total knee replacement. *J Arthrosc Rel Surg* 1989; 5:294–297.

81. Waters RL, Perry J, Conaty P, et al: The energy cost of walking with arthritis of the hip and knee. *Clin Orthop* 1987; 214:278–284.

82. Watkins MP, Haris BA, Wender S, et al: Effect of patellectomy on the function of the quadriceps and hamstrings. *J Bone Joint Surg (Am)* 1978; 60A:664–674.

83. Werner F, Foster D, Murray DG: The influence of design on the transmission of torque across knee prostheses. *J Bone Joint Surg (Am)* 1978; 60A:342–248.

84. Winter DA, Fatla AE, Frank JS, et al: Biomechanical walking pattern changes in the fit and healthy elderly. *Phys Ther* 1990; 70:340–347.

Chapter 19

Knee Injuries: A Rehabilitation Perspective

Karen A. Knortz, Ph.D., P.T.

ANATOMY AND PHYSIOLOGY

Osteology

Components

The knee is the largest synovial joint in the body and is subclassified as a simple hinge joint.[69] Yet to those practitioners who specialize in assessment and treatment of knee disorders, the knee joint is complex in design and is magnificently suited to the stresses put upon it. Nonetheless, it has been estimated that knee injuries account for 23% to 25% of athletic injuries[49] and degenerative arthritis occurs the knee with a frequency surpassed only by the spine and hip.[35]

The femur, which is the largest bone in the body, runs inferiorly and medially, and forms a 6-degree angle with the vertical plane,[34] which accounts for a certain degree of physiologic valgus. This valgus angle may be exaggerated by a wide pelvis, resulting in a naturally greater valgus angle for females than males. At its distal end, the femur forms two rounded ends, or condyles, which articulate with the tibia. Anteriorly, the condyles form the trochlear groove, which articulates with the patella.

The proximal end of the tibia comprises two condylar plateaus, which are concave in shape. They are divided by the intercondylar eminence, which provides additional bony stability to the femorotibial joint.

The patella has five articulating surfaces: the medial, lateral, superior, inferior, and odd facets.[5] The trabecular orientation of the retropatellar surface varies for each of the facets, with the trabeculae organized perpendicularly for the lateral facet, while the organization is more oblique medially; centrally, the trabecular organization is horizontally arranged, making it susceptible to damaging forces.[66]

Biomechanics

The femorotibial articulation, with the convex condyles approximating the concave tibial plateau, is responsible in part for the geometric stability of the knee joint. Likewise, the patellofemoral articulation augments stability of the patella as it tracks through the trochlear groove, permitting the patella to function as a fulcrum for the extensor mechanism.

The femorotibial articulation follows the convex-concave rule,[33] which describes translatoric gliding. The rule states that if the moving surface is concave, such as is the case in the knee joint, then the translatoric gliding that takes place in the joint will occur in the same direction of the moving joint surface. Thus, the tibia moves posteriorly as the knee joint moves from a position of extension to flexion. Conversely, the tibia moves anteriorly as the joint goes from a position of flexion to extension.

Helfet[27] described the rotatory motion of the femorotibial joint as the screw home motion, meaning that the tibia rotates externally as the knee joint goes from flexion into extension. Conversely, the tibia rotates internally as the knee joint goes from an extended to a flexed position.

In full extension, the patella sits slightly lateral.

As the knee goes into flexion, the patella becomes centered in the trochlear groove and until approximately 90 degrees, the patella is centered in the groove. Thereafter, the patella tracks laterally again, so that in full flexion the patella sits lateral to the groove and the medial femoral condyle is almost exposed.[59]

Ligaments and Tendons

Components

The cruciate and collateral ligaments are the primary static stabilizers of the knee joint. Both the anterior and posterior cruciate ligaments are intra-articular, while the medial and lateral collateral ligaments are extra-articular. While the cruciate ligaments stabilize the femorotibial joint in an anterior and posterior direction, the collateral ligaments stabilize the joint in a medial and lateral direction. The most important tendons crossing the knee joint are the patellar tendon anteriorly, and the hamstring tendons posteriorly.

The anterior cruciate ligament runs superiorly and laterally and is attached proximally to the intercondylar notch of the femur. The distal attachment is on the anterior intercondylar fossa of the tibia. When the knee is in full extension, the anterior cruciate ligament prevents excessive internal tibial rotation, but its major function is control of anterior tibial translation.

The posterior cruciate ligament arises posterior to the femoral attachment of the anterior cruciate ligament in the intercondylar notch and runs anteriorly, medially, and obliquely. The distal attachment is on the posterior aspect of the posterior intercondylar fossa of the tibia. Because of its orientation, this ligament also prevents excessive medial rotation of the tibia, but its primary function is to control posterior translation of the tibia.

The medial collateral ligament, larger of the two collateral ligaments, runs obliquely and anteriorly, from the medial aspect of the medial femoral condyle to the medial aspect of the tibia. The posterior fibers of the medial collateral ligament blend with the medial capsule and the medial border of the medial meniscus. That is why injuries to the medial collateral ligament often involve medial meniscal pathology. The primary role of the medial collateral ligament is to control valgus stress at the femorotibial joint, though it also acts as a constraint for excessive lateral rotation of the tibia.

The lateral collateral ligament is attached proximally at the posterior aspect of the lateral femoral condyle and has its distal attachment at the head of the fibula. The fibers run inferiorly and posteriorly; thus, its alignment crosses the orientation of the medial collateral ligament. Control of varus forces is the primary function of the lateral collateral ligament; however, it also serves as a passive restraint in excessive medial rotation of the tibia.

The patellar tendon is broader superiorly than inferiorly and attaches proximally to the inferior pole of the patella. The distal attachment is on the tuberosity of the tibia. Thus it comprises the distal end of the extensor mechanism, anchoring the quadriceps muscles distally and contributing to the action of the quadriceps muscles in extension of the knee, with anterior translation of the tibia.

Three hamstrings tendons, arising from the semimembranosus, semitendinosus, and biceps femoris, attach distally to the tibia. These tendons provide dynamic assistance to the anterior cruciate ligament in preventing anterior translation of the tibia, while also serving as prime movers for knee flexion and tibial rotation.

Histology

Ligaments and tendons are composed of regularly arranged, dense, ordinary connective tissue.[22] The regular arrangement of ligaments and tendons is accounted for by alignment of collagen fibers in more or less the same plane or direction. The cells of regularly arranged, dense, ordinary connective tissue are nearly all fibrocytes, and can be found between parallel bundles of collagen fibers.[26]

It is within the fibrocyte that procollagen and subsequently collagen are formed. Collagen accounts for approximately 70% of the dry weight of ligaments and tendons.[1] Proteoglycan found in various connective tissue is relatively uniform chemically.[23] The proteoglycan aggregate is a hydrophilic subunit of a core protein with protein linked glycosaminoglycan (GAG) chains. The main component GAG of ligaments and tendons is dermatin sulfate[32]; however, hyaluronic acid, chondroitin-4-sulfate and chondroitin-6-sulfate are also found.[1] It is interesting to note, however, that water accounts for 60% to 80 percent of the total wet weight of ligaments and tendons.[22]

Four histologically distinct layers comprise the ligament-bone complex.[12] In the ligament proper, parallel collagen fibers are interspersed with fibroblasts. In the next layer approaching the ligament-bone attachment is a zone of fibrocartilage with chondroblast-like cells embedded in the extracellular matrix. Yet closer to the bone is a zone of mineralized cartilage hydroxyapatite crystals within the matrix. Lastly, collagen fibers of a mineralized fibrocartilage layer blend with the collagen network of bone.

Nutrition and Innervation

The insertion sites are nearly avascular in most ligaments; however, sparse vascularity has been observed in extra-articular ligaments.[1] Ligaments derive most of their vascular supply from periarticular plexuses. Nutrients and metabolic waste products diffuse from ligament tissue in proximity to the vessels to avascular segments of ligament.[1]

Nerves supplying muscles send branches to nearby ligaments. Pain is mediated through numerous free nonmyelinated and finely myelinated nerve fibers. Ligaments also contain specialized encapsulated nerve endings, including pacinian, Ruffini's, and Golgi-Mazzoni corpuscles, which mediate position sense and speed of movement.[1] Specialized tension-sensitive Golgi tendon organs located in muscle tendons mediate a protective reflex arc, which prevents damage associated with overstretching.

Function

Ligaments connect bone to bone, while tendons connect muscle to bone. Ligaments are noncontractile, providing static stability to joints, while contractile tendons provide dynamic support. Multiple ligaments and tendons surrounding a single joint act collectively to guide bony displacement during normal motion, while limiting the extremes of displacement. The orientation of collagen fibers permits some passive elongation of these tissues accompanied by a decrease in collagen fiber diameter, much like a net being stretched.[22]

Growth

Collagen is a stable protein in a dynamic state of turnover, which is the sum of synthesis and degradation. After fibroblasts synthesize proteoglycan and collagen they deteriorate, releasing lysosomal enzymes. Partial extracellular matrix breakdown is followed by endocytosis of fragments by fibroblasts. Inside the fibroblasts these fragments of extracellular matrix are recycled into new matrix.[22]

Repair

When the structural integrity of ligaments is damaged by injury, wound healing proceeds via the inflammatory response and structural repair. The inflammatory process predominates for 1 to 7 days after injury[1] and can occur in extra-articular ligaments

and tendons because of their vascularity, sparse as it may be. Thereafter, fibroblasts proliferate between 2 and 3 weeks after injury, forming loose and disorganized scar tissue approximating the ends of the tear.[1, 8] Once this has occurred, the maturation phase ensues and matrix alignment begins, reaching a histologic end point after around 18 months.[1] While healing does occur in vascularized extra-articular ligaments, little healing, if any, occurs in intra-articular ligaments because of their avascularity.[1] Moreover, functional alignment of collagen during scar formation is enhanced by some degree of stress that mimics that which occurs with normal joint motion.[1, 20, 65]

Articular Cartilage

Histology

Articular cartilage, also known as hyaline cartilage, is a specialized, semirigid connective tissue lining the articular surfaces of the bony components of the knee. Its thickness may be as great as 5 mm.[3, 14] Articular cartilage contains a moderate amount of collagen,[32] arranged in a tangential fashion.[26] A relatively small number of chondrocytes are embedded in a proteoglycan matrix.

Chondrocytes synthesize the proteoglycan matrix and collagen fibrils. Collagen is arranged in tangentially oriented fibrils[32] and is homogeneous, consisting of type II collagen.[41] Type II collagen accounts for 40 percent of the dry weight of articular cartilage.[32]

Proteoglycan aggregates, which provide the rigidity associated with articular cartilage, are composed of a hyaluronic acid core with attached chains of GAGs radiating outward. The hydrophylic nature of the proteoglycan aggregate accounts for the fact that 70% to 80% of the wet weight of articular cartilage is water.[26, 41]

Though articular cartilage may appear smooth to the eye, microscopically, depressions and undulations may be seen. These surface irregularities may play a role in lubrication by trapping synovial fluid close to the cartilage surface.[3]

Nutrition

Articular cartilage is avascular, aneural, and alymphatic.[3, 26, 32, 41] The relatively great amount of water bound to proteoglycan aggregates serves as a medium permitting gases, nutrients, and waste products to diffuse between the capillaries outside the cartilage and the chondrocytes residing in the lacunae within the cartilage matrix.[26] The nutrients are carried via the synovial fluid from the highly vascularized synovial lining to the surface of articular cartilage.[26]

Joint movement flushes synovial fluid through the joint and thereby facilitates passage of nutrients into cartilage and catabolites from cartilage to fluid.[30, 41] This is a very long pathway for nutrients and waste products and may account, in part, for the limited healing capacity of articular cartilage. There is also evidence that nutrition can occur from diffusion through the underlying vascular bone.[41] This has been shown to occur only in the young, however, because in the adult, heavy deposition of apatite in the calcified zone acts as a barrier to the cartilage-bone interface.[3] Weight bearing also plays a role in cartilage nutrition through an alternating flux of fluid in and out of cartilage in response to the pressure gradient caused by loading and unloading of the joint.[11]

Function

Hyaline cartilage is essential for the longitudinal growth of bones at epiphyses.[32] It provides a protective covering for articular bones and facilitates joint motion by virtue of its smooth, lubricating properties.

Repair

Since articular cartilage lacks the blood supply necessary for the inflammatory process, very little healing of superficial lesions takes place, and that which does is "intrinsic" in nature.[3, 22] In animals it has been demonstrated that chondrocytes have a limited ability to revert to chondroblasts in response to surgically induced partial-thickness lesions.[56] Immediately following trauma chondrocytes adjacent to the wound margin die, but 24 hours later adjacent cells show increased mitotic activity.[7] This activity ceases after 2 weeks and the defect remains stable with time.[64]

If a chondral lesion penetrates full thickness into the underlying bone, then the blood supply of the subchondral bone is exposed and wound healing, via inflammation, proliferation, and maturation, can occur.[3] Scar tissue formed by scar tissue proliferation is initially vascular and loose, but becomes less vascular and dense with time.[3, 56] Surviving chondrocytes revert to chondroblasts and undergo mitosis, but this response is minimal.[7] The repair tissue is mixed histologically and contains fibrous, chondroid, and intermediate cells.[3, 50] Some investigators believe that this tissue is not well suited to joint function and eventually undergoes degeneration.[56]

Fibrocartilage

Histology

Fibrocartilage, with features intermediate between dense connective tissue and articular cartilage, is found in the menisci of the knee joint. Like ligament and articular cartilage, menisci consist of a tissue fluid held in a proteoglycan and collagen matrix. The extracellular matrix has a dense network of collagenous fibers, similar histologically to the collagen of ligaments and tendons, and these fibers are oriented in a circumferential manner, with some radially directed fibers.[3] Cells of the menisci have characteristics of both fibroblasts and chondrocytes since they produce proteoglycan that is similar to that of cartilage and collagen similar to that of ligaments.[32]

The proteoglycan aggregate of the meniscus consists of the same GAGs found in articular cartilage, but dermatin sulfate accounts for 20% of the GAGs in the former while it is not present at all in the latter.[3] In fact, proteoglycan content is far less for menisci, approximately one eighth of that found in articular cartilage.[3]

Nutrition

The menisci are vascularized during growth, but by middle to late adolescence become avascular.[3] Branches of arteries supplying the joint form premeniscal capillaries which provide the blood supply of the periphery of the menisci. The remainder of the menisci derives its nutrition from the synovial fluid in much the same manner as articular cartilage.[3]

Function

The function of the meniscus is twofold. First, it serves a protective function by absorbing and distributing shock to decrease bone and joint stress during weight bearing.[3] The second function is to assure joint congruity and guide the motion that occurs between articulating bones.[34]

Growth and Repair

Vascularity appears to be the determining factor in meniscus growth and repair.[2, 28] If the lesion communicates with the capillary bed, normal wound healing will occur and a fibrous scar may fill in the defect.[3] Total meniscectomy in animals has resulted in formation of a fibrous pseudocartilage devoid of cartilage cells within 12 weeks.[13] In human knees, fibrocartilaginous pseudocartilage has been observed after total meniscectomy with subsequent arthrotomy.[68]

Muscles

Components

While the clinician often focuses rehabilitation efforts on the quadriceps and hamstrings muscle groups, four other muscle groups cross the knee joint and contribute to normal joint function. These include the sartorius, gracilis, popliteus, and gastrocnemius muscles. Indeed, these muscle groups should not be overlooked in the rehabilitation process.

The quadriceps is the largest muscle group, contributing to knee function and dynamic stability. This group comprises the rectus femoris, vastus intermedius, vastus lateralis, and vastus medialis.

The hamstring muscle group serves an equally important role as the quadriceps in terms of function, but is smaller in terms of bulk. Components of the hamstring muscle group include the biceps femoris, semitendinosus, and semimembranosus.

Functional Anatomy and Biomechanics

Of the four quadriceps muscles, only one, the rectus femoris, crosses two joints. The proximal attachment of the rectus femoris is on the anterior superior iliac crest of the pelvis, with a distal attachment on the superior pole of the patella. It is a bipenniform structure, with most of the muscle fibers oriented in an inferior and central direction. Its function is twofold, as it contributes in both knee extension and hip flexion. As such, when a lack of flexibility is noted in this muscle, a deficit in knee flexion is noted when the hip is in the fully extended position.

The vastus muscles attach proximally just inferior to and anterior to the trochanter of the femur. The vastus intermedius lies under the rectus femoris and is not easily palpable, with most of the fibers arranged in a vertical direction, while the vastus lateralis and medialis muscle fibers are oriented in a diagonal direction. The fibers of the vastus lateralis are oriented in an inferior and lateral-to-medial direction, while the fibers of the vastus medialis are oriented medial to lateral with an inferior slant. The vastus lateralis interdigitates with the superficial fibers of the lateral retinaculum and serves the function of lateralizing the patella in the trochlear groove while assisting in knee extension. Though the vastus medialis also contributes to knee extension, it counterbalances the lateral pull of the vastus lateralis by dynamically pulling the patella medially during knee extension.

The role of the vastus medialis obliquus (VMO) with regard to patellofemoral dynamics is to centralize the patella in the trochlear groove during knee extension. This muscle is active throughout the entire range of motion from flexion to extension[38] and is not selectively active during terminal extension. Because of this, the VMO is an important muscle group deserving much attention in the case of lateral maltracking problems.

The hamstring muscle group is attached proximally at the ischial tuberosity, with the distal attachment differing for each of the three components. The biceps femoris has two heads, the short and the long head. The long head attaches proximally to the ischium; however, the short head attaches to the linea aspera on the posterior surface of the femur. Together they join at the lateral condyle of the femur and attach distally to the fibular head. Because of the orientation of this muscle, it serves as both a knee flexor and external rotator. The semimembranosus and semitendinosus comprise the medial hamstrings, with the former lying deeper and attaching more proximally and medially on the distal femur. Although both muscles act primarily as knee flexors and internal rotators, they also serve as hip extensors because of their proximal attachment to the ischial tuberosity.

The gastrocnemius muscle, while a prime mover for ankle plantar flexion, also serves an important role in stabilizing the knee during both weight-bearing and non–weight-bearing activities because of its proximal attachment on the distal femur. During non–weight-bearing activities the gastrocnemius functions as a knee flexor, but during weight-bearing activities it is most effective in terms of contributing to knee extension when ankle plantar flexion is fixed.

The gracilis is usually classified as a hip adductor, but because it has attachments to both the pubic ramus and medial aspect of the proximal tibia, it also contributes to knee flexion. When the limb is in a non–weight-bearing position, it serves as in internal rotator of the tibia as well.[69]

The popliteus is a small but important muscle. The proximal attachment is on the lateral condyle of the femur and the distal attachment on the posteromedial aspect of the tibia. Concentric contraction of this muscle results in knee flexion and internal tibial rotation. When contracting eccentrically, the popliteus helps to control deceleration of knee extension.

The sartorius muscle, the longest muscle in the body, has its proximal attachment on the anterior superior iliac spine, with its distal attachment on the anteromedial aspect of the proximal tibia. It is a long, ribbonlike muscle that curves posterior to the medial condyle of the femur before making attachment on the tibia. Because of this orientation, the sartorius serves as a hip flexor as well as knee flexor and internal rotator.

EVALUATION OF THE KNEE JOINT

Patient History

Once an orthopedic and medical diagnosis has been identified, the rehabilitation professional must perform a thorough evaluation of the patient in order to determine individual needs and goals of rehabilitation. Gathering a history enables the clinician to appreciate the nature and progression of the pathology. Many geriatric patients with knee pathologies report that the onset of symptoms was a long time ago—sometimes 30 or 40 years ago! This is because so many of the knee dysfunctions observed in geriatric patients are progressively destructive in nature.

The natural history involves deterioration of all of the aforementioned anatomic structures, not only as the result of microtrauma and macrotrauma, but also as a result of normally occurring changes in these tissues as a result of aging. This combination often brings about a series of pathologic events that disable the patient functionally and precede the patient's decision to seek medical and orthopedic evaluation. Therefore a complete medical and orthopedic history provide the rehabilitation specialist with valuable information regarding length and progression of pathology.

Lower Extremity Mechanics

Function of the knee joint is dependent on both static, or noncontractile, structures and dynamic structures such as muscles. Static evaluation includes assessment of lower extremity biomechanics, while dynamic assessment addresses abnormalities during movement. It is of little value to the rehabilitation specialist to establish a care plan based on what is observed when the patient is immobile. Once changes in movement patterns are integrated with characteristics of static alignment, the clinician has the information to make a good clinical judgment about which of these factors can be altered. In this way, assessment of lower extremity mechanics contributes to the establishment of an individualized care plan.

Static Assessment

Much information can be gained from observation of the patient's lower extremity alignment, assessed in both a weight-bearing and non–weight-bearing position. In the standing position, the patient is assessed from the front, the rear, and the side. The patient is instructed to assume a natural weight-bearing posture while the clinician observes limb alignment.

When observing lower extremity alignment anteriorly, the clinician should assess symmetry of posture starting at the pelvis and ending at the foot. Visual observation of a discrepancy in height of the anterior iliac crests should be noted. The position of the femurs may be assessed by palpation of the medial and lateral femoral condyles. If, in the frontal plane, the medial condyle is posterior to the lateral condyle, then the femur is anteverted. Bulk of the quadriceps muscles is observed, comparing the involved to the uninvolved side. Patellar position can be assessed by visual inspection of orientation. The patella is in one of three positions: parallel to the frontal plane, in a "squinting" (turned-in) posture, or in a "grasshopper eye" (turned-out) posture. Tibial alignment is determined by the relative position of the proximal and distal segments. The position of a line oriented perpendicular to the proximal tibial crest is compared with that of a line drawn perpendicular to the plane formed by the medial and lateral malleoli. When the angle formed is greater than 15 degrees, external tibial torsion is a component in the patient's knee pathology.[31]

Attention is then directed at the subtalar joint. The clinician palpates the talus both medially and laterally with the fingers to assess position; if more of the talus can be palpated medially than laterally, then the subtalar joint is pronated.[45] Similarly, the subtalar joint is in a supinated position if more of the talus is palpated laterally than medially. The feet should be assessed in the standing position for callus formation. When a callus located at the first metatarsophalangeal joint is evident, then the clinician should suspect abnormal medial weight bearing. If callus formation is palpated laterally, then abnormal lateral weight bearing should be suspected.

In observing the patient from an anterior view, it is also useful to note the patient's posture when asked to place the feet together. Patients with excessive genu valgum have great difficulty in achieving this position, while those with genu varum do so easily.

The patient is also observed systematically from the rear, again starting at the pelvis and ending at the foot. Symmetry of the posterior inferior iliac crests is evaluated. Relative height of the popliteal crease is likewise assessed for symmetry. Lastly rearfoot position is evaluated by measuring the intersection of a line drawn from the midline of the gastrocnemius to the axis of the subtalar joint with a line drawn from the midline of the calcaneus to the axis of the subtalar joint. When the line of the calcaneus lies lateral to the line of the gastrocnemius, then the rearfoot is in pronated position; conversely, if the line of the calcaneus is medial to the line of the gastrocnemius, the rearfoot is supinated.

When observing the patient from the lateral side, anterior or posterior pelvic tilt may be observed. In addition, the clinician should assess the degree of genu recurvatum in this position. The iliotibial band, when tight, will form a septum that clearly separates it from the vastus medialis muscle when observed from this position, especially when the patient is asked to place the feet together.[44]

Dynamic and Functional Assessment

Dynamic assessment involves observation of movement, particularly functional movement, such as gait and negotiation of a stair step. In terms of gait assessment, the clinician should note any asymmetry in stride length or time spent weight bearing on the extremity during stance phase, with or without an assistive device. The distance the patient is able to negotiate prior to fatigue must be noted. Videotape analysis can be most helpful in gait analysis, both for the clinician and the patient. Aberrations in gait patterns become more apparent when viewed in slow motion and the patient can become aware of such abnormalities with the help of a rehabilitation professional who can analyze gait patterns. Again, evaluation should be systematic, starting at the trunk and pelvis and ending at the foot. Common observations in the patient with a long history of dysfunction include a Trendelenburg shift to compensate for weak hip abductors, excessive internal or external rotation of the femur on heel strike, an abnormal dynamic Q angle during stance phase, and abnormal foot pronation or supination. Often gait analysis with recognition of the abnormality by the patient is the first step toward improvement in function via an appropriate care plan.

Patients should be observed in performance of several functional activities in addition to gait.[44] For example, the patient should be observed for symmetry and muscle control while performing a step-down from a block that is 2 to 6 inches high. The quality of movement is assessed with attention to

pelvic and quadriceps control. Noting that this is an advanced functional activity for some geriatric patients, the rehabilitation professional should base such evaluations of dynamic control on the abilities of the patient.

Range of Motion

Normal active and passive range of motion of the knee is 0 degrees of extension (full extension) to about 135 degrees of flexion, depending on the muscle bulk of the hamstrings and gastrocnemius muscles.[31] The end feel of extension should be hard or bony, while the end feel of flexion is soft owing to the fact that range of motion in flexion is limited by soft tissue approximation.[15] Depending on the end feel, as described by Cyriax,[15] the clinician can identify factors restricting range of motion. The position in which range of motion is measured can affect passive and active measurements. Much information can be gained from measuring range of motion in differing limb positions.

For example, when passive range of motion is measured in the long sitting position, tight hamstrings or posterior capsule contracture may be limiting factors. If range of motion in extension is equally restricted in both the long sitting and supine positions, then the posterior capsule is a contributing factor in restriction of range of motion in extension. If, on the other hand, range of motion in extension is greater in the supine than the long sitting position, then hamstrings tightness is a contributing factor in restriction of range of motion in extension.

Similarly, range of motion in flexion should be evaluated in several different positions. If the same amount of passive flexion is observed when the patient is in the supine as in the prone position, then muscle inflexibility can be eliminated as a source of restriction. When flexion is less in the prone than supine position, then the rectus femoris is a contributing factor in range of motion restriction, since it is the only quadriceps muscle that crosses both the hip and the knee. In the former case, the possible contributing factors include lack of component mobility, infrapatellar adhesion formation, mechanical blockage, or adhesions in the collateral ligaments.

Strength and Endurance

It has been shown that strength of knee musculature in 70- to 86-year-old men is 55% to 65% of that observed in 20- to 35-year-old men.[48] The decline in muscle strength and endurance has been attributed to selective atrophy of fast-twitch muscle fibers,[37, 50] which have low endurance properties with relatively high tension production. Slow-twitch muscles, with high endurance and low tension development, appear to be less affected by age. Therefore, the geriatric rehabilitation professional should suspect deficits in muscle strength, but should not rule out endurance deficits resulting from a decrease in activity level secondary to injury or surgery.

Activities of Daily Living

Activities of daily living (ADL) should be a priority in assessment of the geriatric patient, in both cases of chronic dysfunction and following orthopedic surgery. Performance of ADL should be evaluated by a team of rehabilitation professionals, including the physician, physical therapist, occupational therapist, and rehabilitation nurse. Improvement in the ability to perform ADL fosters independence and adds greatly to the quality of the patient's life.

Assessment should include an overview of the patient's daily activities from waking in the morning to going to bed at night. Structural characteristics of the home environment must be considered. Difficulties with transfers, mobility or ambulation, and feeding deserve a great deal of attention. In some cases, assistive devices can be extremely helpful in improving the patient's level of independence in ADL.

In the case of the postoperative knee patient, preparation for the demands of daily activities prior to discharge can make the difference between success and failure. It must be remembered that, to the patient, success is improvement in independent performance of functional ADL tasks. Assessment of the patient's home situation and need for assistive devices can be key factors in the patient's postoperative recovery.

A simple but good example of the importance of this sort of early postoperative assessment of ADL involves the frustration felt by by both the patient and the home health care professional. Too often, the patient is discharged from the acute care facility, where all daily needs are provided by a staff of rehabilitation professionals, to a home environment where an elderly and sometimes uneducated spouse assumes responsibility for the care and recovery of the patient. Day-to-day problems arise in such situations and rehabilitation professionals have a responsibility for evaluating and dealing with such dilemmas.

For example, too often the patient is sent home with an assistive ambulation device, such as an adjustable walker, that has been set on its lowest possible height setting. Since the changes associated with aging include a decrease in height, it would make more sense that the patient be provided with a walker that can be set so that *decreasing* height can be accommodated. While simple, this example reemphasizes the need for the rehabilitation professional to consider the specific needs of the individual patient.

REHABILITATION: GENERAL CONSIDERATIONS

Foundations

Rehabilitation of the knee should be founded on an understanding of the joint's anatomy, mechanics, arthrokinematics, kinesiology, and pathophysiology. The long-term goal of rehabilitation should be to return the patient to the highest possible level of activity. Short term goals postinjury or postsurgery include control of pain and effusion, restoration of mobility, and muscle reeducation. A great deal of emphasis should be placed on functional activities that are introduced in a logical progression for each individual patient.

Factors Contributing to Joint Loading

Contributing factors that increase joint loading must be addressed in the rehabilitation process. Obesity is one of these factors. It has been shown in the literature that joint loading and joint reaction forces are directly proportional to an individual's body weight.[21, 29, 40] As an example, consider the case of a geriatric patient who reported to our clinic with a diagnosis of osteoarthritis of the right knee and a chief complaint of pain on ambulation of graded surfaces. In gathering the history of the patient's symptoms, the patient admitted that he had experienced the very same symptoms some 5 years earlier while hiking in the Rocky Mountains. He had taken along his 5-year-old grandson, who weighed about 50 lb, and the child, being unable to negotiate uphill grades, requested that "Grandpa" carry him. This, he reported, brought on the same symptoms he was experiencing now. When asked how much weight he had gained over the past 5 years, the patient stated that he had gained 10 lb/year, for a total of 50 lb over the previous 5 years. In effect, he had added the equivalent weight of his grandson to his joint-loading forces and the logical conclusion was that a weight loss and maintenance program should be an important part of his care plan.

The Team Approach

When establishing a rehabilitation plan for the geriatric patient, health care professionals must operate as a team. The physician serves the role of providing the orthopedic and medical diagnosis, which guides the rehabilitation team in choosing an appropriate care plan and mechanism for recovery. Communication between the physician, rehabilitation professional, and patient is of paramount importance.

TREATMENT GOALS

Treatment goals should be specific to the needs of the patient, as identified during the initial and ongoing assessment. It must be kept in mind that aging is accompanied by a general decline in strength, endurance, and flexibility, along with a propensity for medical problems such as diabetes and heart disease. These factors must be carefully considered in establishing a treatment plan for the geriatric patient.

Control of Pain and Effusion

Pain and effusion have a tremendous influence on muscle function. The effect of these factors on muscle inhibition is so significant that they must be monitored on a regular basis and should act as a yardstick for determining an appropriate level of rehabilitation and ADL. Several investigators have demonstrated that even small amounts of knee joint effusion result in reflex muscle inhibition.[16, 61]

Pain has an equally disabling effect on muscle function. Pain inhibition is a well-known phenomenon and has been documented in recent literature.[61, 63] The presence of pain with activity can significantly reduce the ability of a patient to recruit muscles during rehabilitation exercises.

Considering the amount of pain and effusion that may accompany knee injury and surgery, clinicians should have a great deal of respect for these two factors and their influence on function of the lower extremity. Reducing the negative influence of these factors should be a priority for the rehabilitation professional. Measures that tend to control pain

and effusion have great merit in the rehabilitation process.

Effusion is best controlled by ice, elevation, and compression. Ice can be applied via cold packs or compresses for 20 minutes as often as every hour if necessary. It must be explained to the patient that elevation means raising the knee joint higher than the heart. If no contraindications exist, the patient can obtain good elevation simply by placing 2-inch blocks under the bedposts at the foot of the bed. A thigh-length high-compression stocking with a compression gradient greater distally than proximally assists with control of effusion and soft tissue swelling of the lower leg and should be applied routinely as part of the postoperative care plan.

Restoration of Mobility

Gaining range of motion in the knee following injury or surgery can be most difficult for both the patient and the physical therapist. For the patient, range-of-motion activities are often dreaded and elicit a typical pain response of muscle guarding accompanied by great pain and anxiety. The physical therapist finds it frustrating to "push" motion and see little in the way of permanent gains in range of motion. This can be avoided through a thorough evaluation of the joint with identification of the factors restricting mobility. Most people would never consider going to their dentist and having their teeth pulled without the benefit of anesthesia and they certainly should never be subjected to painful passive manipulation of the knee without anesthesia. Passive manipulation through a painful arc does nothing to benefit the patient or the clinician. The pain and joint irritability created by such intervention only increases the likelihood of muscle inhibition and further delays the recovery process.

Factors Restricting Range of Motion

In evaluation of factors restricting range of motion, one must consider normal arthrokinematics of the knee joint. Three component movements occur as the knee goes from extension to flexion and vice versa. Component movements consist of involuntary motions of the articular surfaces, including rotation, rolling, and translation.[33, 39, 46] Flexion is accompanied by internal tibial rotation, caudal patellar glide, and posterior tibial translation, while extension is accompanied by external tibial rotation, cephalad patellar glide, and anterior tibial translation. If any of these components of motion is restricted, range of motion will be limited. Patellar mobility should be of great concern to the physical therapist because of the tendency for rapid adhesion formation in the infrapatellar area following surgery or trauma. The physical therapist should target restricted components and utilize passive mobilization to restore mobility based on a thorough assessment. Grade four mobilizations, which involve small oscillations at the end range, are highly effective (Figs 19–1 and 19–2). These maneuvers are not painful to the patient and therefore rarely increase joint irritability.

Sometimes mobility is restricted owing to the formation of adhesions between the collateral ligaments and the underlying femoral condyles.[5] Normally these ligaments glide over the condyles as the knee goes into flexion from a position of extension; however, when adhesions prevent normal gliding of the collateral ligaments, pain over the site of the adhesion will restrict the ability to achieve full flexion. The affected area will be tender to palpation and the patient will report pain over the site of the adhesion at the end range of flexion. This problem can be resolved by deep friction transverse massage, which actually teases the ligament away from the underlying bone and tears the restricting adhesions, thus restoring normal glide of the collateral ligaments.

Soft-tissue contracture can be another pertinent factor in restriction of joint mobility. Most commonly, flexion is prevented by soft-tissue contracture of the extensor mechanism, while extension is prevented by contracture of the gastrocnemius-soleus complex and hamstrings or by posterior capsule tightness. Once the soft tissue accounting for the restriction in motion is identified via evaluation, *gentle*

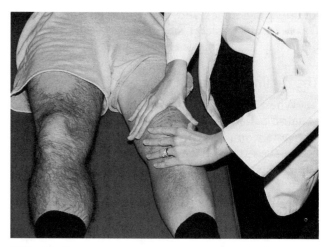

FIG 19–2.
Patellar mobilization cephalad and caudal. Grade 4 mobilizations are utilized initially.

soft tissue stretching activities should be introduced. It is extremely important that the physical therapist approach this in a slow and controlled fashion to avoid activation of muscle guarding in response to pain. It has been shown that slow, sustained, low-intensity stretching is more effective than quick and painful passive manipulation of the joint.[57] Use of modalities such as moist heat or ultrasound directed at the areas of contracture can increase soft tissue pliability prior to stretching and make such maneuvers more effective.[57]

Gaining Range of Motion in Flexion

When the problem is gaining range of motion in flexion, the extensor mechanism should be stretched by positioning the patient in hip extension, then applying a low-intensity stretch into flexion. By doing so, the rectus femoris, which crosses two joints, is the target of the stretching. Proprioceptive neuromuscular techniques, more specifically the hold-relax method, are most effective. The patient actively flexes the knee by firing the hamstring muscles then relaxes all muscles as the end range of motion is met. This is followed by an isometric contraction of the quadriceps muscles at end range while the physical therapist provides manual resistance. It is extremely effective when the physical therapist also physically blocks the posterior aspect of the lower leg so that there is no danger of the joint being pushed into passive flexion beyond the patient's pain tolerance (Fig 19–3). This serves to decrease the tendency for anxious anticipation of pain in the event that the patient cannot sustain an isometric quadriceps contraction against resistance.

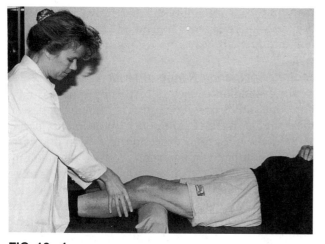

FIG 19–1.
Mobilization procedure for posterior tibial glide. Grade 4 mobilizations are utilized initially.

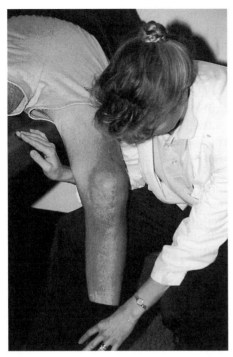

FIG 19–3.
Position for stretching the quadriceps muscles to gain range of motion in flexion.

The rationale for this procedure is well founded. Maximal contraction of the hamstrings results in inhibition of the quadriceps muscles, therefore allowing the patient the benefit of maximal pain-free flexion.[36] After the relaxation phase, the isometric quadriceps contraction causes internal elongation of the connective tissue framework restricting soft tissue mobility as the muscle fibers contract. It should be emphasized that this approach to soft-tissue stretching should be done within the patient's pain tolerance, which should be determined by the patient, not the physical therapist.

Another way to improve range of motion in flexion is to strengthen the hamstring muscle group actively. This may be done via use of manual resistance or isotonic training. Whatever the method, the patient should be encouraged to flex the joint to a tolerable end range with every repetition. From a neurologic perspective, this makes sense because maximal contraction of the agonist (hamstrings) results in relaxation of the antagonist (quadriceps) thus avoiding activation of a muscle guarding response. Patients can be taught to maintain relaxation of the quadriceps muscles via biofeedback training, either with manual or EMG feedback.

Activation of the muscle-guarding response can also be avoided by use of self-ranging activities, with

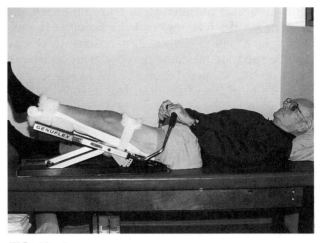

FIG 19–4.
Patient performing self-ranging activity with the Genuflex to stretch the posterior capsule.

the patient in full control of the range-of-motion activity. A manual continuous passive motion (CPM) device such as the Genuflex (New Concepts, Springville, Utah) can be of great assistance (Figs 19–4 and 19–5). These devices can be rented to patients for use at home.

Another approach would be to use a stationary bicycle for "freewheeling" without resistance. The patient is instructed to slowly pedal forward, controlling the motion with the uninvolved side until a good stretch is felt on the involved side at the end range of flexion. After a brief stretch at the end range (5 or 10 seconds), the patient then pedals backward, again controlling the motion with the uninvolved lower extremity until a good stretch is felt on the involved side at the top of the stroke. This

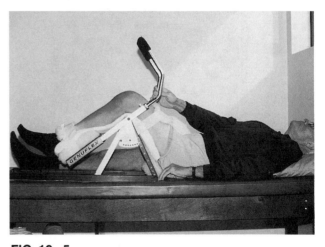

FIG 19–5.
Patient performing self-ranging activity with the Geneflex to stretch the hamstring muscles.

can be repeated for intervals of 5 to 15 minutes, depending on the tolerance and the needs of the patient. The Kinetron (Cybex, Ronkonkoma, NY) may also be used for the same purpose. The device can be set so that the pedal excursion is equivalent to the patient's available range of motion (Fig 19–6). The speed of isokinetic exercise can be adjusted and slow speeds are recommended so that the patient can better control the motion and gain a strengthening benefit at the same time. The patient can be challenged to achieve greater flexion angles by gradually lowering the seat height throughout the exercise interval. This activity can be performed for intervals of 5 to 15 minutes, depending on the patient's tolerance and needs.

Gaining Range of Motion in Extension

Gaining range of motion in extension can pose an even greater problem than restrictions in flexion because of the need for full extension during functional activities. Factors restricting extension include loss of component mobility, loss of flexibility in the gastrocnemius-soleus complex or hamstring muscles, posterior capsule contracture, and loss of quadriceps control. Again, it is extremely important that the physical therapist base the approach to gaining extension on the findings of the evaluation. In this

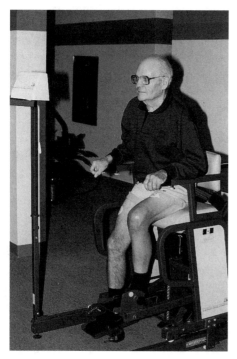

FIG 19–6.
Patient utilizing the Kinetron to gain strength, endurance, and range of motion.

manner the most important factors restricting extension can be identified and targeted for treatment.

In some cases extension is restricted by the formation of scar tissue in the anterior joint space. This connective tissue can be compressed by prolonged passive extension, but the patient will note that although full extension can be achieved after range-of-motion activities, the knee tends to "drift" back into a position of flexion within 20 or so minutes. This is the typical finding in a patient who is experiencing proliferation of adhesions in the anterior joint space. This is most commonly seen in cases where the distal portion of the extensor mechanism has been subject to trauma, but it can also occur as a result of prolonged immobilization in flexion. Keeping in mind that the "angry" and inflamed knee seeks the position of comfort; it should be no surprise that a resting position of 20 degrees of flexion is the position of maximal joint capacity, accommodating gross effusion. Flexion contractures can occur even in the absence of trauma to the distal extensor mechanism. Fortunately, connective tissue tends to align itself according to the stresses imposed on it, much like osseous tissue. Therefore, low-intensity, sustained stretching into extension can result in consolidation and shrinking of scar tissue restricting range of motion in extension. It is very important that the development of such scar tissue be recognized and dealt with immediately. The longer the physical therapist waits to address scar tissue formation of this nature, the more likely that it will proliferate and cause a permanent flexion contracture.

One of the most effective ways to prevent formation of scar tissue in the infrapatellar area is to mobilize the patella passively and actively. Passive patellar mobilization cephalad and caudad should be done immediately postoperatively, or posttrauma in such cases, using grade 4 oscillations, when restriction in patellar mobility is noted (see Fig 19–2). Quadriceps activity via quadriceps setting provides active mobilization of the patella and is of great benefit in preventing infrapatellar adhesions. In the event that the patient is unable to activate the quadriceps mechanism sufficiently to actively mobilize the patella, then electrical muscle stimulation (EMS) of the quadriceps is very helpful. This is not, however, the treatment of choice, as EMS bypasses the central nervous system and thus does not reinforce neuromuscular control. When the patient is instructed to overlay a volitional quadriceps contraction in synchrony with the electrical stimulation, use of EMS can be quite effective. Nonetheless, if the patient demonstrates good quadriceps control and recruitment, then active contractions are preferred over passive activation via EMS because of the additional benefit of reinforcement of the neural pathway.

Flexibility activities directed toward the gastrocnemius-soleus and hamstrings complex can be of great merit when attempting to improve range of motion in extension. Such therapeutic interventions may be preceded by use of modalities such as moist heat or ultrasound when indicated. The stretch may be applied either manually or by self-stretching activities. Whatever the case, the stretch should be applied within the patient's pain tolerance in order to avoid stimulation of the muscle spindles, which will result in reflex contraction of the muscles being stretched. A low-intensity, sustained stretch is more effective than vigorous short-term stretching. It is recommended that the low-intensity, sustained stretch be held for intervals of at least 5 minutes for maximal results.

When the posterior capsule is the primary factor restricting range of motion in extension, the same principles apply. Stretching of the posterior capsule can be achieved by a number of therapeutic approaches.

If the patient demonstrates a fair amount of hamstrings guarding on stretching activities directed at gaining extension, then self ranging activities are recommended. The Genuflex can be very beneficial in such cases. This device permits the patient to manually perform self-ranging activities so that the patient can determine the end range, thus eliminating the possibility of exceeding the pain tolerance of the patient. For posterior capsule stretching the device should be set so that the patient performs self-ranging through an arc of motion from 20 degrees to full passive extension (see Fig 19–4). When the device is set at greater flexion angles, the hamstrings offer passive resistance to extension before any stretch is felt in the posterior capsule (see Fig 19–5). Positioning the patient in a semireclining posture also helps eliminate passive restraint of the hamstrings.

Another method of stretching the posterior capsule is to utilize a low-intensity sustained stretch preceded by application of moist heat or ultrasound to the capsule. Prone stretching with the pelvis stabilized and the lower leg supported permits a gravitational stretch to the posterior capsule. Patients who have difficulty maintaining pelvic stabilization can achieve a similar effect by lying supine with the lower extremity in neutral rotation while the heel is propped by a rolled towel or bolster. These activities

should be performed within the patient's pain tolerance for intervals of 5 to 15 minutes.

Proper limb positioning during the patient's daily activities can also be highly effective in treatment of range-of-motion restrictions. The patient who has a flexion contracture should be advised not to support the posterior aspect of the knee with pillows or bolsters while resting or sleeping. Such patients should be encouraged to position the limb in full available extension for prolonged intervals frequently throughout the day. Similarly, patients with range-of-motion restrictions in flexion should be advised to position the knee at the end range of available flexion for prolonged intervals frequently throughout the day. Since geriatric patients tend to be fairly inactive, particularly following injury or surgery, the natural tendency is to assume positions of flexion. These patients need strict guidelines with regards to proper positioning, including instructions with respect to time out of the reclining and sitting position.

While the goal of the aforementioned range-of-motion techniques is to achieve full passive extension, the physical therapist should place great emphasis on gaining extension actively as well. It does not serve any useful purpose to restore full passive extension without muscle control of the motion gained. Dynamic stabilization of the joint via muscle control should be done throughout the full arc of motion—particularly terminal extension, as this is often the position of the knee joint during functional activities.

The patient Incentive Dynamometer (Techdyne, Inc., Silver Springs, Md) can be used for this purpose. The Incentive Dynamometer consists of an air-filled bolster connected by a hose to a dynamometer, which registers the pressure exerted against the bolster. When the device is used to gain active range of motion in extension, it is placed against the posterior knee with the patient in the supine or standing position (Fig 19–7). When done standing the patient positions the hip and heel of the involved side against a wall, with the bolster between the posterior aspect of the knee and the wall. The patient is then instructed to actively push backwards into the wall for a 5-second contraction. The amount of pressure exerted will be monitored by the dynamometer so that the patient receives valuable feedback. In performing this activity, the patient activates both the hip extensors (gluteus maximus and hamstrings) and the knee extensors (quadriceps). The standing position is preferred, as it involves weight bearing and is more functional than the supine position. The

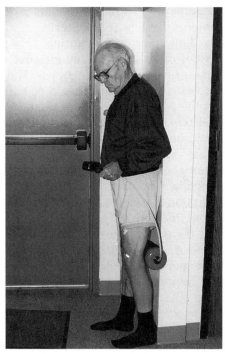

FIG 19–7.
Use of the Techdyne incentive dynamometer to improve quadriceps strength in terminal extension while weight bearing.

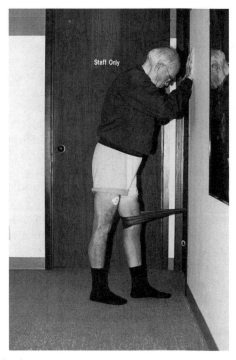

FIG 19–8.
Use of Theraband to improve quadriceps strength in terminal extension while weight bearing (stove pipe extension).

feedback provided by the dynamometer provides the patient with some incentive for greater effort and can be extremely helpful in terms of motivating patients.

Another rehabilitation activity that encourages active terminal extension in a functional manner is similar to the activity described above, but requires little in the way of equipment. This exercise, "stove pipe extension," is done with the patient in the standing position. Resistance is applied either manually or with an elastic band to the posterior aspect of the knee as the patient works from a position of knee flexion to knee extension (Fig 19–8). Patients often compensate for inadequate quadriceps control by shifting the center of gravity backwards when performing this activity; therefore, it is important that patients be instructed to keep the hip and ankle aligned while performing the motion at the knee joint only. The number of recommended repetitions depends on the patient's ability to perform the exercise properly. When the patient starts to fatigue, compensation will be evident, and regardless of the number of repetitions, the exercise should be terminated for that particular rehabilitation session.

A simple activity directed at restoration of active quadriceps control in terminal extension is backward

walking. The patient is instructed to step backward with the involved limb, planting the foot flat with the heel in contact with the floor. After a weight shift onto the involved limb, the patient concentrates on achieving full available active extension by contracting the knee and hip extensors simultaneously as the uninvolved limb is reached backwards and planted next to the involved extremity. When the patient is no longer able to demonstrate good quadriceps control, the exercise is terminated for that session.

It should be noted that all rehabilitation activities that require quadriceps control in terminal extension are effective measures to gain active range of motion in extension. The activities described above can be particularly effective; however, restoration of motor control during functional activities, which is the goal of muscle reeducation, is equally effective.

Muscle Reeducation

Strength vs Motor Control

There is a distinct difference between strength and motor control,[19] although the two terms are somewhat related. Strength is defined as the amount of force that a muscle can exert, while motor control involves the quality of the contraction.[6, 58]

Strength training should involve motor control, but the body's ability to substitute inappropriate motor programs to achieve a strength task is simply amazing. In other words, in the injury or postsurgical state, the patient learns to compensate quite effectively for weak muscles by activating strong muscles in order to complete functional demands placed on the extremity.

At our facility, where approximately 70% of our case load involves knee patients who are posttrauma or postsurgery, we instituted a clinical study (still in progress) investigating quadriceps muscle activity during functional tasks such as stair negotiation and ambulation. Surface EMG electrodes were placed on the quadriceps muscles bilaterally using a dual-channel EMG (M44 Dual Channel EMG, Davicon, Inc., Burlington, Mass). Patients were asked to perform step-downs from a four-inch block while maximal quadriceps output (measured in microvolts) was observed (Figs 19–9 and 19–10). Although the patients were able to perform exactly the same functional task, the EMG output for the quadriceps muscles on the involved side was typically only one half the output for the uninvolved side. When patients were monitored for EMG output during ambulation, the results were quite similar. In fact, we have moni-

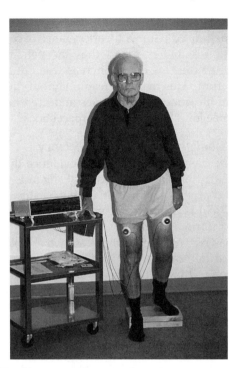

FIG 19–10.
Use of electromyography to monitor quadriceps recruitment of the involved extremity during a step-down from a 3 in. block.

tored EMG activity in the quadricep bilaterally for every rehabilitation activity aimed at strengthening and have found drastic differences in output, despite the fact that the patient is performing the same activity with the lower limbs.

Most surprising is our observation of the difference in EMG output between the involved and uninvolved sides during unilateral leg press. While the patient can effectively push exactly the same amount of weight to complete the repetitions requested, the EMG output of the involved quadriceps can be as low as one tenth of the EMG output observed for the uninvolved extremity. We are learning that patients can perform many strengthening activities by substituting strong muscles for the weak ones, particularly for the quadriceps muscles, which are most affected by pain inhibition after trauma such as injury or surgery.

Fortunately, patients are able to institute changes in their motor programs by volitional effort with the aid of biofeedback training. With biofeedback, patients can recognize appropriate motor patterns and learn to recruit motor units that have previously been dormant. We have noted that some patients have been able to double their EMG output for the quadriceps muscles in just one session of biofeedback train-

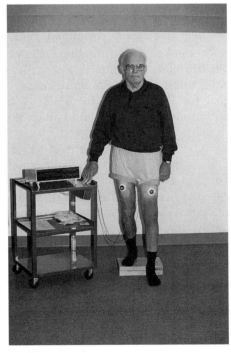

FIG 19–9.
Use of electromyography to monitor quadriceps recruitment of the uninvolved extremity during a step-down from a 3 in. block.

ing. It is interesting to note that many of our patients who experienced pain with performance of certain rehabilitation activities report that the pain is eliminated when they are able to increase their quadriceps EMG output. This makes sense in light of the contribution of the quadriceps muscles in decreasing stress to the knee joint by absorbing impact shock.

Vastus Medialis Obliquus Insufficiency

There has been some recent evidence that EMG activity of the vastus medialis obliquus muscle (VMO) compared with that in the vastus lateralis muscle (VL) is different for subjects with knee pain than for normal subjects.[42, 52, 54, 60, 68, 70] While our study has not yet been completed, we are observing a marked decrease in the EMG output of the VMO compared to that of the vastus lateralis during functional tasks. This is likely the result of selective VMO inhibition by pain and effusion, as mentioned previously.[16, 61] The net result is a tendency for lateral tracking of the patella, which results in excessive patellofemoral joint contact forces, with subsequent inflammation and inhibition of the VMO. Therefore patellofemoral dysfunction is a common complication following injury or surgery and must be addressed in the rehabilitation process.

VMO reeducation can be facilitated by the use of patellar taping to improve patellar orientation. McConnell describes four components of patellar malalignment that are identified by clinical assessment of patellar orientation, and proposed a treatment approach having its basis in patellar taping and muscle reeducation activities.[43] The taping procedure is then used in accordance with the findings of the clinical evaluation. It is easy to apply and patients can be taught how to use the tape on a home basis. Taping to improve patellar orientation is used on a short-term basis, daily for 10 to 14 days. When used appropriately, the reduction in the patient's pain on functional activities is remarkable. Taping is *not*, however, the key to treatment of patellar maltracking. The key factors are restoration of static and dynamic mobility of the patella through stretching of tight lateral structures and reeducation of the VMO. Since the VMO is selectively inhibited by pain, use of the tape to control pain facilitates reeducation of the VMO.

Biofeedback training is most effective in teaching patients how to activate the VMO. With an electrode directly over the muscle belly of the VMO, patients receive visual and/or auditory feedback when they activate the muscle. Early in training, it may be necessary to use facilitation techniques, such as simultaneous activation of the VMO and gluteus medius muscles. Once the patient demonstrates good VMO control in a seated position with the knee slightly flexed and the foot flat on the floor, then training is done in functional positions, such as standing with the knee slightly flexed as weight shifts are performed. Eventually patients progress to VMO training during ambulation and stair negotiation. The progression to functional training should be based on the activity needs of each individual patient. The number of repetitions or length of muscle reeducation sessions is also individualized, and is based on the patient's ability to maintain good VMO control. When fatigue becomes apparent, the training session is over. For this reason, it is recommended that patients perform VMO training frequently throughout the day, rather than in just one session. Biofeedback units such as the Myotrac (Thought Technology, Toronto, Ontario, Canada) may be dispensed for home use, or the patient can be taught to utilize manual feedback during VMO training activities.

Total Limb Rehabilitation

Many of the orthopedic knee pathologies observed in the geriatric patient are progressive in nature, resulting in gradual degeneration of function in all joints of the affected extremity. The clinician must keep in mind that compensation for an injured or painful knee joint must necessarily involve the hip and ankle; therefore, peripheral joints should never be overlooked as contributing factors to abnormal lower extremity function.

Rehabilitation of the total limb should be a primary goal for the physical therapist. A thorough evaluation of lower extremity mechanics, both static and dynamic, should be followed by a care plan aimed at functional improvement of the entire extremity. Since most functional activities involve both concentric and eccentric muscle contractions of the lower extremity, rehabilitation activities that mimic these functional demands are very appropriate.

Recently, there has been a renewed interest in the use of closed kinetic chain rehabilitation activities because of their similarity and carryover to activities of daily living such as ambulation and stair negotiation. Closed kinetic chain exercises are defined as activities that involve a total limb movement with the distal end of the extremity fixed in space.[24, 51, 62] By nature, there is a concentric and eccentric phase during closed chain activities as long as they are isotonic in nature. While all closed kinetic chain activities involve a total limb movement, some total limb movements can be performed in an open kinetic chain. For example, stair climbing or descent is a closed-chain activity because the foot is planted against an unmoving step; however, use of certain types of leg press apparatus, where the pedal planted against the foot moves while the body remains stationary, is not considered a closed chain activity because the foot is planted against a movable surface. Both examples, however, involve total limb movements with concentric and eccentric contractions. Since both activities are total limb movements and are quite functional in nature, it makes sense to this author that rehabilitation professionals focus on total-limb movements instead of isolated joint movements, rather than basing rehabilitation exercise judgments on closed- vs. open-chain activities.

Therefore, total limb movements and isolated joint movements necessarily involve both concentric and eccentric muscle contractions as long as they are isotonic, and not isometric or isokinetic in nature. During the eccentric phase, the contribution of muscles to dynamic stability of the limb reverses itself.[24] For example, during a step-down, the action of stair descent, the quadriceps are active as the knee flexes, the gluteus maximus and hamstrings are active as the hip flexes, and the gastrocnemius muscle is active as the ankle dorsiflexes. In this manner all of the aforementioned muscles serve to decelerate movement in the opposite direction of their concentric action. It makes sense, then, that all of these muscle groups should be trained eccentrically in order to mimic functional demands.

The importance of concentric contractions should not be overlooked, however. One must remember that the patient must have some means of returning to starting position after an eccentric contraction, and that is accomplished by concentric contractions of the very same muscle groups, now acting as prime movers. The way to accomplish both is through total-limb movements, which require a quick reversal from concentric to eccentric contraction.

Isolated limb movements should not be completely abandoned as a means of improving function. If a normal firing pattern of muscle activity cannot be achieved through total limb training, which should include biofeedback training, then isolated joint training can be very useful. When employing this method, proper stabilization makes it virtually impossible for the patient to substitute inappropriate muscles to complete the task. For example, if the patient cannot learn to activate the quadriceps during step-downs, then isotonic leg extension may be utilized to isolate the quadriceps, demanding both a

concentric and eccentric muscle contraction. Thus, while total limb movements may be considered more functional, isolated joint movements have great merit in cases where the patient cannot overcome an abnormal motor program that involves substitution of the wrong muscles at the wrong time. Once adequate motor control of the affected muscle is restored, functional (total limb) training should be initiated.

Functional Rehabilitation

Functional rehabilitation activities should follow a logical progression. Lead-up activities directed at achievement of functional tasks are similar to skill drills introduced to athletes in training for sport activities with high physical demands. The only difference is that the activity of high physical demand for the geriatric patient may be a motor skill as rudimentary as arising from the seated position, or ambulation on level surfaces.

Take, for example, the musculoskeletal demands placed on the lower extremity for sitting and standing. The physical therapist could start by monitoring the quadriceps EMG output bilaterally during quadriceps setting done seated with the foot planted on the floor. If the patient learns to improve motor unit firing of the quadriceps in this position, then training could proceed to the standing position during weight shifts. Once good quadriceps control is achieved, the next step might be to work on quadriceps control with biofeedback during a mini–step-down and step-up, performed in an arc between 20 degrees of flexion and full extension. Once this can be achieved with good quadriceps control, the patient's regimen would be advanced to minisquats performed in an arc between 45 degrees of flexion and full extension. Ultimately the patient would advance to full squats through an arc of motion from 90 degrees of flexion to full extension. If at any point in this progression the patient demonstrates failure to improve quadriceps EMG output with EMG training, then isolated joint movement such as isotonic leg extension exercises should be initiated until eccentric and concentric control is noted. While there is no solid clinical evidence that there is carryover in muscle recruitment from isolated joint training to total limb training, it makes sense that motor units that are not being recruited via total limb activities (as a result of substitution) will not be strengthened via such activities. If isolated joint training is introduced at this point in rehabilitation, the possibility of substitution is reduced and the patient is forced to recruit the specific motor units required to perform the open chain task, provided that proper stabilization accompanies the activity. Once the patient demonstrates the ability to produce similar EMG output with the involved extremity as compared with the uninvolved extremity, then the patient could return to working on the functional progression, as the ultimate goal of rehabilitation is restoration of *function.*

Balance and Proprioception

When considering function in the rehabilitative plan, balance and proprioception come to mind as factors that can undermine function in even the strongest patient.[4, 10, 25] Strength and muscle control are important to function, but cannot prevent potentially disastrous falls resulting from loss of joint proprioception. Balance activities such as unilateral stance and biomechanical ankle proprioception (BAPS Gray, Inc., Adrian, Mich) training are also extremely important and should be included in the rehabilitation process. Balance activities that mimic the demands posed on the patient during daily activities such as getting in and out of a bathtub should be part of the rehabilitation program. In addition, patients should be given the opportunity to practice negotiation of uneven surfaces during ambulation training in order to prepare them for the real environment and prevent falls.

REHABILITATION FOLLOWING INJURY OR SURGERY

The Osteoarthritic Knee

In establishing a rehabilitation plan for the patient with an osteoarthritic knee, the physical therapist must consider the extent and location of degenerative changes. If the joint degeneration involves primarily the medial compartment, for example, rehabilitation activities should be performed in the limb position that poses the least amount of stress to the joint, namely a position of foot pronation that serves to "unload" the medial side of the joint. If the patient has an osteochondral defect, the painful arc that accompanies joint loading should be identified and avoided. The ultimate orthopedic solution for the severely degenerated joint is total knee replacement, but high tibial osteotomy is sometimes an intermediate solution, especially for patients who are under 55 years of age and are still quite active.[7]

High Tibial Osteotomy

Following surgery, the patient who has undergone high tibial osteotomy is usually immobilized in a plaster cast for 4 to 6 weeks, depending on bone healing as assessed via roentgenography by the orthopedic surgeon. Weight bearing with crutches may be initiated as early as 2 weeks postoperatively, as weight bearing can actually serve to compress the osteotomy and facilitate the reparative process.

While the patient is still in the cast, every effort should be made to prevent atrophy of the muscles at the hip, knee, and ankle. This may be accomplished safely in the non–weight-bearing phase by quadriceps setting, straight leg raising, and isolated hip and ankle strengthening performed against resistance in non–weight-bearing positions.

Once the orthopedic surgeon has full confidence that bony repair has occurred, the patient may progress to a full weight-bearing gait pattern. The rehabilitation specialist can then progress the patient through activities directed at restoration of mobility and strength during functional activities in accordance with the guidelines described above.

Total Knee Arthroplasty

When the patient with an osteoarthritic knee is functionally disabled by pain, total knee arthroplasty is often the best therapeutic choice provided that other medical complications do not supersede the surgical procedure. Indeed, there are many total knee arthroplasty patients who can testify to the benefits of this procedure with regards to diminution of their pain, and improvement in their activity level. Nonetheless, total knee replacement is not without risks, and as such, is considered by some to be an end-stage procedure for the osteoarthritic knee. It is a decision that can only be reached with the professional guidance of the orthopedic physician who is acting in the best interests of the patient.

Range-of-Motion Goals

After the surgery has been completed, the fate of the patient lies in the hands of the patient and the team comprising the surgeon and the rehabilitation professionals, most likely the physical and occupational therapists. One of the most important postoperative goals with regard to physical therapy is restoration of range of motion in both flexion and extension. It is this author's experience that this goal is more easily accomplished when the patient goes into the procedure with good range of motion; therefore preoperative rehabilitation should be a priority with such patients. The next most important goal is restoration of functional strength, and this, too, should be addressed preoperatively. The merit of this approach has been recognized in athlete patients who choose to undergo surgical procedures aimed at ligament reconstruction after an acute injury; the concept applies equally as well to the geriatric patient with a long history of progressive degeneration in muscle function secondary to pain and disuse.

Immediately postoperatively—within 24 hours—rehabilitation should be initiated. Use of continuous passive motion may be considered for some patients for whom it is indicated, but it has been found by at least one investigator that the range-of-motion outcome 6 months postsurgery is the same for patients after total knee replacement, regardless whether continuous passive motion was utilized.[55, 67] The problem with motorized continuous passive motion is that the patient has no control of range of motion and can easily be forced into extremes that elicit the guarding and pain response. Therefore, use of a manual continuous passive motion device such as the Genuflex can be extremely useful in the early postsurgery phase because it permits the patient to control the range of motion and thus eliminates the possibility of muscle guarding in response to pain.

Great emphasis should be placed on early restoration of range of motion in patients who have undergone total knee replacement. In fact, many orthopedic surgeons require that their patients achieve 90 degrees of flexion prior to discharge from the hospital after total knee replacement. Equal attention should be directed at restoring range of motion in extension, as full active extension is important in performance of functional activities. The physical therapist should avoid the urge to get overzealous regarding range-of-motion activities when treating the immediately postoperative total knee replacement patient, however. Factors such as pain and effusion should be monitored, and range-of-motion activities should be done within pain-free limits in order to avoid an increase in joint irritability, effusion, and muscle guarding.

Patellar Malalignment

Patellofemoral dysfunction is the most common source of dissatisfaction following total knee arthroplasty.[9, 11, 18, 23, 47] Selective inhibition of the quadriceps muscles—in particular the VMO—occur commonly in total knee arthroplasty patients owing to the joint trauma that accompanies the surgical procedure. Attention should be directed to stretching of tight lateral structures and to reeducation of the quadriceps muscles, with emphasis on the VMO. The McConnell approach can be quite useful in treatment of this postoperative complication.[43]

Gait Training

Gait training is another important aspect regarding rehabilitation after total knee arthroplasty. Weight bearing status depends on the nature of the arthroplasty fixation. When cement is utilized, full weight bearing can be accomplished as early as 4 to 6 weeks postoperatively.[17] On the other hand, use of a cementless prosthesis requires some time for bony ingrowth to completely stabilize the prosthesis, and a partial weight-bearing gait may be required for 10 to 12 weeks in order to accommodate bony proliferation. Should this be the case, proper gait training with an assistive device such as crutches or a walker is an important part of the patient's care plan. Even when the patient requires an assistive device for ambulation, every effort should be made to normalize the gait pattern. Problems such as shortened stance phase on the involved extremity, lack of adequate push-off, and inadequate knee flexion during swing through phase should be addressed immediately. Correction of these gait abnormalities prevents reinforcement of inappropriate motor patterns, and makes ambulation a therapeutic activity in and of itself.

Functional Rehabilitation

The approach to rehabilitation of total knee arthroplasty patients should be directed at functional improvement of strength, balance, and proprioception as well. Functional progressions should be utilized and the individualized needs of the patient should be considered. The general rehabilitation guidelines mentioned above have great application in patients who have undergone total knee arthroscopy. It should be kept in mind by the clinician, however, that these patients typically have a history of progressive functional disability over a period of perhaps 20 or 30 years; therefore, improvement in terms of activity level may be quite slow. Nonetheless, functional improvement is the goal of rehabilitation and patients who have been properly rehabilitated should be able to return to a level of activity beyond their preoperative status.

Patellar Fracture

Because of the tendency for loss of balance among the elder population, fracture of the patella resulting from a fall is fairly common. Sometimes this injury can be treated nonsurgically by a period of immobilization with the knee in full extension for periods of 4 to 6 weeks. In other cases, the fracture is more extensive, requiring open reduction with internal fixation. The general criterion for deciding which of the two methods is the best intervention is the amount of displacement of the fracture. When the displacement for a transverse fracture is greater than 1 cm between the superior and inferior poles of the patella, then open reduction is usually the treatment of choice. While the prognosis for the patient with a simple fracture is quite good, the prognosis for the patient who requires open reduction may be guarded.

When the articular cartilage on the retropatellar surface has been compromised by trauma, osteoarthritis of the patellofemoral joint ensues. Though measures aimed at centralization of the patella in the trochlear groove may result in some improvement in pain and function, excessive patellofemoral joint-loading forces will always pose a problem for such patients. In particular, loading the joint in positions of flexion, such as during stair negotiation or squatting, tends to increase the patient's pain. Leg extension exercises also tend to load the patellofemoral joint and should be avoided.

Such patients should be treated exactly the same way as normally active, healthy persons with patellofemoral dysfunction. A thorough assessment of lower extremity mechanics is necessary in order to identify static and dynamic factors that contribute to the patient's dysfunction. In this author's experience, if patients can be taught to maintain good quadriceps control during functional (rehabilitation) activities, their pain is reduced, and their level of function is augmented. In this regard, biofeedback training can be very useful to the clinician.

Sepsis

Joint sepsis, no matter what measures medical professionals take to avoid it, can indeed occur. It can happen in two situations. The first is the case of the nonoperative patient who develops an infection secondary to bacteremia or following minimally invasive procedures such as joint aspiration. In the case of a patient undergoing open reduction, sepsis may be inadvertently introduced as a result of intraoperative contamination. No matter the case, joint sepsis is a serious complication.

Treatment with antibiotics is sometimes effective; however, in most cases the infiltration of bacteria is so widespread that surgical interventions including joint debridement and drainage are required.[53] It must be kept in mind that the infected joint is inflamed and extremely irritable, therefore any rehabilitation activities aimed at restoring range of motion or strength should be performed gently, so that joint irritation is not augmented. In fact, placing the patient in charge of such activities is the treatment of choice. The patient can be taught to effectively improve range of motion and strength without increasing joint irritation via use of self-ranging activities and strengthening exercises done within the patient's tolerance. This is one occasion where the rehabilitation professional can do *more* by doing *less*. An educated patient can have greater success than the rehabilitation specialist in the case of knee sepsis, provided that the patient is well instructed and motivated toward compliance.

SUMMARY

The knee joint is magnificently suited for normal function by virtue of its histologic characteristics and arthrokinematics. However, changes occurring with age and trauma can severely alter joint mechanics and function. Many of the orthopedic pathologies observed in the geriatric patient are the result of a long natural history of deterioration of anatomic components.

Rehabilitation of the geriatric patient with knee pathology involves a team approach, including the primary care physician, orthopedic surgeon, physical therapist, occupational therapist, and rehabilitation nurse. Assessment of the patient should focus on individual needs. Successful rehabilitation is founded in an understanding of anatomy, joint mechanics, arthrokinematics, kinesiology, and pathophysiology.

The paramount concern of the rehabilitation professional is the return of the patient to the highest possible level of independent function. Realistic goals must be set and a logical progression of rehabilitation activities should be established. Rehabilitation professionals must acknowledge the contribution of pain and effusion in limiting joint function and should use these signs and symptoms as a guide in the rehabilitation process. Gaining range of motion must be approached in a manner that identifies restricting factors so that treatment is specific to them. In this manner, increasing pain and effusion can be avoided. Restoration of normal motor control and balance contributes highly to improvement of the patient's functional abilities. Special considerations related to the nature of the patient's pathology influence the rehabilitation approach and improve the opportunity for a successful outcome.

Successful rehabilitation of the geriatric patient is most satisfying for all members of the rehabilitation team. Although geriatric patients present a challenge, improvement in the quality of their lives is the reward both the patient and the rehabilitation team receive as a result of careful planning and efforts directed toward individual needs. Nothing is more professionally rewarding to this author than the appreciation expressed by a geriatric patient who believes that rehabilitation after injury has truly enhanced the quality of life!

REFERENCES

1. Akeson WH, et al: The biology of ligaments, in Hunter LY, Funk JS (eds): *Rehabilitation of the Injured Knee.* St Louis, Mosby-Year Book, 1984, pp 93–147.
2. Arznozcky SP, Warren RF: The microvasculature of the human meniscus. *Am J Sports Med* 1983; 10:90–97.
3. Arznozcky SP, Tortilli PA: The biology of cartilage, in Hunter LY, Funk JS (eds): *Rehabilitation of the Injured Knee.* St Louis, Mosby-Year Book, 1984, pp 148–209.
4. Barrack P, et al: Proprioception of the knee joint. *Am J Phys Med* 1984; 63:175–181.
5. Blackburn TA, Craig E: Knee anatomy—a brief review, *Phys Ther* 1980; 60:1556–1560.
6. Brooks V: Motor control. *Phys Ther* 1983; 63:664–673.
7. Brueckmann FR, Kettelcamp DB: Proximal tibial osteotomy. *Orthop Clin North Am* 1982; 13:3–16.
8. Bryant WM: Wound healing, *Clin Symp* 1977; 29:2–36.
9. Cameron HV, Fedorkow DM: The patella in total knee arthroplasty. *Clin Orthop* 1982; 165:179–199.
10. Clark L, et al: Role of intramuscular receptors in the awareness of limb position. *J Neurophys* 1985; 54:1529–1540.
11. Clayton MI, Thirupathi R: Patellar complications after total condylar arthroplasty. *Clin Orthop* 1982; 170:152–155.
12. Cooper RR, Misel S: Tendon and ligament insertion. *J Bone Joint Surg* (Am) 1970; 52:1–8.
13. Cox JS, et al: The degenerative effects of partial and total resection of the medial meniscus in dogs. *Clin Orthop* 1975; 109:178–183.
14. Crelin ES: Development of the musculoskeletal system. *Clin Symp* 1981; 33:3–24.
15. Cyriax J: *Textbook of Orthopedic Medicine,* ed 7. London, Brailliere Tindall, 1978.
16. DeAndrade JR, Grant C, Dixon AS: Joint distension and reflex muscle inhibition in the knee. *J Bone Joint Surg* (Am) 1965; 47:313–322.
17. Ecker ML, Lotke PA: Postoperative care of the total knee patient, *Orthop Clin North Am* 1989; 20:55–62.
18. Figgie HE, et al: The influence of tibial-patella femoral mechanical axis on patella femoral function in the

19. posterior stabilized condylar knee prosthesis. *J Bone Joint Surg* (Am) 1986; 68:1035–1040.
19. Fox EL, Matthews DK: *The Physiological Basis of Physical Education and Athletics,* ed 3, Philadelphia, CBS College Publishing, 1981.
20. Frost HM: *Orthopedic Biomechanics.* Springfield, Ill, Charles C Thomas, 1973.
21. Fulkerson JP, Hungerford DS: *Disorders of the Patellofemoral Joint,* ed 2. Baltimore, Williams & Wilkins, 1990.
22. Gamble JG, Edwards CC, Max SR: Enzymatic adaptations in ligaments during immobilization. *Am J Sports Medicine* 1984; 12:221–228.
23. Goldberg VM, Figgie HE, Figgie MP: Technical considerations in total knee surgery—management of patellar problems, *Orthop Clin North Am* 1989; 20:189–199.
24. Gray GW: *Chain Reaction,* Adrian, Mich, Wynn Marketing, 1991.
25. Grigg, P, Finerman GA, Riley LH: Joint position sense after total hip replacement. *J Bone Joint Surg* (Am) 1973; 55:1016–1025.
26. Ham AW, Cormack DH: *Histophysiology of Cartilage, Bone and Joints.* Philadelphia, JB Lippincott. 1979.
27. Helfet AJ: *The Management of Internal Derangements of the Knee,* Philadelphia, JB Lippincott, 1963.
28. Helfet AJ: Anatomy and mechanics of movement in the knee joint, in Helfet AJ (ed): *Disorders of the Knee.* Philadelphia, JB Lippincott, 1982, pp 1–18.
29. Henry JS: Patellofemoral problems. *Clin Sports Med* 1989; 8:17–23.
30. Honner R, Thompson R: The nutritional pathways of articular cartilage. *J Bone Joint Surg* (Am) 1971; 52:742–748.
31. Hoppenfeld S: *Physical Examination of the Spine and Extremities.* New York, Appleton-Century-Crofts, 1976.
32. Junquiera LC, Cuniero J: *Basic Histology.* Los Altos, Calif, Lange Medical Publications, 1980.
33. Kaltenborn FM: *Manual Therapy for the Extremity Joints,* ed 2. Oslo, Olaf Norlis Bokhandel, 1976.
34. Kapandji IA: *The Physiology of the Joints,* vol 2. New York, Churchill Livingstone, 1970.
35. Kettelkamp DB, Colyer RA: Osteoarthritis of the knee, in Moskowitz RW, et al (eds): *Osteoarthritis Diagnosis and Management,* Philadelphia, WB Saunders, 1984, pp 403–421.
36. Knott V, Voss M: *Proprioceptive Neuromuscular Facilitation,* New York, Harper & Row, 1968.
37. Larsson L, Grimby G, Karlsson J: Muscle strength and speed of movement in relation to age and muscle morphology. *J Appl Physiol* 1979; 46:451–456.
38. Lieb F, Perry J: Quadriceps function. *J Bone Joint Surg* (Am) 1968; 50:1535–1548.
39. Maitland GD: *Peripheral Manipulation,* ed 2. London, Butterworths, 1977.
40. Mangine RE: Physical therapy of the knee. *Clin Phys Ther* 1988; 19:7–15.
41. Mankin HJ, Brandt KD: Biochemistry and metabolism of cartilage in osteoarthritis, in Moskowitz RW, et al (eds): *Osteoarthritis Diagnosis and Management.* Philadelphia, WB Saunders, 1984, pp 43–80.
42. Mariani P, Caruso I: An electromyographic investiga-

tion of subluxation of the patella. *J Bone Joint Surg (Am)* 1979; 61:169–171.

43. McConnell JS: The management of chondromalacia patella: A long term solution. *Austral J Physiother* 1986; 32:215–223.

44. McConnell JS: *McConnell Patellofemoral Treatment Plan Course Notes.* Santa Ana, Calif, 1991. Unpublished data.

45. McPoil TP, Broccato ML: The foot and ankle, in Gould J (ed): *Orthopedic and Sports Physical Therapy,* ed 2. St Louis, Mosby-Year Book, 1990, pp 313–341.

46. Mennell JM: *Joint Pain.* Boston, Little, Brown, 1964.

47. Merkow Rl, Soudry M, Insall JN: Patellar dislocation following total knee replacement. *J Bone Joint Surg (Am)* 1985; 67:1321–1327.

48. Murray MP, et al: Strength of isometric and isokinetic contractions. *Phys Ther* 1980; 60:412–419.

49. Nicholas JA, Scott WN: Major knee injuries in contact sports, in Helfet AJ (ed): *Disorders of the Knee,* ed 2. Philadelphia, JB Lippincott, 1982, pp 391–402.

50. Orlander R, et al: Skeletal muscle metabolism ultrastructure in relation to age in sedentary men. *Acta Physiol Scand* 1977; 101:351–361.

51. Palmitier RA, et al: Kinetic chain exercises in knee rehabilitation. *Sports Med* 1991; 11:402–413.

52. Petsching R, et al: Objectivation of the effects of knee problems on vastus medialis and vastus lateralis with EMG and dynamometry. *Eur J Phys Med Rehab* 1991; 2:50–54.

53. Rand JA, et al: Management of infected total knee arthroplasty. *Clin Orthop* 1986; 205:75–85.

54. Richardson C: The role of the knee musculature in high speed oscillating movements of the knee. *MTAA 4th Biennial Conference Proceedings,* Brisbane, Australia, 1985, pp 59–70.

55. Romness DW, Rand JA: The role of continuous passive motion following total knee arthroplasty. *Clin Orthop* 1987; 226:34–37.

56. Salter R, et al: The biological effects of continuous passive motion on the healing of full thickness defects in articular cartilage. *J Bone Joint Surg (Am)* 1980; 62:1232–1251.

57. Sapega A, et al: Biophysical factors in range of motion exercise, *Phys Sportsmed* 1981; 9:57–65.

58. Schmidt RA: *Motor Control and Learning,* ed 2 Champaign, Ill, Human Kinetics Publishers, 1988.

59. Scott NR, et al: *Principles of Sports Medicine,* Philadelphia, WB Saunders, 1984.

60. Souza DR, Gross MT: Comparison of vastus medialis obliquus: Vastus lateralis muscle integrated electromyographic ratios between healthy subjects and patients with patellofemoral pain, *Phys Ther* 1991; 71:310–316.

61. Spencer J, Hayes K, Alexander I: Knee joint effusion and quadriceps reflex inhibition in man. *Phys Med* 1984; 65:171–177.

62. Steindler A: *Kinesiology of the Human Body Under Normal and Pathological Conditions,* Springfield, Ill, Charles C Thomas, 1973.

63. Stokes M, Young A: Investigations of quadriceps inhibition, *Physiotherapy* 1984; 70:425–428.

64. Thompson RC: An experimental study of surface injury to articular cartilage and enzyme responses within the joint. *Clin Orthop* 1975; 107:239–246.

65. Tipton CM, et al: The influence of physical activity on ligaments and tendons. *Med Sci Sports Exerc* 1975; 7:165–175.

66. Townsend P, et al: Biomechanics of the human patella and its implications for condromalacia. *J Biomech* 1977; 10:403–407.

67. Traina SM, et al: Continuous passive motion following total knee arthroplasty. *Am J Knee Surg* 1991; 4:137–143.

68. Wells KF, Luttgens K: *Kinesiology,* ed 6. Philadelphia, WB Saunders, 1976.

69. Wigren A, Kolstad K, Brunk V: Formation of new menisci after polycentric knee arthroplasty. *Acta Orthop Scand* 1978; 49:615–621.

70. Voight ML, Wieder DL: Comparative reflex response times of vastus medialis and vastus lateralis in normal subjects and subjects with extensor mechanism dysfunction. *Am J Sports Med* 1991; 19:131–136.

Chapter 20

Leg and Ankle Injuries: An Orthopedic Perspective

Robert Karpman, M.D.

When a senior adult has lower extremity problems, attention is usually directed to the hip or knee joint: the hip owing to the possibility of fracture caused by decreased bone mass, and the knee primarily related to the likelihood of changes in the articular surfaces. However, "leg pain" is a common complaint among senior adults and its diagnosis and treatment are frequently more complex than attending to these frequently occurring hip or knee problems. This is true primarily because of the variety of sources from which the leg pain can derive, including neurologic, vascular, and musculoskeletal etiologies. In some instances more than one source can be responsible, such as vascular claudication occurring in addition to spinal stenosis, making the diagnosis even more confusing. It is therefore mandatory that a careful history and physical examination be performed in patients presenting with leg pain and efforts made to differentiate the multiple causes.

As with other problems of the anatomy, the leg is not immune to systemic changes. This is particularly true of the skeletal system, where bone mass decreases on a yearly basis beginning at age 30. A variety of factors are responsible for osteopenia, among them menopause, inadequate calcium intake, vitamin D deficiency, and use of alcohol or steroids. The result is increased bone fragility and likelihood of fracture, particularly in the areas of the distal radius, vertebral bodies, and proximal femur. We have also noted in our institutionalized, nonambulatory population that fractures of the tibia, fibula, and distal femur occur in almost the same frequency as fractures of the hip. Little research, however, has been directed in these anatomic areas in reference to bony architecture and the biomechanical stresses that would make these regions more vulnerable to fracture.

In the more active person, osteopenia can lead to other injuries such as stress fractures in the proximal tibia and calcaneus. Therapy is obviously directed toward increasing total bone mass or at least prevention of further bone loss both by pharmacologic means such as estrogens, calcium, vitamin D, and fluoride, as well as through increased exercise.

Other systemic factors of aging that predispose older patients to injury of the lower limb include decreased muscle strength, poor vision, and abnormal gait and posture.

Cybex testing has demonstrated significant changes in lower extremity muscle strength of senior adults compared with younger adults.[2, 5] With a decrease in muscle mass and response time, a person becomes more prone to injury from a fall since he or she cannot adequately respond by protecting the limb or provide adequate strength to prevent the fall. Brown,[1] Morey et al,[6] and Hopkins et al[3] have demonstrated, however, that exercise can indeed improve muscle strength in older people, perhaps leading to a decreased risk of injury.

Other systemic changes occurring with age that can impair or delay healing of injuries include immune compromise with increased risk of infection, diabetes, and vascular disease. All of these entities must be taken into account on managing a patient with lower extremity injury.

The etiology of leg pain can be divided into three

major categories: musculoskeletal, neurogenic, and vascular. Perhaps the easiest of the three to diagnose and treat is musculoskeletal pain, since the source and result are frequently visible (a history of trauma with an abnormal x-ray). Leg pain derived from neurogenic and vascular causes may be more insidious and difficult to distinguish, as will be discussed later.

MUSCULOSKELETAL PAIN

Specific injuries related to the musculoskeletal system include fractures, rupture of the Achilles tendon, bursitis and tendinitis, rupture of popliteal cyst, and osteonecrosis. Arthritis, which is frequently seen in other joints of the lower extremity, is rare in the ankle unless related to antecedent trauma. Diagnosis and management of arthritic joints is discussed in other chapters.

Fractures

As mentioned previously, osteopenia leads to increased bone fragility and fracture. The fact that bone mass is decreased also makes the management of fractures difficult in that internal fixation devices that rely on solid bony architecture are inadequate and must be supplemented with other materials including bone cement. In addition, the needs of the older patient with a fracture are much more significant than those of a younger patient. Of particular significance is early mobilization to prevent sequelae of bed rest, including pneumonia, incontinence, mental confusion, and death. Treatment must therefore be geared to allowing early mobilization of the patient.

Although the diagnosis of a fracture of the lower extremity is usually obvious on the basis of history and physical examination in some cases it may be more difficult to discern, particularly in patients with impaired cognitive function, where obtaining an adequate history of trauma is difficult and examination is complex. If a fracture is suggested by the presence of increasing pain, swelling, and/or deformity, radiographs of the involved bones are required, as well as of the bones immediately adjacent to the area of suspected fracture. In some cases, pain associated with lesions around the hip and femur may be referred to the lower extremity and a careful examination including radiographs of the entire

lower extremity may be indicated. Difficulties in interpretation of the radiographs can arise when the fracture is not obvious. Impacted fractures of the tibial plateau in a severely osteopenic patient may be misdiagnosed, as well as stress fractures in the midtibia, fibula, or calcaneus. Radioisotope bone scans may be useful in identifying a stress fracture when radiographs are inconclusive. An area of fracture will "light up" on bone scan.

The management of lower extremity fractures in the older patient will depend upon the type of injury, configuration of the bony fragments, but most importantly the overall physical and mental condition of the patient. We have found that in severely demented, nonambulatory patients the management of the lower extremity fracture in a routine cast or splint is extremely difficult and may lead to skin breakdown from the cast, not only in the injured extremity, but also in the normal extremity because of pressure and irritation from the casting materials. Also, care of a patient in a cast, particularly personal hygiene, is difficult owing to muscle and joint contractures; the result may be open skin ulcerations and infection. In some instances amputation of the limb, although considered to be extremely aggressive, has provided the optimum treatment, allowing for alleviation of pain, easy mobilization of the patient, perineal care, and prevention of serious infections. These, however, are rare instances; in most cases the standard principles of fracture care are used, including restoration of normal joint alignment, either through closed methods or open reduction and internal fixation. As mentioned previously, fixation of fractures in osteopenic bone can be difficult and may require augmentation with bone cement or external support. A thorough vascular examination of the lower extremity must also be done prior to operative intervention in order to assure that proper healing of the wounds can occur. A vigorous program of muscle strengthening and range of motion exercises should be performed immediately postoperatively. Various therapeutic modalities are discussed in Chapter 21.

Osteonecrosis

Another bony source of leg pain that must be considered in the elderly patient is osteonecrosis of the femoral condyle and/or tibial plateau. The diagnosis of osteonecrosis is often missed and the lesion often mistaken for arthritis of the knee or an internal derangement. Patients usually present with a history of increasing knee pain with ambulation, usually along the medial side of the knee. A history of specific trauma may or may not be obtained. Examination of the extremity demonstrates exquisite tenderness to palpation along either the medial femoral condyle or tibial plateau rather than along the joint line. X-rays may show some mild degenerative arthritis of the knee but are otherwise unremarkable. Bone scans are the best means of confirming the diagnosis. They initially will show increased uptake, followed by a loss of uptake as the disease progresses. Treatment is addressed to the symptoms and includes partial weight bearing and immobilization in a soft brace. Symptoms usually improve in 3 to 6 months; operative treatment is rarely indicated. Occasionally severe destruction of the distal femur or proximal tibia develops, leading to significant degenerative arthritis ultimately requiring total joint replacement.

Soft-Tissue Sources

Other musculoskeletal sources of leg pain are derived from soft tissues; they include ruptures of the Achilles tendon and plantaris tendon, popliteal (Baker's) cyst rupture, tendinitis, and bursitis.

Patients with a ruptured Achilles tendon or Baker's cyst tend to present with acute onset of pain and swelling in the calf. These conditions are often confused with deep venous thrombosis and patients are mistakenly given anticoagulant therapy. Achilles and plantaris tendon ruptures tend to occur in active people, particularly those involved in racquet sports. The diagnosis of an Achilles tendon rupture is made on the basis of history and a careful evaluation of the calf. Often a defect is present demonstrating a discontinuity of the Achilles tendon as well as a positive Thompson test result, in which the examiner squeezes the involved calf and the foot does not plantar flex. (In an intact tendon, squeezing of calf will cause plantar flexion of the foot.) A rupture of the plantaris tendon can present with similar complaints; however, the physical findings are more subtle. The treatment of Achilles tendon rupture remains controversial. Immobilization in a long leg cast has led to equivalent results as operative treatment; however, in most centers, complete ruptures, particularly in active people, tend to be treated operatively. A plantaris tendon rupture can be managed with partial weight bearing, progressing to a heel lift, in the involved extremity for 6 to 8 weeks. In either case, a vigorous physical therapy program must

follow in order for the patient to regain muscle strength and prevent future injury.

In the case of a ruptured Baker's cyst, the patient will not have a history of acute onset of pain following physical activity; however, the symptoms and signs will be acute, particularly swelling in the calf. As mentioned previously, this condition is often confused with deep venous thrombosis. The diagnosis can be made on the basis of an arthrogram of the knee demonstrating the presence of a Baker's cyst frequently with a leak of contrast into the soft tissues. A deep venous thrombosis can be ruled out easily with duplex ultrasonography or a venogram. Treatment of the popliteal rupture consists of rest and use of compressive stockings, followed by progressive weight bearing and activity.

Tendinitis in the Achilles tendon can be diagnosed on palpation of the tendon and occasionally calcifications are seen on plain radiographs. Treatment should consist of rest and use of a heel lift followed by progressive activity. Nonsteroidal anti-inflammatory drugs are often used; however, an injection of corticosteroids into the tendon or tendon sheath is *absolutely* contraindicated. Several reports of rupture following steroid injections into the tendon have been reported in the literature.[4] If necessary, surgical release of the tendon sheath can be done with minimal morbidity. In some patients, it is difficult to differentiate Achilles tendinitis from calcaneal bursitis. In calcaneal bursitis there is swelling and pain at the attachment of the Achilles tendon with the swelling more profound between the tendon and the calcaneus, rather than uniform pain and swelling along the tendon sheath. Aspiration of the bursa is possible. An injection of steroid into the bursa can be performed; however, extreme caution should be used to assure that the steroid is not placed into the tendon or tendon sheath.

Night Cramps

The final musculoskeletal source of leg pain is night cramps. The cause of this condition is extremely difficult to diagnose and treatment may not be effective. It is important to differentiate chronic leg cramps from other sources of leg pain, particularly those of neurogenic or vascular origin, and the diagnosis is usually one of exclusion. Leg cramps are usually treated with some type of quinine derivative; most patients' symptoms demonstrate improvement. In some patients, however, quinine causes gastrointestinal problems, making treatment difficult. Some physical therapy modalities, including heat and calf stretching, may be beneficial.

VASCULAR PAIN

Vascular sources of leg pain include either arterial insufficiency, resulting stenosis of the vessels to the lower extremity, or venous insufficiency leading to stasis with progressive swelling of the lower extremity and ulceration. Patients with arterial claudication will have a history of progressive cramping with ambulation relieved by rest. In extreme cases, the cramping will be present even at rest.

The diagnosis of vascular claudication can be made on the basis of history as well as a physical examination demonstrating decreased peripheral pulses. A simple technique to determine the severity of the illness is the ischemic index, in which sequential blood pressure readings are taken of the lower extremity and compared with those of the upper extremity. This can help delineate the area of stenosis and is also quite predictive in terms of wound healing following operative intervention for any lower extremity problem.[3, 7]

The treatment of vascular claudication is dependent upon the area of stenosis and may include bypass, angioplasty, use of vasodilators, and in severe cases amputation. It is important to note at this point that patients who are elderly and have below- or above-knee amputations can function quite well with lower extremity prostheses given appropriate rehabilitation. Age should not be considered a contraindication to providing prosthetic rehabilitation in elderly lower extremity amputees.

NEUROGENIC PAIN

Patients with leg pain of neurogenic origin also have a history of cramping and pain with progressive ambulation. This is particularly true in cases of spinal stenosis.

Leg pain from a neurogenic origin often presents with symptoms and findings similar to those found in vascular occlusion. Patients complain of increasing pain in the leg and calf that is often relieved by rest. In patients with spinal stenosis symptoms can also be relieved with flexion of the spine. Patients with severe spinal stenosis tend to ambulate in a flexed position. Pain is also increased on extension of the spine. Unlike radiculopathy, the pain resulting from spinal stenosis is aching in origin and may not radiate. A careful neurologic examination may demonstrate decreased strength in both lower extremities as well as hyporeflexia and hypesthesias. The symptoms and signs do not occur in any specific nerve root distribution and are frequently bilateral.

Radiographs of the lumbosacral spine demonstrate increased degenerative changes as well as narrowing of the spinal canal. The most definitive method of confirming the diagnosis is with a computed tomographic (CT) scan demonstrating the presence of stenosis in the central portion of the canal or in the lateral gutters near the neural foramina.

Treatment of severe spinal stenosis is surgical and requires decompression of the spinal cord. Less severe cases can be treated with nonsteroidal anti-inflammatory drugs, therapy, and occasionally epidural steroid injection.

Other neurogenic causes of leg pain include lumbosacral radiculopathy and peripheral neuropathies.

The most common peripheral neuropathy is associated with diabetes. Patients complain of hypesthesias or anesthesia in the feet. A careful evaluation should be performed to rule out diabetic neuropathy. A careful examination of the foot is mandatory in patients with peripheral neuropathy in order to rule out any skin irritation not perceived by the patient, which might ultimately lead to infections. The best method of treatment for these problems is prevention. All patients with peripheral neuropathy should be instructed on careful routine evaluation of their feet.

More infrequent peripheral neuropathies include Charcot-Marie-Tooth disease and idiopathic peripheral neuropathies, all leading to decreased sensation with the potential for injury and infection. A careful neurologic examination as well as electromyograms (EMGs) and nerve conduction velocity tests can confirm the diagnosis.

As mentioned previously, most peripheral neuropathies cannot be treated specifically; however, the underlying disorder should be evaluated. In particular, determining the presence of diabetes and protection of the feet are of utmost importance in order to prevent injury and infections. Once a complication has developed the morbidity rate is extremely high.

SUMMARY

In summary, leg pain is a common complaint among senior adults. A careful evaluation should be performed to determine the exact etiology of the leg pain, particularly whether it is of musculoskeletal, vascular, or neurologic origin. A careful history and physical examination can frequently lead to the correct diagnosis. Obviously, the treatment of the disorders will depend upon their etiologies. Several basic principles should be utilized, however, including early mobilization of the patient in order to prevent the sequelae of chronic bed rest as well as careful evaluation of the skin in order to prevent the possibility of ulceration and infections.

REFERENCES

1. Brown MH: Effects of a low intensity exercise program on selected physical performance characteristics of 60 to 71 year olds. *Aging* 1991; 3:129–139.

2. Gersten JW: Effect of exercise on muscle function decline with aging. *West J Med* 1991; 154:579–582.
3. Gibbons GW, et al: Noninvasive prediction of amputation level in diabetic patients. *Arch Surg* 1979; 114:1253–1257.
3. Hopkins DR, et al: Effect of low-impact aerobic dance on the functional fitness of elderly women. *Gerontologist* 1990; 30:189–192.
4. Karpman R, McComb J, Volz R: Tendon rupture following local steroid injection. *Postgrad Med* 1980; 68:169–174.
5. Laforest S, et al: Effects of age and regular exercise on muscle strength and endurance. *Eur J Appl Physiol Occup Physiol* 1990; 60:104–111.
6. Morey MC, et al: Two year trends in physical performance following supervised exercise among community-dwelling older veterans. *J Am Geriatr Soc* 1991; 39:549–554.
7. Wagner FW Jr., Buggs H: Use of Doppler ultrasound in determining healing levels in diabetic dysvascular lower extremity problems, in Bergan JJ, Yao JST (eds): *Gangrene and Severe Ischemia of the Lower Extremities.* New York, Grune & Stratton, 1978, pp 131–138.

Chapter 21

Leg and Ankle Injuries: A Rehabilitation Perspective

Perry S. Esterson, M.S., P.T.

Marc O. Meadows, P.T.

This chapter's area of focus is the active older adult and the rehabilitation of orthopedic injuries in this population. The fitness boom of the 1970s and 1980s has led to greater numbers of older adults participating in athletic activities. Older people have traditionally played golf and tennis. The popularity of organized running, walking, swimming, and cycling competition has brought forth opportunities for a more active life style.[28, 32, 38, 51, 60] We now have professional masters golf and tennis, and senior adult baseball, softball, and soccer leagues. This new, or renewed, interest in fitness has also brought about an increase in orthopedic injuries.

While many older persons have health problems related to their age, they are just as reluctant to give up their pursuit of exercise activities as their younger counterparts. The older adult may have previous experience to guide his or her exercise program, but this apparent advantage may also be diminished by prior injuries. Physical training practices that were advocated in the past, such as "ballistic" stretching, "don't drink water when playing," or "no pain, no gain," are now considered incorrect or even dangerous. A review of the body's changes with aging, particularly changes relating to the lower extremity, will further better understanding of the prevention and treatment of orthopedic injuries in this population.

Many orthopedic injuries of the lower extremities, in both young and old persons, result from errors in exercise programs. These mistakes include exercising too fast, too often, or too rapidly increasing in pace or distance.[18] Any of the above changes in the exercise program may result in loading the musculoskeletal system above its ability to respond to stress without breakdown. Long-distance runners are particularly susceptible to overuse injuries because of the tremendous demands on their lower extremities. Up to 250% of body weight is absorbed by the musculoskeletal system at heel strike.[22, 35, 36] Foot strike will take place between 800 and 2,000 times per mile while running.[12, 22, 35] Indeed, it is easy to imagine the overload of the musculoskeletal system that can take place with exercise at a high intensity. Progressive loading of stress leads to strengthening the components of the musculoskeletal system. Overloading or overuse of the body leads to a chain of events resulting in increased inflammation of soft tissues and possible bone fracture.

ANATOMIC REVIEW

The leg is composed of the tibia, fibula, and talus, and the ligamentous, nervous, and circulatory tissues contained within the skin.

The tibia begins with its concave tibial condyles separated by the intercondylar eminence and centered between anterior and posterior intercondylar areas.[24] The condyles, smooth with a covering of hyaline cartilage, are protected from great weight-bearing stress by the medial and lateral fibrocartilag-inous menisci which are positioned to move with the tibia in flexion and extension, but also allow movement on the tibial condyle.

Numerous ligaments attach to the tibia in this area. The anterior and posterior cruciate ligaments insert anterior and posterior to the intercondylar eminence. Medially and wrapping posteriorly just inferior to the medial flange of the condyle, the medial collateral ligament inserts to help with valgus restraint. The lateral collateral ligament inserts on a small area on the head of the fibula to restrain against varus force.

The tibia articulates with the articular facet of the upper end of the fibula posterolaterally and inferior to the lateral tibial condyle. The fibula continues distad to articulate again with the tibia along its distal and most lateral surface and then protrudes further outward to form the lateral malleolus. The body of the tibia continues cylindrically distal, gradually flaring to form a medial malleolus, and articulating with the fibula forms the mortise for the ankle joint. A site of numerous ligamentous attachments, these will be examined more closely below.

Muscular insertion, as it defines lower extremity function, is extensive about the leg. The quadriceps gains insertion to the proximal anterior tibia, albeit with a rather short moment arm, into the tibial tuberosity. This tuberosity acts with the patella to greatly increase the moment arm of the extensor mechanism. Inferiorly and medially to the tuberosity of the tibia is the combined insertion of the three slender tendons that comprise the pes anserine muscle group that originates on the pelvis insertion. The most medial, the semitendinosus, is followed next laterally by the gracilis and sartorius. These three muscles help to flex and internally rotate the tibia on the femur. On the medial side of the tibial spine, running distal from the tibial tuberosity, the tibialis anterior has an origin nearly two thirds the length of the tibia.

The extensor musculature, important for dorsiflexion of the foot, preceding both the heel strike and swing phases of gait, has its origin high and along the mid third of the fibula and interosseous membrane. The extensor digitorum longus, by exerting an eversion moment by passing lateral to the subtalar joint of the foot, helps to counteract the inversion moment of the tibialis anterior and produce straight dorsiflexion. Lateral to this extensor musculature, the peroneal group of evertors has its origins solely upon the fibula. Starting superiorly, just distal to the fibular head, the peroneus longus originates,

followed by the peroneus brevis, and lastly by the peroneus tertius, slightly medial, and occasionally inserting with the extensor group.

The bony architecture of the tibia continues much as in the anterior tibia with the exception of a notable soleal line running distal and medial marking the origin of the soleus. At the distal end of the tibia a medial flaring of the medial malleolus serves as a fulcrum for several tendons of the posterior musculature. This malleolus also serves as a site of insertion for the deltoid ligament complex medial at the ankle.

The posterior musculature can be seen first with the insertions of the hamstring group. Medially the semimembranosus, just distal to the medial tibial condyle, can exert rotatory force. Laterally, near the posterior aspect of the fibular head, the biceps femoris gains its insertion into the leg where it exerts a rotatory force upon the knee if isolated in function. Distally, the popliteus muscle gains insertion onto the leg from its origin at the lateral femoral epicondyle. This muscle flexes and internally rotates the knee while running broadly and distally on the tibia. The deepest of the musculature of the leg includes the tibialis posterior, flexor digitorum longus, and flexor hallucis longus.

The tibialis posterior originates from medial about the posterior aspect of the tibia, the interosseus membrane, and the medial aspect of the fibula to course posterior to the medial malleolus of the tibia and insert upon the plantar aspect of the midfoot. This muscle is important in gait, both to invert and plantarflex the ankle, but more important it helps to control the pronation of the midfoot as it progressively accepts more force in gait. The flexor digitorum longus originates at the mid third of the posterior tibia and its tendon courses posteriorly around the medial malleolus to run through the plantar surface of the foot to its insertion upon the plantar base of the distal phalanx. The flexor hallucis longus, originating solely at the posterior fibula, crosses the posterior surface medially to also course posterior to the medial malleolus before its tendon runs again through the plantar surface of the foot to the base of the first phalanx.

The posterior musculature is composed of, in succeedingly superficial layers, the soleus and the gastrocnemius. The soleus originates medial to the soleal line on the tibia and immediately distal to the insertion of the popliteus muscle, and laterally about the proximal one fourth of the fibula. Distally, its fibers insert into the Achilles tendon, and further distally this tendon inserts into the posterior aspect of the calcaneus. Its function of plantarflexion of the ankle is aided by the gastrocnemius which, being longer through its origins posteriorly at the medial and lateral femoral condyles, adds great strength to plantarflexion. Since it originates proximal to the knee, the gastrocnemius is also active in knee flexion, though its poor leverage prevents primary function here. The plantaris muscle closely parallels the gastrocnemius, but owing to its small size contributes little to function.

Of concern in the leg neurologically is the sciatic nerve which forms from branches L4–S1 of the lumbar plexus. As it nears the leg, the common peroneal nerve is given off to course lateral to the knee until it branches into the deep peroneal and superficial peroneal nerves. The deep peroneal provides immediate innervation to the tibialis anterior muscle before becoming sensory distally and medially. The superficial peroneal nerve, distal to the deep nerve, courses around the head of the fibula and provides motor innervation to the peroneal group.

The tibial nerve continues distally to innervate the gastrocnemius, soleus, and deep flexor musculature before coursing posteriorly around the medial malleolus to provide innervation to the foot.

The arterial supply to the leg arrives posterior to the knee through the popliteal artery and anteriorly through a smaller-diameter anterior tibial artery. Distal to the knee, the popliteal artery becomes the posterior tibial artery and provides circulation to the posterior and medial musculature before coursing inferomedially to the ankle on approaching the foot. The anterior tibial artery provides circulation to the extensor musculature before crossing the ankle as the dorsalis pedis artery before entering the foot.

It appears that as form dictates function, no further musculature originates on the tibia as we follow the bone distally. The musculature presented here so far as necessary in proper gait would not be afforded appropriate leverage with any further distal origin. The muscles and their tendinous portions must function with appropriate leverage over the articular function of the ankle and subtalar joints to be effective in gait.

The trochlea of the talus, the only bone to support all of the body weight, provides articulation with the tibia and fibula at the medial and lateral surfaces of the talus. Root et al[52,53] describe the axis of the ankle joint passing from medial to lateral as follows: lateral, plantar, and posterior to medial, dorsal, and anterior. Joint motion about the ankle ranges from dorsiflexion, or eversion, to plantarflexion, or inversion.[67] The talus is wider transversely

and anteriorly than posteriorly, limiting dorsiflexion and allowing a greater degree of movement on plantarflexion. Upon the talus, there are sites of ligamentous attachment medially for the deltoid and the talofibular complexes. The talus, positioned medially upon the calcaneus, provides passage for the previously mentioned tendons and neurovascular structures.

The subtalar joint is the talar articulation with the calcaneus. Motion about this joint is triplanar owing to the alignment of the joint axis. The joint axis is positioned 42 degrees from the horizontal and 16 degrees medial to the sagittal plane (when the foot hits the ground) to provide inversion and eversion to a greater extent than in dorsiflexion and plantarflexion.[53, 67]

The calcaneus provides three convex facets[59] to the articulation, an anterior, middle, and posterior facet, to articulate with three corresponding facets on the inferior surface of the talus. Connecting the two bones and guiding movement of the joint is the interosseous talocalcaneal ligament. As the talus abducts and adducts with motion during gait, the articular surfaces and ligamentous structures limit eversion and inversion of the calcaneus. The subtalar joint has been found to be an integral part of the hindfoot's capacity to transmit torque between the leg and foot.[47] Compensatory mechanisms demanded as a result of abnormal leg or foot biomechanics can place great stress upon the subtalar or any lower extremity articulations and lead to degeneration.

EFFECTS OF AGING ON THE LOWER EXTREMITY

Aging is a complex process that is affected by both activity and inactivity. Changes in flexibility, bone density (osteoporosis), and muscle mass have been documented.[6, 8, 41, 56, 61] A decrease in lower extremity flexibility may lead to a short stride.[49] Tight or inflexible Achilles tendons cause an elevated calcaneus on heel strike leading to an increase in compensatory pronation. Related injuries include plantar fasciitis, posterior tibial tendinitis or periostitis (shin splints), and peroneal tendinitis.[22, 25]

As collagen fibers age, they become less compliant owing to a decrease in water content. Menard and Stanish[41] have shown that physical training increases the strength of collagenous fibers such as muscle and tendon. A decrease in flexibility results from less flexible ligaments and tendons. Hagen,[23] using the sit-and-reach test, demonstrated that women maintain better low back and hamstring flexibility by losing 0.15 cm/year vs. 0.2 cm/year in men. Nicholas and colleagues[45, 46] presented a skeletal linkage system to demonstrate that flexibility in one part of the body can affect another part.

The causes of osteoporosis in women are multiple. Many women lose more than 30% of their bone mass before the age of 70 years, whereas men rarely have osteoporotic problems until their eighth decade.[8, 41, 56, 61] Activity has been shown to hypertrophy bone when sufficient stress is applied.[56] Thus physical activity may contribute positively to bone density, but overloading of the skeletal system may lead to breakdown.

The decline in exercise capacity during aging can be caused by decrease in blood flow to skeletal muscle, changes in fatigue perception, decrease in lean body (muscle) mass, and decrease in physical activity.[6, 62] Significant strength gains using progressive resistance exercises have been demonstrated in people from 50 to 96 years old.[13, 19, 20, 48] In a group of veterans aged 65 to 74 years, improvements in cardiovascular function and flexibility gained in the early stages of an exercise program were maintained for at least 2 years.[43]

CLINICAL EXAMINATION

A systematic and detailed evaluation is the foundation of all treatment. A thorough review of the patient's history and subjective complaints will guide the examiner in the objective section of the evaluation. Based on the subjective and objective assessment, the treatment program is conceived and then constantly reevaluated as treatment progresses.

History

The patient's history is obtained to elicit any activities that may have caused the injury or problem that brought him or her to the practitioner. Specific questions should include:

- How did the injury occur (the exact mechanism if possible)?
- Over what length of time did the injury develop (acute or chronic)?

- Has the injury lessened or worsened?
- Has the injury moved or expanded into another body part?
- What makes the injury worse?
- What makes the injury less severe?

The patient's general health is reviewed to obtain a holistic view. Conditions such as diabetes, cardiovascular heart disease, and osteoporosis need to be identified as they may affect treatment of the older patient. The practitioner should identify prior injuries that may influence the current problem. Finally, the examiner will inquire about medications the patient is using.

The short- and long-term goals of the patient should be assessed and compared with the objective findings and the proposed treatment plan. In this manner, the practitioner becomes aware of the patient's time frame and the patient understands the medical and rehabilitation requirements for a successful return to activity.

Objective Signs

Following the history and subjective information obtained from the patient, the examiner should obtain reproducible or objective data. The evaluation of the leg and ankle will take place both in the weight-bearing and non–weight-bearing position. Evaluating the injured part statically and dynamically will give the examiner a better idea of the functional level of the patient. Case[14] has listed the following items for assessment:

Posture
Weight-bearing status
Sensation and skin changes
   Areas of pain
   Areas of numbness
   Areas of hypersensitivity
   Skin color
Measurements
   Range of motion
   Strength
   Joint play
   Stability
   Alignment
   Gait
   Balance
   Footwear

When necessary, the examiner may palpate the femoral, popliteal, posterior tibial, and dorsalis pedis pulses to determine circulatory status. The joints above and below the affected part should be screened to rule out referred symptoms. If available, a slow-motion video camera will enable the examiner to more fully evaluate gait, both walking and running.

TREATMENT AND PROGNOSIS

Tibial Stress Syndrome

This syndrome is a continuum of injuries ranging from posterior tibial tendinitis and periostitis to stress fracture. Pain is present distal to the knee and proximal to the ankle. Persons participating in weight-bearing aerobic exercise such as running, walking, or aerobic dance may sustain these injuries. Pain presents in the distal third of the medial tibial ridge. A careful analysis of the exercise program will often reveal either a too rapid progression in running, an increase in speed, or an increase in downhill impact loading.[57] In the first case, the patient is unprepared to exercise at the chosen level of intensity or frequency and overstress of the medial tibial border results. The last two cases both lead to increased pronation which exerts excessive pull of the posterior tibialis at its insertion into the tibia.[37] A tight gastrocnemius-soleus complex will also elevate the calcaneus in heel strike leading to compensatory increased pronation exacerbating this syndrome.[25,40]

If allowed to continue, traction on the tibia will lead to a stress fracture.[1, 25, 37] The differential diagnosis includes tendonitis, periostitis, and stress fracture. Point tenderness is present at the insertion of the posterior tibialis into the tibia. Manual muscle testing will be normal. Flexibility of the gastrocnemius-soleus muscle group will often be limited. To check for tightness of this muscle group the patient should fully squat, maintaining the feet in parallel and in contact with the floor. If tightness is present, the heels will rise off the floor or the patient will fall backward. Some older patients may lack adequate range of motion in the hips, knees, or ankles to perform this test. Radiographs are often negative for weeks in revealing a stress fracture or periosteal reaction. A bone scan will make the definitive diagnosis.

Another form of shin splint is pain in the anterior leg, but the mechanism of injury is different. In this condition, there is a relative imbalance between the plantar- and dorsiflexors, with the former being much stronger. Treatment is aimed at strengthening the tibialis anterior, extensor digitorum, and extensor hallucis longus using either weights or latex tubing for resistance. A neoprene sleeve on the lower leg will support the inflamed area, and stretching exercises of the posterior musculature will maintain flexibility. Ice may be applied to the anterior muscle group to reduce inflammation.

A complete examination must include a biomechanical evaluation of the foot in relation to the leg. The patient is viewed while bearing weight and the feet are observed for excessive pronation or supination. The height of the medial arch is compared to that in the non–weight-bearing position. The extent of varus or valgus angulation and the internal or external rotation of the foot in relation to the leg are checked. Evaluating the walking and running gait from anterior and posterior using video or film analysis with slow motion will aid in detecting abnormalities not easily seen at normal speeds. The use of a treadmill has been validated for this purpose.[11] In the midstance phase, the heel should be everted approximately 10 degrees or less. The examiner should be directly behind the patient to make this determination to avoid evaluating foot position in a tangential view. The plantar surface of the foot should be inspected for callus formation indicating areas of increased weight-bearing stress. Callus in a flexible foot that pronates excessively will be found under the second and third metatarsal heads and the medial great toe. A more rigid foot will demonstrate callus under the first and fifth metatarsal heads with minimal callus under the central metatarsal heads.[26] For a more complete review of the biomechanical evaluation of the foot, ankle, and leg, see Hunt[26] and McPoil and Brocato.[39]

Treatment should be directed to both the symptoms and causes. Correcting flaws in the exercise program will reduce the excessive load in the tibia. Because of the more brittle and inelastic nature of collagen in the older patient, a longer recovery period may be anticipated.[41] Reducing exercise intensity and duration, and changing from a hard to a soft surface will reduce stress to an acceptable level. Alternative exercises, such as biking, swimming, running in a pool, or water aerobics, may be substituted as long as no pain is present during these activities.[9, 12]

To correct overpronation, which is the biomechanical cause of the stress, support is provided to the longitudinal arch either by taping (Fig 21–1) or orthosis (Fig 21–2).[22] Often, immediate pain relief is achieved by taping the longitudinal arch of the foot.

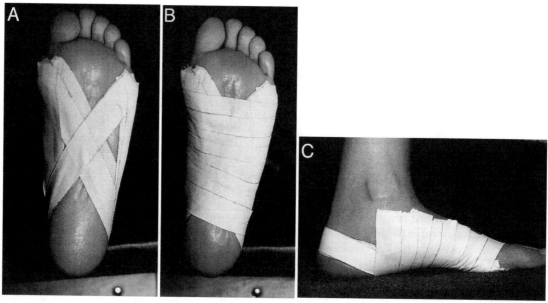

FIG 21–1.
A, longitudinal arch taping; base strips starting at first and fifth metatarsal heads. **B,** longitudinal arch taping; lateral-to- medial arch support strips. **C,** longitudinal arch taping; medial view.

However, Ator et al[3] found that support from adhesive taping of the medial longitudinal arch was significantly diminished after 10 minutes of exercise.

Proper athletic shoes will add to the successful return of the athlete. When overpronation is present, shoes with stiff and long medial counters and good medial foot support should be worn. For this condition, a straight lasted shoe will provide more support than one with a curved last. An inexpensive shoe with little support or shock absorption will often exacerbate the problem.

The active older adult must follow a comprehensive flexibility program of prolonged and gentle stretching of the lower extremities and low back. These muscle groups include the gastrocnemius and soleus, quadriceps, hamstrings, iliotibial bands, and low back extensors and thoracolumbar fascia (Figs 21–3 to 21–5). Stretching of each muscle group should be done without pain and with a sensation of a mild stretch. Each stretch should be maintained for a minimum of 30 seconds to help overcome the inelasticity in the collagen of the older adult. The exercising adult should warm up with light exercises or calisthenics before stretching and not use stretching as a substitute for warm-up exercises.

Additional pain relief can be achieved with the use of nonsteroidal anti-inflammatory agents and either moist heat or ice applications. Wallace[64] has found microampere electrical stimulation to effectively decrease inflammation and pain in both acute and chronic conditions. The key to successful return is the progressive loading of stress in the patient's exercise program. Pain should be monitored as the duration of exercise is increased. The presence of pain indicates that the level of intensity needs to be reduced. Full return to prior levels of activity can be expected.

Stress Fractures

Stress fractures result from the bone's inability to withstand the forces placed upon it. The metatarsal shafts, distal fibula, and proximal tibia are the

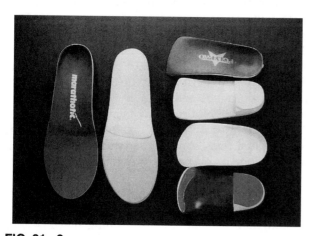

FIG 21–2.
Various orthotic devices.

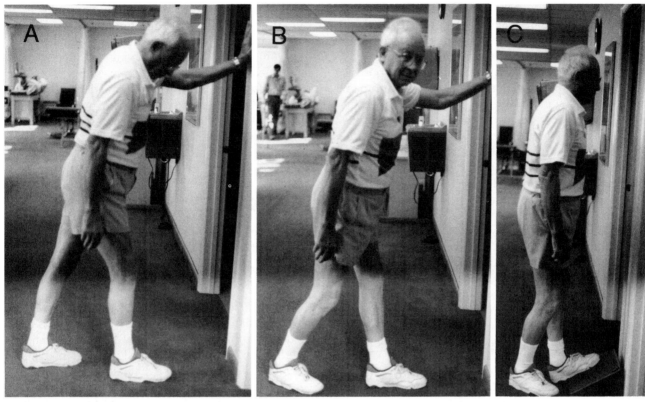

FIG 21–3.
Flexibility exercises. **A,** gastrocnemius stretch (back leg). **B,** soleus stretch (back leg). Note that knee is flexed to relax gastrocnemius. **C,** gastrocnemius stretch using wedge board.

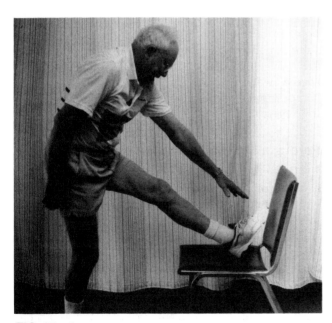

FIG 21–4.
Flexibility exercises: hamstring stretch.

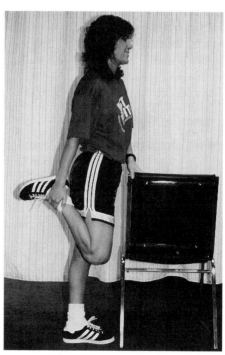

FIG 21–5.
Flexibility exercises: quadriceps stretch.

most common sites.[12] The site of the stress fracture will be point-tender. Plain films in the first month may be inconclusive. A bone scan can be used to make a definitive diagnosis. Healing fractures will show new periosteal bone formation. Osteoporosis is a significant problem in the older woman and pain over a bony site must be carefully evaluated. A complete history and detailed review of the patient's training and competitive program is required to determine the level of intensity to which he or she can return. If exercise-related errors are present, a presumptive diagnosis of stress fracture may be made. Percussing the affected bone at a site away from the painful part (the tap test) may elicit pain.[2, 55] The older adult who is relatively inflexible and has a rigid, high-arched foot has a decreased ability to absorb shock. These persons are at higher risk of stress fractures. The presence of callus formation over the lateral border of the foot and over the first and fifth metatarsal heads demonstrates the small area of contact in these feet. This patient requires more cushioning in the exercise shoe or the use of a soft accommodative orthosis to help absorb shock.

Return to activity is gradual and must be without pain. A recovery period of 4 to 6 weeks may be expected. Treatment follows a program of relative rest. Running or walking on land that produces pain is not permitted, but running or walking in a swimming pool is acceptable as there is no overloading impact to the lower extremity. Running vests are used to support the body while in water that is over the runner's head. Normal land running may be started when there is no pain or tenderness over the bone.

Compartmental Syndromes

Increased pressure within the fascial compartments of the leg can produce symptoms of pain and tightness during and after exercise. This condition must be differentiated from shin splints and stress fractures. Pain in any of the anterior, lateral, or posterior compartments of the leg usually starts during exercise. Rest may relieve the discomfort, but often symptoms may be present for hours after exercise is completed. Weakness, tenderness, a sensation of tightness of the dorsiflexors, or numbness in the anterior leg indicates involvement of the anterior compartment. Similar symptoms in the peroneal musculature are present in the lateral compartmental syndrome. Pain felt medial and deep to the tibia indicates a problem in the posterior compartment.

The increased pressure within a muscle compartment leads to a local ischemia resulting in pain. Various authors have described techniques to measure intramuscular pressure to diagnose a compartmental syndrome.[4, 54, 68] Treatment should be directed at relieving excessive compartmental pressure. Deep connective tissue massage may facilitate decreasing compartment pressure by making the overtight fascia more elastic and allowing expansion of the compartment during exercise. Also, altering the exercise program to reduce intensity, duration, and pace may enable the patient to continue, as compartmental pressures are proportional to walking speeds.[34] If conservative measures fail, then a fasciotomy may be performed. After soft tissue healing, a progressive return to exercises and running is started. Full range of motion and strength should be restored before returning to prior activity levels.

Intermittent Claudication

Pain that develops with activity but diminishes or disappears with rest is indicative of intermittent claudication. The posterior tibial, dorsalis pedis, and femoral pulses should be palpated bilaterally and compared for strength and vigor. The popliteal pulse is often difficult to palpate and is therefore an unreliable indicator. Obstruction of the femoral artery has been found by one of us (P.S.E.) both in the proximal femur and distally in the popliteal fossa. Referral to a vascular specialist is required to determine the extent of the obstruction or occlusion. Exercise has been shown to increase collateral circulation.[66] Some investigators suggest walking to the point of severe claudication, resting until the pain subsides, then returning to walking, and repeating this cycle for 20 to 30 minutes.[5] Graded exercises such as walking, biking, running, or swimming may be appropriate if the intermittent claudication is not too severe.

Peroneal Tendinitis

Caused by excessive shearing stresses,[63] or subluxating or dislocating tendons, peroneal tendinitis will present with pain and focal tenderness about the lateral malleolus. Pain is produced with either resistance or stretching of the peroneals, and crepitus is present in the tendon sheaths. In a chronically unstable ankle, the evertors of the foot may become overstressed by functioning as a secondary lateral stabilizer of the ankle. In the acute phase, treatment includes icing, anti-inflammatory drugs, and a rehabilitation program to strengthen the lateral muscles. This can be accomplished with rubber tubing exercises, balance board activities, or by moving the ankle through motions in a container of rice. Orthotic control to place the foot in a neutral position may also help reduce compensatory stresses.[22] Peroneal tendons that remain unstable around the lateral malleolus will require surgical intervention. Athletic taping or commercial ankle braces will not keep the peroneal tendons in a reduced anatomic position.

Achilles Tendon Problems

Problems of the gastrocnemius-soleus complex are common injuries in active older adults. The most serious of these injuries is rupture of the Achilles tendon, most often found in athletes over 30 years of age.[7, 29] Partial tears of the Achilles tendon and medial head of the gastrocnemius at the muscle-tendon junction or complete rupture of the plantaris tendon is less severe but frequently sustained. Achilles tendinitis is also common, and may require a long recovery period.[33, 44]

Rupture.—The cause of Achilles tendon rupture remains unresolved. Fox et al[21] suggest that repetitive microtrauma causes chronic degeneration in the tendon. Chronic degeneration typically is found in an area 2 to 6 cm above the calcaneus.[21] Inglis and Sculco[27] postulated that the tendon rupture was a malfunction of the normal inhibitory mechanism in the musculotendinous unit which prevents failure from excessive or uncoordinated muscle contraction. Corticosteroid injections have been implicated as a predisposing cause of rupture.[31] Beskin et al[7] reported that 3 of 42 patients with ruptured Achilles tendons had been injected 3 to 6 weeks before the time of rupture. With a complete rupture, most patients complain of being hit by a "bullet" on the back of their leg and are unable to continue with their activity.[10] The patient is unable to push off on the affected foot or stand on the toes. Using Thompson's test, the examiner squeezes the calf and looks for a resultant plantarflexion of the foot (Fig 21–6). When positive, plantarflexion is absent.[50, 55] Manual muscle testing will reveal absent or extremely weak plantarflexion. Swelling and tenderness in the area of the rupture are present. Magnetic resonance imaging has been shown to clearly delineate between hemorrhage and soft tissue structures and define the condition, separation, and orientation of the ends of a torn Achilles tendon.[30] Standard radiographs demonstrate soft tissue swelling, calcium deposition, or a traction spur on the superior aspect of the calcaneus extending into the substance of the tendon.[30, 33]

Orthopedic consultation is necessary as either surgery or immobilization will be the treatment of choice. Casting in the equinus position has been suggested for as little as 6 to 8 weeks, with extended protection against dorsiflexion for an additional 12 weeks.[7, 10] Gentle active range-of-motion exercises may be started upon cast removal and progressive return of dorsiflexion over the course of 6 to 8 months is expected. Excellent return of strength has been found by Beskin et al[7] and Bradley and Tibone,[10] but the latter noted a decrease in endurance testing. The latter also found that those patients with a longer course of physical therapy had better endurance scores. Maintaining aerobic conditions on the stationary bike or in the swimming pool is essential. Full return to preinjury activity level is not expected for 12 months.

Partial Tear.—Although less severe than a complete rupture, a partial tear will still require several months for complete recovery. The initial symptoms will be the same as above except that Thompson's test will be negative. Immobilization may be used, again in the plantarflexed position, to reduce tension on the tendon. Because of the lengthened tendon, there may be residual weakness in the plantarflexors. Once adequate healing has taken place, vigorous strengthening of all the plantarflexors is essential for safe and effective return to sports. Heel lifts up to ⅜ in. may be used to provide biomechanical support.

Partial Tear of the Medial Head of the Gastrocnemius and Plantaris Rupture.—Both of these injuries produce pain in the posterior calf, but generally heal rapidly. The patient will feel as though the calf has been hit sharply, but active plantarflexion is present. Pain is usually present anywhere along the length of the plantaris tendon. Initial treatment consists of compressive wrapping, icing, and agents to reduce inflammation. Crutches may initially be used to reduce pain on ambulation. Active range-of-motion and light resistive exercises may be instituted as soon as pain allows.

Tears of the medial head of the gastrocnemius will present with pain at the musculotendinous junction. Local swelling and ecchymosis may be present and a rent at the site of the injury may be palpated. Active plantarflexion is intact. Thompson's test is negative. Magnetic resonance imaging can be used to differentiate between a plantaris and medial head gastrocnemius rupture.[42] Treatment is the same as for the plantaris rupture with the addition

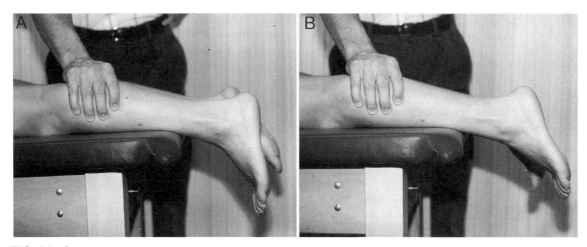

FIG 21–6.
Thompson's test. **A,** positive test results with no plantar flexion as the examiner squeezes the calf. **B,** negative test results with plantar flexion as the examiner squeezes the calf.

of massage over the site of injury to prevent excessive scarring. With symptoms of calf pain, phlebitis must be ruled out before initiating rehabilitation.

Achilles Tendinitis and Tenosynovitis.—Pain in the Achilles tendon affects both the sedentary person and the trained athlete. The intensity of the patient's activity level may be too advanced or strenuous for his or her musculoskeletal condition. For walkers and runners, a change in terrain or shoes will bring about this problem.

Nelen et al[44] describes Achilles tendinitis as presenting in three stages. In the first stage, the peritendinous tissue is thickened and may be adherent to the tendon. In some cases, there may be a fluid exudate around the tendon. The second stage consists of tendinosis and is characterized by degenerative and inflammatory change of the tendon itself. In the final stage there is visible disruption of the tendon either at the periphery or in the central part. Symptoms of either tendinitis or tenosynovitis will start with stiffness or pain after a workout. In acute tendinitis, there will be pain on active plantarflexion, on dorsiflexing the tendon, and on direct palpation. The tendon may appear fusiform with swelling.[33] With tenosynovitis, the peritenon sheath will be inflamed and swollen, but stretching of the tendon does not usually cause pain. Fine crepitus or "creaking" will be palpated about the tendon. It is important to treat this condition early; otherwise a chronic problem will develop.

In acute cases, rest and refraining from running until the symptoms abate are necessary. Swimming pool activities or bicycling is allowed if pain-free.

Anti-inflammatory medication is a useful adjunct. A ¼-in. heel wedge will reduce tension in the tendon. At this time, stretching the Achilles and soleus musculature is to be avoided as this will increase the inflammatory process.[15] Once the symptoms are quiescent, activities at a less intense level than prior to

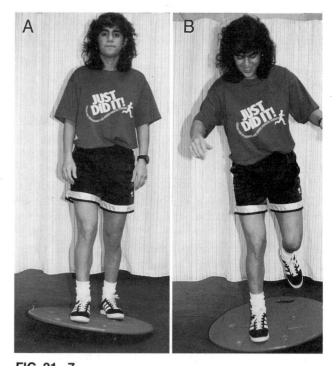

FIG 21–7.
BAPS board (Biomechanical Ankle Platform System). **A,** Early stage with both feet on platform, back foot assists in balance and control. **B,** Late stage for proprioception training.

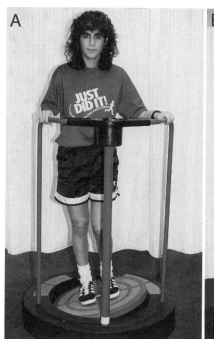 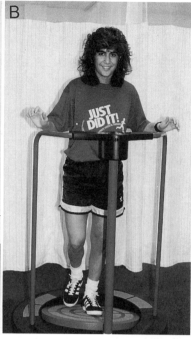

FIG 21–8.
KAT platform (Kinesthetic Ability Training). **A,** early training to increase range of motion. Patient can use digital display for objective biofeedback to enhance range of motion. **B,** Later stage using one leg. An inflatable bladder under the platform can be adjusted to vary stability.

the injury may be resumed. Stretching of the calf muscles as well as strengthening the dorsiflexors with latex tubing will serve to prevent further injury. As symptoms decrease, the heel lift should be discontinued or reduced to allow for full flexibility in the Achilles tendon and gastrocnemius-soleus complex.

Progress to an asymptomatic state in difficult cases may take weeks or months. Pain and stiffness may decrease as the patient warms up, but these symptoms will return after running. Scarring in the tendon perpetuates the pain-inflammation-pain cycle. Cross-fiber friction massage, as advocated by Cyriax,[16] is often helpful at breaking down the scar tissue formed by the chronic inflammation. Orthotic intervention is necessary if biomechanical foot imbalances exist.[22] Patients can maintain aerobic conditioning by biking, swimming, walking, or running in the swimming pool while allowing rest of the injured part.

Ankle Sprains

Over 80% of all ankle sprains occur in the lateral joint with the foot plantarflexed and suddenly inverted.[14, 55] The anterior talofibular ligament is most commonly involved in inversion sprains. With in-creased force, this becomes a two-ligament injury as the calcaneofibular ligament is stressed. Medial ankle sprains happen infrequently as this affects the stronger deltoid ligament. This eversion-type injury occurs with abduction, eversion, and dorsiflexion of the foot. Because of the strength of the deltoid ligament, this injury is often associated with tears of the tibiofibular ligament, interosseus membrane, or fracture of the fibula.[55] Motions involving extreme valgus angulation with external rotation, as in changing direction with the foot plantarflexed, can result in significant injury. Disruptions of the syndesmosis and interosseus membrane will lead to severe pain about the lower leg, and instability about the ankle mortise.

Ankle sprains demand accurate diagnosis and early treatment. The nonoperative phase of treatment, discussed below, can be divided into four phases: the acute phase, protective phase, functional phase, and preventive phase.[14] The goal of nonoperative treatment is to first control inflammation and swelling and as rapidly as possible move the patient through a functional progression of exercises leading to an ankle that is stable under active conditions.

Acute Phase.—During the first 24 to 48 hours, ice, compression, and elevation make up the imme-

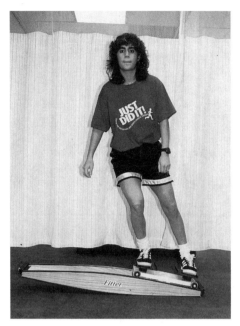

FIG 21–9.
Fitter provides progressive lateral motion exercises for strengthening lower extremity musculature

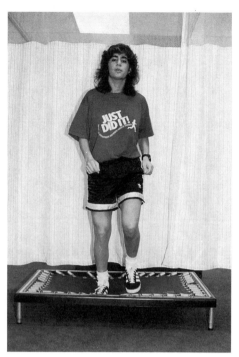

FIG 21–10.
Minitrampoline is used as a precursor to running.

diate treatment. Crutches may be used in a non–weight-bearing gait on the affected side to reduce excessive stress across the joint. Walking without assistive devices while limping appears to prolong this phase of recovery. In the following 3 to 7 days, physical agents, such as microampere electrical stimulation, may be used to reduce inflammation.[64] Ice should be applied for 15 to 20 minutes three to four times daily as long as there is greater warmth in the injured area than on the contralateral side. Changing to heating modalities too early increases the risks of increasing edema and prolonging recovery.[65] Care should be taken to avoid frostbite in patients with a history of circulatory problems. In

this initial phase, the clinician should obtain baseline measurements of range of motion, girth in a figure-of-8 configuration,[17] stability, strength, and balance (if the patient can stand adequately on the injured ankle). Gentle active range-of-motion exercises may be started, with emphasis on plantarflexion and dorsiflexion.

In the following week, gentle stretching exercises of the gastrocnemius-soleus muscle group can be started in weight bearing. The use of a BAPS board (Camp International, Jackson, Miss.) or KAT platform (Breg Inc., Vista, Calif.) facilitates range of motion and proprioception (Figs 21–7 and 21–8). Stationary bicycle riding can be started if the ankle is

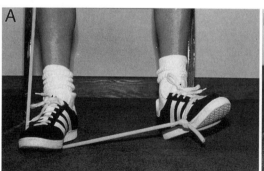
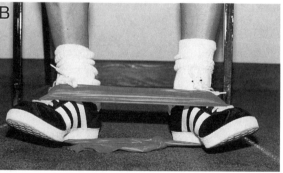

FIG 21–11.
A, latex tubing used for ankle exercises. **B,** Theraband used for strengthening the evertors of the ankle.

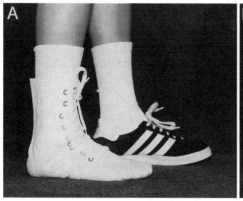
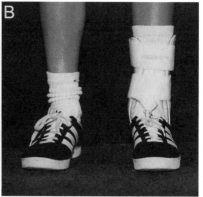

FIG 21–12.
A, Swede-O ankle brace can be worn early in rehabilitation or during athletic activities. **B,** Aircast stirrup can be worn in athletic shoe; the bladder inside the brace may be inflated or deflated to adjust the level of support required.

sufficiently pain-free. Modalities to control pain and swelling are used as necessary. Pain-free motion is required before resistive exercises are started.

Protective Phase.—During the next 2 to 4 weeks, more aggressive and controlled exercise may be initiated. Progressing from simple range-of-motion exercises, the BAPS board or KAT platform can be utilized to progressively increase the stresses across the ankle in all planes of motion. Strength and proprioception can be developed by increasing the size of the disc in the BAPS board or by altering the pressure in the KAT system. Other devices, such as slide boards, the Fitter (Fitter International Inc., Calgary, Alta., Canada) and the minitrampoline will provide functional exercises to develop balance, stability, and strength in weight-bearing positions (Figs 21–9 and 21–10). Latex tubing or Theraband can be used for home strengthening exercises (Fig 21–11).

During this phase and the initial phase, the ankle may require external support to protect healing ligaments and maintain compression about the ankle. The Swede-O (Swede-O-Universal, North Branch, Minn.) or Duo-Loc (Omni Scientific, Inc., Martinez, Calif.) ankle brace, and the Air Stirrup (Air Stirrup Inc., Summit, N.J.) provide excellent support while the patient is fitted in a shoe to allow weight bearing (Fig 21–12).

Functional Phase.—Functional activities and return to normal activities are stressed in this phase. Progressive return to prior activity levels is allowed provided no limp or gait deviation is present. External supports can be discontinued as the patient demonstrates adequate control, full range of motion, and normal strength and balance.

Prevention Phase.—Maintaining appropriate aerobic conditioning will help the patient to avoid fatigue and reduce the risk of reinjury. Stretching the gastrocnemius and soleus muscles will maintain the dorsiflexion necessary for walking and running. Finally, selecting shoewear that is appropriate for the activity will protect the foot and ankle by providing cushioning of the forefoot and heel and stability in the heel counter. Shoes that are wornout in either the upper portion or sole should not be used.

SUMMARY

Injuries to the leg and ankle in the older patient do not necessarily signal the end of an active lifestyle. Aggressive treatment based on an accurate diagnosis will allow the most rapid return to activities. Care should be taken to allow for decreased flexibility, osteoporosis, circulatory impairment and other health problems that may be present in this population.

REFERENCES

1. Andrish J, Work JA: How I manage shin splints. *Physician Sportsmed* 1990; 18:113–114.
2. Arnheim DD: *Modern Principles of Athletic Training.* St Louis, Mosby–Year Book, 1989.
3. Ator R, Gunn K, McPoil TG, et al: The effect of adhesive strapping on medial longitudinal arch support before and after exercise. *J Orthop Sports Phys Ther* 1991; 14:18–23.
4. Awbrey BJ, Sienkiewicz PS, Mankin HJ: Chronic exercise-induced compartment pressure elevation

measured with a miniaturized fluid pressure monitor. *Am J Sports Med* 1988; 16:610–615.

5. Barnard RJ, Hall JA: Patients with peripheral vascular disease, in Franklin BA, Gordon S, Timmis GC (eds): *Exercise and Modern Medicine*. Baltimore, Williams & Wilkins, 1989, pp 107–117.

6. Bell AT: The older athlete, in Sanders, B (ed): *Sports Physical Therapy*. Norwalk, Conn, Appleton & Lange, 1990, pp 159–184.

7. Beskin JL, Sanders RA, Hunter SC, et al: Surgical repair of Achilles tendon ruptures. *Am J Sports Med* 1987; 15:1–8.

8. Beyer RE, Huang FC, Wilshire EB: The effect of endurance exercise on bone dimensions, collagen and calcium in the aged rat. *Exp Gerontol* 20:315–323.

9. Bishop PA, Frazier S, Smith J, et al: Physiologic responses to treadmill and water running. *Physician Sportsmed* 1989; 17:87–94.

10. Bradley JP, Tibone JE: Percutaneous and open surgical repairs of Achilles tendon ruptures. *Am J Sports Med* 1990; 18:188–195.

11. Brandell BK, Williams K: An analysis of cinematographic and electromyographic recording of human gait, in Nelson R, Morehouse C (eds): *Biomechanics IV*. Baltimore, University Press, 1974.

12. Brody DM: Running injuries. *Clin Symp* 1980; 32:2–36.

13. Brown AB, McCartney N, Sale DG: Positive adaptations to weight-lifting in the elderly. *J Appl Physiol* 1990; 69:1725–1733.

14. Case WS: Ankle injuries, in Sanders, B (ed): *Sports Physical Therapy*. Norwalk, Conn, Appleton & Lange, 1990, pp 451–464.

15. Curwin S, Stanish WD: *Tendinitis: Its Etiology and Treatment*. Lexington, Mass, Collamore Press, 1984.

16. Cyriax J: *Textbook of Orthopaedic Medicine: Diagnosis of Soft Tissue Lesion*, ed 7. London, Bailliere Tindall, 1975.

17. Esterson PS: Measurement of ankle joint swelling using a figure of 8. *J Orthop Sports Phys Ther* 1979; 1:51–52.

18. Esterson PS: Leg injuries in the older athlete. *Top Geriatr Rehabil* 1990; 6:59–64.

19. Fiatarone MA, Marks EC, Ryan ND, et al: High-intensity strength training in nonagenarians. *JAMA* 1990; 263:3029–3034.

20. Fisher NM, Pendergast DR, Calkins E: Muscle rehabilitation in impaired elderly nursing home residents. *Arch Phys Med Rehabil* 1991; 72:181–185.

21. Fox JM, Blazina ME, Jobe FW, et al: Degeneration and rupture of the Achilles tendon. *Clin Orthop* 1975; 107:221–224.

22. Gross ML, Davlin LB, Evanski PM: Effectiveness of orthotic shoe inserts in the long-distance runner. *Am J Sports Med* 1991; 19:409–412.

23. Hagen RD: The kinematics of aging, in Nelson CL, Dwyer AP (eds): *The Aging Musculoskeletal System*. Lexington, Mass, Health, 1984.

24. Hollingshead HW: *Textbook of Anatomy*, ed 3. Philadelphia, Harper & Row, 1974.

25. Hughes LY: Biomechanical analysis of the foot and ankle for predisposition to developing stress fractures. *J Orthop Sports Phys Ther* 1985; 7:96–101.

26. Hunt, GC: Examination of lower extremity dysfunction, in Gould J (ed): *Orthopaedic and Sports Physical Therapy*. St Louis, Mosby–Year Book, 1990, pp 395–421.

27. Inglis AE, Sculco TP: Surgical repair of ruptures of the tendo Achilles. *Clin Orthop* 1981; 156:160–169.

28. Jobe FW, Schwab DM: Golf for the mature athlete. *Clin Sports Med* 1991; 10:269–282.

29. Jozsa L, Kvist M, Balint BJ, et al: The role of recreational sport activity in Achilles tendon rupture. *Am J Sports Med* 1989; 17:388–443.

30. Keene JS, Lash EG, Fisher DR: Magnetic resonance imaging of Achilles tendon ruptures. *Am J Sports Med* 1989; 17:333–337.

31. Kleinman M, Gross AE: Achilles tendon rupture following steroid injection. *J Bone Joint Surg [Am]* 1983; 65:1345–1347.

32. Leach RE, Abramowitz A: The senior tennis player. *Clin Sports Med* 1991; 10:283–290.

33. Leach RE, Schepis AA, Takai H: Achilles tendinitis: Don't let it be an athlete's downfall. *Physician Sportsmed* 1991; 19:87–92.

34. Logan JG, Rorabeck CH, Castle GSP: The measurement of dynamic compartment pressure during exercise. *Am J Sports Med* 1983; 11:220–223.

35. Lutter LD: Foot-related knee problems in the long distance runner. *Foot Ankle* 1980; 1:112–116.

36. Mann RA, Baxter DE, Lutter LD: Running symposium. *Foot Ankle* 1981; 1:190–244.

37. McKeag DB, Dolan C: Overuse syndromes of the lower extremity. *Physician Sportsmed* 1989; 17:108–123.

38. McLennan JC, McLennan JC: Cycling and the older athlete. *Clin Sports Med* 1991; 10:291–300.

39. McPoil TG, Brocato RS: The foot and ankle: Biomechanical evaluation and treatment, in Gould J (ed): *Orthopaedic and Sports Physical Therapy*. St Louis, Mosby–Year Book, 1990, pp 293–321.

40. Melillo TV: Gastrocnemius equinus: Its diagnosis and treatment. *Arch Podiatr Med Foot Surg* 2:159–205, 1975.

41. Menard D, Stanish WD: The aging athlete. *Am J Sports Med* 1989; 17:187–196.

42. Menz MJ, Lucas GL: Magnetic resonance imaging of a rupture of the medial head of the gastrocnemius muscle. *J Bone Joint Surg [Am]* 1991; 73:1260–1261.

43. Morey MC, Cowper PA, Feussner JR, et al: Two-year trends in physical performance following supervised exercise among community-dwelling older veterans. *J Am Geriatr Soc* 1991; 39:986–992.

44. Nelen G, Martens M, Burssens A: Surgical treatment of chronic Achilles tendinitis. *Am J Sports Med* 1989; 17:754–759.

45. Nicholas JA, Friedman MJ: Orthopedic problems in middle aged athletes. *Physician Sportsmed* 1979; 11:39–46.

46. Nicholas JA, Grossman RB, Herschman EB: The importance of a simplified classification of motion in sports in relation to performance. *Orthop Clin North Am* 1977; 8:499–532.

47. Olerud C, Rosendahl Y: Torsion-transmitting properties of the hind foot. *Clin Orthop* 1987; 214:285.

48. O'Shea JP: Masters power weight training. *Physician Sportsmed* 1981; 9:133–137.

49. Perry J: Gait characteristics, in *Therapeutic Considerations for the Elderly.* New York, Churchill Livingstone, 1987.

50. Peterson L, Renstrom P: *Sports Injuries.* St Louis, Mosby–Year Book, 1986.

51. Richardson AB, Miller JW: Swimming and the older athlete. *Clin Sports Med* 1991; 10:301–318.

52. Root ML, Orien WP, Weed JA, et al: *Biomechanical Examination of the Foot.* Los Angeles, Biomechanics Corp, 1971.

53. Root ML, Orien WP, Weed JA: *Normal and Abnormal Function of the Foot.* Los Angeles, Biomechanics Corp, 1977.

54. Rorabeck CH, Bourne RB, Fowler PJ, et al: The role of tissue pressure measurement in diagnosing chronic anterior compartment syndrome. *Am J Sports Med* 1988; 16:143–146.

55. Roy S, Irvin R: *Sports Medicine: Prevention, Evaluation, Management, and Rehabilitation.* Englewood Cliffs, NJ. Prentice-Hall, 1983.

56. Smith EL: Exercise for prevention of osteoporosis: A review. *Physician Sportsmed* 1982; 10:72–79.

57. Stamford B: What is interval training? *Physician Sportsmed* 1989; 17:193.

58. Subotnick SI: Equinus deformity as it affects the forefoot. *J Am Podiatry Assoc* 1971; 61:423–427.

59. Subotnick SI, Jones R, in Subotnick SI (ed): *Sports Medicine of the Lower Extremity.* New York, Churchill Livingstone, 1989.

60. Ting AJ: Running and the older athlete. *Clin Sports Med* 1991; 10:319–325.

61. Twomey L, Taylor J: Age changes in lumbar intervertebral discs. *Acta Orthop Scand* 1985; 56:496–499.

62. Van Camp SP, Boyer JL: Cardiovascular aspects of aging (part 1 of 2). *Physician Sportsmed* 1989; 17:121–130.

63. Viel ER, Desmarets JJ: Mechanical pull of the peroneal tendons on the fifth ray of the foot. *J Orthop Sports Phys Ther* 1985; 7:102–106.

64. Wallace LA: My-O-Matic clinical effectiveness on 1531 musculoskeletal patients, unpublished data, 1990.

65. Wallace L, Knortz K, Esterson P: Immediate care of ankle injuries. *J Orthop Sports Phys Ther* 1979; 1:46–50.

66. Ward A, Taylor P, Rippe JM: How to tailor an exercise program. *Physician Sportsmed* 1991; 19:64–76.

67. *When the Foot Hits the Ground, Everything Changes.* Course Notes: American Physical Rehabilitation Network, 1988.

68. Whitesides TE, et al: Tissue pressure measurements as a determinant for the need of fasciotomy. *Clin Orthop* 1975; 113:43–51.

Chapter 22

Foot Injuries: An Orthopedic Perspective

Robert Karpman, M.D.

Foot problems, one of the most common complaints in the senior adult, are often given low priority as a health care concern.[3, 11] The majority of these complaints arise from three or four major sources: (1) skin and nails, (2) bony deformities, (3) soft tissue problems, particularly on the plantar surface of the foot, and (4) inadequate footwear. Injuries to the foot tend to be less common in older as compared with younger persons because of decreasing activity; however, some chronic problems, particularly ruptures of the posterior tibial tendon, are directly related to recurrent rather than acute trauma.

On examination of the feet, it is imperative that the patient be seen ambulating both with and without shoes. Often gait changes that are directly related to inappropriate footwear, such as inadequate support or inadequate flexibility to the shoe will be noticed. In a recent study performed at our institution,[8] we found that more than 50% of patients residing in long-term care facilities do not have adequate footwear, particularly of a sort providing any type of support. The majority of patients had only one pair of shoes, which were slippers. These are obviously easy to apply, but provide little protection of the foot and often do not have rubber soles, which prevent sliding and falls.

SKIN AND NAIL PROBLEMS

The majority of skin problems around the foot are primarily related to footwear. Frequently, patients do not wear shoes that are of appropriate size, particularly in width and height. This leads to irritation over bony prominences, such as bunions on the medial side of the foot and corns dorsally. Inadequate subcutaneous tissue over the heel and metatarsal region can lead to increased callus formation and pain. Nail deformities are quite common, particularly those resulting from fungal infections of the nails.

Careful neurologic and vascular evaluation is also of extreme importance as problems in the foot can reflect systemic disease, particularly peripheral neuropathies resulting from diabetes or vascular insufficiency. Pain resulting from vascular insufficiency and neurogenic origins has been discussed in the prior chapter. It should be stressed, however, that patients with peripheral neuropathy *must* examine their feet on a daily basis in order to alleviate any pressure ulcers and potential infection.[2, 5]

The majority of skin problems can be managed with modifications of footwear. These involve obtaining a shoe with a wide and high toe box. Several soft pads have been developed that also help relieve pressure areas. Women with wide feet should be advised to purchase men's shoes. A Hoke ball and socket stretcher is extremely useful in that shoes can be rapidly stretched in one area to decrease pressure and skin irritation. The majority of surgical procedures can be avoided with appropriate shoewear.

Nail deformities can be treated with adequate trimming. Nails should not be trimmed proximal to the lateral nail bed. It is extremely difficult to manage nail deformities resulting from fungal infections, as topical ointments are of little use. Systemic antifungal agents such as griseofulvin can be utilized; however, the fungal infections will return shortly after cessation of the drug. Fungal infections of the nail should be left alone and are primarily a cosmetic problem. If the deformity continues to cause irritation or recurrent infections, then removal of the nail and matrix is required. This is done in an outpatient setting with minimal risk as long as a careful vascular evaluation has been done prior to surgery.

Like skin problems, a majority of bony deformities of the foot, particularly the forefoot, are related to inadequate or inappropriate footwear. Most bunion deformities are a direct result of footwear and correction is indicated only when there is chronic pain that cannot be corrected with shoe modifications. Similar findings are noted with hammer toe deformities.

In order to provide a more detailed review of the foot in the elderly patient, a review of the problems by anatomic region is advised.

HINDFOOT AND ANKLE

The hindfoot and ankle are areas where there can be acute bony injuries. These include ankle fractures as well as stress fractures of the calcaneus. The management of ankle fractures in older persons is no different than in younger individuals. Cases of severe displacement are managed with open reduction and internal fixation. As mentioned in the previous chapter, internal fixation can be difficult in some instances because of severe bone loss, and extreme caution must be taken in reducing these fractures and providing adequate fixation. Fractures of the talus are quite rare except in motor vehicle injuries and can be easily diagnosed on radiographic evaluation. Calcaneal fractures are often missed in the older patient and are frequently misdiagnosed as plantar fasciitis or calcaneal spurs. Radiographs frequently do not demonstrate the presence of a fracture, so that a bone scan is required to make the diagnosis. Treatment of a stress fracture of the calcaneus consists of a padded splint until the swelling has subsided, followed by a well-padded cast with progressive ambulation. A heel cup can then be utilized to provide continued padding for the patient.

Heel pain is often a difficult problem to manage as there are several etiologies. As mentioned above, a stress fracture of the calcaneus should be ruled out. Other sources of heel pain include plantar fasciitis, calcaneal spurs, and various compression neuropathies. It is difficult to differentiate the sources of heel pain; however, selective injections of lidocaine may be helpful. It should also be noted that the presence of a calcaneal spur does not necessarily mean that that is the source of the problem. It has been this author's experience that up to 50% of patients over the age of 50 years have calcaneal spurs present on x-ray. Spurs tend to be symptomatic primarily in patients who have atrophy of the heel pad. In the majority of patients for whom the diagnosis of a heel spur is made, pain is related to plantar fasciitis. With time, microscopic tears of the plantar fascia develop, leading to inflammation, particularly at the origin of the plantar fascia on the medial side of the calcaneus. This results in extreme pain, particularly after periods of rest. Patients complain of marked pain when arising in the morning that tends to improve as the day progresses. The symptoms tend to worsen following a sustained period of rest.

In 90% of cases, patients with plantar fasciitis can be managed nonoperatively. Treatment includes plantar fascia stretching exercises, use of nonsteroidal anti-inflammatory drugs, Achilles tendon stretching exercises, and occasionally immobilization in a walking cast. If previous treatments have failed, an injection of hydrocortisone in the area of inflammation is helpful. Repeated injections should not be done as they lead to further heel pad atrophy, which can aggravate the condition.

Entrapment neuropathies must also be considered as a possible source of heel pain, including entrapment of the posterior tibial nerve in the area of the tarsal tunnel, the sural nerve on the lateral side of the calcaneus, and the nerve to the abductor digiti quinti muscle on the medial side of the heel at the level of the abductor hallucis muscle.

Diagnosis of entrapment neuropathy can be made clinically with the presence of a positive Tinel's sign or symptomatic improvement following injection of local anesthetics. Nerve condition velocity tests may be helpful but are often nondiagnostic, particularly in compression neuropathies of the smaller nerves. Should symptoms persist, decompression of the nerve may be warranted. This should be utilized only in extreme cases.

Another hindfoot problem that may be related to recurrent trauma is sinus tarsi syndrome. In this case, patients complain of pain in the area of the tarsal sinus along the lateral aspect of the hindfoot. There may or may not be a history of trauma, but often a history of an ankle sprain can be elucidated.

On examination, patients will have tenderness

in the area of the tarsal sinus that can be differentiated from a chronic ankle sprain by its location. Ligamentous injuries tend to be more posterior, particularly those around the calcaneal fibular ligament or anterior involving the talofibular ligament. An injection of local anesthetic in the tarsal sinus often relieves the patient's symptoms. In rare cases, repeated injections are necessary and occasionally a surgical procedure, which removes the content of the tarsal sinus including the fat and other debris, will relieve the patient's symptoms.

MIDFOOT PROBLEMS

A diagnosis that is often missed in the geriatric patient is a rupture of the posterior tibial tendon. Patients present with a 6-month to 1-year history of pain along the medial side of the foot as well as a progressive unilateral planovalgus deformity. They deny any history of acute trauma.

Examination may or may not demonstrate tenderness along the posterior tibial tendon; however, patients are unable to raise a single toe on that extremity as compared with the normal side. This is pathognomonic for a rupture of the posterior tibial tendon. Radiographs may show some arthritic problems in the subtalar joint from chronic impingement as a result of the heel valgus. Severe deformities can lead to arthritis in the subtalar, talonavicular, and calcaneocuboid joints.

Another diagnostic procedure that may be helpful is magnetic resonance imaging, which can show degenerative tears within the tendon and perhaps a complete rupture.

Management of this problem is extremely difficult. If patients have developed severe deformity with arthritis, a subtalar and perhaps talonavicular fusion is necessary in order to place the foot in a plantigrade position and relieve symptoms. In less severe cases, reconstruction of the tendon utilizing the flexor digitorum longus tendon can be done to improve the longitudinal arch and prevent further deformity.[7] As mentioned previously, the disease is often missed and patients can develop severe deformity prior to diagnosis.

Other causes of severe collapse of the midfoot are related to Charcot's foot and result from severe peripheral neuropathy. Patients complain of swelling and redness and specifically deny any history of trauma. It is untrue that Charcot joints are nonpainful; pain may be a reason for seeking physician assistance.

Radiographs demonstrate severe bony destruction and new bone formation in any of the midtarsal joints.[6] Charcot's foot is often confused with osteomyelitis; however, unless there are open lesions or a history of infection, the more likely diagnosis is Charcot's joint. Management of this disease includes elevation to decrease swelling followed by protection of the foot in a total contact cast or protective shoes.[1, 4, 5, 9] To date, there are no specific treatments for this disease other than protection from further trauma and deformity.[10, 11] Patients with severe deformity eventually must undergo amputation.

PROBLEMS OF THE FOREFOOT

As mentioned previously, the majority of forefoot problems are related to inappropriate footwear. Several of these problems can be resolved with corrective shoes and/or appropriate padding of the foot. Surgery should be utilized only in cases that do not respond to conservative management. Surgical correction of forefoot deformities should not be extensive. For example, in a case of severe bunion deformity and hallux valgus, a simple removal of the exostosis can result in symptomatic relief, without need for a more extensive procedure to realign the great toe. Similar procedures can be used to remove bony prominences that cause hard and soft corns. However, even with the simplest procedure a careful vascular examination must be done preoperatively to assure that wound healing will not be obstructed.

SUMMARY

In summary, acute injuries of the foot and ankle are uncommon in the older patient; however, the sequelae of recurrent trauma are present particularly in disease entities such as a ruptured posterior tendon, plantar fasciitis, and Charcot's foot. The majority of foot problems can be managed nonoperatively with appropriate footwear modification.

REFERENCES

1. Brower AC: The acute neuropathic joint. *Arthritis Rheum* 1988; 31:571–573.
2. Coleman WC: Footwear in a management program of injury prevention, in Levin ME, O'Neal LW (eds): *The Diabetic Foot*, ed 4. St Louis, Mosby–Year Book, 1988, pp 293–310.
3. Gould N, Schneider W, Ashikaga T: Epidemiological survey of foot problems in the continental United States 1978–1979. *Foot Ankle* 1980; 1:8–10.
4. Greene DA: Neuropathy in the diabetic foot: New concepts in etiology and treatment, in Levin ME, O'Neal LW (eds): *The Diabetic Foot*, ed 4. St Louis, Mosby–Year Book, 1988, pp 76–82.
5. Harrelson JM: Management of the diabetic foot. *Orthop Clin North Am* 1989; 20:605–798.
6. Harris JR, Brand PW: Patterns of disintegration of tarsus in the anaesthetized foot. *J Bone Joint Surg (Br)* 1966; 48:4–16.
7. Johnson K: Tibialis posterior tendon rupture. *Clin Orthop Rel Res* 1983; 177:140–147.
8. Karpman R, Wolfe K: Shoewear in the Institutionalized Elderly, presented to Gerontological Society of America, Nov 1992.
9. Lang-Stevenson AI, et al: Neuropathic ulcers of the foot. *J Bone Joint Surg (Br)* 1985; 67:438–442.
10. Mooney V, Gottschalk F, Powell H: The diabetic foot ulcer: Treating one, preventing the next. *Clin Diabetes* 1985; 3:177–179.
11. Pawlson LG, Bernstein LC: Dysmobility in aging and clinical practice—Musculoskeletal Disorders. Igaku Shoin, 1988, p 130.
12. Sloman-Kovacs SD, Braustein EM, Brandt KD: Rapidly progressing Charcot arthropathy following minor joint trauma in patients with diabetic neuropathy. *Arthritis Rheum* 1990; 33:412–417.

Chapter 23

Foot Injuries: A Rehabilitation Perspective

Jennifer M. Bottomley, M.S., P.T.

Hollis Herman, M.S., P.T.

Modification of foot dysfunction and malalignment may be accomplished through the use of foot orthotics, orthotic materials, podiatric products, shoes, and shoe modifications. The provision of orthotics and shoes in the management of foot problems in the elderly is only one facet of conservative rehabilitative intervention. Numerous other forms of treatment are available to supplement and enhance the overall outcomes of treatment, including manual therapies such as joint and soft-tissue mobilization, Buerger-Allen exercise, therapeutic exercise, muscle strengthening, stretching, range-of-motion exercises, and massage. Modalities such as electrical stimulation (high galvanic, interferential, and direct currents), heat and cold, paraffin, and ultrasound can be used. In addition, gait training, graded walking programs, and patient education are vital components to comprehensive treatment programs for foot problems in the elderly.

If properly employed in conjunction with muscle strengthening and joint and soft-tissue mobilization, orthotics and shoe modifications help accomplish the transfer of pressure from sensitive to more tolerant areas by reducing friction, shock, and shear forces, and modifying weight transfer patterns. All of these modalities are used to relieve pain and improve balance and function during standing and ambulation. Manual therapies, physical modalities, and muscle strengthening assist in breaking up adhesions, realigning the joints of the foot, and providing supporting musculature to promote those structural alter-

ations. Orthotics serve to reposition flexible deformities, accommodate fixed deformities, and limit motion of painful, inflamed, or unstable joints, promoting better healing and protection of these areas.

The focus of this chapter is common foot dysfunctions and injuries related to aging. Rehabilitative approaches for management of "normal" and pathologic changes are presented as suggestions for conservative intervention for foot problems in the elderly.

ANATOMIC AND PHYSIOLOGIC CHANGES IN THE FOOT WITH AGING

The "normal" aging process involves a degeneration in the health and quality of skin, fat, muscle, and osseous structures of the foot. Vascular and nutritional changes occur, leading to changes in the integrity of the skin and muscle-force production in the foot. The plantar fat pads atrophy. Muscle fibers are fewer in number, decrease in size, and are often replaced by fat, causing intrinsic muscle weakness of the foot. Common orthopedic deformities lead to abnormal pressure points, changes in joint mobility owing to capsular changes, subluxation of the metatarsophalangeal joints with resulting toe deformities, overlapping toes, and a decline in muscle-force production. Changes in sensory input lead to abnormal weight-bearing patterns. Disuse or immobility complicates and compounds the varied factors associated with aging and pathologies limiting ambulation. Helfand states that "ambulation is many times the key or the catalyst between an individual retaining dignity and remaining in a normal living environment or being institutionalized."[23] Foot care is a vital adjunct for the maintenance of functional ambulation in the elderly.

Foot Contour

Few persons retain the same shoe size throughout adult life. Morphologic changes occur with static and dynamic loads imposed on the feet during normal activities of daily living (ADL). Foot structure is also altered by ill-fitting shoes and unforgiving walking surfaces. The foot becomes wider and width is often further increased by metatarsal deformities such as hallux valgus or the lowering of the transverse or longitudinal arches. Foot height increases with lesser toe deformities or an equinus deformity at the ankle from chronic use of triangular toe box and high-heeled shoes. The overall result is a change in the contour of the feet with age.

The normal physiologic changes seen in the foot with age include atrophy of the plantar fat pads. The metatarsal pad shifts distally and the heel pad atrophies and shifts laterally. The shifting of the pads away from bony prominences leads to microtrauma, often resulting in further bony malalignment. Calluses form as a protective mechanism with repeated stress. If callus formations become too large and thick, they no longer provide protection; in fact, they cause problems by inducing added frictional stress. Ulceration can form at the interface of the thickened callous tissue and the thinner epithelium below. Excessive callus formation under the metatarsal heads and heel can make weight bearing very painful and alter the contour of the foot.

Edema caused by circulatory changes or inflammatory diseases distorts the foot shape. Donning shoes can cause discomfort and shearing occurs around the collar of the shoe. Velcro-closure sandals or sneakers are often advised to allow for accommodation to a changing foot contour resulting from swelling.

Obesity also influences the foot contour. Overweight persons commonly have broad feet with dorsal enlargement and fat deposits. The plantar surfaces usually show excessive thickening of tissues in response to greater loads. The transverse arch is decreased if not flattened by extra weight and the weight-bearing alignment is usually one of pronation with a valgus heel.

Connective Tissue Changes With Aging

Collagen is the basic protein component in fibrous connective tissue, including bone, tendon, ligament, and cartilage.[18, 22] Strands of procollagen group together to form mature collagen fibers.[7] Cross-linkage of collagen fibers increases with "normal" aging. Increased cross-linking results in shortening and distortion of collagen fibers, which in turn results in contractures with progressive restriction in tissue and joint mobility.[22] The foot and ankle is one place in the body where slight tissue restrictions have enormous functional manifestations. Diminished talocrural joint mobility may lead to excessive stresses on the first metatarsophalangeal joint during push-off or plantar fascia stretching during midstance.

Fibrinous adhesions resulting in foot and ankle dysfunctions are common in sedentary elderly people. With limited or reduced activity levels, complete breakdown of insoluble fibrin may not occur, leading to extracellular accumulation of this substance and strands of fibrinogin consolidate. Together these substances result in adhesions that restrict movement.[37]

Articular cartilage is found at most articular joint surfaces. With aging, cartilage tends to dehydrate, stiffen, and thin out in weight-bearing areas. Erosion and degeneration of the joint surfaces are often advanced before symptoms of pain, crepitation, and limitation of movement are detected because cartilage has no nerve innervation and limited blood supply.

Restriction in the talocrural or subtalar joint motion increases the stresses on the forefoot. Excessive subtalar eversion decreases metatarsophalangeal flexion, which increases the stresses on the metatarsal heads. Hypermobility or hypomobility of the joints in the feet can lead additionally to skin changes owing to persistent shear stresses resulting from ill-fitting shoes, repetitive stresses, or arthritic changes.

Osteoporosis

Osteoporosis will be covered in depth in Chapter 25. It is important to realize that osteoporosis primarily equates with fracture, especially in women.

Fracture prevention can focus on biologic remediation but should include safety during ambulation. Adequate lighting, safe flooring, and prominent handrails will assist in preventing fracture, in conjunction with prescriptions for estrogen, calcium, phosphorus, and exercise.[38, 39]

Muscle Changes With Aging

The most notable changes in body composition and weight with aging occur with the body's fat and water content. There is a decrease in body lean-muscle tissue while there is an increase in fat concentration. Decreases in muscle mass occur with old age, with proximal muscles of the lower extremity particularly affected. This decrease in muscle mass results from a decrease in both fiber number and diameter. No change in the number of motor neural fibers has been found, but the size of the motor unit decreases owing to the loss of muscle fibers. The preponderance of evidence based on enzyme histochemistry and physiologic properties suggests a greater loss in the fast type II fiber. The ability to rapidly adjust the foot to changing ground contours, rug heights, and curbs when walking is significantly impaired; this, in combination with visual impairments, is a reason for falls in the elderly.

Vascular Changes With Aging

Peripheral vascular resistance is increased with aging owing to a loss of elasticity and vessel narrowing. Factors affected by both "aging" and inactivity include a decrease in available oxygen and cardiac reserve and a diminished endocrine performance. There is a decrease in cardiac output at rest, a decline in the cardiovascular system's response to stress, an increase in the systolic blood pressure, and a progressive increase in peripheral vascular resistance. The overall result is a decreased vascularization, with the distal vessels undergoing the most pronounced changes,[11, 48] increasing the likelihood of injury and poor healing. These biologic and structural changes result in physiologic and functional alterations of the cardiovascular system, all potentially affecting the blood flow to the foot.

Skin Changes With Aging

The skin is a very important element in the ability to sense touch. The dermis thins, loses elasticity, and has a diminished vascularity in old age. Loss of tissue support for remaining capillaries results in fragility and easy bruising (senile purpura).

The most common appearance of aging skin is dryness, scaling, and an atrophic appearance.[23] These changes may be related to systemic disease or functional problems but are considered to be a part of the "normal" process of aging. The changes are associated with diminished sebaceous activity, a decrease in hydration of the horny layers, alterations in the metabolic and nutritional components associated with skin production and repair, and a dysfunction in keratin formation. Hair loss is related to vascular insufficiency. The skin of the foot loses its elasticity. The associated involvement of the peripheral arterial and venous systems produces pigment changes and an increased deposit of hemosiderin in the soft tissues, adding to the disturbed keratin formation. In general, the skin of the older foot appears dry and yellowish with a wrinkled, inelastic, and parchment-like appearance. The decline in cellular division with age results in a slower rate and efficiency of tissue repair following any trauma.[26]

Peripheral receptors provide the neurosensory input for the sense of touch. As with the other senses, touch acuity declines with age. Specific receptors for touch, pressure, pain, and temperature are found within the dermis and epidermis of the skin. Receptors can be freestanding or arranged in small corpuscular masses. Meissner's corpuscles (touch-texture receptors), pacinian corpuscles (pressure-vibration receptors), and Krause's corpuscles (temperature receptors), as well as peripheral nerve fibers are noted to decline in transmission. Sensitivity to touch, temperature, and vibration frequently decline with age. The ability to sense pain remains intact because few age-related changes occur in the free nerve endings. The elderly person must take special care to avoid injury to the foot from concentrated pressures or excessive temperature on the skin.[19, 25]

Nail Bed Changes

Nail changes in aging include a thickening and an increase in the brittleness of the nail. These changes are accentuated in the presence of severe trauma or repeated microtrauma. Nails tend to grow more slowly with age. Nail changes can occur in relation to infections, dietary deficiencies, drug reactions, circulatory changes, diabetes mellitus, and degenerative changes associated with aging. The toenail may atrophy as a result of a disturbance of nutrition, infection or injury to the nail, or disturbances in peripheral circulation seen in occlusive arterial disease or in diabetes. The nail appears disorganized and in some cases avulsed. There is generally an appearance of regrowth, but the original texture of the nail tends to be lost. Alterations may occur in the shape and the thickness of the nail. There is generally no pain involved.[23]

The longitudinal ridging (onychorrhexis) that occurs in the toenails reflects the aging process. This striation may be accentuated, in combination with discoloration, in certain systemic diseases such as diabetes and peripheral vascular insufficiency.

Hypertrophic changes in the nail are common in the elderly. Excessive activity of the matrix, either induced by systemic disease or traumatic injury, may produce hypertrophic nail changes. The nail increases in bulk and hardness and becomes enlarged and/or grossly deformed. The most common etiologic factor when one or two nails are involved is repeated microtrauma (such as ill-fitting shoes). If all the nails are affected, the condition is associated with a systemic disorder that disrupts the normal vascular supply to the nail plate, nail bed, and matrix. Pain is not generally a major factor; however, as hypertrophy continues to evolve, the pressure in the nail bed can give rise to discomfort in the elderly person.

The contour of the nail changes as a result of the influence of the hyperkeratotic barrier. When injury only affects one side of the matrix, there tends to be a sideways growth of the nail plate. The appearance of a "ram's horn" or "club" nail may result. It is often seen that neglect of this problem increases the deformity. The deformity itself is not generally painful, but the pressures induced by footwear on the deformity may create a painful situation.

Nail changes occurring in elderly persons may be related to disease or the aging process itself. Nonetheless, they do not represent a "normal" condition and require appropriate and periodic management by a podiatrist to prevent a more serious problem or deformity from occurring.

Peripheral and Vestibular Sensory Changes

Proprioception and kinesthesia are affected by changes in the neurosensory mechanisms. Though a greater degree of sensory-perceptual loss results from local system changes (e.g., impaired vision from increased lens density), cerebral cortex cell loss may result in less cellular availability for sensory interpretation. This is important when evaluating an elderly person's gait pattern and foot placement. Peripheral vascular disease and diabetes may affect proprioceptive input. Vibratory sense is diminished or lost in the early stages of type II diabetes.

Degeneration occurs in the sensory receptors in both the otoliths and semicircular canals affecting the vestibular system. The function of this system is to monitor head position and to detect head movements. When a person is deprived of visual and lower extremity somatosensory information, the vestibular system is left to control balance. Healthy young adults are able to balance without meaningful visual or support surface information. Healthy elderly persons with "normal" amounts of vestibular degeneration lose their balance and are at risk for falls when vestibular input is the only spatial orientation information available. Diseases of the neuromuscular system further compound this problem. Balance problems or the "fear of falling" may severely compromise ambulatory capabilities in elderly persons. Ankle sprains, stubbed toes, and fractured hips are the result of this diminished input.

NUTRITIONAL CONSIDERATIONS

Nutritional requirements are influenced by heredity, metabolic rates, reaction to stress (including surgery), and environmental factors. Nutritional deficiencies in elderly persons can result in poor skin condition, ulceration, slow healing times, and inadequate metabolism to meet physiologic demands following foot or ankle injuries. Poorly fitting dentures or loss of teeth, decreased smell and taste, changes in postural alignment resulting from osteoporosis or neuromuscular pathologies, or gastrointestinal problems may inhibit eating and lead to nutritional deficiencies in aged persons. An elderly person's nutritional status may be compromised because of the inability to physically get out to obtain food or inability to afford food. Chronic diseases such as diabetes or peripheral vascular disease can impede nutrition. It has been shown that the basal metabolic rate decreases with age, further compromising nutritional status by preventing efficient use and absorption of metabolic substrates.

Interaction between nutrients and drugs may also adversely affect the elder's nutritional status. Diuretics increase the urinary excretion of potassium, chlorides, calcium, magnesium, and zinc; antacids decrease iron absorption; hormonal drugs decrease vitamin B_6 levels, increasing the chance of developing neuropathies; and alcohol decreases the absorption of many nutrients, especially folates, zinc, and magnesium, leading to vitamin B_1 deficiency and neuritis. Smoking depletes levels of vitamin C, which has an effect on blood vessel fragility and is essential for collagen production and wound healing.

Overall, changes in nutrition related to aging result in an alteration of blood vessels and nerves, keratin production dysfunction, thickening of the skin, and changes in the nail beds. Therapeutic nutritional intervention may include several supplements. Vitamins C, B_1, and B_6 as well as zinc enhance the integrity of blood vessels and nerves and improve wound healing. Vitamin C also lessens capillary fragility (i.e., reduces petechiae, ecchymosis, and hematoma) and aids in collagen production, facilitating the formation of connective tissue for joint integrity and wound healing. Zinc is additionally necessary for bone growth, wound healing, and strength of muscle contraction.[45] A common nutritional deficiency in diabetes is thiamine (B_1), a coenzyme in carbohydrate metabolism. Tong[44] showed a significant increase in the nerve conduction velocity of the lateral popliteal and posterior tibial nerves with a well-balanced diet of vitamins B_1, B_6, and B_{12} in diabetic elderly persons. Vitamin B_6 alone was demonstrated by Jones and Gonzales[27] to improve diabetic neuropathies, which so often are manifested in the elder foot.

DISUSE

The expression "use it or lose it" can readily apply to joint changes in the immobile and sedentary person. Deprivation of normal weight-bearing stresses alters the morphologic, biochemical, and biomechanical characteristics of various components of synovial tissues. Alterations are manifested as proliferation of fibrofatty connective tissue within joint spaces, adhesions between synovial folds, adherence of fibrofatty connective tissue to cartilage surfaces, atrophy of cartilage, ulceration at points of cartilage-cartilage contact, disorganization of cellular and fibrillar ligament alignment, weakening of ligament insertion sites owing to osteoclastic resorption of bone and Sharpey's fibers, regional osteoporosis of the involved extremity, reduced energy-absorbing capacity of the bone-ligament-bone complex, 10% decline in collagen mass; increased collagen turnover with accelerated degradation and synthesis, and increase in collagen cross-linking.[1, 30, 46, 47]

GENDER DIFFERENCES

By the year 2030 the elderly in North America will account for 18% to 20% of the total population and a majority will be women. Other than differences in bone rate demineralization at the time of menopause (discussed under the heading of osteoporosis), are there specific musculoskeletal differences between men and women? Studies of isokinetic muscle strength of the ankle revealed that gender was not a significant factor affecting strength scores.[42] Isokinetic peak torques of the ankle plantar flexor muscles occurred in the supine position with 0-degree knee extension angle in both males and females. There was no correlation found between calf circumference and plantar flexor muscle strength in either males or females.[42]

There is no significant difference in the passive stiffness of ankles in healthy women associated with age or knee positioning.[9] If an age-related increase in passive joint stiffness does exist, such as that shown in studies[9] of the finger and knee, the phenomenon may be joint specific. Even though decreases in contractile tissue occur with aging, the noncontractile tissues around the ankle joint do not seem to exhibit similar changes in the mechanical behavior within the functional range of motion in women.[9]

EVALUATION

Though there are many technologically sophisticated methods of objectively evaluating gait and weight transfer patterns, the least expensive method is a thorough biomechanical assessment and observation of gait. A thorough evaluation and interpretation of the findings are vital to the establishment of an effective, targeted treatment program. Examination of the foot and lower extremity includes medical history (symptoms), visual inspection, palpation, sensory and proprioception tests, determination of range of motion and joint mobility, muscle strength testing, and gait assessment. Often muscle testing positions must be modified for the elderly patient who cannot assume the prone or supine position because of respiratory or cardiopulmonary difficulties, hiatal hernias, or spinal problems. Assessment of joint end feel can be performed in other positions but grades will be more often zero, one, or two out of Maitland's scale of zero to six, reflecting the hypo-mobility between joint surfaces and the stiffer surrounding capsular-ligamental tissues. Verbal testing instructions to an elderly patient should be clear and uncomplicated. A learning effect may produce significantly different test results so it is advised that a number of trials be performed first before recording the grades of strength or range of motion.

With all elderly patients we test sensation using the Symmes-Weinstein filaments, vibration (tuning fork), light touch, and temperature. Particularly important in the diabetic patient, this information on sensory deficits is needed for safety instruction and for determination of the best shoe to fit the foot.

Dynamic footprints, if available, are an inexpensive means of determining abnormal weight distribution and joint restriction. This evaluation utilizes ink-based mats upon which the patient steps barefooted during gait. The darker the ink, the greater the pressure. Other means of determining weight-bearing patterns include the use of chalk, water, or pressure-sensitive paper to record gait. Foot angle, width, stride length, and cadence can be objectively measured using these simple methods. The elderly patient should be observed with shoes on to determine whether shoe fit is a contributing factor to foot pathology. The shoe should be inspected for abnormal wear patterns on the sole and heel, distortion of the toe box or heel counters, wrinkles or creases in the toe box, and pressure points (especially along the shoe seams) that may cause irritation or enhance deformity. Proper shoe size and width should be checked in relation to the foot. The insole should be inspected for abnormal wear patterns by the toes, metatarsal joints, and heel. Deeper indentations will reflect heavier pressures and most often will be correlated with callus and corn formation on the foot.

When orthotic intervention is prescribed, it should first be determined whether the orthotic is to be functional or accommodative. A functional orthotic enhances present foot function and is commonly used in younger persons, very active elders, or athletes. An accommodative orthotic "accommodates" fixed deformities and provides a cradle or padding that enhances functional mobility by redistributing weight-bearing pressures by providing total-contact on the plantar surface for shock absorption.

Careful examination of the foot to identify the pathology and/or mechanical problems involved in a particular condition provides the basis for specific use of manual and physical modalities, orthotic materials, podiatric products, and shoe intervention. The following section of this chapter presents gen-eral and specific considerations in the aging foot, treatment objectives and corresponding therapeutic interventions, orthotic and shoe considerations for conservative management of the pathomechanical elderly foot.

GENERAL CONSIDERATIONS IN TREATING THE AGING FOOT

Treatment time frames for the elderly patient may be extended beyond those of the younger patient for a number of reasons. Transportation may be a significant problem. The patient may no longer drive a car and need to rely on friends and family to get to therapy. Scheduling may be difficult for all parties involved and allowances should be made for treatment flexibility. Clinically, we find it advantageous to have a spouse, relative, or neighbor accompany the patient to therapy even if the patient can drive. Having another person involved seems to ensure better compliance, recollection, and follow-through with home programs. Insurance coverage may be limited to a dollar amount or a certain number of visits. We circumvent the problem of limited patient visits by seeing patients only once a week for an extended time frame. Change in tissue structure may be slower in elders owing to changes in hyaluronic acid, contractile proteins, collagen, and elastin production. Extending the treatments over many weeks enables tissue modifications to be made slowly and new problems to be handled as they come up. Increasing the length of treatment sessions ensures sufficient patient education time and write out all instructions for the patient to take home.

CONSERVATIVE INTERVENTIONS FOR FOOT PATHOLOGY IN THE ELDERLY

The most common foot disorders in people aged 65 and over include hallux valgus and deformities of the lesser toes, degenerative joint diseases, circulatory changes, and neurologic changes related to diabetes and peripheral vascular disease.[20, 29] All of these foot problems require conservative intervention to prevent loss of function resulting from pain and the possibility of ulcerations, compromised circulation, or insensitivity.

Arthritis

Rheumatoid Arthritis

Deformities and inflammation resulting from arthritic changes in the foot can affect single joints, as in osteoarthritis or traumatic arthritis, or can systemically affect all the joints of the foot, as in cases of rheumatoid arthritis. It is estimated that 89% of patients with rheumatoid arthritis have problems with their feet.[28]

Evaluative Findings.—In the early stages of rheumatoid arthritis, the joints become inflamed with marked thickening of synovial tissue and the accumulation of panus covering the articular surface of the joint. This results in pain and swelling of the joints limiting motion and causing muscle atrophy and weakness. These periods of inflammation result in damage to the articular surfaces leading to progressive deformities. The affected joints become fibrotic from long periods of immobility, losing joint mobility and range of motion. Most commonly, these deformities involve the first metatarsal (hallux valgus or hallux limitus), the lesser toes (hammer, claw, mallet, and overlapping toes), and severe rearfoot deformities. Valgus deformity of the hindfoot in rheumatoid patients results from exaggerated pronation forces on the weakened and inflamed subtalar joint. These forces are caused by alterations in gait secondary to asymmetric muscle weakness and the compensatory efforts of the patient to minimize pain in the feet. The patient fails to roll over the forefoot during late stance and stride length, velocity, and efficiency are diminished.[28] As the disease progresses, the destruction of the joint tissues and loss of muscle strength leads to more pain in the forefoot seen as subluxation of the metatarsophalangeal and midtarsal joints and ankylosis of the ankle. Radiographs suggest an association between valgus deformity of the feet and valgus deformity of the knees in rheumatoid patients.[28] The skin of the rheumatoid arthritis patient takes on a characteristic translucence and becomes smooth, glossy, tender, and "tissue-paper" thin. Other clinically significant findings, especially in rheumatoid arthritis, include arthritic nodules, and inflamed bursal sacs at the heel.[34] Alternative interventions will be discussed in greater detail in subsequent sections of this chapter relating to specific foot deformities.

Treatment Suggestions.—General objectives in treating the rheumatoid arthritic foot include decreasing pain and swelling through heat modalities and grade 1 joint mobilization oscillations; increasing and/or maintaining range of motion and joint mobility at the ankle through stretching and mobilization techniques; stabilizing the forefoot and midfoot through stretching of the antagonistic muscles and strengthening of the agonistic muscles; and protection of the vulnerable skin. Paraffin (Fig 23–1) is an excellent means of obtaining uniform heating of the foot. Talar rocking (Fig 23–2) and long-axis distraction are mobilization techniques that are particularly successful in improving range of motion at the talocrural and subtalar joint. Stretching ligamentous structures of the midfoot, forefoot, and toes will lessen developing or developed deformities. Strengthening exercises should be targeted toward the weakened, elongated muscles. For instance, in a hammer or claw toe it is important to strengthen the toe extensors; strengthening of the toe flexors would only increase flexion deformities of the lesser toes.[4] Strengthening dorsiflexors of the ankle counters plantar flexion deformities.

Osteoarthritis

In osteoarthritis, the most common of the various forms of arthritis affecting humans, the joints of the foot may be enlarged with extra bony growth but are rarely swollen with fluid. Primary osteoarthritis (having no known cause) of the foot usually involves the first metatarsophalangeal joint. Secondary osteoarthritis (anatomic or pathophysiologic causes are known) may affect any joint.[17]

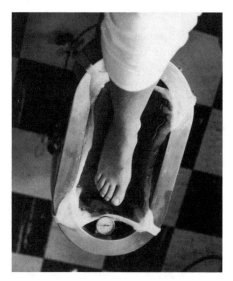

FIG 23–1.
Paraffin bath provides uniform heating of the foot.

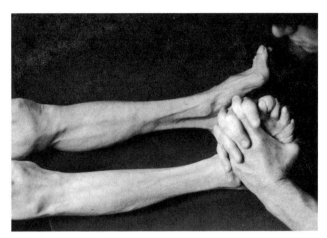

FIG 23–2.
Talar rocking mobilization technique.

Osteoarthritis is a process that involves articular cartilage and subchondral bone. Breakdown of cartilage leads to fissuring, pitting, and erosion of the cartilaginous surfaces. The body then responds with proliferation of cartilage and bone, usually at the joint periphery. This leads to bone spurs. Release of enzymes from chondrocytes may lead to some inflammation when the repair process breaks down.

Evaluative Findings.—Osteoarthritis of the subtalar joint begins with hindfoot pain and instability in walking. The first metatarsocuneiform joint may have degenerative changes with dorsal exostosis making shoe fit difficult. Enlargement, limited range of motion, and pain in the metatarsophalangeal joint are common. Mallet or hammer toe deformities may develop secondarily.

Treatment Suggestions.—Treatment for pain control may include use of modalities such as heat, cold, (TENS), ultrasound, and paraffin. Splinting, casting or bracing may be employed when biomechanical correction is necessary to diminish abnormal stresses on joints. Orthotic intervention with accommodative devices to pad areas of pressure and provide shock absorption are recommended. Materials such as PPT, Sorbathane, and Spenco inserts in the shoes will diminish impact-loading forces. Movement of the joint surfaces can be increased with joint mobilization, long-axis distraction, and grade 3 and 4 oscillations. Friction massage, deep muscle massage, hold-relax proprioceptive neuromuscular facilitation (PNF) techniques, passive stretching, and active stretching exercises are used to decrease soft-tissue contractures and promote range of motion. It is important to evaluate for and prescribe range-of-motion techniques for joints up the *entire* kinetic chain of the lower extremity, including the sacroiliac joint, for first metatarsophalangeal biomechanical correction. Limitations in the motion of the hip may be manifested by excessive hypermobility stresses on the joints of the foot.

Gouty Arthritis

True gouty arthritis is caused by monosodium urate crystals in the joint. Clinically, it is an acute, intermittent, monoarticular or oligoarticular arthritis with pain so severe the patient can not tolerate weight bearing, no matter how slight, on the affected joint.

Evaluative Findings.—In 75% of cases, the first metatarsophalangeal joint of the foot is the joint affected. Secondarily, the midfoot, ankle, and heels are affected. Tophi may become calcified and extra articular erosion of the bony cortex may progress. In the acute phase involved joints are swollen, hot, reddened, and incapable of tolerating any degree of pressure. In chronic phases involved joints present with limited range, impaired function, and aching. Joint mobility is often severely restricted secondary to calcification and joint erosion.

Treatment Suggestions.—Acute attacks are treated with nonsteroidal anti-inflammatory drugs (NSAIDS). It is important to encourage the continuation of ambulation. Shoes and orthotic provisions should be designed to relieve pressures in order to enhance ambulation. Application of ice followed by grade 1 oscillations is helpful in reducing swelling and pain during the acute phase of gouty arthritis. In the chronic phase use of allopurinol to inhibit xanthine oxidase and block uric acid synthesis is indicated. Accommodative orthotics are recommended to protect the involved joints and provide total contact of the uninvolved plantar surface to evenly distribute the forces of weight bearing. Active exercises to maintain range of motion and function are necessary. The patient can be instructed in the use of heat, self-mobilization, stretching, and muscle strengthening.

General Treatment Suggestions: Arthritic Conditions

In all forms of arthritis, the patient needs to be instructed in the importance of a balance between rest and activity. The patient should be taught principles of ergonomics to ensure joint protection during lifting and carrying loads. A graded walking program is advised to maintain ambulation but avoid undue stress to acutely inflamed joints. Strengthening exercises should be geared toward the maintainance of functional ADL. Rather than having the patient do short-arc quadriceps exercises or straight leg raising, have the patient practice rising slowly from sit to stand, and stand to sit ten times. Rocking chairs are good for maintaining ankle mobility and assist in improving circulation as well as strengthening the lower leg and ankle.

The orthotic objectives in treating the foot deformed by rheumatoid arthritis, osteoarthritis or gouty arthritis include the prevention or limitation of painful joint motion, accommodation of deformities, and cushioning during impact loading. A total-contact orthotic is best for protection of the involved joints. If sensation is intact enough to permit heat molding, the foot should be positioned optimally in subtalar neutral. If sensation is impaired, the foot should be protected from the heat by additional sock layers. A semirigid material on the bottom layer controls foot position, and Plastazote no. 1, Aliplast XPE, PPT, or Plastazote no. 3 cushions sensitive areas on the top layer.

Shoes prescribed for the arthritic person should provide a reinforced heel counter to limit subtalar motion. High-top sneakers or a special high collar added to the shoe can serve to control excessive ankle motion. An extra-depth shoe such as P. W. Minor's Extra-depth Thermold shoe has a wide, rounded toe box, which accommodates toe and midfoot deformities and provides the room needed for the orthotic insert. The thermally moldable leather enables the shoe to be altered in specific places by using a ball-and-socket device or shoe stretcher. The shoe can be placed in a convection oven at 130 degrees to stretch and mold it further. A rocker-bottom sole added to the shoe for the arthritic foot can improve push-off during ambulation. This type of sole shortens the distance between the heel and the metatarsophalangeal joints and reduces the ankle motion required for push-off. A SACH heel may be added to the shoe to further absorb shock at heel strike and limit ankle and subtalar joint motion. A flared heel (such as the Thomas heel) can reduce medial-lateral movement at the subtalar joint and prevent or limit motion into excessive varus or valgus.

Diabetes

To the experienced clinician, the term *diabetes* automatically suggests *foot problems.* The pathologic processes of neuropathy and macrovascular and microvascular disease are common to the lower extremity of the diabetic patient. These processes may occur individually or together, placing the patient at increased risk for morbid conditions such as ulceration, gangrene, and infection.[43] The metabolic effects of diabetes are profound and insidious, affecting all parts of the body. The peripheral vascular system commonly develops arteriosclerosis obliterans and the nervous system deteriorates leading to diminished sensation and peripheral neuropathy.[31] The elderly diabetic patient is usually more susceptible to infection and has associated avascularity, atrophy of tissue, neuropathic changes, and the general lack of concern for foot health that appears to be an endemic situation.[23]

Evaluative Findings.—Protective sensation defined by Nawoczenski et al[36] is 5.07 g of pressure using the Symmes-Weinstein monofilaments. Specific evaluation of the entire plantar surface of the foot will designate areas of sensory loss vulnerable for breakdown. Vibratory and temperature sense is diminished very early in the disease process, compromising proprioception, kinesthesia, and awareness of temperature gradients. The skin of the diabetic is often dry, scaly, and fissured, further increasing susceptibility to breakdown. Muscular strength is decreased owing to poor nerve conductivity, decreased energy utilization by muscle cells, altered and inefficient biomechanical gait patterns, and inactivity.

Friction and pressure forces combine as shear force during dynamic walking. At heel contact there is a direct downward force of the body weight through the heel and an upward ground reactive force into the heel. The foot contacts the ground in supination and during the first 25% of stance pronates with the leg and thigh internally rotating. The foot is fixed on the ground by the body weight pushing downward and ground reactive forces pushing upward. Shear force results from parts of the body sliding relative to each other in a direction parallel to their plane of contact. Shear force is believed to be the force most responsible for tissue breakdown in the insensitive foot.[21]

The diabetic foot is special because of concurrent neurologic and circulatory involvement. Alterations of sensory impulses are evidenced by absent vibratory, pinprick, and pressure sensation. Motor involvement accompanies sensory involvement with muscular atrophy and weakness, leading to cocked-up toes, prominent metatarsal heads, intrinsic muscle wasting, equinus deformity, varus position of the hindfoot, and proximal malalignment. The intrinsic muscles function to stabilize the metatarsophalangeal joints during midstance immediately before push off. Extensor hallucis longus muscle weakness allows hammering of the hallux by the overriding pull of the long flexors.

Atrophy or distal deformation of the protective subcutaneus fat pad leads to soft-tissue trauma and breakdown under the metatarsal heads. Preexisting deformity and abnormal foot function will be accentuated, leading to tissue ulceration. A long, short, or plantar-flexed metatarsal produces excessive pressure owing to repetitive trauma at a site that the patient will not feel. Symmes-Weinstein monofilament testing along with vibratory testing is an essential part of diabetic foot evaluation for determination of impaired pressure, pain, and protective sensation.

Foot lesions account for 20% of all diabetic hospitalizations and 50% to 70% of all nontraumatic amputations performed yearly.[2] Removal of one of the lesser toes because of irreversible soft-tissue and bony destruction has little effect on the posture and function of the foot. Ablation of the hallux and metatarsal head has a dramatic effect on function of the foot in gait. As the weight-bearing surface area beneath the foot decreases, the pressure on the remaining weight-bearing surface area increases. Identical pressure on a diminished surface area can cause rapid soft-tissue breakdown. With amputation of the hallux, the forces at push-off are transmitted laterally to the lesser digits through the long flexor tendons, causing hammering of the toes. Ulceration at previous ulcer sites is unfortunately all too common an occurrence in the diabetic person.

Treatment Suggestions.—The major objective of treating the diabetic foot is to prevent tissue ulceration. This can best be accomplished through patient education in regard to adequate nutrition, skin care, and safety. For instance, a diabetic elder should use a thermometer or ask a nondiabetic relative or friend to measure water temperature in a bath before immersing the feet in water that may be too hot. The feet should be checked nightly for reddened areas using a mirror under the plantar surface or with help from another person. Establishment of a full-time podiatry clinic enabled Grady Memorial Hospital in Atlanta to reduce the amputation rate of its diabetic population by 24% within the first year of operation.[5]

The major objectives in treating the diabetic foot are to protect the plantar surface of the foot from repetitive microtrauma and accommodate deformities that could be traumatized by excessive shoe pressures resulting in ulceration and amputation. Total-contact full-foot orthotics using soft, shock-absorbing materials helps to distribute weight-bearing pressures over the entire plantar surface of the foot away from the vulnerable bony prominences. A Thermold leather shoe is recommended for the insensitive diabetic foot.

Peripheral Vascular Disease

Peripheral vascular disease results in increased peripheral vascular resistance owing to narrowing and loss of elasticity in the vessel walls. Peripheral arterial insufficiency is present in most elderly individuals in varying degrees.

Evaluative Findings.—Indications of poor circulation in the feet include absence of the dorsal pedal and posterior tibialis pulses, muscle fatigue, cramps in the foot and leg, intermittent claudication, pain, burning, coldness, pallor, paresthesias, atrophy of soft tissues, nail bed alterations, and trophic dermal changes such as dryness and loss of hair. Prime significance should not be placed upon absence or presence of pedal pulses, however. Pulses may not be palpable at pressures between 70 to 100 mm Hg and are usually absent below 70 mm Hg. The ankle brachial index may be lower in some patients with palpable pulses resulting from hypertension than in normotensive patients with lower ankle pressures and nonpalpable pulses.[33] Decreased vascularization increases the likelihood of injury owing to fragility of the tissues to normal stresses. Delayed and inadequate healing results because there is a decrease in the oxygen supply to tissues. Assessment of the two separate vascular beds in the lower extremity should include the major arterial system and small arteries, arterioles, capillaries, and venules that nourish the skin. In most cases the small vessels are dependent on the flow in the major vessels; however, in chronic occlusive vascular disease in which partial or complete occlusion of the major vessels occurs, the blood supply to the tissues may be adequate owing to extensive collateral arterial circulation developed by the body as a defense to the slowly progressing ischemia.

Treatment Suggestions.—The objectives in conservative rehabilitative intervention include improving circulation by promoting smooth-muscle strength in the vessels for more efficient oxygenation, skin care, decreasing edema associated with decreased circulatory efficiency and inactivity, and increasing over-all cardiovascular endurance.

The most effective vasodilators of these collateral vessels are locally produced metabolites, which accumulate during exercise or ischemia. It is clear then that the best vasodilator of vessels within skeletal muscles is exercise.[33] Clinically, the use of Buerger-Allen exercises has been found to be very effective in enhancing peripheral circulation. These exercises consist of a series of positional changes in the following sequence: the lower extremities are supported in an elevated position at an angle of 45 degrees for 30 to 180 seconds or for the minimum time required to produce blanching (Fig 23–3, A). Next, the legs are lowered to a horizontal position for 2 to 3 minutes (Fig 23–3, B) or until blanching recedes. This is a modification in the original Buerger-Allen regimen to prevent adverse cardiovascular reactions in the elderly. Following the horizontal position, the feet are permitted to hang down in a dependent position over the edge of the bed for 2 to 3 minutes (Fig 23–3, C). Once hyperemia or rubor has appeared, the feet are kept dependent for 1 extra minute. The last position change in the sequence is a return to the horizontal position (Fig 23–3, B). The entire sequence is repeated three to five times depending on patient tolerance. Throughout the exercise sequence, the patient is encouraged to dorsiflex, plantarflex, and circle the feet to further promote circulation by active muscle contraction. A Jobst compression pump or stockings are alternatives to providing management of lower extremity edema and enhancing circulation; however, these authors have observed clinically that the latent effects of Jobst compression are not long-lived, based on circumferential measurements and skin color, and that high

levels of compression are not well tolerated by elderly persons. Jobst stockings, while effective in controlling edema, are very difficult for most elderly individuals to don. Massage, high-galvanic electrical stimulation, and active resistive exercise can enhance peripheral circulation. Ambulation is encouraged to facilitate overall cardiovascular health and maintain strength in the lower extremities.

Orthotic and shoe intervention in the elderly individual with peripheral vascular disease are identical to those presented in the management of the diabetic foot. Compression stockings are recommended to decrease edema provided they will not cause excessive pressures or compromise the cardiovascular system. Elastic laces in the shoes are used to accommodate varying levels of edema. The patient is instructed in elevation of the legs at rest and in proper skin care. To control for the possibility of excessive sweating with orthotic wear (which is a confounding problem in peripheral vascular disease), the patient is also instructed in frequent sock and shoe changes to prevent hyperhydration and skin breakdown.

Cerebral Vascular Accidents

The residual deficits of a cerebral vascular accident (CVA) involve muscle weakness, muscle tone changes (i.e., hypotonus or hypertonus), loss of proprioception and sensation in the involved lower extremity, and problems with coordination and balance. All of these factors have a direct effect on the biomechanical components of gait.

Evaluative Findings.—The most significant finding influencing foot and ankle functioning following

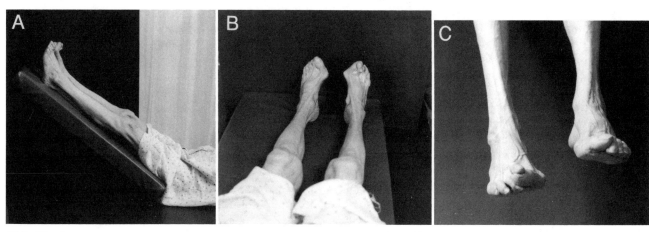

FIG 23–3.
Buerger-Allen exercises. **A,** legs elevated. **B,** legs horizontal. **C,** legs dependent.

a CVA is alteration in the neuromuscular status. With extensor spasticity, plantar flexors and invertors of the foot and ankle generally have an increased tone with consequential equinus and varus deformities overriding the ability to dorsiflex the foot. In the event of flaccidity, a weakness in the dorsiflexors and evertor muscles will be seen. In combination with proprioceptive and kinesthetic losses, the involved extremity in both spasticity and flaccidity is usually unstable and ineffective in propulsion during gait. Primitive reflexes such as flexor withdrawal or crossed extension may be present, interfering with the ability of the patient to bear weight on the leg without eliciting flexor or extensor synergies, respectively. Tone changes severely alter the biomechanic functioning of the foot, often rendering the donning of shoes intolerable. Peripheral vascular changes in the CVA patient are consistent with those found in peripheral vascular disease and the same assessment principles need to be applied.

Treatment Suggestions.—Muscle strengthening and reeducation is a primary focus in treatment following a CVA. This can best be accomplished by functional mobility therapeutic techniques such as proprioceptive neuromuscular fascilitation (PNF), neurodevelopmental techniques (NDT), and active muscle strengthening. An adjunct to strengthening exercises may be electrical stimulation; this modality greatly assists in muscle reeducation.

The objectives in prescribing orthotics in an individual with a CVA include controlling the foot and ankle despite tone changes, accommodating fixed deformities, and cushioning impact loading. A two-ply orthotic using semirigid materials like Aliplast XPE will control foot position and a softer top layer will cradle and protect the foot. It has been clinically observed that accurate placement of a metatarsal bar aids in controlling muscle tone. A metatarsal bar placed slightly proximal to the metatarsal heads enhances plantar flexion, while a metatarsal bar placed slightly distal to the metatarsal heads produces dorsiflexion in some individuals. When tone is controlled, accommodation of foot deformities with the orthotic is more easily managed. In the flaccid lower extremity, accommodation of the foot may need to include an ankle-foot orthoses (AFO) or short leg brace with the orthotic inserted in the shoe.

A reinforced heel counter helps to limit subtalar motion and stabilize the foot on heel strike. A flared heel is often recommended to provide better foot placement. A rigid shoe shank may be required for better control, especially with lower extremity brac-

ing. A high-top shoe may provide the needed ankle control for foot placement. In the presence of an equinus deformity, a heel lift on the shoe provides total contact during weight bearing and facilitates stability and aids in decreasing excessive stress on the gastrocnemius-soleus muscle complex. In severe deformities of the foot or ankle, a custom-molded shoe may be the only effective alternative.

REARFOOT PROBLEMS

Ankle Sprains

Too often the fibular bone and cuboid bone are ignored when a lateral sprain occurs. If the fibula or cuboid have been displaced inferiorly they will impede dorsiflexion at the talocrural joint. Natural joint play of tibiofibular distraction and superior gliding of the fibula do not occur and gliding of the talus is limited, producing pain, pressure, and decreased ankle movement. Severe ankle sprains necessitating surgical tendon and ligament repair will compromise the mobility of the talocrural, subtalar, and midtarsal joints.

Enwemeka[15] states that as prolonged immobilization is the major cause of complications following tendon repair, the challenge in rehabilitation is to safely limit the period of immobilization in order to permit therapeutic motion. Biochemical changes that occur with immobilization include a decrease in glycosaminoglycans and water content, which leads to alterations in the viscous nature of connective tissue causing an increase in the stiffness of the joint.[13] Latest research indicates that three weeks of immobilization induces progressive disorganization of tendon collagen and a decline in the size of collagen fibrils.[15] Rapid muscle atrophy, not scar tissue formation, poses a major hindrance to rehabilitation after surgical repair of the Achilles tendon. More than 40% atrophy was demonstrated in the soleus muscle after 3 weeks of immobilization in a cast without a tenotomy, and this percentage was increased with tenotomy. Thus prolonged cast immobilization may weaken tendons and muscles. Enwemeka suggests that tendon healing has, in addition to a 5-day inflammatory phase, a fibroplasia and fibrillogenesis phase from day 7 onward, and remolding phase from day 8 to day 21, as well as two additional processes of collagen synthesis and organization. Perhaps with prolonged immobilization metabolically active fibroblasts in areas of disorganized collagen are involved in active degradation of the collagen matrix. Muscle lengthening by serial casting produces a temporary but significant reversal of progressive atrophy but when the muscle was kept at the same length for longer than 3 weeks, reversal of atrophy was not observed. In summary, the therapist should be familiar with the biologic time frame following injury and repair to maximize the rehabilitative program. Excessive stresses too early in the biologic healing process can be harmful, as can too little too late.

Evaluative Findings.—The most consistent findings in acute ankle sprains are pain, swelling, and discoloration. The ankle is unstable and joint motion very painful. The force of muscle contraction may be decreased secondary to inhibitory influences created by extracellular effusion, further increasing the instability of the ankle joint.[12] In subacute ankle sprains there is often tenderness along the involved tendons and ligaments. Joint mobility is restricted by discomfort and fibrinogen deposition related to the healing process.[8, 13] Postsurgically, scarring may also be a factor limiting both joint and soft tissue mobility.

Treatment Suggestions.—Fibular mobilization, cuboid realignment, and tibiofibular distraction will restore full dorsiflexion at the talocrural joint (Fig 23–4). All treatment plans should involve control of edema, protection of the joint, and rehabilitation of the muscles and tendons. Control of swelling requires immediate consideration since effusion and hemorrhage distend the joint and favor formation of adhesions, which delay healing. Ice, elevation, compression, pulsed ultrasound, electrical stimulation, and limited weight bearing are prescribed in acute and subacute conditions.

Use of cold has been shown to to decrease vasodilator metabolism, encourage vasoconstriction, and increase blood viscosity.[16] Massage is reported to enhance venous and lymphatic drainage of the lower extremity.[16]

Use of high-galvanic electrical stimulation may alter hemodynamics. Animal experiments concluded that such stimulation decreased the protein leakage from blood vessels by an unknown mechanism. Decreased protein leakage allows the lymphatic system to remove excess fluid in the tissues and prevent further increase in fluid migration into the surrounding cells.[16] Clinically, the most effective electrode placement for general ankle and foot effusion and contusions is to use four leads criss-crossing the electrodes to bisect the ankle medially and laterally (Fig 23–5). As severe swelling causes an acid tissue environment, the desired polar effect of electrical stimulation is to create a negative electrical field. In a lateral ankle sprain, the two negative leads should be placed laterally and the positive leads medially (Fig 23–6). The negative field produces an alkaline environment and softens tissue.[24] The ultimate effect of high galvanic or interferential electrical stimulation is to reduce pain, reduce swelling, increase circulation, and soften scar tissue so that it can be remolded more effectively. Transcutaneous electrical nerve stimulation (TENS) is another electrical modality that is effective in controlling pain, especially in the acute phases of ankle sprain. The control or relief of pain is explained by theories that the stimulation of cutaneous sensory fibers may inhibit the perception of pain and/or stimulate the release of beta-

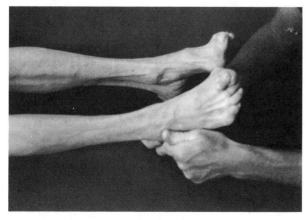

FIG 23–4.
Fibular mobilization technique.

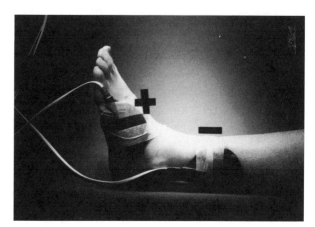

FIG 23–5.
Four leads transecting the ankle to reduce effusion and contusion.

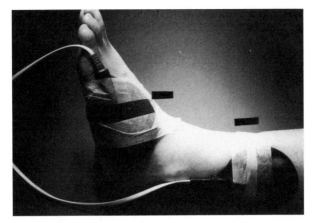

FIG 23–6.
Creating a negative electrical field in lateral ankle sprain.

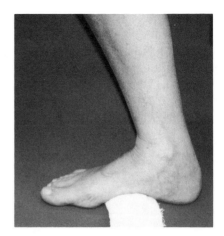

FIG 23–7.
Proper stretching of the gastrocnemius-soleus locking mid-tarsal joint.

endorphin substances that inhibit the transmission of pain.

Toe curling and extension exercises assist in stabilizing the whole foot and ankle complex through active exercise. Ankle dorsiflexion, plantar flexion, and inversion-eversion exercises are also recommended to improve muscle strength and eliminate muscle imbalances in function. Taping the ankle is a means of providing additional support to the ankle when instability exists; it should only be used as a temporary measure, as improved muscle strength is the best ankle stabilizer.

Joint mobilization techniques are sometimes helpful in restoring adequate joint play motions between the distal tibiofibular, talocrural, subtalar, and intermetatarsal joints. Distal tibiofibular joint mobilization consists of anterior and posterior glides of the tibia on the fibula. Superior gliding of the fibula will help restore pain-free eversion motions. Talocrural joint mobilizations consist of anterior and posterior glides of the tibia and fibula on the talus and long axis distraction of the talocrural joint. Subtalar joint mobilizations include: calcaneal distraction, calcaneal rocking, and talar rocking. Intermetatarsal mobilizations consist of superior and inferior glides of the metatarsals on one another and rolling of the forefoot. Mobilization treatments begin with oscillatory forces of grade 1 and progress to grade 4. Joint mobilization is purported to stimulate production of glycosaminoglycans, thereby increasing the water content of connective tissue.[16] Breaking of abnormal collagen cross-links and stimulation of proper collagen fiber orientation have been reported.[41]

To perform gastrocnemius-soleus stretching correctly the patient must keep the subtalar joint in a supinated position; otherwise it will allow the mid-tarsal joint to unlock and the stretching of the plantar fascia will occur, rather than calf muscle stretching (Fig 23–7). The patient holds the stretched position for 10 seconds for ten repetitions, six times a day. Resistive exercises using an elastic material for resistance (Theraband) consists of eversion, plantar flexion, inversion, and dorsiflexion for 20 repetitions, six times per day (Fig 23–8). Patients are encouraged to use ice immediately after exercising to decrease swelling and pain.

Painful Heel Pad

A painful heel pad, the most common rearfoot problem seen in the elderly population, is caused by cumulative repetitive impact loading at heel strike, prolonged weight bearing, obesity, and atrophy of the fat pad of the heel.

Evaluative Findings.—Tenderness is located at the center of the heel. Pain is increased with heel rather than toe weight bearing. X-ray findings are usually negative for central calcaneal calcification on the plantar aspect of the bone. Palpation generally

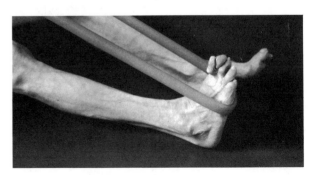

FIG 23–8.
Resistive ankle exercises using Theraband resistance.

reveals that the fat pad of the heel has migrated laterally and that the calcaneal tuberosities (lateral and medial) are prominent.

Treatment Suggestions.—In the presence of acute heel pad pain, rest is recommended. Ice is used to decrease swelling and pain. In subacute and chronic cases, deep friction massage may be employed to decrease the scarring of tissues over the painful area.[6] Interferential current or pulsed ultrasound is helpful for releasing or reducing tissue adhesions.

Orthotic intervention may be utilized to provide shock-absorbing materials at the heel. In the acute phases, the heel pad may be excavated beneath the painful area to further diminish the stress forces producing the discomfort.

Arthrodesis

Arthrodesis is a surgically induced fixation of a joint (most commonly the ankle) by fusion of the joint surfaces.[34]

Evaluative Findings.—In arthrodesis joint mobility is completely restricted. As a result, pain is often reported secondary to shock-absorptive forces at that joint or hypermobility (overuse) pain is reported at the neighboring joint (either superior or inferior). The foot is unable to accommodate to the ground surface during the pronation phase and cannot absorb the ground reaction forces, which are often transmitted up the kinetic chain to the sacroiliac or lumbar joints. Lack of supination-pronation and the absence of dorsiflexion and plantar flexion promote marked substitution patterns during gait. Soft tissues are restricted owing to postsurgical scarring. Muscle force production is diminished owing to altered biomechanics and immobility. Mild to moderate edema is chronically present around the fused joint.

Treatment Suggestions.—If the arthrodesis is properly fused nothing can be done from a therapeutic perspective to alter bony alignment, but muscle reeducation is an important component of working with arthrodesis. As the muscle pull is usually redirected from its original orientation, the patient must relearn effective muscle contraction. This is best accomplished through active assistive, active, and active resistive exercise. Electrical stimulation is helpful in improving patient awareness of muscle function. Deep friction massage is employed to decrease the scarring and enhance the mobility of the surrounding soft tissues. Joint mobilization of the adjacent joints may be indicated to restore full flexibility for functional activities during gait. For instance, if the subtalar joint is fused, talarcrural and midtarsal mobilization assists in providing additional mobility. Muscle reeducation is required to produce an efficient gait pattern. Physical modalities may be used to eliminate edema and promote circulation, though they are contraindicated in the presence of metallic (rather than bony) fixation devices. Proper skin care and joint protection is important. In the presence of permanent bony restriction the treatment of choice to protect the joint is accommodative orthotics and shoes.

The objectives in orthotic management of a patient with an arthrodesis are to absorb shock at heel strike, improve comfort and efficiency at push-off, and accommodate the residual equinus deformity. A total-contact orthotic with a heel lift will accommodate Achilles tendon shortening or residual equinus. The heel should be cushioned and elevated to absorb shock and simulate plantar flexion after heel strike. A metatarsal pad helps to redistribute the pressures on the metatarsal heads, which bear most of the weight during stance owing to the equinus deformity.

A reinforced heel counter, high-top shoe, or medial-lateral flared heel is recommended for added heel stability. A SACH heel helps to absorb shock and simulate plantar flexion after heel strike. A rocker-bottom sole assists dorsiflexion.

Achilles Tendinitis, Bursitis, Haglund's Deformity

Achilles Tendinitis

Achilles tendinitis is a painful inflammation of the peritenon without tendon inflammation. Acute cases of Achilles tendinitis involve the peritenon, which surrounds the Achilles tendon. In chronic cases there may be nodule formation (scarring) on the tendon itself. The causes are usually related to trauma, chronic overstress, accumulated impact loading (i.e., prolonged standing or walking), mechanical irritation from shoe friction, inflammatory diseases, metabolic disorders, or infectious diseases.

Evaluative Findings.—Evaluation of acute tendinitis reveals severe pain, swelling, and discoloration along the Achilles tendon especially at the tendon's insertion. Dorsiflexion, both passive and active, is extremely uncomfortable. Tenderness is present at the junction of the Achilles with the calcaneus and along the tendon's course. In subacute and chronic Achilles tendinitis, nodular formations may be palpated on the tendon itself. Muscle strength is diminished in the gastrocnemius-soleus group and pain is elicited with both active and passive dorsiflexion. Weight bearing on the toes produces pain in the contracting Achilles muscle complex. Soft tissues surrounding the tendon are adhered secondary to immobility and the mobility of the peritenon is decreased as a result of scarring.

Treatment Suggestions.—Alternative rehabilitative interventions, in addition to orthotic and shoe modifications, include rest, heat or cold, anti-inflammatory medications, stretching, and soft-tissue mobilization. It is important that proper stretching be performed as shown in Figure 23–7 to eliminate midtarsal joint motion and focus the stretching to isolate the gastrosoleus muscle complex and talocrural joint. Deep friction massage is helpful in mobilizing scar tissue and improving circulation.[6] Ice is recommended to reduce swelling and provide a better environment for healing. Ultrasound and interferential current are helpful in mobilizing tissue adhesions and promoting blood flow to assist in localized healing of the tissues. In addition, electrical stimulation may be used to facilitate muscle contraction. Pulsed ultrasound is recommended for the local effects of mobilizing extracellular fluid and thereby decreasing edema and mobilizing adhesions in tissues surrounding the achilles tendon. Strengthening exercises in all planes of motion of the ankle are important to correct muscle imbalances.

Achilles Bursitis

Achilles bursitis can involve either or both of the bursae. The retrocalcaneal bursa is located between the Achilles tendon and the posterosuperior angle of the calcaneous, and the precalcaneal bursa is between the Achilles tendon and the skin. The most common cause of Achilles bursitis is repeated mechanical stress (i.e., irritation from shoe friction) irritating these bursae. Other causes may include metabolic or inflammatory diseases and tightness of the gastrocnemius-soleus muscle.

Evaluative Findings.—Achilles bursitis is positively identified by swelling and pain in the bursae. Tenderness to palpation is present superior to the Achilles-calcaneal junction. Active and passive dorsiflexion elicit pain at the same site. The patient often reports a decrease in discomfort when a small heel lift is provided.

Treatment Suggestions.—Treatment is similar to that employed in the treatment of Achilles tendinitis. Massage is particularly helpful in relieving pain, mobilizing soft tissue, and reducing the swelling and induration following soft-tissue trauma associated with bursitis. Iontophoresis, using ethyl alcohol or a procaine ointment, helps to decrease the localized pain. Aspirin helps to decrease the inflammation of the bursae. Taping the ankle into equinus may alleviate the irritation to the bursa or a heel lift may help reduce stresses. Stretching a tight gastrocnemius-soleus muscle complex is an important adjunct to maintaining the positive, pain reducing effects of intervention.

Haglund's Deformity

Haglund's deformity, commonly called the "pump bump," is an enlargement of the posterior superior aspect of the calcaneous at the attachment of the Achilles tendon. This is most commonly found as a result of mechanical friction stresses from shoes or from excessive rearfoot varus.

Evaluative Findings.—On evaluation, a visible calcification is present at the posterosuperior angle of the calcaneus. This "lump" may or may not be painful to palpation; however, the patient will report marked irritation with prolonged shoe wearing. Haglund's deformity is palpated as a dense nodule with surrounding soft-tissue restriction. Frequently, dorsiflexion may be restricted as a result of scarring at the Achilles-calcaneal junction.

Treatment Suggestions.—Successful treatment encompasses ultrasound, soft-tissue mobilization, elimination of shoe irritation, and neutral positioning of the subtalar joint with orthotics.

Reducing the tension on the Achilles tendon, providing dorsiflexion assistance at heel strike and toe-off, reducing the tendency of the foot to pronate, and reducing the friction (shear) force at the insertion of the tendon on the calcaneus are the major objectives in prescribing orthotics and shoes for Achilles tendinitis, bursitis, and Haglund's deformity (pump bump). The orthotic should provide a heel lift to reduce tension on the Achilles tendon. A longitudinal arch support with medial posting at the heel and metatarsal heads will assist in reducing pronation. A higher-heeled shoe helps to reduce dorsiflexion and a long medial shoe counter will limit subtalar motion. It is recommended that a longer shoe size, foam cut-out, or a backless shoe be utilized to reduce the pressure resulting from compression on the insertion of the Achilles tendon at the calcaneus.

REARFOOT/MIDFOOT PROBLEMS

Pes Planus (Flexible)

Pes planus involves the flattening of the medial longitudinal arch and a valgus deflection of the heel secondary to hypermobility. This deformity is commonly seen in the rheumatoid arthritic foot or in neurologic deficits with posterior tibialis or peroneus longus muscle weakness. In the absence of pathology the causes of pes planus are usually related to heredity or years of walking on unyielding surfaces with stiff, "non–user-friendly" shoes. Hard surfaces reduce the function of intrinsic foot muscles and the result is eventual muscle weakness and atrophy.

Evaluative Findings.—Muscle imbalances involve the posterior tibialis muscle, which is important in maintaining the arch and providing inversion of the foot. Associated problems include plantar faciitis, shin splints, and patellofemoral disorders related to hypermobility of the foot. Joint play is excessive in the midfoot and rearfoot articulations. Flatfootedness is increased in the elder with a hallux valgus deformity and a concomitant decreased transverse arch. Pain and aching are often reported along the longitudinal arch. In severe cases, hyperkeratotic formation may actually occur over the medial navicular bony prominence as a result of direct weight-bearing pressures. During ambulation, supination of the foot for heel strike is not attained. On heel strike, the foot immediately pronates. Heel strike may be completely absent and the individual may land in a flatfooted, plantar-flexed position prior to assuming severe pronation during midstance. Push off is usually absent as well. Instead, the individual rolls laterally on the ball of the foot, furthering the hallux valgus deformity forces.

Treatment Suggestions.—Muscle strengthening and reeducation inclusive of the toes, midfoot, posterior tibialis, and peroneus longus is important in conservatively managing a flexible pes planus. Exercises could include digital contraction using a towel or small object (such as a marble) to grasp, walking on the outer borders of the feet, a tiptoe inverted gait, rocking on the toes and heels (such as in rocking-chair exercises) and progressive resistive exercises using Theraband. Deep friction massage is helpful in mobilizing the tissues that become stiffer and unyielding from the body's attempts to stabilize the unstable midfoot. Electrical stimulation may be employed to facilitate stronger contractions of the plantar flexor, peroneus longus, and posterior tibialis muscles.

Orthotic prescription principles of managing a flexible pes planus (flatfoot deformity) include reducing the amount of pronation from heel strike to midstance, correcting calcaneal eversion, relieving excessive strain on the posterior tibialis tendon, and reducing excessive ligamentous strain. Use of a medial heel wedge will correct calcaneal eversion and reduce pronation. A heel cup will hold the calcaneus in vertical alignment and stabilize the subtalar joint in neutral. The heel cup also serves to reinforce the heel counter of the shoe. A medial longitudinal arch support made of rigid or semirigid material (Aliplast XPE, Nickleplast) will assist in reducing excessive pronation.

A reinforced medial heel counter is needed in severe deformity. A Thomas heel with a medial extention or a firm wedge sole will help to stabilize the subtalar and ankle joint in neutral and take the stress off of the posterior tibial tendon and excessive ligamentous strain. A straight-last shoe will serve to control the midtarsal joint by blocking pronation. In severe cases a custom-molded shoe may have a medial heel wedge and a flared medial heel to correct calcaneal eversion and excessive pronation.

Pes Planus (Rigid)

A rigid pes planus is a result of chronic flatfootedness (flexible pes planus) as described above.

Evaluative Findings.—Mobility between the midtarsal joints is severely restricted; commonly they are fused. Discomfort and pain is reported in the longitudinal arch with hyperkeratotic formation over the navicular and under the metatarsal heads owing to excessive friction and shear forces encountered secondary to altered biomechanics of gait. Heel strike is absent during gait and the individual lands flat on the foot. Push-off is usually absent as a result of midtarsal joint restriction. Posterior tibial muscle weakness is a concomitant finding in the rigid pes planus deformity.

Treatment Suggestions.—Joint mobilization and modalities like interferential current or ultrasound may be effective in promoting motion in semirigid joints of the midfoot. Muscle reeducation is an important adjunct to treating the rigid midfoot as posterior tibialis weakness can lead to accompanying ankle, knee, and hip problems. Gait training is essential. Tiptoe walking with inversion and lateral-foot walking assist in overemphasizing a correct gait pattern. The patient should be instructed to attempt a "neutral" heel strike and maintain a lateral weight-bearing pattern throughout the stance phase of gait. If this is not actively possible, the use of corrective orthotics and shoes may be needed to facilitate a more effective heel strike, midstance, and toe-off pattern during ambulation.

With a condition of rigid pes planus the orthotic objectives will serve to accommodate the deformity, rather than reposition the foot, relieve ligamentous strain, relieve arch pain by providing shock-absorptive materials, and correct eversion. The shoe should have a broad shank (extra width at the midfoot) and a straight last. A long medial counter modification of the shoe will assist in controlling excessive calcaneal eversion. A medial wedge sole will reduce the load on the metatarsal heads, stabilize the midtarsal joint and provide dorsiflexion assist when ambulating.

Pes Equinus (Flexible)

Pes equinus is most frequently seen in women who have worn high-heeled shoes throughout life. It is also seen with extensor hypertonicity related to neurologic problems such as CVA and is commonly the final result of an Achilles tendinitis or avulsion of the Achilles with surgical repair.

Evaluative Findings.—The most notable result is a shortening of the Achilles tendon and the gastroc-nemius-soleus muscle group. The patient is unable to wear flat shoe gear as this causes too much strain at the posterior attachment of the Achilles tendon to the calcaneus. Usually the patient reports pain or strain at the insertion of the Achilles or in the muscle bellies of the gastrocnemius or soleus muscle. In many cases, there is hypermobility in the subtalar joint and the individual pronates excessively in an attempt to compensate for the equinus deformity. Restriction of the distal tibiofibular joint is common preventing splay and blocking the talus thereby limiting dorsiflexion.

Treatment Suggestions.—The goals of conservative intervention should be directed toward relieving the mechanical stress, balancing muscle pull, and stabilizing the subtalar and midtarsal joints.

Modalities such as hot packs, ultrasound, or hydrotherapy provide some relief. Deep friction massage, stretching of the Achilles and gastrocnemius-soleus muscle complex, and joint mobilization

techniques assist in gaining mobility and decreasing the discomfort associated with equinus deformity. A joint mobilization technique termed "calcaneal distraction" (Fig 23–9) is helpful in promoting increased motion at the limited talocalcaneal joint. Fibular bone mobilization is essential in allowing the distal fibulotibular joint to splay to allow the talus to move freely through the ankle mortise during dorsiflexion. Muscle reeducation to correct muscle imbalance assists in the return of the heel to a foot-flat stance position.

Objectives for orthotic prescription in a flexible pes equinus deformity include reducing ankle plantar flexion, reducing the load on the metatarsal heads, and stabilizing the subtalar joint. This can be accomplished by providing a total-contact orthotic for accommodation and stability and lowering the heel either intrinsically via the orthotic or extrinsically by lowering the heel of the shoe. A rocker-bottom sole will assist dorsiflexion and reduce the load on the metatarsal heads.

Pes Equinus (Rigid)

Evaluative Findings.—A rigid pes planus deformity is the end result of severe extensor hypertonicity. It is commonly seen in the bedridden elderly owing to blanket pressures, immobility, and infrequent weight bearing. Dorsiflexors are weakened and dorsiflexion is impossible in the fixed deformity. Weight bearing is painful as the individual must bear all of his or her weight on the metatarsal heads. Barefooted weight bearing is often necessary owing to the inability to fit the rigid pes equinus deformity into standard shoe gear.

Treatment Suggestions.—A rigid pes equinus deformity is treated much like a surgically induced

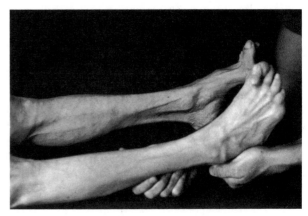

FIG 23–9.
Calcaneal distraction mobilization technique.

arthrodesis. There is only minimal allowance for joint mobility; thus, joint mobilization techniques need to be concentrated on the surrounding joints. Modalities employed are those used with the flexible pes equinus pathology. The goal of using modalities is to relieve pain and mobilize the soft tissues to prevent current and future strain. Muscle reeducation is vital in maintaining stability, and the focus of treatment should be on gait training to eliminate excessive stresses on other joints from limitations of motion in the fused joints. The goal of conservative intervention should be to protect the ankle joint and promote the most efficient gait pattern possible. This is best accomplished through orthotic and shoe intervention.

With a fixed or rigid pes planus deformity, a posterior heel lift will raise the rearfoot during heel strike and midstance, provide a dorsiflexion assist at toe-off, keep the foot in the shoe, reduce the load on the metatarsal heads, and in the case of unilateral involvement (such as that seen in a CVA), equalize the leg length difference through all phases of gait. The orthotic should provide a posterior heel elevation of up to ⅜ in. inside the shoe and shock-absorbing metatarsal pads placed to relieve the pressures during weight bearing.

A Cuban-heeled shoe provides an adequate platform for heel strike and midstance. A deeper quarter-heel counter or a high-top shoe may assist in stabilizing the ankle and subtalar joint. Flat shoes can be modified by providing a posterior heel elevation. Placing a heel elevation on the contralateral shoe will facilitate the swing phase of the involved limb and reduce pelvic obliquity by improving swing clearance.

Pes Cavus

Pes cavus is the exaggerated height of the long arch of the foot. This can be congenitally present or neurologically induced.

Evaluative Findings.—Patients with pes cavus present with a rigid midtarsal joint and hyperextension at the metatarsophalangeals. As a result of increased tension on the flexors, toe deformities are frequently a concomitant problem. There is often a complaint of dorsal midfoot discomfort as a result of shoe pressures across the instep.

Treatment Suggestions.—It is rare that this deformity is not a fixed deformity; however, treatment in the case of flexible deformity includes stretching of the muscles in the arch and mobilizing the sur-

rounding soft tissue. Joint mobilization, deep friction massage, and muscle reeducation are essential components in treating the pes cavus deformity. The primary intervention in pes cavus deformity is an accommodative orthotic and custom-molded shoes.

In the pes cavus, or high arch, deformity the objectives of orthotic intervention should include providing a broader plantar heel platform for greater stability; reducing impact loading on the heel, lateral foot border, and metatarsal heads; and the accommodation of the foot within the shoe. The orthotic should be a shock-attenuating total-contact orthotic with metatarsal padding to reduce the load to the bony prominences. It should have a medial longitudinal arch support to assist in equally distributing weight-bearing pressures over the entire plantar surface.

The shoe should have a firm heel counter to maintain rearfoot stability. It may be necessary to provide a shoe with a modified curved last to accommodate the shape of the foot. Custom-molded shoes are recommended in very severe cases. The shoe can be modified by laterally flaring the heel to provide a platform for greater stability. A cushioned sole absorbs the shock on the heel and metatarsal heads. A metatarsal bar will serve to shift the weight off of the metatarsal heads and assist in push-off during gait.

Plantar Fasciitis/Heel Spurs

Plantar fasciitis is an inflammation of the plantar fascia and short flexors of the foot at their insertion to the calcaneus. It is usually an overuse syndrome and in elders is seen more frequently in women than in men. Causes may be from prolonged standing, excessive weight gain, shifting or atrophy of the heel fat pad, joint limitations at the talocrural joint necessitating repeated stretch on the plantar aspect of the sole during walking, or athletic strain.

Evaluative Findings.—Symptoms include a sharp pain at the insertion of the plantar fascia on weight bearing, increased discomfort with passive dorsiflexion of the toes, and local tenderness at the insertion of the plantar fascia and the short flexors of the foot. Occasionally the individual will complain of heel pain radiating into the arch of the foot. Upon palpation, pain will be elicited along the course of the plantar fascia. Excessive pronation is a characteristic finding in patients with plantar fasciitis. Clinically, there is associated weakness of the posterior tibialis, peroneus longus, and anterior tibialis muscles.

Treatment Suggestions.—Treatment objectives are to reduce the inflammation, transfer pressure from the painful area to more tolerant areas, reduce tension on the plantar fascia and the Achilles tendon, control pronation from heel strike to midstance, and to maintain subtalar joint neutral position.

Inflammation can be reduced by pulsed ultrasound to the calcaneal insertion of the plantar fascia, ice massage to the calcaneal tuberosities where soft tissues insert including the surrounding plantar surface, interferential current using the small pinpoint applicator to the fascial insertion (Fig 23–10), or high galvanic electrical stimulation with two negative leads (one electrode anterior to the calcaneus; one electrode proximal to the metatarsal heads) attached to the plantar surface (Fig 23–11), or four leads surrounding the ankle and heel (Fig 23–12) with the positive leads on the Achilles and plantar facial insertion. A posterior heel lift with an excavated area under the spur enables transfer of pressure from the painful to less painful area of the heel.

Reduction of tension on the plantar fascia and Achilles tendon is best accomplished by correct stretching of the gastrocnemius-soleus muscle complex (see Fig 23–7) to gain dorsiflexion at the talocrural joint. This is accomplished by stabilizing the midtarsal joint using a towel roll. This isolates the stretch to the gastrocnemius-soleus muscles and talocrural joint and eliminates midtarsal substitution. Deep friction massage helps to reduce fibrotic adhesions in the fascia (Fig 23–13). Interferential current, as demonstrated in Figure 23–10, in combination with deep friction massage (see Fig 23–13) has been found to assist in breaking up noncalcified heel spurs. Taping of the foot in slight equinus and inversion is another method of relieving the tension

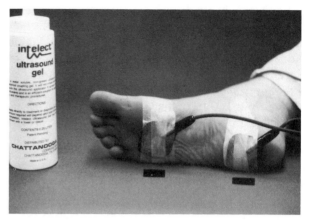

FIG 23–11.
High glavanic electrical stimulation to plantar fascia.

on the plantar fascia and the Achilles tendon. Controlling pronation and maintaining subtalar joint neutral position is accomplished by orthotic and shoe modifications, in addition to muscle strengthening of the posterior tibialis, peroneus longus, and anterior tibialis muscles.

The transfer of pressure from the painful to tolerant areas of the foot is the major objective in treating plantar fasciitis. This can be accomplished by reducing the tension on the plantar fascia and Achilles tendon, controlling pronation from heel strike to midstance and maintaining the subtalar joint in a neutral position. By providing an orthotic with a posterior heel elevation the tension is reduced on the plantar fascia as well as the Achilles tendon. The orthotic can be excavated (relieved) under the "center" of pain to unload (relieve) the painful area. A medial longitudinal arch support with the apex under the tubercle of the navicular helps to control pronation. Clinical observation indicates that posting

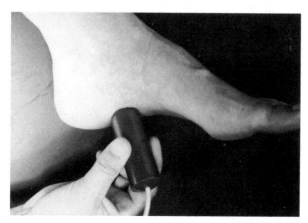

FIG 23–10.
Localized inferential current for plantar fasciitis.

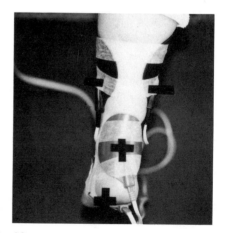

FIG 23–12.
High galvanic current in the treatment of plantar fasciitis.

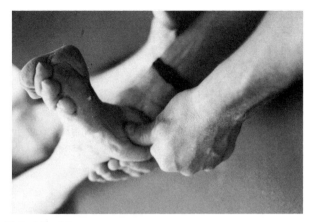

FIG 23–13.
Deep friction massage assists in breaking up noncalcified heel spurs.

under the cuboid serves to reduce the tension on the plantar fascia in some cases. The orthotic materials should be a combination of semirigid materials with shock-absorbing materials.

A long medial heel counter in the shoe will help to limit calcaneal valgus. A higher heel will aid in reducing the tension on the plantar fascia and Achilles tendon by placing the foot into plantar flexion. It has also been observed that a longer shoe serves to reduce the pressure owing to compression on the fascia, and, in combination with the above described orthotic, promotes supination from midstance to toe-off.

FOREFOOT PROBLEMS

Callusing in the Forefoot

Callusing on the plantar surface of the foot, especially in the metatarsal area can be quite painful. Thick calluses are formed as a response to mechanical stress, and are the body's attempt to protect the area.

Evaluative Findings.—The presence of a hyperkeratotic area is indicative of biomechanical, frictional, or shear stress. The underlying joint mobility should be assessed. Callusing in the forefoot on the plantar surface may be the result of the distal shifting of the fat pad into the sulcus of the toes. Callusing medially on the first metatarsal head or laterally on the fifth metatarsal head is unusual, but can be the result of shoe irritation. Shoes should be evaluated for unequal sole wear and distortion of the toe box consistent with callus location.

Treatment Suggestions.—Calluses can be softened by the use of skin creams that do not contain alcohol. The most effective treatment for dense callusing is debridement by a podiatrist and subsequent protection and realignment to prevent reoccurance.

The simple provision of a shock-absorbing material such as PPT or Plastazote, cut to fit inside the shoe, can provide shock absorption necessary to decrease the discomfort and repetitive trauma to poorly protected bony prominences on the plantar surface of the foot. Metatarsal pads or cushions are available in different shapes, sizes and thicknesses. Soft polyfoam, Plastazote, foam rubber, or felt pads are either affixed directly to the foot with rubber cement or tape, or have a self-adhesive backing so they can easily be attached within the shoe. Forefoot cushions or metatarsal pads are designed to provide padding for the metatarsal heads and are indicated for temporary relief of plantar forefoot pain. Both orthotic shock-absorbing materials and metatarsal cushions or pads are especially helpful for protecting sensitive plantar keratoses and preventing the speed at which they recur once debrided by a podiatrist.

Metatarsalgia

Metatarsalgia is a nonspecific diagnosis referring to pain in the metatarsal heads. In the elderly, it is usually secondary to atrophy of the protective fat pad and resultant weight bearing directly on the metatarsal heads.

Evaluative Findings.—Hallux valgus deformity and deformities of the lesser toes where the digits are contracted in an extended, dorsally directed position cause the metatarsal shafts to plantar flex, driving the metatarsal heads downward. Painful calluses and corns usually develop. Abnormal pressures can cause an acute bursitis or capsulitis or eventually lead to arthritic changes in the joint surrounding the metatarsal head. Palpation elicits pain surrounding the involved metatarsal head. Hypermobility is often found in the subtalar and midtarsal joints in conjunction with metatarsalgia.

Treatment Suggestions.—Treatment objectives in this condition include reduction of inflammation, realignment of the joint surfaces, transfer of pressure from painful areas to more tolerant areas, reducing friction by stabilizing the metatarsophalangeal joint, and stabilizing the rearfoot and midfoot to reduce pressure on the metatarsals.

Ice, pulsed ultrasound, or grade 1 joint mobilization oscillations to the joints will help reduce inflammation. Joint mobilization using a metatarsal roll or splay (Fig 23–14), dorsal glide of the metatarsal head on the phalanx, or volar glide of the phalanx on the metatarsal head will realign the joint surfaces. Patients can mobilize their metatarsal joints themselves by rolling the foot over a tennis ball while sitting. Following mobilization, the joints can be held in alignment with pads under the metatarsal heads to assist in maintaining the splay (separation) of the heads and providing shock absorption in place of the atrophied or absent anatomical fat pads.

Stabilization of the metatarsophalangeal joints by flexor strengthening exercises can be performed using resistive elastic or surgical tubing or gripping a towel or marbles with the toes.

The transfer of pressure from painful and sensitive areas to more tolerant areas, the reduction of friction by stabilizing the metatarsophalangeal joint, and stabilizing the rearfoot and midfoot to reduce pressures on the metatarsal heads are the primary objectives in orthotic prescription for metatarsalgia. These objectives can best be accomplished by padding placed proximal to the metatarsal heads. This redistributes forces from the metatarsal heads to the metatarsal shafts when using a soft-tissue supplement (e.g., PPT, Plastazote) for shear attenuation and shock absorption.

A wider-width shoe helps to reduce pressure on the transverse arch. A longer shoe helps to eliminate jamming of the metatarsophalangeal joint, and subsequent plantar flexion and subluxation. A cushioned sole assists in shock absorption, and a high toe box allows adequate forefoot flexion and extension within the shoe. A long medial counter should be provided in the shoe to stabilize the rearfoot. By

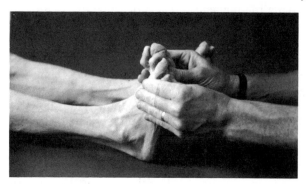

FIG 23–14.
Splaying of metatarsal heads.

lowering the heel of the shoe, pressure is reduced on the metatarsal heads. Thermally moldable leather shoes are recommended to accommodate toe deformities. A transverse metatarsal bar placed on the sole of the shoe will further assist in redistributing the pressure from the metatarsal heads to the metatarsal shafts, and shorten stride length to reduce over stretching of the gastrocnemius-soleus complex during push-off. Rocker-bottom soles serve to reduce the motion of the painful joint.

Sesamoiditis

Sesamoiditis is an inflammatory process caused by microtrauma to the sesamoid bones beneath the first metatarsal head.

Evaluative Findings.—Inflammation involves the tendon as well as the osseous structures. There is marked soft-tissue suppuration, resulting in a great deal of pain on weight bearing.

Treatment Suggestions.—Treatment objectives for sesamoiditis include reduction of inflammation and redistribution of weight-bearing forces from the first metatarsophalangeal joint and sesamoids to the long medial arch and shafts of the lesser metatarsals.

Ice massage, pulsed ultrasound and grade 1 joint mobilization oscillations promote reabsorption of excess fluids and reduce swelling. Deep friction massage may release adhesions formed in the connective tissues as a result of microtrauma and promote relaxation of hypertonic musculature. Joint mobilization may realign the sesamoids, and provide more movement in the first metatarsophalangeal joint.

The primary objective in managing sesamoiditis is to redistribute weight forces from the first metatarsophalangeal joint and sesamoids to the long medial arch and the shafts of the lesser metatarsal. Prefabricated "bat mats" or "dancers pads" provide a relief directly under the first metatarsophalangeal joint and sesamoids and are easily glued directly to the foot or affixed within the shoe.

The principles of shoe modifications are similar to those discussed under metatarsalgia. A transverse metatarsal bar will redistribute pressure from the metatarsal heads to the metatarsal shafts and shorten stride. Again, a rocker-bottom sole will reduce the motion of the painful first metatarsophalangeal joint and prevent undue pressure on the sesamoids.

Morton's Syndrome

Morton's syndrome involves hypermobility of the first metatarsophalangeal joint and shortening of the first metatarsal ray. This anatomic condition is usually a result of hereditary factors.

Evaluative Findings.—Morton's syndrome is recognizable clinically because the second digit is longer than the hallux. The normal foot parabola is disturbed owing to the shortened first ray causing abnormal pronation at the subtalar joint. Excessive subtalar joint pronation results in hypermobility of the first ray during weight bearing. As a result, weight is shifted onto the second metatarsal head, creating symptoms similar to those of metatarsalgia.

Treatment Suggestions.—Treatment objectives for this condition are the same as for the condition of metatarsalgia. The goal of treatment is to mechanically redistribute weight-bearing pressures to provide a more normal metatarsal balance.

The objectives in orthotic prescription in Morton's syndrome are to redistribute the weight from the lesser metatarsals (primarily the second and third metatarsals) and from the proximal phalanx of the hallux, stabilize the rearfoot by maintaining subtalar joint in a neutral position and to accommodate forefoot varus (dorsiflexed first metatarsal). Orthotic intervention includes a metatarsal pad proximal to the second and third metacarpophalangeal joints to redistribute the weight, and a Morton's extension (platform) under the first metacarpophalangeal joint to accommodate the dorsiflexed first ray and varus forefoot. The objective is to redistribute weight from the proximal phalanx of the hallux. This is supplemented by providing a long medial arch support with a medial heel wedge to maintain subtalar neutral and limit excessive pronation.

The shoe prescribed should provide a long medial counter for rearfoot support and stability. It is recommended that a straight or flared shoe last be used to accommodate the foot shape. A high, wide toe box will reduce the compressive forces across the transverse metatarsal arch. Shoes need to be sized to accommodate the longer second toe. A Thomas heel or wedge sole will facilitate the support of the medial longitudinal arch.

Morton's (Interdigital) Neuroma

Morton's neuroma is the end result of repetitive microtrauma and compression of the interdigital nerves as they traverse between the metatarsal heads. Interdigital peripheral nerve entrapment can occur between any of the metatarsal heads.

Evaluative Findings.—The most prominent evaluative finding is pain elicited by palpation of the involved interdigital space. Local inflammation occurs in the acute phases. Restricted mobility is often present between the involved metatarsal heads owing to soft-tissue adhesions related to the entrapment and scarring around the nerve.

Treatment Suggestions.—Conservative treatment objectives for this condition are similar to those for metatarsalgia. TENS is helpful in eliminating the perception of pain. Cold packs assist in reducing local inflammation and pain. Ultrasound and massage are employed to mobilize adhesions of the nerve sheaths as they course between the metatarsal heads. If a neuroma is problematic enough to necessitate surgical removal, postsurgical electrical stimulation in conjunction with controlled exercise is recommended for reinnervation and muscle strengthening. Joint mobilization techniques as described in the discussion of metatarsalgia are useful in splaying the metatarsal heads (Fig 23–14).

The orthotic objectives in treating Morton's Neuroma are to relieve the pain and burning in the third interspace of the metacarpophalangeal joint and to reduce the compression of the digital nerve as it passes between the heads of the third and fourth metatarsal heads. A metatarsal pad may be placed proximal to the neuroma to open the interspace. A medial longitudinal arch support immobilizes the metatarsals and compensates for skeletal abnormalities such as pes planus. A prefabricated splint provides Morton's (platform) extension for the first ray. A toe crest distal to the neuroma helps to redistribute weight forces and dorsiflex the metatarsophalangeal joint.

The shoe needs to be wider to eliminate transverse compression of the metatarsal heads and longer to reduce plantar flexion of the metacarpophalangeal joint. A long medial counter will serve to reduce excessive pronation. In addition, the sole should be cushioned to absorb shock and the heel lowered to unload the pressure on the metatarsal head. Elastic laces are recommended to allow expansion of the forefoot. Padding of the tongue of the shoe takes the pressure off of the instep and assists in stabilizing the foot within the collar of the shoe. Extrinsically, a metatarsal bar on the shoe helps to elevate the metatarsals and redistribute the weight to the rearfoot. A metatarsal rocker bar serves to immobilize the metatarsals and assists in push-off.

Metatarsalgia of the Fifth Metacarpophalangeal Joint

Metatarsalgia is frequently isolated at the fifth metatarsophalangeal joint. The etiology is as previously described.

Evaluative Findings.—The most common biomechanical cause of inflammation of the fifth metatarsophalangeal joint is excessive supination of the subtalar joint. The propulsion forces during gait are directed laterally causing excessive weight forces on the fifth metatarsal head. This condition is most commonly seen in athletes who run on the outside of their feet or in the neurologically involved patient whose spasticity pattern causes inversion of the calcaneous during ambulation. Metatarsalgia of the fifth metatarsophalangeal is frequently seen in persons with the pes cavus deformity.

Treatment Suggestions.—Treatment objectives for this condition are similar to metatarsalgia. The modalities employed are the same.

A lateral platform proximal to the fifth metatarsal head helps to redistribute the weight to the fifth metatarsal shaft and provides a broader base of support along the lateral boarder of the foot. These are the objectives of orthotic intervention with metatarsalgia of the fifth metacarpophalangeal joint.

Shoes should have a rigid lateral last to accommodate the lateral aspect of the foot and the 5th metatarsal shaft. With this diagnosis it is recommended that the shoe have a firm lateral counter and a firm leather or rubber sole. The shoe can be modified by providing a flared lateral heel and sole ending proximal to the fifth metatarsal head thereby providing a broader base of support. Lateral heel and sole wedges may also be used in the flexible foot.

Hallux Rigidus (Limitus)

Restriction of extension in the first metatarsophalangeal joint is termed hallux limitus. If ankylosis of the joint occurs, totally preventing movement, it is described as hallux rigidus. Hallux limitus/rigidus is commonly the result of hypermobility of the first ray with concomitant eversion of the rearfoot secondary to subtalar pronation; a long first metatarsal shaft; and a hyperextension or crush injury to the first metatarsophalangeal joint.[40] The

biomechanical etiology results from an inability of the first metatarsophalanx to move below the transverse plane of the lesser joints.

Evaluative Findings.—Symptoms include pain in the first metatarsophalangeal joint, restricted first metatarsophalangeal joint extension, and increased lateral drifting on the affected side. The patient often complains of discomfort at the cuneonavicular and talonavicular joints, most likely as a result of hypermobility in these joints as these articulations attempt to compensate for the restricted mobility of the first metatarsophalangeal.

During gait the first metatarsophalangeal joint is required to extend approximately 65 degrees in order to provide adequate push-off.[35] In hallux limitus/rigidus, extension at the first metatarsophalangeal is either quite restricted or impossible, making ambulation very uncomfortable.

Treatment Suggestions.—Treatment objectives are to reduce pain and discomfort in the first metatarsophalangeal joint, increase movement of the first ray, reduce inflammation, and reduce pressure to the dorsal and plantar aspects of the hallux and first metatarsophalangeal joint.

Ice massage, grade 1 joint mobilization oscillations, and pulsed ultrasound will reduce the edema, swelling, and pressure felt with this condition. Dorsal and volar glides of the first metatarsal bone on the cuneiform will enable the metatarsal to plantar flex as needed to get increased dorsiflexion at the first metatarsophalangeal joint (Fig 23–15). Strengthening of the peroneus longus muscle will assist in plantar flexion of the first ray and increase range of motion at the joint.

The effect of heat on connective tissues is to de-

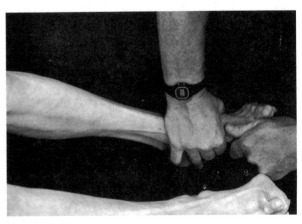

FIG 23–15.
Dorsal and volar glides of first metatarsal head.

crease their viscosity, which helps with contractile movements and consequently reduces the stiffness in the underlying joint. Elevated tissue temperatures in conjunction with stretching may cause plastic deformation in connective tissues.[32] Elevated tissue temperatures may also increase oxygen uptake and blood flow to the heated tissues, making more nutrients available to damaged tissues and enhancing the healing process.[32]

The orthotic objectives in managing hallux rigidus (limitus) are to limit the motion of the hallux and first metatarsophalangeal joint. In addition, it is desirable to reduce the pressure to the dorsal and plantar aspect of the hallux and the first metatarsophalangeal joint. A total contact orthotic insert is recommended to redistribute weight forces from the first metatarsophalangeal to more tolerant areas. A medial longitudinal arch support helps to make the foot plantar flexed, diminishing the forces on the hallux and first joint.

Recommendations for shoes include a high and wide toe box in Thermold shoes or soft leather uppers to accommodate the hallux and associated toe deformities. A steel shank from the heel to the phalanx of the hallux helps to immobilize the first metatarsophalangeal joint. A rigid rocker-bottom sole compensates for heel elevation for push-off during gait and helps to drop the heel for heel strike.

Hallux Valgus (Bunions)

The primary deformity in hallux valgus is a lateral drifting of the first digit with secondary deformities of a dorsal medial bunion and overlapping toes. Hallux valgus is caused by a progressive subluxation of the first metatarsophalangeal joint. The proximal phalanx is displaced laterally as a result of abnormal subtalar joint pronation, creating a hypermobile first ray; progression leads to a metatarsus primus adductus of the first metatarsal shaft. Contributory factors for formation of hallux abductor valgus (HAV) include ill-fitting shoes, heredity, metatarsus primus adductus, structure of the metatarsal head,[10] and a long first metatarsal bone.[14]

Evaluative Findings.—Evaluative findings in HAV include keratosis located medially on the first metatarsal head and commonly, bursitis of the first metatarsophalangeal joint. Plantar tylomas (calluses) at the distal interphalangeal joint and under the second metatarsal head are associated with hallux valgus, in conjunction with displacement of the second digit and prolapse of the metatarsal heads resulting

from continued microtrauma. Symptoms include pain over the dorsal medial aspect of the first metatarsal head or over the bunion deformity. The first toe becomes enlarged and is tender to palpation. The second toe may cross over the first digit, causing callusing under the second metatarsal head. Radiographically, the first metatarsal head is frequently enlarged with osseous proliferation and degenerative joint changes. Excessive mobility of the subtalar joint is a concomitant finding in HAV deformities.

Treatment Suggestions.—Objectives for physical therapy treatment of HAV should include reduction of pain and discomfort in the first metatarsophalangeal joint, reduction of inflammation, reduction of friction and pressure to the first metatarsophalangeal joint, reduction of excessive pronation from heel strike to midstance, correction of eversion and reduction of ligamental and muscular imbalance.

To reduce pain, discomfort and inflammation, ice massage, pulsed ultrasound, grade 1 joint mobilization oscillations, and massage are effective treatment techniques. Deep massage to the lumbrical and interosseus muscles between the hallux and second digit helps relieve the hypertonicity and subsequent aching.

For normal gait to occur at least 65 degrees of motion is necessary in the first metatarsophalangeal joint.[3] Controlling excessive pronation at the subtalar joint is necessary to prevent further HAV deformity. Goals of treatment are to increase the mobility of the first metatarsophalangeal to 65 degrees of extension, reduce edema and pain, and stabilize the subtalar joint.

Ice and massage reduce the edema and promote tissue mobilization, enabling adequate nutrition to the joint. Long axis distraction mobilizations release adhesions and help realign collagen fibers to appropriate lines of stress. Temporary orthotics are meant to decrease the excessive pronation in the subtalar joint, thereby reducing the stresses on the first metatarsophalangeal joint. Progression in treatment should include: superior gliding of the proximal phalanx of the hallux on the first metatarsal, gastrocnemius-soleus muscle stretching, metatarsophalangeal stretching (lifting up of the heel while the hallux is on the ground) while standing, and semirigid orthotics.

Stretching out the medial toe box, padding the shoe, and buying shoes with rounded toe boxes are effective means of reducing friction and pressure to the first metatarsophalangeal joint. Orthotic fabrication with the subtalar joint in neutral, and strengthening of the peroneus longus and anterior tibialis muscles will reduce the tendency for excessive pronation. Range of motion exercises, contract-relax and hold-relax proprioceptive neuromuscular facilitation (PNF) techniques should be utilized to promote external rotation if lower extremity limitations exist. Strengthening of the external rotator muscles of the hip brings the lower limb into a position that promotes foot and ankle supination rather than pronation.

The reduction of friction and pressure to the first metatarsophalangeal joint is a primary objective in orthotic fabrication for an HAV deformity. It is important to eliminate the pressure from narrow-fitting shoes, to reduce the excessive pronation from heel strike to midstance, to correct forefoot eversion, and to relieve the stress on the posterior tibial tendon and the strain on the ligaments. Excavation of the orthotic material under the "center" of the painful area helps to unload the first metatarsophalangeal joint. A medial longitudinal arch assists in decreasing excessive pronation. A total-contact orthotic with a deep heel cup limits subtalar motion. Providing a soft, shock-absorbing surface serves to cushion sensitive areas. A hallux valgus splint may be utilized to promote alignment of the first metatarsophalangeal joint while sleeping. Additional padding may be provided by prefabricated bunion protectors. Toe separators can control any overlapping of the lesser digits and protect the digits. Compensatory anomalies that may be associated with hallux valgus include pes planus, metatarsalgia, hammer toes, and claw toes. These all need to be considered when prescribing an orthotic for a hallux valgus deformity.

Shoes should provide a high, wide toe box. Thermold shoes or soft leather uppers are recommended to protect the hallux valgus and accompanying deformities. A combined last with an increased width in the toe box and a smaller heel will assist in maintaining a neutral subtalar position. A longer and wider shoe helps to accommodate the deformity. Lowering the heel serves to reduce forefoot pressure. Reinforcing the medial heel counter assists in preventing excessive pronation.

Hammer Toes, Claw Toes, Mallet Toes, Overlapping Toes

Toe deformities are common in the elderly. These deformities include hammer toes, claw toes, mallet toes, and overlapping toes. These problems often result from wearing shoes that are too short and narrow, or from weakness or imbalance of the intrinsic muscles of the foot.

The hammer toe deformity consists of a flexed proximal interphalangeal joint, a compensatory hyperextension of the distal interphalangeal joint, and hyperextention of the metatarsophalangeal joint. It is the result of changes in the intrinsic musculature over a long period of time. Once the intrinsic muscle stability is compromised, the function of the long flexor muscle and its tendon is altered. This produces a buckling at the metatarsalphalangeal and proximal interphalangeal articulations. The long and short extensor muscles accommodate by contracting. If this contraction persists there is a concomitant shortening of the surrounding dorsal capsule of the metatarsophalangeal and proximal interphalangeal joints. Because the intrinsic muscles fail to stabilize the metatarsophalangeal joints of the lesser toes, the proximal phalanx becomes displaced dorsally on the metatarsal and the intermediate phalanx becomes plantar flexed in relation to the proximal phalanx. If left untreated, these joints eventually fuse. A related dysfunction is seen with dorsal subluxation of the proximal phalanx. This subluxation pulls the plantar fat pad from beneath the metatarsal head into the sulcus of the foot. Metatarsalgia and hyperkeratosis are resultant problems.

Claw toes differ from hammer toes in that the distal interphalangeal joint is flexed. The metatarsophalangeal is extended and the proximal interphalangeal is flexed. The etiology of claw toes is similar to that of hammer toes, though there is an increase in the shortening contractures of the flexor muscles of the toes.

A mallet deformity consists of a flexion contracture of the distal interphalangeal joint only. Combined with flexion contractures of the proximal and distal interphalangeal joints, this results in a deformity similar to the hammer toe with the exception that weight bearing is on the distal tip of the toe. The etiology of a mallet toe is one of muscle imbalance involving excessive contraction of the flexor tendons of the toe. The tissue of the toe pulp is not capable of withstanding stresses induced by weight bearing. As a result, distal callusing and possible ulceration are a problem in the mallet toe deformity.

Overlapping toes result when these deformities, especially in combination with a hallux valgus deformity, progress. The metatarsal heads are compressed as a result of shoe pressures and become subluxed. In severe cases, toes may actually dislocate and become flail, rendering them useless.

Evaluative Findings.—The primary problem associated with hammer, claw, mallet, and overlapping toe deformities is dorsal interphalangeal joint skin lesions resulting from abnormal shoe pressures. A secondary problem is the prominence of the metatarsal heads from plantarflexion of the metatarsal heads and dislocation of the plantar fat pad with breakdown at these sites. These problems are usually successfully managed by appropriate orthotic and foot wear.

Treatment Suggestions.—If the toe deformities are flexible, the treatment objectives are to reduce the inflammation, realign the joint surfaces, balance the surrounding musculature, and promote full and pain-free range of motion. If the deformities are fixed, the treatment objectives are to protect the joints and skin from breakdown in addition to the above-stated objectives.

Ice massage, ultrasound, grade 1 joint mobilization oscillations, and padding the area reduce inflammation. The joint surfaces can be realigned through long axis distraction (Fig 23–16) and dorsal and volar glides. Splaying the metatarsals by dorsal pressure applied to the plantar surface with thumbs can realign the joints and straighten out a distal hammer or claw deformity (see Fig 23–14).

Friction massage to the proximal tendons, interdigital musculature, and collateral joint ligaments can mobilize tissue adhesions, promote range of motion, and enhance circulation. Muscle strengthening of the intrinsic musculature should be attempted in efforts to utilize the muscles in correct spatial and temporal sequences.

Fixed deformities require accommodation and protection to avoid breakdown of the skin. Stretching the shoe, padding the shoe, foam toe sleeves slipped over the digit, lamb's wool between digits, taping digits together, and full-contact orthotic fabri-

cation may be indicated. Patients must be educated in how to buy a shoe that fits correctly, as these toe deformities are largely a result of shoes that were too short, too narrow, or too pointed.

There are two objectives in managing deformities of the lesser toes. First, it is important to transfer the pressure from the metatarsal heads, proximal interphalangeal joints and distal phalanx joints. Second, an orthotic should encourage flexion of the metatarsophalangeal joint and extension of the proximal interphalangeal joints. Metatarsal pads help to reduce pressure to the metatarsal heads. Toe crests, pads, or slings act as a fulcrum to help extend the proximal interphalangeal joint and flex the joint in a flexible foot. They also serve to accommodate the deformity and redistribute weight from the distal end of the phalanges to the toe sulcus in a rigid foot. Prefabricated splints can be used to promote extension while cushioning the metatarsal heads and "toe combs" will aid in relieving the pressure to the inner space between the toes. Other prefabricated devices that serve to protect the bony prominences of toe deformities include toe protectors or toe sleeves.

Recommendations for shoes include a high, wide toe box such as Thermold shoes or soft leather uppers, and a longer shoe to promote flexion of the metatarsophalangeal joint and extension of the proximal interphalangeal joint. A soft, cushioned outer sole and a lower heel help to reduce pressure to the metatarsal heads. Extrinsically, a metatarsal bar affixed to the shoe sole helps to reduce pressure to the metatarsal heads by increasing weight bearing to the metatarsal shafts. A rocker bar or rocker-bottom sole accommodates rolling over on a fixed deformity and facilitates the stance phase of gait.

CONCLUSION

The focus of this chapter has been on common foot dysfunctions and injuries related to anatomic and physiologic changes associated with aging. Suggestions for conservative, nonsurgical intervention have been presented for management of common foot problems in the elderly.

Providing conservative foot care for the elderly is essential in preventing disuse and progression of foot dysfunction. Many orthopedic conditions arise from biomechanical imbalances. Ill-fitting shoes are common in the elderly patient and interfere with functional mobility. The same modalities can be used with

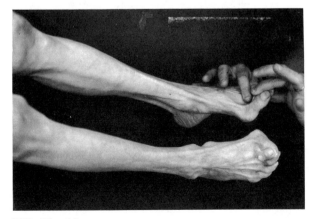

FIG 23–16.
Long-axis distraction of the lesser toe.

elderly patients as would be used for a younger patient, with precautions discussed in this chapter related to medical status, nutritional status, medications, and the age-related changes in skin condition and integrity, sensation, muscle changes, bone density, tissue compliance, and cardiovascular endurance. The major differences in treating the elderly foot with respect to anatomic, physiologic and biologic age changes are diminished tissue elasticity, muscle strength, and joint mobility. Other consid erations in therapeutic intervention and exercise prescription in the elderly should include balance, posture, vision, cognition, and environmental restrictions. All of these factors may affect safe and efficient ambulation.

The provision of orthotics and shoes in the management of foot problems in the elderly is a vital component of conservative rehabilitative intervention. Other treatment techniques and protocols that supplement and enhance the overall outcomes of intervention in the foot include manual therapies such as joint and soft tissue mobilization, Buerger-Allen exercises, therapeutic exercise, muscle strengthening, stretching, range-of-motion exercises and massage. Modalities such as electrical stimulation (high galvanic, interferential, and direct currents), heat and cold, paraffin, and ultrasound are very effective. In addition, gait training, graded walking programs, and patient education in foot care are vital components to comprehensive treatment programs for foot problems in the elderly.

The therapist may have to alter the time frame of intervention (i.e., length of treatment sessions and overall duration of intervention) and instructions given (i.e., providing written follow-up instruction), and enlist family members' and friends' assistance for compliance in exercise and orthotic and shoe prescription. Emphasis should be on patient education to prevent the debilitating effects of unchecked foot problems and consequential disuse. It is important to determine what is appropriate to the patient's level of education, native language, and motivation. The health care provider should make a realistic assessment of an elderly individual's ability to fit exercise and treatment regimens into daily life and provide functionally directed exercises and activities that enhance daily activities of living.

Foot problems affecting the older adult are often undetected until they lead to debilitating pain and loss of functional ambulation or loss of limb. Many foot deformities can be minimized or prevented by early detection, regular podiatric and physical therapy care, and provision of proper shoe gear and orthotics. Foot care is a unique medical specialty that contributes to the total health of the elder individual, physically, psychologically, and socially. Delivery of comprehensive, conservative intervention reduces the problems associated with foot deformity, injury, and pain, and the secondary problems associated with lack of ambulation and immobility.

Much emphasis has been placed on prevention in this chapter. As a wise old woman once said, "We must protect what we can't replace." Prevention is the key.

REFERENCES

1. Akeson WH, Amiel D, Abel MF, et al: Effects of immobilization on joints. *Clin Orthop* 1987; 219:28–36.
2. Bailey TS, Yu HM, Rayfield EJ: Patterns of foot examination in a diabetes clinic. *Am J Med* 1985; 78:371–374.
3. Biossonault W, Donatelli R: The influence of hallux extension on the foot during ambulation. *J Sports Phys Ther* 1984; 5:240–243.
4. Bruno J: Physical therapy for elderly patients with foot conditions, in Helfand AE (ed): *Clinical Podogeriatrics.* Baltimore, Williams & Wilkins, 1981, pp 122–153.
5. Canter K: Podiatric health planning for the aging veteran. *J Am Pod Med Assoc* 1986; 76:47–51.
6. Chamberlain GL: Cryiax's friction massage. *J Sports Phys Ther* 1982; 4:16–22.
7. Chapman EA, DeVries HA, Swezey R: Joint stiffness: Effects of exercise on young and old men. *J Gerontol* 1972; 27:218–221.
8. Cherry DB: Review of physical therapy alternatives for reducing muscle contracture. *Phys Ther* 1980; 60:877–881.
9. Chesworth B, Vandervoort A: Age and passive ankle stiffness in healthy women. *Phys Ther* 1989; 69:217–224.
10. Clough J, Marshall H: Etiology of hallux abducto valgus. *J Am Podiatr Assoc* 1985; 75:238–243.
11. Cotton R, Wartman WB: Endothelial patterns in human arteries, their relation to age, vessel site and atherosclerosis. *Arch Pathol* 1961; 2:15–24.
12. deAndrade JR, Grant C: Joint distention and reflex muscle inhibition in the knee. *J Bone Joint Surg (Am)* 1965; 47A:313–322.
13. Donatelli R, Owens-Burkart H: Effects of immobilization on the extensibility of periarticular connective tissue. *J Sports Phys Ther* 1981; 3:67–71.
14. Duke H, Newman L, Bruskoff B, et al: Relative metatarsal length patterns in hallux abducto valgus. *J Am Podiatr Assoc* 1982; 72:1–5.
15. Enwemeka C: Connective tissue plasticity: Ultrastructural, biomechanical and morphometric effects of physical factors on intact and regenerating tendons. *J Sports Phys Ther* 1991; 14(5):198–211.
16. Garbalosa J: Physical therapy, in Donatelli R (ed): *Biomechanics of the Foot and Ankle.* Philadelphia, FA Davis, 1990, pp 217–247.
17. Gerber LH: The foot in arthritic diseases, in Hunt GC

(ed): *Physical Therapy of the Foot and Ankle.* New York, Churchill Livingstone, 1988, pp 91–108.

18. Goldberg AL, Goodman HM: Effects of disuse and denervation on amino acid transport by skeletal muscle. *Am J Physiol* 1975; 216:1116–1119.

19. Goldman R: Decline in organ function with age, in Rossman I (ed): *Clinical Geriatrics,* ed 2. Philadelphia, JB Lippincott 1979, pp 112–146.

20. Gould N, Schneider W, Ashikaga T: Epidemiological survey of foot problems in the continental United States—1978–1979. *Foot Ankle* 1980; 1:8–10.

21. Habershaw G, Donovan J: Biomechanical considerations of the diabetic foot, in Kozar GP, Hoar CS, Rowbotham JL, et al (eds): *Management of Diabetic Foot Problems.* Philadelphia, WB Saunders, 1984, pp 32–44.

22. Hamlin CR, Luschin JH, Kohn RR: Aging of collagen: Comparative rates in four mammalian species. *Exp Gerontol* 1980; 15:393–398.

23. Helfand AE: Podiatric management of the diabetic foot in the elderly, in Helfand AE (ed): *Clinical Podogeriatrics.* Baltimore, Williams & Wilkins, 1981, pp 106–121.

24. Helfand AE, Bruno J: Therapeutic modalities and procedures. III. Kinetic procedures, surgical considerations, direct and alternating currents. *Clin Podiatry* 1984; 1:323–341.

25. Hole JW: *Human Anatomy and Physiology.* William C. Brown, 1988.

26. Jacobs R: Physical changes in the aged, in O'Hara-Devereaux M, Andrus LH, Scott CD (eds): *Eldercare.* New York, Grune & Stratton, 1981, pp 31–48.

27. Jones CL, Gonzales V: Pyridoxine deficiency. *J Am Physiol Assoc* 1978; 68:651–652.

28. Keenan M, Peabody T, Gronley J, et al: Valgus deformities of the feet and characteristics of gait in patients who have rheumatoid arthritis. *J Bone Joint Surg (Am)* 1991; 73A:237–247.

29. Kessler R, Hertling D: The ankle and hindfoot, in Kessler R, Hertling D (eds): *Management of Common Musculoskeletal Disorders: Physical Therapy Principles and Methods.* Philadelphia, Harper & Row, 1983, pp 178–192.

30. Klein FA, Rajan RK: Normal aging: Effects on connective tissue metabolism and structure. *J Gerontol* 1985; 40:579–585.

31. Kozak GP, Rowbotham JL: Diabetic foot disease, in Kozak GP, Hoar CS, Rowbotham JL, et al (eds): *Management of Diabetic Foot Problems.* Philadelphia, WB Saunders, 1984, pp 1–8.

32. Lehman J, Warren C, Scham S: Therapeutic heat and cold. *Clin Orthop* 1974; 99:207–209.

33. Lyons D: Vascular anatomy of the lower extremity and its clinical relevance. *Contemp Podiatr Physiol* 1991; 7:11–15.

34. Mattei FA: Orthopaedic surgical considerations of the aged, in Helfand AE (ed): *Clinical Podogeriatrics.* Baltimore, Williams & Wilkins, 1981, pp 44–49.

35. McPoil TG, McGarvey TC: The foot in athletics, in Hunt GC (ed): *Physical Therapy of the Foot and Ankle.* New York. Churchill Livingstone, 1988, pp 199–230.

36. Nawoczenski D, Birke J, Graham S, et al: The neuropathic foot—a management scheme. *Phys Ther* 1989; 69:287–291.

37. Pickles LW: Effects of aging on connective tissues. *Geriatrics* 1983; 38:71–78.

38. Pogrund H, Bloom R, Menczel J: Preventing osteoporosis: Current practices and problems. *Geriatrics* 1986; 41:5:55–71.

39. Riis B, Thomsen K, Christiansen C: Does calcium supplementation prevent postmenopausal bone loss? *N Engl J Med* 1987; 316:173–177.

40. Root ML, Orien WP, Weed JH: *Normal and Abnormal Function of the Foot,* vol II. Los Angeles, Clinical Biomechanics, 1977, pp 36–102.

41. Sapega A, Quedenfeld T, Moyer R: Biophysical factors in range of motion exercises. *Phys Sports Med* 1981; 9:57–61.

42. Seymour R, Bacharach D: The effect of position and speed on ankle plantarflexion in females. *J Soc Phys Ther* 1990; 12:153–156.

43. Spencer F, Sage R, Graner J: Incidence of foot pathology in the diabetic population. *J Am Podiatr Med Assoc* 1985; 75:590–592.

44. Tong HT: Influence of neurotrophic vitamins on the nerve conduction velocity in diabetic neuropathy. *Ann Acad Med* 1980; 9:6.

45. Valente LA: A nutritional overview for the podiatrist. *Curr Podiatr Med* 1987; 25–27.

46. Viidik A: Function properties of collagenous tissue. *Int Rev Connect Tissue Res* 1982; 6:127–215.

47. Walker J: Connective tissue plasticity: Issues in histological and light microscopy studies of exercise and aging in articular cartilage. *J Sports Phys Ther* 1991; 14:189–197.

48. Yin FCP: The aging vasculature and its effects on the heart, in Weisfeldt ML (ed): *The Aging Heart,* vol 2. New York, Raven Press, 1980; pp 27–41.

Chapter 24

Geriatric Amputee and Prosthetic Training

Teri Nishimoto, P.T.

Most of the amputees a physical therapist will encounter are from the geriatric population. Approximately 50% to 75% of amputees are over the age of 61 and most of those amputations are disease related.[5, 20, 39] Men have about three times as many amputations as women, about 90% of them occurring in the lower extremity. Distribution of lower extremity amputations reveals 2.6% Syme's amputation, 53.8% below-knee amputations, 0.7% knee disarticulations, 32.6% above-knee amputations, and 2.0% hip disarticulations.[20] A myriad of medical problems are associated with this population, most stemming from cardiovascular and respiratory disorders,[14] in particular peripheral vascular insufficiency secondary to diabetes, arteriosclerosis, Buerger's disease, embolism, massive arterial thrombosis, and arteriovenous aneurysm.[7, 14, 20, 37] Because of this high predominance of cardiovascular disease, 33% lose the opposite limb within 5 years.[22, 28, 41] To summarize, the clinical profile of an amputee is that of a man 61 years of age or older with a history of peripheral vascular disease resulting in a below-knee or above-knee amputation. This chapter will focus on the effects of normal aging and rehabilitation of the lower extremity geriatric amputee.

EFFECTS OF NORMAL AGING

Cardiovascular Implications

Cardiovascular changes that occur with normal aging compound the problems of an amputee with vascular problems. In the elderly there is a decrease in cardiac output and an increase in diastolic and systolic blood pressure. This results in a decrease in cardiac efficiency. What this means to an amputee with peripheral vascular disease is a slower rate of healing, a potentially longer period of hospitalization, and further vascular complications.

Respiratory Implications

The effect aging has on the respiratory system is a reduction in oxygen to healing tissue and an increase in energy cost, resulting from the loss of elasticity in the lung tissue and a reduction in maximum voluntary ventilation. With the amputation of a lower limb the energy cost can increase to as much as 65% in an above-knee amputee.[37] This amount decreases as the level of amputation lowers. Studies have shown that a key factor in successful rehabilitation is the preservation of the knee joint.[4, 29, 36, 45]

Muscular Implications

Strength declines in elderly persons because of a decrease in muscle contractile force, decrease in size and number of fast-twitch fibers, and increase in fat cells and connective tissue within the muscle. In most limbs with vascular insufficiency disuse atrophy is already evident, resulting from pain and ulceration. Add to that the normal reduction in strength and the result is a significantly weakened person. Flexibility of soft tissue also diminishes with age. Combine this factor with a flexed position of comfort in a painful limb and it is not long before contractures arise. In the amputee, severe hip and knee flexion contractures are detrimental to successful rehabilitation.[8, 37, 42]

Skeletal Implications

The risk for lower extremity fracture secondary to falls in elderly persons is high. Many amputees after initial loss of a limb experience phantom sensation and often try to step on the residual limb. This can be tragic in the already osteoporotic older adult. Suspension of a cast if the femur is fractured is almost impossible and an osteoporotic limb cannot be internally fixated. If the geriatric amputee is confined to bed rest, a vicious cycle of bone loss and deconditioning results. Secondary postural changes that occur within the skeletal structure also contribute to the increase in energy demand.

Sensory Implications

Sensory changes that occur with age include a deterioration of visual, auditory, proprioceptive, and vestibular systems. When a limb is lost because of vascular insufficiency, the ability to don, doff, and use a prosthesis is further compromised. Diabetic neuropathy results in the loss of sensation. It is therefore critical to train the amputee in the proper care of the insensitive residual and intact limb.[34]

Neurologic Implications

The decrease in nerve conduction velocity and impulses across the synapse retards the reaction time and reflex responses in the older amputee. It is important to incorporate equilibrium and balance reactions into the rehabilitation program.

Other Implications

The ability to fight infection diminishes with age. Unfortunately, the most prevalent postoperative complication in amputation is stump infection. Besides the physical stress, the older adult also sustains the psychological stress of adjusting to the last stages of life. Depression is common in elderly persons[35] and with the loss of an extremity it is intensified. Much of this depression can be prevented by preoperative and postoperative explanation[14] and involvement with decision making.[5] Many amputees with vascular conditions, however, are more prepared for the loss of a painful limb and the reassurance of their life being saved by the surgery.[13] Social support is vital to permit the older adult to maintain independence. This is even more critical with an amputee who may be a borderline prosthetic candidate. Financially, amputation can be devastating. The majority of amputations are done as a result of failed bypass grafts or as a last resort.[34] This means multiple surgeries and huge expenses are incurred, even without taking into account the cost of a prosthesis.

Rehabilitation Outcomes

Normal physiologic changes that occur with aging complicated by amputation can lead to a "presumed outcome" of dependency by the patient and health professional.[30] Studies indicate that there is a correlation between the decline in functional outcome and an increase in age.[22, 29] Most researchers indicate that age alone is not a barrier to successful prosthetic use.[18, 29, 36] A large percentage of geriatric amputees—68% to 79%—were found able to use their prosthesis at the time of discharge.[11, 18, 36] Follow-up studies on the continued use of a prosthesis after 1 to 5 years, which was described as "everywhere"[30] to use up to 8 hours,[36] averaged a 71% success rate.[1, 18, 30, 49]

Extensive research has been done on predicting functional outcome of the geriatric amputee.[1, 22, 29, 36, 37, 42] A plethora of factors that have positive and negative effects on the successful rehabilitation of older amputees are suggested. Positive factors include the importance of a multidisciplinary team approach; prompt and aggressive postoperative management, including immediate postoperative prostheses (IPOP) and prevention of contractures; and the preservation of the knee joint.[14, 16, 34, 36] Negative factors in successful prosthetic management are mental deterioration, poor motivation, class 4 cardiac disease, and the lack of social support.[8, 25, 34, 42, 47] A study done by Medhat et al on the types of activity achieved by amputees showed activities of daily living (ADL) that were difficult for most amputees were yard care, shower bathing, and gardening.[30] Kegel et al confirmed that 55% of amputees had difficulty in bathing.[22] Both these studies were conducted on a relatively young age group, 58 and 45 years of age, respectively, but this can give us some indication of problem areas in the elderly.

POSTOPERATIVE MANAGEMENT OF THE GERIATRIC AMPUTEE

Evaluation

As discussed earlier, to maximize functional outcome of the geriatric amputee several essential factors must be addressed. Components of an amputee evaluation are illustrated in Figure 24–1. Of particular importance are the sections on range of motion and strength, condition of intact and residual limb, and functional status.

Range of Motion and Strength

Knee and hip flexion contractures in the residual limb greater than 15 degrees make the limb difficult to fit in a prosthesis and achieve a safe, functional gait.[34] Many vascular amputees develop flexion contractures prior to amputation because of positions they have maintained to compensate for a painful limb with limited weight-bearing ability. Strength in all extremities is crucial for independent mobility.

Intact Limb

In the diabetic amputee with vascular insufficiency the intact limb is of major importance because of the high incidence of contralateral amputation.[42, 47] If edema or open wounds are apparent steps should be taken to promote healing and prevent amputation by early intervention.

Residual Limb

The primary goal with the residual limb is wound healing.[4] Factors that delay this are edema and infection. Malone et al found immediate postoperative prosthetic use to be effective in improving healing rates and decreasing rehabilitation time.[27] Other physical agents can be used as well, such as a modified hyperbaric chamber,[15] Jobst pump, electrical stimulation, or some type of occlusive dressing.

The secondary goal with the residual limb is shaping. The ideal is to achieve a conical shape. Measuring the circumference at 1-inch intervals helps determine when a limb has reached a plateau. This is one factor in determining prosthetic readiness. If an immediate postoperative prosthesis is used, measurements can be taken at cast changes, which occur approximately every 2 weeks.

Pain can be a contributing factor to dependency in the elderly.[47] Amputees can experience a variety of pain. Pain within the healing stump resulting from incision may be described as an ache or hypersensitivity. Phantom pain is actual pain perceived as coming from the amputated foot. Bony prominences such as the distal end of the tibia and fibula are often described as sensitive and do not tolerate pressure upon palpation. Bony spurs can also develop in these areas if surgery was not properly done. Neurologic pain resulting from a neuroma is common at the level of the peroneal nerve near the distal fibula. Descriptions often associated with a neuroma are a sharp, shooting, stabbing, or burning feeling.[17] Phantom limb sensation is nonpainful and primarily gives the amputee a feeling of having the limb still intact.[17] This can be detrimental in the early stages of recovery; the patient may try to stand on the limb during a transfer and fall, injuring the stump. In a study done by Jensen et al, 84% of the amputees had a sensation of phantom limb, 72% phantom pain, and 57% stump pain 8 days after surgery. After 6 months, the incidences were 90%, 67%, and 22%, respectively.[17]

Functional Status

Functional status assessment is well understood and the achievement of independence without a prosthesis is another important factor in identifying a prosthetic candidate.

Treatment Plan

Preprosthetic rehabilitation of the geriatric amputee follows four basic principles, regardless of level of amputation.

1. Wound healing and residual limb shaping
2. Range of motion and strengthening
3. Pain management
4. Functional mobility training.

The overall goal is to prepare the amputee to achieve the highest possible level of independence. Not all patients benefit from a prosthesis, although use of a prosthesis is an ideal goal for most patients. Prosthetic candidacy will be discussed later.

Wound Healing and Residual Limb Shaping

The geriatric amputee with vascular disease is in a compromised state of healing because of the aging and disease processes. Important factors in wound management include clean surgical procedure, controlling edema and hematoma formation, and immobilization of tissue.[4] The current and most effective

VI.   Residual Limb Examination _____

Circumference and Length of Residual Limb(s)

	Circumference			Length	
	Left	Right		Left	Right
Date _____			AK length from ischial tuberosity _____		
Initial _____					
			BK length (from distal end of patella) _____		

Measured from:

Residual Limb Examination

Edema _____   Bony prominences _____

Color _____   Sensation _____

Wound Healing _____   Scars _____

Temperature _____   Pain _____

VII.   Functional Status

Wheelchair Management _____

Wheelchair Mobility _____

Transfers: WC—Bed/Mat. _____   Gait _____

Bed Mobility: Supine—Sit _____

Sit—Stand _____

Rolling _____

Coordination _____

Balance: Sit Static _____   Stand Static _____

Sit Dynamic _____   Stand Dynamic _____

VIII.   Endurance (circle one):   Poor   Fair   Good

Equipment Needed _____

IX.   Assessment _____

_____

X.   Treatment Plan _____

Goals: Short-Term _____

Long-Term _____

Signature _____

FIG 24–1.
Amputee evaluation form for physical therapy.

means of immobilization is a closed rigid dressing, applied directly after amputation.[4, 27] The immediate postoperative prosthesis is a cast socket with a pylon and foot attached to the distal end, suspended by a waist belt. Pressure relief is incorporated into the socket to prevent tissue breakdown over bony prominences.[2] A load cell, a device that monitors the amount of weight bearing with an audible tone, is sometimes incorporated into the IPOP. Initially a patient with peripheral vascular disease is only allowed to place 20 to 25 pounds of weight on the amputated limb.[21] There is some controversy about the use of an immediate postoperative prosthesis because it does not readily provide visual inspection and can cause tissue breakdown in patients with poor sensation, which can lead to higher levels of amputation. Weinstein et al supported the use of an immediate postoperative prosthesis but suggested patients with a life-threatening extremity infection resulting in amputation be observed closely. They also recommended the prosthesis be removed earlier to ensure good wound healing.[46]

Another type of rigid dressing developed by Wu, the removable rigid dressing, is an alternative to the immediate postoperative prosthesis. As its name suggests, it is a rigid cast that can be removed to inspect the residual limb.[48] The fabrication of the dressing is relatively simple and poses less risk than the immediate postoperative prosthesis of healing complications if not applied properly.[12] As the limb decreases in size, additional stump socks are used to take up the shrinkage. Gradual weight bearing is also part of the protocol and begins 10 to 14 days postamputation.[48]

The most common form of dressings are the elastic wrap (Ace) bandage and stump shrinkers. The elastic wrap can be highly effective if managed properly. A 4-inch wide bandage at least 10 yards in length is used with below-the-knee amputations and a 6-inch wide bandage at least 20 yards in length is best for above-knee amputees. The best method of wrapping is the figure-8 wrap, where pressure begins distally and is projected proximally on a diagonal (Fig 24–2). This procedure must be repeated several times a day to ensure an accurate pressure of between 15 and 20 mm Hg. With the geriatric amputee, consistent independent management is often difficult because of decreased visual and tactile senses. Assistance in compliance with bandaging instructions may not be available, and if available, may not be adequate enough to maintain safe use. If a bandage is applied with pressure in excess of 25 mm Hg, tissue damage can result.[19] In many instances in which a patient is unable to manage an elastic bandage safely and with most above-knee amputees, a stump shrinker is prescribed. It is critical in the above-knee amputee that the entire residual limb be encompassed to properly shape it. Adductor rolls often develop because adductors are not included, making prosthetic fitting nearly impossible. The stump shrinker is easily donned and can provide a fair amount of edema reduction. Its major drawback is its lack of graded pressure.

Other types of residual limb shaping and healing appliances are the controlled environment, in which ambient pressure, temperature, sterility, and humidity can be controlled; air splints with a metal cone of aluminum frame with a solid ankle cushion heel (SACH) foot; inflatable splints; and Unna paste. Problems with the air pressure units are sweating beneath the splint and the need to carefully monitor the pressure.[19]

Range of Motion and Strengthening

The maintenance of full range of motion in the residual limb can be compromised by positioning, poor surgical technique, or high flexor tone. To avoid contractures, amputees must be instructed in prone lying two to three times a day for 20 minutes each session. When a below-knee amputee is up in a wheelchair, the residual limb must be elevated and in knee extension. If the limb is allowed to remain flexed, dependent edema and contractures can ensue. A removable elevating leg rest is easily obtainable and can meet these objectives. Another alternative is to fabricate a seat and leg board out of ¼-in. plywood. The seat dimension is dependent on the wheelchair. A normal adult seat is 18 × 16 in.; a narrow adult seat is 16 × 16 in. The leg board is usually 9 × 32 in. (Fig 24–3). If a cushion is added to the seat the leg board must also be padded. The two separate units allow an amputee to conveniently remove the board prior to transfer. If the patient is using an immediate postoperative prosthesis the knee is already casted in knee extension, lacking approximately 20 degrees of extension for comfort,[2] but still requires elevation.

In order for the patient to functionally ambulate with and without a prosthesis, strength and endurance should be in the good to normal range in all extremities. Upper extremities become important to an amputee whose base of support has been reduced. Shoulder depressors and extensors are key muscle groups to address. Exercises such as wheelchair pushups, latissimus dorsi pulls, rickshaw, and

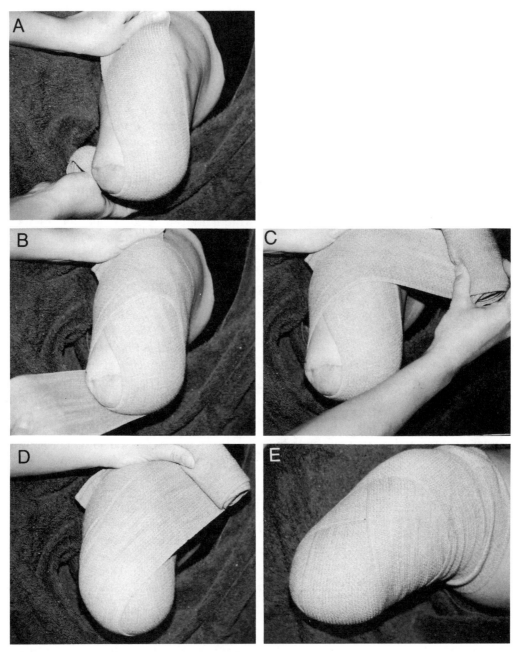

FIG 24−2.
A−D, using an elastic bandage to wrap a below-knee residual limb. **E,** the entire limb should be covered; compression should be centripedal and extend above the knee.

pushup blocks (Fig 24−4) focus on these areas. In the lower extremity, strengthening is even more essential. The use of a prosthesis requires more energy and greater muscle activity than normal walking. Instead of the alternating contraction and relaxation of muscle groups, Kegel et al found that there is more simultaneous contraction in the residual limb.[23] Their study investigated the effects of isometric muscle training in the residual limb, in strength,

control of prosthesis, and gait pattern. The results suggested that by actively contracting the anterior tibialis and gastrocnemius, amputees could improve their muscle mass, prosthetic retention, and velocity in gait.[23] In the hip, all muscles should be strengthened, especially the extensors and abductors (Fig 24−5, A and B). During ambulation with a prosthesis, hip and knee extensors are actively used to maintain stance and the abductors prevent a Tren-

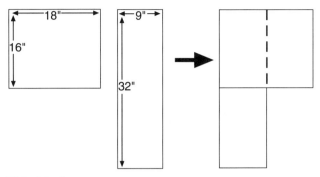

FIG 24–3.
Example of dimensions for fabricating a seat and leg board out of ¼-in. plywood. The seat dimension is dependent on the dimensions of the wheelchair seat.

delenburg deviation. Knee extensors and flexors are difficult to address in the below-knee amputee because of the short lever arm and the difficulty with weight suspension. In most instances it can be incorporated into hip exercises such as straight leg raises and hip extension with the knee in extension. Isometrics can be used immediately postoperatively or with arthritic joints, but whenever possible isotonic strengthening throughout the arc of motion should be instituted. Theraband is an excellent resistance tool used with the elderly in independent exercise programs (Fig 24–5, C). Cardiovascular training is essential in building the older amputee's endurance to sustain the increase in energy demand. Upper extremity ergometers, wheelchair mobility, or a modified form of circuit training can be implemented. In her article on aging and the cardiovascular system, Lewis recommends that the older adult has the same needs as the younger and should be exercising at 60% to 80% of maximum heart rate. In the more deconditioned elderly, she suggests beginning at 40% to 60% of maximum heart rate.[26] Often, medication can interfere with heart rate; in these cases different methods, such as perceived exertion, may be used to monitor cardiovascular training.

Pain Management

As discussed earlier, pain in the amputee can originate from a variety of sources: stump pain, phantom pain, phantom limb sensation, bony spurs and prominences, and neuromas. It has been reported by Jensen et al that stump pain decreases within the first six months.[17] Phantom pain declines as well, but to a lesser degree. Sherman in his study of American veterans found that 80% of respondents experienced significant phantom pain.[40] Various techniques have been used to address phantom pain: biofeedback, surgical intervention, electrical

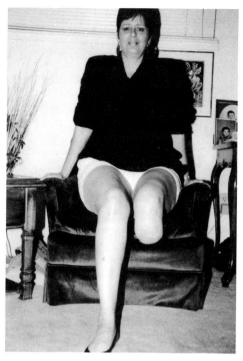

FIG 24–4.
Armchair pushups.

stimulation, and transcutaneous electrical nerve stimulation (TENS).[10, 41] Sherman et al expressed the opinion that a majority of the techniques based their success prematurely because they lacked appropriate long term follow-up studies.[41] TENS is a physical therapy modality which has been successful in the reduction of phantom pain. Peripheral nerves lacking sensory feedback are stimulated and block the pain through inhibition.[10] A study by Carabelli et al achieved similar positive results by stimulating the contralateral extremity.[6] Surgical removal of bony spurs is done when prosthetic accommodation is not met with favorable results. Neuromas are the result of a nerve wrapping around itself and creating a sensitive mass. They only create problems when they are superficial. TENS or ultrasound can be beneficial but in most instances surgical transection is the only method of pain relief.

Functional Mobility Training

The positive effects of early mobilization on postoperative illness, mortality, and long-term survival are well known. Regarding the geriatric amputee with vascular insufficiency, early mobility training is even more crucial to prevent secondary problems such as thrombus, pneumonia, and pressure sores. Osterman et al believed that ambulation is integral in the geriatric population to prevent con-

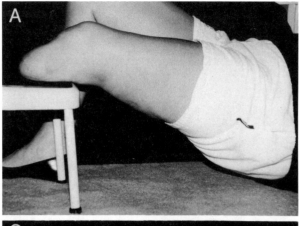

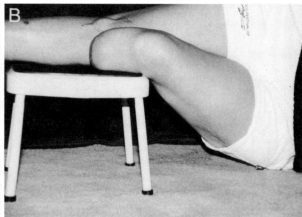

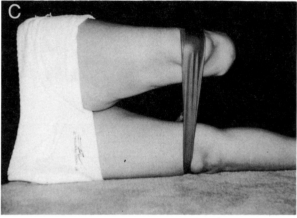

FIG 24–5.
A, one-legged bridging. **B,** dynamic hip abduction. **C,** Theraband used for resisted lower extremity exercise.

tractures and disuse atrophy secondary to a sedentary life-style.[34]

Most unilateral amputees are able to perform stand pivot transfers. Bilateral amputees or unilateral amputees with a neurologic disorder may do better with sliding board transfers. For most bilateral above-knee amputees straight-on and back-off transfers are easiest and do not require a transfer board.

Balance and gait training should also be included in the treatment plan. Sit-to-stand activities are usually progressed to hopping in the parallel bars and with a wheeled walker. Pickup walkers and crutches are more difficult for elderly persons to use unless they have had experience with them prior to amputation. It appears that with these devices the amputee experiences unilateral weight bearing when the device is advanced, decreasing balance. Knee walking or patterns on hands and knees can further challenge a below-knee amputee's balance. These skills are also important in recovery from a fall.

Home Health and Long-Term Care Physical Therapy

Many amputees are not hospitalized for the entire rehabilitation process. Often, they are discharged as soon as they are medically stable. Some are sent to rehabilitation centers; others are sent home or to long-term care facilities until their wounds have healed. It is critical that the physical therapist address as many functional skills as possible to equip the patient and caretaker with maximum functional ability. Home health and long-term care facility therapists do not have access to equipment that may be present in a hospital. Creative use of rails, countertops, beds, and dining room tables can be incorporated into the balance and gait-training phase. Cans of food, dried beans, or reclosable bags filled with water can be used for strengthening. The advantages of having therapy at home or using "home made" devices are that patients can train using practical situations. Ensuring follow-through can be difficult in these settings but constant verbal and written training can promote consistency. The physical therapist in many instances must be an advocate for the geriatric amputee to receive a prosthesis and training if he or she demonstrates the potential to benefit from one.

Prosthetic Candidacy

Factors that must be considered when recommending a patient for a prosthesis are medical history, cognition, condition of the residual limb and other extremities, functional status, energy cost, patient's motivation and goals, and the patient's support system.

Medical History

The medical history of a geriatric amputee, as discussed earlier, is quite extensive; cardiopulmonary and cerebrovascular disease is apparent as well as vascular diseases. Moore et al suggested older above-knee or bilateral amputees with coronary artery disease be further evaluated by a cardiologist before prescribing a prosthesis because many will not use a prosthetic device. Cerebrovascular accidents are common in the elderly population. When a stroke is further complicated by an amputation, the outcome depends on the extent of the neurologic impairment and side and level of amputation.[5] Hemiplegia was not found to be a contraindication to prosthetic use, but outcome was poor in hemiplegic patients over 60 years of age.[44]

Cognition

Cognition can be a major discriminating factor in successful prosthetic use. Short-term memory is often affected by the normal aging process. Alone, this does not affect the outcome of learning to don, doff, and use a prosthesis; however, if memory impairment is compounded by dementia, potential for prosthetic candidacy is reduced.

Condition of Residual Limb and Other Extremities

An optimal length for a below-knee amputation is 6½ to 7 inches measured from the distal patella; the longer the length, the better the patient's control. Other important conditions of a residual limb are a conical shape, well-healed surgical site, absence of adhesions along scar tissue, good pain control, and essentially intact sensation. Other extremities should have adequate range of motion, strength, and sensation.

Functional Status

The higher the previous and present functional status, the greater the level of outcome. The ability to ambulate with an assistive device is viewed as a good indication of prosthetic rehabilitation.

Energy Cost

A study by Waters et al on energy cost of amputees indicated the higher the level of amputation, the greater the energy cost and the lower the velocity.[45] Patients modified speed in an effort to maintain heart rates at a pace similar to their normal walking.

These researchers also discovered that amputees use less effort to walk with a prosthesis than without a prosthesis, except for those with above-knee amputations. A patient with bilateral below-knee amputations uses 20% less energy than one with a unilateral above-knee amputation.[45] Many studies have found that older above-knee amputees do better with wheelchair mobility than with prosthetic use.[28, 32, 33, 47]

Patient Motivation and Goals

Realistic goals coupled with a high level of motivation increase the geriatric amputee's suitability for prosthetic candidacy. Depression, common with aging and exacerbated by the additional trauma of limb loss, can sometimes affect motivation. This may only be a problem initially. Many older, noninstitutionalized amputees are quite adamant about walking again and are incredibly motivated to achieve this goal. There has been limited research on institutionalized geriatric amputees and functional outcome. Weiss et al investigated factors that predict a bad outcome in lower-extremity amputees and found that dependence increased with confinement to an institution.[47]

Support Systems

If cognition is impaired or physical assistance is required, a support system is essential for successful prosthetic use. The geriatric population in general have a narrowing circle of social support. Variations do exist but normally older persons have lost siblings, spouses, and friends through death and illness. Children become primary caretakers in some situations but most are unable to take on additional responsibilities.[35] With the increasing longevity of the elderly, many of their children are in their 60s or 70s and may suffer from multiple medical problems as well. Some long-term–care facilities now offer a continuum of care, providing a variety of levels of assistance with ADL. This type of care can be an alternative for the older, affluent amputee. For many institutionalized elders, individualized attention may not be available. Recent federal mandates regulating the quality of life in nursing home facilities may, however, encourage the kind of support needed to promote prosthetic use.

To summarize, consideration for a prosthesis should take into account the patient's:

- Medical history—for neurologic or cardiovascular limitations

- Cognition—the ability to learn how to use a prosthesis
- Limb condition—presence of adequate strength, range of motion, shaping, and healing
- Functional status—ability to demonstrate a moderate to high level of functional independence and when possible the ability to use a trial or temporary prosthesis[1]
- Energy cost—using a prosthesis is advantageous because it reduces the energy demand, except in above-knee amputations
- Patient motivation and goals—a realistic set of goals with high motivation
- Support system—a supportive environment to assist the amputee in prosthetic use.

PRINCIPLES OF AMPUTATION

Many of the complications that can lead to poor prosthetic outcome can be prevented by proper surgical amputation. Bone that is clean cut, smooth, and free of fragments can eliminate pain associated with bony spurs and infection resulting from osteomyelitis and allow easy prosthetic fitting. In the below-knee amputee, beveling the distal anterior aspect of the tibia and shortening the distal lateral fibula can also promote fit and comfort in a prosthesis. Stabilization of muscle can pad the distal ends of the amputated bone and ensure muscle balance in the residual limb. It also preserves stump circulation. Nerve transection, properly done by using a sharp scalpel while applying gentle traction, encourages the nerve to withdraw into the soft tissue. This can minimize pain from neuromas. Cauterized blood vessels prevent hematoma formation. The use of a drain can discourage exudate from pooling within the limb and encourage wound healing.[3]

LEVELS OF AMPUTATION AND PROSTHETIC PRESCRIPTION

In the majority of amputees with vascular problems, the affected limbs have had a series of amputations. Vascular insufficiency first appears in the most distal segment of the body, the toes.[11, 31]

Toe

Amputations of the lesser four toes do not pose a major disability, although these patients are at risk for valgus deformities. Absence of the great toe can affect push-off and rollover.[4] Padding attached to a firm shank can be inserted into the shoe to maintain foot positioning.

Partial Foot

Partial foot amputations occur mainly between the transmetatarsals and the tarsals—the procedure often referred to as Lisfranc's amputation. Anything proximal to this, such as Chopart's midtarsal amputation, is discouraged because of resulting muscle imbalance and varus deformity. Prosthetic prescription is similar to that of toe amputation: a firm filler with a reinforced shank to allow more rollover during toe-off.

Syme's

Syme's amputation or ankle disarticulation is favorable for prosthetic use. It allows end–weight bearing, provides a long lever arm for control and good suspension, and requires minimal energy cost for the geriatric amputee. The prosthesis is a below-knee socket with a medial wall opening to allow the bulbous end to pass through. It is suspended by the malleoli or femoral condyles. A SACH foot is the most common terminal device used. Some persons find a rocker bottom, similar to a peg leg, advantageous because of its durability. The major drawback of a Syme's amputation is its cosmetic value; the wide ankle region distorts the leg's natural appearance.

Below Knee

Transtibial or below knee is the most common and desired level of amputation in geriatric amputees with vascular insufficiency because of the preservation of the knee joint. The optimal terminus is the middle one third of the tibia. The weight-tolerant areas are the patellar tendon, medial, lateral, and posterior regions of the lower leg, and proximal to the femoral condyles in the femur. These areas provide the major suspension in the below-knee amputee. Most residual limb receptacles or sockets are total-contact with pressure relieved in some areas to prevent skin breakdown. The medial and lateral tibial flares, fibular head, anterior shaft of the tibia, and patella are pressure-relief sites. A survey of prosthetic clinics conducted by Fishman et al found the most commonly used prosthesis in the below-knee amputee is the patellar tendon bearing type with a soft insert, exoskeletal shank and SACH foot suspended by a supracondylar cuff (Fig 24–6).[11] McCollough et al suggested a supracondylar suspension for patients with unilateral and bilateral below-knee amputations. The socket extends above the femoral condyles and is suspended by a medial supracondylar wedge (Fig 24–7). Advantages are ease in donning and doffing, improved medial and lateral knee stability, and cosmetic superiority.[28]

Above Knee

In their study on incidences of amputation, Kay and Newman found that there was a decrease in the number of above-knee amputations performed, as opposed to below-knee amputations.[20] Clearly, the advantages of maintaining the knee joint along with improved surgical techniques and evaluative tools have contributed to this change. Knee disarticulations were often used in amputees with peripheral vascular disease in an attempt to salvage length, but because of recent advances, many of these candidates undergo below-knee amputation.[4] The ideal length of an above-knee amputation is midthigh or 4

inches above the knee.[37] High energy demand is a major limiting factor in effective prosthetic use. Every effort is made to minimize the weight of a prosthesis and maximize stability when prescribing for an older above-knee amputee. A typical prosthesis used in an above-knee amputee are a total-contact quadrilateral socket with full or partial suction, suspended by a waist belt or silesian bandage, having a single axis, constant friction knee, and SACH foot.[11] Recently, changes in prosthetic components have made available lightweight carbon feet and shanks. Pneumatic or hydraulic knees add weight but provide grading of knee movement. Many of these knee innovations are expensive and require high maintenance. Developments that are beneficial to the geriatric amputee are narrow mediolateral and wider anterior posterior sockets as used in the contour adducted trochanteric–controlled alignment method (CAT-CAM),[38] which contains the ischium and prevents the socket from shifting laterally as in the quadrilateral socket. This improves the muscular control of the prosthesis. The quadrilateral socket al-

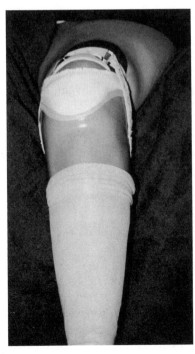

FIG 24–6.
Patellar tendon bearing with a supracondylar cuff.

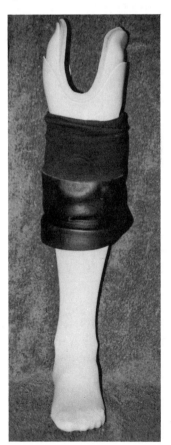

FIG 24–7.
Patellar tendon bearing with supracondylar suspension (medial wedge).

lows ischial weight bearing at the posterior brim causing more mediolateral movement. A safety knee is another important component for the elderly above-knee amputee. The tendency for most above-knee amputees is to decrease stance time on the prosthetic side because of a lack of knee control. The safety knee is designed like a brake system, allowing weight bearing on a flexed knee up to 25 degrees without buckling. This can be of great advantage for short persons or people with hip flexion contractures or weak extensors. It was once supposed that locked knees are less energy demanding then unlocked; study results show that there is no difference.[43] New advances in energy-storing feet have not been thoroughly studied with the geriatric population. One study suggested these feet have too much resistance to plantar flexion making it difficult for elderly persons to weight shift.[9] The least complicated, most inexpensive, and most functional foot used for the geriatric amputee is the SACH foot. Elderly persons do not do well with a prosthesis for amputations higher than the knee because of the physical demands required.[4]

Bilateral Amputation

In bilateral amputees, decreased weight and increased stability are again major factors in component selection. Feet are usually one size larger than the normal shoe size and aligned outset to broaden the base of support. Their center of gravity is lowered by decreasing leg height to again provide more stability. Firmer SACH feet and patellar tendon bearing (PTB) supracondylar suspension is most often used in the bilateral amputee.[28]

PROSTHETIC TRAINING

Several studies have suggested that prosthetic training is most successful when undertaken on a daily basis in a rehabilitation unit.[8, 14, 30] Zenman et al suggested outpatient programs were more appropriate than inpatient because of the short life expectancy of an amputee. Of the 48 subjects located after 5 years, 56% had died.[49] An outpatient program could prove to be more cost effective with the skyrocketing costs of health care. In their study on rehabilitation of the elderly lower-limb amputee,[14] Hamilton and Nichols felt that three or four short walking sessions were more suitable than two long

ones for the geriatric amputee. They referred to a study done by Walder that indicated peripheral vascular disease blood flow stops completely during walking but increases after activity.[14]

Donning and Doffing

Early in rehabilitation it is important to teach proper donning and doffing of the prosthesis. The limb is always inspected prior to placing the nylon or Daw sheath on. The amputee should be taught this skill with a mirror to check for breakdown. The sheath reduces the ? shearing force between the skin and sock. Stump socks are made of wool and come in various thicknesses, single-, three-, and five-ply. It is important to have at least three of each thickness so that all combinations can be made to accommodate the loss of edema. No matter how much edema is lost with stump shaping, an amputee almost always loses more once using a prosthesis. Socks should be donned one at a time, checking for wrinkles and making sure seams are not on bony prominences. Then the soft liner, hard socket, and suspension should be secured. Care must be taken to line up the residual limb and prosthesis and that the suspension is snug enough to prevent pistoning. Patients must also be instructed in cleaning their socks and socket daily.

Alignment

The alignment can vary greatly from one amputee to another. The main point is to check the patient's general balance, static and dynamic, so the base of support and knee movements provide stability and smooth symmetry. The socket in a below-knee amputation will be flexed between 5 and 15 degrees to promote patellar tendon bearing. The knee joint in an above-knee amputation should be positioned ½ in. posterior of the hip and midshank to promote knee extension.

Weight Shifting

The amputee needs to feel transference of weight from one side to the other and from the heel to the toe. Many attempt to weight shift by keeping the amputated side in extreme extension and leaning the trunk forward. Proprioceptive neuromuscular facilitation at the pelvis is an excellent method in achieving proper weight shift. The patient should be placed in a split stance and made to transfer weight on a diagonal, to simulate gait. After weight shifting the prosthesis should be removed and skin inspected for redness, especially over bony prominences. Redness should dissipate quickly; if it remains, the origin must be ascertained. Wrinkles, seams, or donning the prosthesis inaccurately are common errors.

Gait Training

The same care should be carried out when donning the prosthesis before gait training. Repetition helps reinforce learning, especially with the geriatric amputee. The patient should begin in a split stance with the prosthetic limb advanced and in a relaxed, flexed state. Weight shift should be facilitated by verbal and tactile cues to tighten the quadriceps and hip extensors as the pelvis is coming over the fixed foot. Then the sound limb is allowed to advance and should step beyond the affected limb to facilitate swing. Care should be taken when cueing the patient in advancing the prosthetic side, as hip hiking and circumduction are common deviations. Verbal cues such as "relax the [affected] hip" and "pick up the knee" work well. Another major deviation is asymmetry in stride length: an amputee will tend to take a much larger step with the affected side. This causes difficulty in shifting the weight forward to provide the knee extension moment. They should be encouraged to take a small step on the affected limb so success in weight shift will be more readily achieved. One to two trips in the parallel bars should be taken and then the prosthesis removed for skin inspection. If redness persists over bony prominences, especially the distal anterior tibialis, contact the prosthetist and discuss the situation. Developing a good working relationship with the prosthetist is extremely important in the rehabilitation of the patient and can expand the therapist's prosthetic management skills. Good sock management is essential to the fit of the prosthesis. If too many plies are used weight bearing can occur at the tibial tubercle; if too few plies are used, redness and weight bearing may occur at the distal patella. The clinician should watch for pistoning of the residual limb in the socket, for this indicates the need to add another ply.

LEISURE ACTIVITIES

Prosthetic technology is rapidly improving and adaptations are now available to allow the amputee

a more normal life. In her study Kegel et al found that age and amputation level determined participation in sport. She found the average age at which amputees were not involved with sports was 68.[22] As the population continues to shift to a larger geriatric pool, more people will expect to maintain a normal life-style even with a lower extremity amputation. Physical therapists should be prepared to accept this challenge. Informing patients about alternative prosthetic devices for leisure activities can greatly enrich the quality of their lives.[24]

CONCLUSION

The geriatric lower extremity amputee is faced with many obstacles as they relate to normal aging and the causes of amputation. The physical therapist is an integral part of the rehabilitation team that will facilitate the patient's functional independence. Immediate postoperative management, including range-of-motion exercise, strengthening, residual limb shaping, pain control, and functional training, can prevent the spiraling decline of independence in the elderly. Not all amputees will be prosthetic candidates but many factors can improve their potential. Providing the amputee with a prosthesis and training him or her in its use can greatly improve the psychosocial aspect of the geriatric patient. Expanding that by providing information on advances in prosthetics for leisure activity can only promote the dignity and quality of life of the geriatric amputee.

Further Information

"From the clinic: Fabrication of the removable rigid dressing and supercondylar cuff for the below-knee amputee," a videotape by Bradley Gervais and co-workers, is available through Research Dissemination, Rehabilitation Institute of Chicago, 345 E. Superior, Chicago, IL 60611; telephone (312) 649-6184. For further information call (312) 943-6600.

Bernice Kegel's *Sports for the Leg Amputee* is available from Medic Publishing Company, P.O. Box 89, Richmond, WA 98073-0089; telephone (206) 881-2883.

REFERENCES

1. Anderson AD, Cummings V, Levine SL, et al: The use of lower extremity prosthetic limbs by elderly

patients. *Arch Phys Med Rehabil* 1967; 48:533–538.

2. Burgess EM, Zettl JH, et al: Immediate post-surgical prosthesis. *Orthop Prosthet Appliance J* 1967; 21:105–112.

3. Burgess EM, Romano RL, Zettl JH, et al: Amputations of the leg for peripheral vascular insufficiency. *J Bone Joint Surg (Am)* 1971; 53A:874–890.

4. Burgess EM: Amputations. *Surg Clin North Am* 1983; 1:749–771.

5. Caine D: The Geriatric Amputee. *Bull Prosthet Res* 1972; 10:139–147.

6. Carabelli RA, Kellerman WC: Phantom limb pain. Relief by application of TENS to contralateral extremity. *Arch Phys Med Rehabil* 1985; 66:466–467.

7. Dacher JE: Rehabilitation and the geriatric patient. *Nurs Clin North Am* 1989; 24:225–231.

8. Edelstein JE: Optimizing the function of geriatric amputees. *Phys Occup Ther Geriatr*, 1980; 1:21–41.

9. Edelstein JE: Prosthetic feet: State of the art. *Phys Ther* 1988; 68:1874–1881.

10. Deleted in proofs.

11. Fishman S, Berger N, Watkins D: A survey of prosthetics practice 1973–74. *Orthot Prosthet* 1975; 29:15–20.

12. Gervais B, Parhad A, Wu YC: From the clinic: Fabrication of the removable rigid dressing and supracondylar cuff for the below-knee amputee, videotape. Chicago, Rehabilitation Institute of Chicago.

13. Goldberg RT: Vocational rehabilitation outlook for persons with cancer. *Rehab Lit* 1977; 38:310–321.

14. Hamilton EA, Nichols PJR: Rehabilitation of the elderly lower limb amputee. *Br Med J* 1977; 2:95–99.

15. Heng MCY, Pilgrim JP, Beck FWJ: A simplified hyperbaric oxygen technique for leg ulcers. *Arch Dermatol* 1984; 120:640–645, 1984

16. Hutton IM, Rothnie NG: The early mobilization of the elderly amputee. *Br J Surg* 1977; 64:267–270.

17. Jensen TS, Kichs B, Nielsen J, et al: Phantom limb, phantom pain and stump pain in amputees during the first 6 months following limb amputation. *Pain* 1983; 17:234–256.

18. Katrak PH, Baggott JB: Rehabilitation of elderly lower-extremity amputees. *Med J Aust* 1980; 1:651–653.

19. Kay HW: Wound dressings: Soft, rigid or semirigid. *Orthot Prosthet* 1975; 29:59–68.

20. Kay HW, Newman JD: Relative incidences of new amputations. *Orthot Prosthet* 1975; 29:3–16.

21. Kegel B, Moore AJ: Load cell. *Phys Ther* 1977; 57:652–654.

22. Kegel B, Carpenter ML, Burgess EM: Functional capabilities of lower extremity amputees. *Arch Phys Med Rehabil* 1978; 59:109–120.

23. Kegel B, Burgess EM, Starr TM, et al: Effects of isometric muscle training on residual limb volume, strength and gait of below-knee amputees. *J Am Phys Ther Assoc* 1981; 61:1419–1424.

24. Kegel B: Sports for the leg amputee. Redmond, WA, Medic Publishing, 1986.

25. Kihn RB, Warren R, Beebe GW: The "geriatric" amputee. *Ann Surg* 1972; 176:305–314.

26. Lewis CB: Effects of aging on the cardiovascular system. *Clin Manage* 1984; 4:24–29.

27. Malone JM, Moore W, Leal JM, et al: Rehabilitation for lower extremity amputation. *Arch Surg* 1981; 116:93–98.

28. McColough NC III, Jennings JJ, Sarmiento A: Bilateral below-the-knee amputation in patients over fifty years of age. *J Bone Joint Surg (Am)* 1972; 54A:1217–1223.

29. McKenzie DS: The elderly amputees. *Br Med J* 1953; 1:153–156.

30. Medhat A, Huber PM, Medhat MA: Factors that influence the level of activities in persons with lower extremity amputation. *Rehabil Nurs* 1990; 15:13–18.

31. Mensch G, Ellis PM: *Physical Therapy Management of Lower Extremity Amputations*. Rockville, Md, Aspen, 1984.

32. Moore TJ, Barron J, Hutchinson F III, et al: Prosthetic usage following major lower extremity amputation. *Clin Orthop* 1989; 238:219–224.

33. Mueller MJ, Delitto A: Selective criteria for successful long-term prosthetic use. *Phys Ther* 1985; 65:1037–1040.

34. Osterman HM, Pinzur MS: Amputation: Last resort or new beginning? *Geriatr Nurs* 1987; 8:246–248.

35. Purtillo R: *Health Professional/Patient Interaction*, ed 3. Philadelphia, WB Saunders, 1984.

36. Reyes RL, Leahey EB, Leahey EB Jr: Elderly patients with lower extremity amputations: Three year study in a rehabilitation setting. *Arch Phys Med Rehabil* 1977; 58:116–123.

37. Russek A: Management of lower extremity amputees. *Arch Phys Med Rehabil* 1961; 421:687–703.

38. Sabolich J: Contour adducted trochanteric–controlled alignment method (CAT-CAM): Introduction and basic principles, pp 15–26; John Sabolich, CPO, 1071 NW 10th street, Oklahoma City, OK 73106.

39. Sanders GT: *Lower Limb Amputations: A Guide to Rehabilitation*. Philadelphia, FA Davis, 1986.

40. Sherman R, Sherman C: Prevalence and characteristics of chronic phantom limb pain among American veterans. *Am J Phys Med* 1983; 62:227–238.

41. Sherman RA, Ernst JL, Barja RH, et al: Phantom pain: A lesson in the necessity for careful clinical research on chronic pain problems. *J Rehabil Res Devel* 1988; 25:vii–x.

42. Steinberg FU, Sunwoo IS, Roettger RF: Prosthetic rehabilitation of geriatric amputee patients: A follow-up study. *Arch Phys Med Rehabil* 1985; 66:742–745.

43. Traugh GH, Corcoran PJ, Reyes RL: Energy expenditure of ambulation in patients with above-knee amputations. *Arch Phys Med Rehabil* 1975; 56:67–71.

44. Varghese G, Hinterbuchner C, Mondall P, et al: Rehabilitation outcome of patients with dual disability of hemiplegia and amputation. *Arch Phys Med Rehabil* 1978; 59:121–123.

45. Waters RJ, Perry J, Antonelli D, et al: Energy cost of walking amputees: The influence of level of amputation. *J Bone Joint Surg (Am)* 1976; 58A:42–46.

46. Weinstein ES, Livingston S, Rubin JR: The immediate post-operative prosthesis (IPOP) in ischemia and septic amputations. *Am Surg* 1988; 54:384–389.

47. Weiss GN, Gorton A, Read RC, et al: Outcomes of lower extremity amputations. *J Am Geriatr Soc* 1990; 38:877–883.

48. Wu YC, Keagy RD, Krick HJ, et al: An innovative removable rigid dressing technique for below-the-knee amputation. *Am Correct Ther J* 1980; 34:169–175.
49. Zenman BD, Prakash AS, Adler R: Prosthetic legs revisited. *Med J Aust* 1990; 152:54–55.

APPENDIX 24–1

Amputee Exercise Program

A. Upper Extremity
  1. Wheelchair pushups
  2. Lattisimus dorsi pulls
  3. PNF pattern (D_1 and D_2) with Theraband or wall pulleys
B. Lower Extremity
  1. Straight leg raises
  2. One-legged bridging
  3. Bilateral dorsiflexion/plantar flexion (for below-knee amputees)
  4. Dynamic hip abduction/adduction—side-lying, both limbs up on stool, lift hips up (hip abduction); top leg on stool, bottom leg under stool, lift hips up (hip adduction)
  5. Prone-lying hip extension
  6. Abdominal strengthening
C. Endurance Training
  1. Upper extremity ergometer
  2. Wheelchair mobility—distance training
  3. Gait distance training
  4. One-legged bicycle riding
D. Coordination and Balance Training
  1. One-legged standing and hopping
  2. Hands and knees with PNF patterns to pelvis and shoulders (for below-knee amputees)
  3. Knee walking (for below-knee amputees)
  4. Sitting at edge of mat reaching for objects
  5. Standing catching a ball at different heights

Chapter 25

Osteoporosis: Background and Management

Everett L. Smith, Ph.D.

Catherine Gilligan, B.A.

Beth Spellberg Kwiatkowski, P.T.

Osteoporosis is a loss of skeletal integrity to the point at which atraumatic fractures occur. This disease now affects more than 1.3 million persons in the United States and is a major public health issue. Hip fracture risk increases exponentially after the age of 65.[65, 94] The rapid growth of the population over 65 has increased the population at risk. In addition, the number of osteoporotic fractures is increasing faster than the demographic increase in age.[50, 60]

Osteoporotic fractures are the result of a chronic disease process with multiple contributors. Much of the research on the prevention and treatment of osteoporosis has focused on the cellular imbalance of bone formation (osteoblast) and bone resorption (osteoclast) resulting in a net loss of bone mass and strength. Skeletal strength, however, is only one aspect of fracture risk. The occurrence of a fall and impact on the hip or wrist are frequently the catalyst for fracture. Factors related to the risk of falling or the force of impact when a fall occurs are also important in the etiology of hip and wrist factors. These related risk factors include balance, muscular strength, gait, and reaction time.

BONE CELLS

The skeletal system is a specialized connective tissue made up of cells that produce, maintain, and organize the extracellular matrix. In general, five cells participate in bone turnover and maintenance: preosteoblasts, which determine the number and activity level of the bone-forming osteoblasts; osteoblasts, involved in collagen synthesis and mineralization; osteocytes, the resident cells, which are osteoblasts encased in bone matrix and having decreased metabolic activity; preosteoclasts; and osteoclasts, key cells in bone remodeling. Bone remodeling starts with activation of precursor cells, followed by bone resorption and finally bone formation. Osteoclastic and osteoblastic activity are coupled. Osteoclasts form resorption cavities on bone surfaces and tunnel through cortical bone. Osteoblasts migrate to these cavities and form a collagen matrix that later becomes mineralized. In adults younger than age 30 years, bone formation and resorption are equal.[69] After age 30 to 35 years, the resorption cavity is incompletely filled by mineralized matrix, resulting in a net bone loss.[33]

Bone Resorption

The osteoclast, a large multinucleated cell, is the primary cell involved in bone resorption. The osteoclast precursor is a mononuclear cell (monocyte) that arises from hematopoietic cells in the bone marrow and can circulate in the blood. The precursor cells seem to have no bone resorptive function, while the resultant osteoclasts have ruffled borders with many cellular extensions that interface with the bone surface.[77] Once preosteoclasts are activated in the remodeling process, the resultant osteoclasts are responsible for the dissolution of bone. The osteoclast is activated by hormones, microdamage, and mechanical loading.

Bone Formation

Bone lining cells, found on all surfaces of adult bone, have been classified as quiescent osteoblasts or preosteoblasts.[54] They are thin and elongated.[77] Preosteoblasts, arising from mesenchymal stem cells,[88] do not themselves produce bone matrix, but respond to stimuli by cell division and maturation into osteoblasts. The mechanisms by which preosteoblasts are stimulated to produce osteoblasts has not yet been clearly defined, but Lanyon has shown that mechanical loading of bone is one stimulus.[54] Bone formation is induced by proliferation and differentiation of preosteoblasts rather than a direct influence on the already mature osteoblasts.[115]

Osteoblasts have a high metabolic activity, demonstrated by their active nuclei and by the rapid synthesis of protein and polysaccharide by their rough endoplasmic reticula and Golgi apparatus. Bone formation has two phases: production of bone matrix and mineralization. Bone matrix produced by the osteoblast but not mineralized is called the osteoid seam. The osteoid seam is about 8 to 10 μm thick and consists of collagens, proteoglycans, glycoproteins, and other components.[77] The rate of bone matrix formation is related to both the size and number of active osteoblasts on the bone surface.[54] After a time lag, osteoid gradually becomes mineralized.

Osteocytes

Once the osteoblast is surrounded by mineralized bone matrix, it is classified as an osteocyte. It has lower protein synthesis activity than osteoblasts, owing to its role in maintenance rather than formation.

Holtrop[46] reported that osteocytes have both resorptive and formative capacity in response to different hormonal environments. Parfitt[77] reported that the so-called osteocytic osteolysis process is associated only with the perilacunar bone, where the mineral is more soluble and less crystallized. Mundy,[69] however, stated that there is no clear evidence of osteocytic bone resorption.

Whether or how osteocytes respond to homeostatic control mechanisms has not been delineated.

With about 12,000 to 25,000[69, 77] cells/mm^3, and with their linkage by gap junctions, osteocytes seem ideally situated to respond to changes in both the mechanical and biochemical milieus.[54] Gap junctions allow communication and transfer of materials from an osteocyte to other osteocytes and to osteoblasts and lining cells. Gap junctions function not only within an osteon but across cement lines to other osteons.

SKELETAL FUNCTION AND CONTROL MECHANISMS

Bone is subject to both systemic and local control mechanisms. These control mechanisms are specific to two major skeletal functions: (1) metabolically, the skeleton functions as a reservoir for numerous minerals, especially calcium and phosphorus, and (2) the skeleton provides mechanical support for weight-bearing and muscle contraction in movement. Other skeletal functions, such as the protection of vital organs and hematopoiesis, do not appear to be related to the major homeostatic feedback loops controlling bone density.

Hormones, growth factors, and mechanical loads each contribute to the bone's balance between formation and resorption. Bone remodeling has an integral role in maintaining both serum calcium levels and skeletal integrity. Bone remodeling is regulated by hormonal and local stimuli, which affect the cells of the osteoclast and osteoblast lineage. When such stimuli are present, recruitment, replication, and differentiation of precursor bone cells occur. Mechanical loads affect bone to maintain an appropriate level of skeletal integrity to resist the loads applied to the skeleton in activities of daily living (ADL). Skeletal strength is dependent on the quantity, quality, and geometric organization of the skeletal tissue, all of which are responsive to mechanical loads. Both circulating hormones and local growth factors (e.g., insulin-like growth factor, transforming growth factors, platelet-derived growth factor, skeletal growth factor, prostaglandin E$_2$, interleukin-1, growth hormone, calcitonin, and parathyroid hormone [PTH]) play an important role in bone modeling and remodeling.[14] It has been suggested that circulating hormones may directly stimulate bone cells and/or enhance growth factor function. The role of growth factors is still unclear, but some are associated more with fracture healing and bone pathologies than with normal physiologic function of bone.

Calcium Homeostasis

Serum calcium is maintained at a physiologically required level of about 10 mg/dL through regulation of calcium absorption from the gastrointestinal tract, reabsorption by the kidney, and resorption from bone. If serum calcium drops owing to inadequate intestinal absorption or high kidney excretion, parathyroid hormone levels in the serum are increased. This draws calcium from the skeletal reservoir, and increases 1,25-vitamin D, which enhances intestinal calcium absorption and retention of calcium by the kidney. If calcium intake is adequate, calcium intake into the blood is equal to calcium loss (about 200 to 300 mg per day) from the intestinal tract, kidney excretion, and skin. This balance is maintained on the average with a calcium intake of 1,000 mg/day in men and premenopausal women and 1,500 mg/day in postmenopausal women.[42] If serum calcium rises, PTH is decreased and calcitonin increased in order to maintain calcium homeostasis.

Mechanical Homeostasis

Bone cells respond to strain induced by the external and internal forces applied to the bone. Lanyon hypothesized that strain (deformation), unlike external load or stress, is directly related to the number of cells activated and their metabolic activity.[54] Using an in vivo isolated wing model, he showed that bone hypertrophy was related to the strain and to the number of load cycles. Variable (500 to 4,000 microstrain) compressive strains were applied to the bone. Peak strains below 1,000 microstrain resulted in bone loss and strains above 1,000 microstrain resulted in cross-sectional area increases (up to 40%) in proportion to the strain applied.[90] When strain was held constant (at about 2,000 microstrain), as few as four loading cycles prevented disuse atrophy and as few as 36 loadings per day resulted in an increase in cross-sectional area of 30% to 40%. No further hypertrophy was observed if the number of loading cycles was increased to 360 or 1,800 cycles per day at the same strain magnitude.[89]

Neither the osteoblast nor the osteoclast seems to be responsive to mechanical strain but osteocytes seem to be influenced by the magnitude and the distribution of strain in the skeleton.[54] How the osteocyte detects the strain and develops and transmits a message to the preosteoblasts and preosteoclasts is unclear. Preliminary studies have suggested that DNA of the osteocyte must generate a biochemical message or signal that is transmitted to other cells.[54] This message competes with messages generated by hormones and growth factors. The response of the preosteoblast and preosteoclast depends upon their integration of these multiple messages.

The delicate balance between osteoclastic resorption and osteoblastic formation of bone has been defined in terms of systemic and local regulation in which hormonal and local growth factors are known to play a central role. The biochemical message generated by mechanical strain has only recently been suggested as another important regulator of bone remodeling. These local mechanisms may represent another feedback loop in skeletal homeostasis.

CHANGES WITH AGE

Bone Loss

Bone mass peaks in the fourth decade of life for both men and women. Women lose 0.5% to 1% of their bone mass per year starting at about age 30 to 35 years. This loss is accelerated for 3 to 5 years following menopause; some women lose up to 5% per year. Men fare better, losing only about 0.5% per year starting at age 45 to 50 years. There is a faster rate of bone loss in areas with relatively more trabecular bone—the distal radius, femoral neck, and vertebral bodies.

In cortical bone, bone loss results in increased endosteal diameter and increased porosity. In trabecular bone, trabeculae are thinned. The distance between trabeculae increases and entire trabeculae may be resorbed. In the vertebral bodies, there seems to be a preferential loss of horizontal trabeculae, weakening the lattice in the direction of gravity more than would be indicated by the density loss alone.[68] This loss of horizontal support increases the risk for compression fractures.

Osteoporosis has been divided into two syndromes called type I and type II osteoporosis.[82] Type I osteoporosis, also called postmenopausal osteoporosis, is associated with the rapid trabecular bone loss in the distal radius and vertebrae following menopause. The decreased bone mass results in Colles' fractures and vertebral collapse 10 to 20 years postmenopause. Type II osteoporosis is characterized by hip fractures and multiple vertebral wedge fractures, and generally manifests after the age of 70 years. It appears to result from general age-related declines in both trabecular and cortical bone and parallels other age-related declines in physiologic function.

The causes of bone loss with age are numerous. Frequent contributors to bone loss are inadequate mechanical loading and calcium intake, estrogen depletion, and possibly genetic predisposition. Less common conditions leading to osteoporosis are covered later in this chapter.

In women, the most prominent cause of bone loss is estrogen deficiency beginning at menopause. The exact mechanism by which estrogen influences bone is unknown, but estrogen deficiency appears to increase bone turnover from about 2% to 4% of total bone per year.[33] Intestinal calcium absorption is lowered and the requirement for calcium intake to maintain calcium homeostasis is increased.[42] Women experiencing early menopause, either surgical or natural, and untreated with estrogen replacement are at the greatest risk for future fracture owing to the premature onset of the increased skeletal decline. In both premenopausal and postmenopausal women, average calcium intake is inadequate to maintain a positive calcium balance.[40] With age, in both men and women, calcium absorption decreases. Lack of, or a decrease in, physical activity in the average aging person may also be implicated in the loss of bone with age.[100]

Neuromuscular Risk Factors

Age-related changes in neuromuscular function also contribute to the risk of osteoporotic fractures, through their influence on the risk of falls and the force of impact on bone if a fall occurs. These changes include declines in balance, muscle mass, and strength and of speed of reaction, gait, and flexibility (Table 25–1).

OSTEOPOROSIS

Osteoporosis (literally porous bone) is virtually universal in women over age 70 years. The clinical manifestation of osteoporosis is a low-trauma fracture, typically of the wrist, spine, or hip. At the age of 50, a woman has a 15% lifetime risk of hip and Colles' (wrist) fractures[19]; at age 65, the lifetime risk for spine fractures in women is 32%,[64] and the ma-

TABLE 25–1.

Changes in Physiologic Risk Factors for Falls and Fall-Related Trauma With Age

Factor	Change (%)	Group Ages (yr)* Young	Group Ages (yr)* Old
Balance			
Sway[27]	~100	33	73
Single stance time[83]	66	21	69
Muscle mass/strength[37]		30	80
Upper body	30		
Lower body	40		
Reaction time[18, 83, 106]	10–24	18–22	64–69
Gait velocity[44]	29 (women)	29	78
	12 (men)	26	69
Flexibility[99]	0–50	25–35	56–75

*Average age(s) of groups studied.

jority of 80-year-old women have at least one partial fracture of the vertebra.[21] Corresponding to their higher peak bone mass and lower bone loss rates, men at age 50 years have only a 5% lifetime risk of hip fracture and 2% risk of Colles' fracture.[19]

Fractures

Osteopenia resulting from low peak bone mass and age-related bone loss may be considered a primary contributor to fracture risk. Bone mineral density is correlated at 0.85 to 0.90 with bone strength. This relationship is supported by the increased incidence of fractures in subjects with low bone mass. The prevalence of vertebral fractures is under 1% in women with vertebral bone density greater than 1.2 g/cm^3, but over 50% in women with bone density under 0.6 g/cm^3.[63] Similarly, the incidence per person-year of femur fractures is less than 0.1% in women with femur bone density greater than 1.2 g/cm^3, while women with femur density less than 0.6 g/cm^3 have incidence rates of 0.9% for cervical (neck) and 1.8% for intertrochanteric femur fractures.[63] Nevertheless, there is a large overlap in bone density between subjects with and without fractures. This overlap may be partially explained by differences in bone geometry or bone quality not detected by bone density measurements. In addition, fractures may be event-mediated. The vast majority (90%) of hip and Colles' fractures result from a fall.[45] Falls are common among the elderly, especially among women, who fall three times as often as men.[28] About one third of women between the ages of 65 and 74 fall one or more times each year[109] and the risk of falling increases with age. About 5% of falls in the elderly result in fractures.[108] Whether a fall causes a fracture depends upon numerous factors: the ability to break the fall, the forces applied to the bone during the fall, the absorption of impact forces by other tissues (muscle or fat), the force of impact with the ground, and the strength of the bone.

Risk factors for falls include neurologic deterioration or medication-induced sedation and impaired balance, strength, reaction time, gait, and flexibility. Reaction time and strength aid in preventing potential falls and reducing the impact of falls. The risk for recurrent falls in elderly subjects increases as the number of physiologic and functional risk factors increases.[72, 108, 109] Muscular strength of the legs is significantly correlated with balance and the risk of falls.[35, 112] The direction of falls and the impact on the hip are related to gait velocity.[21]

Medications and Diseases That Contribute to the Risk of Fracture

A variety of diseases and medications can induce or increase bone loss. Diseases adversely affecting bone include hyperparathyroidism, diabetes, liver disease, alcoholism, rheumatoid arthritis, hyperthyroidism (either natural or medication-induced), rickets, Paget's disease, certain types of cancer, and poliomyelitis. Prolonged bed rest results in rapid bone loss. Diseases that result in muscle wasting, or spinal cord injuries and other conditions that result in extended bed rest or paralysis also lead to severe osteopenia and osteoporotic fracture. Corticosteroids, anticonvulsants, some estrogen antagonists, catabolic drugs, and chemotherapy have been associated with increased bone loss.

In addition to diseases and medications that compromise bone, factors that increase the risk of falls also may increase the risk of osteoporotic fracture. These include impaired vision, neurologic and neuromuscular disease, and use of psychotropic drugs or alcohol.

EVALUATION FOR SUBJECTS AT RISK

Prevention of osteoporosis is more cost-effective than treatment. Prevention strategies should be based on identifying those at high risk, early diagnosis, and treatments designed to prevent fractures or to reduce the resultant cost, morbidity, and mortality. The choice of methods by which to evaluate a subject on entry to an osteoporosis prevention program should consider (1) patient safety during testing and treatment, (2) fracture risk, (3) cost, and (4) appropriateness of the parameters tested in view of the anticipated treatment. A medical history and physical examination should be obtained for people entering an osteoporosis prevention or treatment clinic. Additionally, nutritional intake (especially calcium intake) and physical activity should be evaluated. Fall history and family osteoporosis history should also be obtained. Bone scans are appropriate for subjects at risk for osteopenia, and roentgenographs for subjects with known or suspected osteoporotic fractures. Gait and balance assessments are important parameters in evaluating the risk of falls. If subjects are to participate in an aerobic exercise program, especially if they have an abnormal electrocardiogram (ECG), high blood pressure, or other cardiovascular limitations, a 12-lead ECG and work capacity test are necessary to ensure patient safety. Strength testing is appropriate if resistance training is contemplated, but is not recommended for subjects with severe osteopenia or prior fracture until a complete assessment of bone mineral density and x-rays are obtained. Range-of-motion evaluation will aid the physical therapist or exercise instructor in determining exercises to address limitations that lower functional capabilities.

Risk factors for osteopenia include female gender, advanced age, small or light build, early menopause, a family history of osteoporosis, and excessive alcohol and/or tobacco use.[23, 41, 93, 97] While it is not necessary to obtain bone density measurements in all subjects, those who are at increased risk of low bone mass should be measured. Subjects with the kyphotic posture typical of those with vertebral fractures, or very low bone density or abnormalities on a bone density scan should also undergo full-spine–length lateral radiography to determine the location, extent, and type of vertebral fractures. This will permit the therapist to design a treatment program to minimize further injury, maximize rehabilitation outcomes, and prevent further degeneration of both bone and muscle.

Fall risk factors include a history of falls as well as impaired balance, gait, reaction time, and strength. For subjects with a history of falls, a careful review of medications and a vision exam including contrast sensitivity and visual field are strongly recommended. Neurologic testing is also appropriate for these subjects.

The following sections are based primarily on

subjects entering an osteoporosis prevention program. Evaluation of subjects recovering from fractures is covered later in this chapter.

OSTEOPENIA AND UNDIAGNOSED VERTEBRAL FRACTURES

Commonly used methods to assess bone include roentgenographs, single photon absorptiometry (SPA), dual photon absorptiometry (DPA), and dual energy x-ray absorptiometry (DEXA).[61, 78] SPA (15 mrem) is typically used for assessing bone density of the distal third and ultradistal of the radius and ulna, while DPA (5 mrem per site) and DEXA (less than 5 mrem) can be used to evaluate bone density in the total body, spine, femur, and tibia. Other methods to measure bone density include quantitative computed tomography (100 to 1,000 mrem), usually applied to the vertebrae, and neutron activation analysis for the whole body.[110] Roentgenographs are used to evaluate the degree of osteophytosis or aortic calcification as well as the presence, location, and degree of vertebral collapse, wedging, or "codfishing," but they are insensitive for quantifying and monitoring bone mineral density. They do provide clear anatomic landmarks useful in the interpretation of the bone mineral densitometric scan. Bone mineral density at a single appendicular or axial site can be used to predict fracture risk, but the discriminatory power of fracture risk indices is moderate at best. Bone mineral density status varies throughout the body; correlations of bone mineral density in one bone to other bones are 0.36 to 0.65, and even two sites in the same bone correlate only at about 0.84.[38]

If the bone mineral density is below the fracture threshold (e.g., 0.75 g/cm^3 for the femur and 0.92 g/cm^3 for the spine[62]), or a patient complains of back pain or has a dowager's hump, it is appropriate to obtain anteroposterior (AP) and lateral spine roentgenographs.

Strength

In patient evaluation and research, dynamometers are often used to assess strength. Depending on the dynamometer available, isometric or isokinetic strength can be measured. Common dynamometers used are the Cybex and Lido isokinetic dynamometers, strain gauges, and hand-grip dynamometers.

One-repetition maximum (1 RM) tests on resistance training equipment can also be used for strength evaluation. The 1 RM tests are a useful way to measure progress if resistance training is included in the treatment protocol; however, there are some drawbacks to 1 RM testing of inexperienced elderly subjects. Resistance training equipment may not have settings or weight increments small enough for use by the frail older adult. Subjects must be familiarized with the movements in a few sessions prior to testing. The recruitment of non–target muscle groups is more likely with this type of equipment than with dynamometers. For testing purposes, range-limiting and stabilization devices are strongly recommended for accuracy of measurement and subject safety. Stroke is a possibility in strength testing of the older adult, although this risk can be reduced greatly by training subjects to breathe properly through the movements.

Strength testing of the trunk is contraindicated for subjects with vertebral fracture as is testing of the hip for subjects with hip fractures. Strength evaluation of these subjects should only be done under the supervision of a rehabilitative physician or physical therapist.

Balance

Balance can be evaluated simply and cheaply by noting how long a subject can stand on one leg,[83] and by use of observational scales. Tinetti[109] developed an observational scale that correlates with faller/nonfaller status. This test consists of 12 items and can be completed in about 10 minutes. The sensitivity of these tests to measure changes in balance is unknown. More sophisticated and costly measures of balance can be obtained by using balance platforms and specially designed platforms that introduce forward, backward, and tilt perturbations. These can measure the area and velocity of sway while standing and in response to the induced perturbations and neuromuscular reactions to the perturbations can be timed.

Gait

In conjunction with the balance evaluation, Tinetti provided a standardized scale to evaluate defects in gait.[109] Shuffling and other gait disorders may predispose subjects to falls or leave the subject ill-prepared to reduce the impact through protective responses. These observations of gait disorders can be inexpensively supplemented by stopwatch measurement of velocity over a fixed distance and measuring stride length by attaching an inked pad to the shoe. At our facility, we use a 40-m course and measure over the middle 20 m to eliminate start-up and slow-down periods. Velocity is an important factor determining whether a person who falls lands on the hands, knees, or hip. More detailed analysis of gait can be obtained by using instrumented force platform walkways and motion analysis and analyzing force and joint ranges of motion. The time and cost of this method, however, generally restrict its use to research studies.

Range of Motion

Measures of available joint range of motion can be performed for almost every joint with a goniometer.[3] Often, a sit-and-reach test is used to evaluate hamstring, hip, and lower back flexibility.[75] Training in flexibility is an important component of any exercise program. Lack of flexibility in the ankle, knee, and hip may compromise gait and balance.

Aerobic Work Capacity

For older subjects, a physical examination and 12-lead ECG are needed prior to work capacity testing. Blood pressure and ECGs should be monitored during the test. Guidelines for ensuring the safety of subjects and protocols for testing are provided by the American College of Sports Medicine.[4] Treadmills and bicycle ergometers are the most common equipment used in aerobic work capacity testing.

Testing may be problematic for subjects recovering from a hip fracture or with back pain from vertebral fractures. These subjects may find it difficult or impossible to perform any meaningful evaluation procedure until the pain is reduced and muscular weakness ameliorated. Once the patient is capable of performing a work capacity test, it may be appropriate to modify treadmill or bicycle ergometer protocols for a more gradual progression.[98] For evaluating elderly subjects in our laboratory, we use a modified Balke protocol on the treadmill, with a speed of 2 mph and progressive increments of 2% in grade every 2 minutes. The work load increases by 0.5 met (1 met = 3.5 mL O_2/kg/min) per grade. The treadmill should be started up at 0 mph and gradually increased to 2 mph at the start of the test. Other options include the chair step test,[101] or for a subject with hip fracture and limited mobility, an arm ergometry test. The chair step test is performed sitting. The subject lifts his or her legs once per sec-

ond, alternating left and right, to 6-, 12-, and 18-in. steps. A final stage adds arm movements to the 18-in. step height.

If the subject's cardiovascular response to exercise cannot be determined, the subject should not be trained aerobically. Instead, exercise should focus on flexibility, regaining mobility, the ability to perform ADL, and maintaining independence.

Heart rate during aerobic training should be kept below that achieved on a work capacity test, whether maximal or submaximal. Maximal tests are preferred, since training heart rates can be more accurately determined for the individual, and medications commonly prescribed for elderly subjects may strongly affect heart rate. However, submaximal tests can be used to estimate the subject's general fitness and to evaluate the cardiovascular response.

PREVENTION AND TREATMENT

Three components are vital to osteoporosis prevention and treatment: adequate dietary intake, muscular strength, and proper body alignment. With rapid bone loss or severe osteopenia or fractures, medications to maintain or possibly increase skeletal mass, such as estrogen replacement therapy (ERT), bisphosphonates, calcitonin, or fluoride, should be considered. (Note that fluoride therapy is still in the research stage and should be prescribed only by experienced specialists. It has numerous side effects, including gastrointestinal upset and joint pain.) The choice of therapy will depend on the individual patient's medical history, the facts available to the physician, and the ability to closely monitor the treatment chosen. Estrogen replacement, bisphosphonates, and calcitonin suppress bone turnover, whereas fluoride stimulates bone formation.[29] As of January 1992, however, the Food and Drug Administration has approved only estrogen replacement and calcitonin for prevention or treatment of osteoporosis among these medications. Secondary osteoporosis induced by pathologic conditions or medications requires careful weighing of the risks of osteoporosis vs. those of the primary disease or the benefits of the medications. Interventions may include reducing dosages of causative medications, countering medication effects on bone with other medications or treatments, or choosing an alternative medication or treatment for the primary condition. Responses to these countermeasures, including calcium balance, should be carefully monitored. Nutrition and physical therapy assessments should be obtained to aid these patients in making nonmedical life-style changes such as increasing calcium intake, modifying poor posture and lifting techniques, and learning methods of falling. The following sections concern exercise or physical therapy strategies for preventing or reversing losses in bone and physiologic and functional abilities associated with fracture risk.

Prevention

Prevention of osteoporosis is a priority because of its irreversible effects and its high rate of prolonged morbidity. The ideal exercise program for prevention of fractures would increase bone mass, balance, strength, gait, flexibility, and speed of reaction, and reduce the incidence of falls. No research to date has addressed these factors in combination. There are indications that each of these parameters can be improved, and fracture risk reduced, through exercise.

Bone Mineral Density

Numerous cross-sectional and intervention studies have reported beneficial effects of exercise on bone mass. Exercise intervention programs have reduced loss or increased arm bone mineral content,[85, 95, 102, 103, 113] total body calcium,[2] spine bone mineral density,[22, 36, 53, 71] calcium bone index (CaBI, a measurement of calcium content by neutron activation analysis of the central third of the body),[16, 17] tibia bone mineral content,[58] and heel bone density and ultrasound attenuation.[52, 91] These studies included both men and women, young and old subjects, and subjects with and without osteoporotic fractures. Exercise intervention studies that measured femur bone mineral density did not report a significant effect,[66, 71, 87] although in cross-sectional studies femoral bone mineral density was higher in athletes than in nonathletes.[10, 43]

The type of exercise optimal for bone has not been determined. Walking or weight-bearing aerobic training accounted for the majority of exercise programs reported to affect spine or lower body bone mineral density.[2, 16, 17, 22, 58, 71, 91] Upper body resistance training affected bone mineral density at the distal third of the radius and ulna and ultradistal radius,[85, 95, 102, 103] but weight-bearing activity alone did not.[2, 79, 92] Studies of other forms of training such as squeezing tennis balls[9] and bicycle ergome-

ter training[48, 66] reported small or insignificant exercise effects at the skeletal sites measured.

Animal studies indicate that bone hypertrophy is directly related to the strain placed on the bone.[90] This hypothesis is supported by cross-sectional studies of athletes; the greatest bone hypertrophy was found in those participating in sports that placed the highest strain on bone.[73] Femur bone mineral density was greater in body builders than in sedentary subjects or other athletes.[10, 43] Studies of athletes have also shown that bone hypertrophy is site specific, as shown by hypertrophy in the dominant vs. nondominant arm of tennis players and baseball pitchers.[47, 49, 51, 67, 68, 78, 111] Intervention studies of resistance training have conflicting results. Two studies reported that adding low-level resistance to aerobic training tended to improve CaBI[17] and radius bone mineral density[85] more than aerobic training alone, although the differences were not significant. In a study combining one-arm resistance training with training on a cycle ergometer, spine bone mineral density increased significantly, femur and training-arm bone density did not change significantly, and non–training arm bone density decreased.[66] A two-year program of spine extension exercises against resistance did not affect spine bone density loss in postmenopausal women.[96] Spine bone mineral density decreased significantly in premenopausal women in a 9-month weight training program and did not change significantly in the control group.[87] Femur bone mineral density did not change in either group. In contrast, exercisers in a different 12-month weight lifting program exhibited significantly improved spine bone mineral density relative to matched-pair controls.[36] In a study of postmenopausal women given estrogen replacement therapy alone or in combination with a weight training program for 1 year, spine, total body, and radius bone mineral density increased significantly in the exercise group while no significant change occurred in the control group.[74]

An exercise program to prevent osteopenia should have exercises to mechanically load and strengthen bones in the three major areas where the risk of fracture is high—the spine, hip, and wrist. The research mentioned above indicates that upper body resistance training should be used for the upper arms and forearms, and weight-bearing exercise, possibly supplemented by resistance training, for the spine. No exercise intervention study has been effective in improving femur bone mineral density; however, one can hypothesize that a combination of weight bearing and resistance training of the muscle groups surrounding the proximal femur should provide improvements in bone mass.

Muscular Strength

Strength training is based on overload, or requiring greater muscular force than the individual's activities habitually demand. This may be 2 to 10 pounds for a frail older adult or multiples of body weight for a young athlete. Strength training is commonly equated with free weights or with resistance training equipment, but other possibilities exist for the frail elderly subject.

In studies using resistance training equipment, older men (aged 60 to 72 years)[32] and very old men and women (mean age, 90 years)[30] had large gains in strength (100%) and also improved muscle mass. Subjects in these studies trained the quadriceps at 85% of their 1RM. Smaller but significant strength gains were reported for elderly subjects trained with activities that provided less resistance and more repetitions,[1, 5, 6, 25] such as wearing light (less than 2 kg) wrist and ankle weights or pulling on elastic tubing. Another possibility for providing the resistance training needed to improve strength is water exercise, although the resistance provided cannot be easily quantified. Water exercise could provide an excellent environment for persons with fear of falling or lower extremity joint limitations. Young women[107] and subjects with multiple sclerosis[34] and rheumatoid arthritis[24] all improved their strength by participation in water exercise programs.

A wide variety of muscle groups may be involved in the prevention of osteoporotic fractures through loads placed on bones, prevention of falls, and/or reduction of impact from falls. The strength of the ankle, knee, and hip musculature is an important component of balance. Hip muscles not only place strain on the femur but are also important in the absorption of energy if a fall occurs. Back and shoulder muscles place strain on the vertebrae and help in maintaining correct upright posture. Arm and shoulder muscles place strain on the humerus, radius, and ulna and help in preventing falls or absorbing the force of impact by protective responses. To maximize the benefits of strength training in an osteoporosis prevention program, both upper and lower body musculature should be trained. It may be impractical for the average elderly subject to properly train all these muscle groups in a session that also includes aerobic activities. No obvious solution to this problem is evident, but a well-rounded program could alternate resistance training days with aerobic/weight-training days, or alternate which muscle groups are trained, while carefully training antagonist muscle groups equally.

Balance

Balance relies on many factors, including vision, proprioception, neurons, muscular strength, and flexibility. Muscular weakness of the leg is implicated in poor balance and the likelihood of falls.[35, 112, 116] Subjects with impaired leg strength may become unsteady in performing simple ADL owing to muscle fatigue.

Cross-sectional studies have indicated that balance is improved by exercise. Active elderly women were able to maintain a one-legged stance significantly longer than inactive elderly women.[83] Lichtenstein et al[56] studied elderly women in a balance training program held 60 minutes per session, 4 days per week for 16 weeks. Each session included stretching, walking, response exercise (maneuvering in response to signals), and static (e.g., standing on one leg) and active (e.g., tandem gait) balance exercises. Biomechanics platform measures of sway improved significantly in exercisers compared with controls for the eyes-open single stance, but controls improved significantly compared with exercisers in the eyes-closed condition. An exercise program consisting solely of walking 30 minutes, 3 days a week for 6 weeks at an aerobic training level significantly improved balance in elderly subjects.[86] Balance was determined by timing how long subjects could hold various stances. Rikli and Edwards[84] also reported increases in stance time. Exercise subjects who participated in a 3-year general exercise program, 3 days a week for 60 minutes, improved significantly compared with controls in single-leg stance time. The increase in balance was accomplished during the first year of the program. The program consisted of 5 to 10 minutes of warm-up, 20 to 25 minutes of aerobic weight-bearing exercise (dancing to music and walking), 20 to 25 minutes of calisthenics designed to affect muscular strength and endurance, balance, and coordination, and 5 to 10 minutes of cool-down.

General principles of physiology and anatomy suggest training specifically for the outcome function of interest. Subjects with impaired balance would probably benefit from practicing activities that stress the neuromusculature and proprioceptors associated with balance. Since strength and flexibility of the lower limbs contribute to balance, activities to improve strength and flexibility may be useful in improving balance; however, few intervention trials have been performed to document these hypotheses.

Gait

Gait, like balance, depends upon a complex of factors that may include strength, flexibility, and aerobic capacity. Although training can improve these factors, it is not known whether gait is affected by exercise training. Jones et al[52] reported that average brisk walking pace improved with a 1-year walking program. Twenty-five women, mean age 44, walked briskly for an average of 159 minutes per week. Their brisk walking pace increased by 10%. No data on walking speed for the control group was reported, and it is unclear whether this pace was ad lib or a result of training progression and measured during the exercise sessions. If impaired strength, flexibility, or aerobic capacity limits gait, correcting these weaknesses would permit improved gait function. Physical habits, however, may persist and subjects may maintain an abnormal gait adopted because of weakness despite amelioration of the problem. An exercise program should include "normal" walking. The instructor should carefully observe the gait of participants and remind them as frequently as necessary of ways to improve their gait and posture. Ironically, fear of falling and thus increased timidity and tentativeness may contribute to a person's gait limitations that increase the risk of falls or hip fracture rather than protect the person.

Flexibility

Various studies have shown that flexibility in elderly subjects can be improved by exercise training.[12, 15, 31, 39, 55, 70, 80] These improvements included trunk, neck, shoulder, wrist, hip, knee, and ankle range of motion. Munns[70] reported upper and lower body range-of-motion improvements of 8% to 48% in elderly (mean age, 72 years) women participating in an hour-long exercise class held 3 days a week for a year. In another study of elderly women (mean age, 71 years), Raab et al[80] reported the effects of a 25-week exercise program of 1-hour sessions three times per week. Elderly women who participated in the program, with or without weights (2 kg), showed improved ankle plantar flexion, shoulder flexion and abduction, and left cervical rotation compared with controls. Exercise subjects did not, however, improve significantly compared with controls in hip flexion, ankle dorsiflexion, wrist flexion and extension, or right cervical rotation.

Flexibility training designed to incorporate the major muscle groups involved in other aspects of the exercise program, such as resistance or aerobic training, helps subjects to avoid injury and perform activities through a normal range of motion. Ankle, knee, hip, and spine flexibility are all important in the maintenance of balance, gait, and posture.

Reaction Time

In cross-sectional studies, both young and old subjects who regularly performed aerobic exercise had faster reactions than their sedentary counterparts.[8, 18, 83, 105, 106] Spirduso[104] hypothesized that aerobic activity improves oxygenation of brain cells and that this increased oxygenation is a possible mechanism for exercise-induced improvements in reaction time. Subjects over 50 who participated in a 16-week aerobic training program improved their reaction time significantly, while subjects in a relaxation program and control subjects did not change significantly.[26] In an attempt to determine whether aerobic training and resistance training differed in their effects on reaction time, Panton et al[76] randomized subjects into control, aerobic, and strength training groups. Reaction time improved similarly in both training groups, but there was no significant difference between the trained groups and controls. Rikli and Edwards,[84] however, found that simple reaction time improved significantly compared with controls in subjects participating in a 3-year general exercise program. Choice reaction time also tended to improve more in the exercise than in the control group, but the difference was not significant.

Since aerobic training was the form of exercise in most studies showing a significant exercise effect, it is the logical choice for inclusion in an exercise program with a goal of improving reaction time.

Exercise Program Summary

Exercise programs for the prevention of osteoporosis should include training of the major muscle groups, weight-bearing exercise (including normal walking), aerobic exercise, and postural alignment. Flexibility should be included in each session both for patient safety and for the benefits increased range of motion confers on the ability to perform ADL. Static and dynamic balance activities should be performed; many of the strength training or weight-bearing exercise routines will incorporate elements of balance.

Falls and Fractures

Falls are a major contributor to hip fractures. Cross-sectional studies have indicated that fallers were less active than nonfallers, and subjects with hip fractures less active in earlier life than subjects without hip fractures.[7, 11] Prospective studies also showed that more active subjects had a lower risk of falls and fractures.[13, 114] These studies are not conclusive, since activity and falls or fractures may both be affected by underlying common factors such as health. No randomized trials of the effects of exercise on falls or fractures have been published.

Treatment of Fractures Related to Osteoporosis

At the University of Wisconsin Osteoporosis Clinic we have developed a program for patients with hip or vertebral fractures or severe osteopenia. The general program consists of a 4- to 6-week physical therapy phase, followed by a graded progressive exercise program. This is an ambitious program, intended not only for regaining full mobility and independence but for increasing fitness in terms of aerobic capacity and muscular strength and reducing the risk of subsequent fractures resulting from falls and/or low bone mineral density.

Physical Therapy Phase

The focus of the physical therapy phase is to aid the subject in regaining mobility and correcting deficiencies in balance, strength, gait, flexibility, and posture that would limit the individual's participation in ADL and exercise.

Vertebral Fractures.—Symptoms of acute vertebral fracture most frequently include sudden onset of back pain in the area of the spinous processes, paravertebral muscle spasm in overstretched muscles from a wedge fracture, and referred pain along the intercostal nerves. Pain is usually absent from the buttock or lower extremities. The symptoms often improve in the horizontal position, either supine or side-lying.

Evaluation of the acute vertebral fracture should include a subjective description of the onset of the pain, including whether there were any predisposing events such as lifting a heavy object or leaning over and pulling on a window or garage door. It is important to determine the severity and location of the pain and to note postural changes. If not already available, an x-ray should be obtained to determine the type and degree of vertebral fracture.

Treatment for the first 1 to 3 weeks is symptomatic; bed rest, pain medications, cold applications the first 2 to 3 days followed by heat applications and light massage to the paravertebral muscles. A

transcutaneous electrical nerve stimulation (TENS) unit may be tried. The patient should be positioned with a low pillow, knee support to avoid strain on the back, and a firm mattress. Precautions must be observed to prevent the formation of decubitus ulcers, pulmonary complications, and loss of active range of motion in the extremities.

Within a week after fracture the patient should be able to tolerate movement. He or she should begin ambulation and be instructed in back protection techniques to minimize trunk flexion, including stiff back postures during bending, lifting, and transfer activities. Recommendations should include the use of low-heeled shoes, soft sole inserts, and a raised toilet seat if needed.

When the patient is ambulatory, a more complete assessment of the patient can be completed:

1. Observe patient for spinal deformities such as kyphosis or lordosis with accompanying overstretching or shortening of paravertebral and sacrospinal muscles.
2. Check head and shoulder position and compensatory changes in lower extremity positioning to maintain balance.
3. Perform as complete an evaluation as the patient can tolerate of range of motion and a manual muscle test of the back extensors, abdominals, neck, shoulders, hip, knee, and ankle muscles.
4. Evaluate the gait pattern, observing for painful secondary joints, balance, speed, stride length, cadence, foot clearance, and need for an assistive device. If the patient is unable to maintain a comfortably erect posture, an orthosis or rigid jacket may be ordered.

Treatment planning must include instructing the patient in pectoral stretches, deep breathing to maintain intercostal mobility, trunk extensor strengthening, isometric abdominal strengthening, and assessment of the home for environmental factors that increase the risk of falling, and of the need for postural and ambulatory assistive devices after discharge. Care must be given when recommending assistive devices; they may initially provide short-term benefits but may accelerate loss of abdominal and back extensor strength because of disuse. In addition, the patient's ambulation posture may change; for example, forward flexion and weight bearing on the arms may increase. The patient will need to maintain as erect a posture as possible to minimize the risk of anterior wedge fractures.

By an average of 6 to 8 weeks after fracture, patients will be relatively pain free and resuming normal activities. They may need short rest periods during the day or need to use an orthosis if still experiencing pain. Trunk strengthening activities and prevention of excessive flexion should continue to be encouraged. Patients also benefit from a comprehensive exercise program geared toward osteoporotics that includes weight-bearing, ambulation, and balance activities to increase mechanical stress on bone and decrease risk factors related to falling.

Complications from severe kyphotic postures include pain, fatiguability from decreased vital capacity, postural changes in the legs and hips from compensatory postures to maintain the center of balance, and increased susceptibility to falling owing to diminished balance.

Hip Fracture.—Evaluation of the hip fracture patient should include the postural, balance, flexibility, strength, and gait evaluations described for vertebral fractures. Treatment of the osteoporotic hip fracture patient must include joint protection techniques, falls prevention, and assessment for vertebral fractures. Patients who experience hip fractures tend to ambulate more slowly and have diminished balance reactions. Any intervention methods that impact on these variables will be of benefit to the patient.

Hip fracture patients have limited range of motion and strength of the hip; however, exercises emphasizing hip abduction and internal rotation, or which apply torsion to the hip, should not be used.

Wrist Fracture.—Wrist fractures are more common than hip fractures in women aged 55 to 65 years. It is hypothesized that persons walking with greater velocity fall forward, breaking their fall with their outstretched hand rather than falling onto the knee and hip. Assessment and treatment planning should be sensitive to other risk factors related to osteoporosis.

Once the cast has been removed, flexibility and strength exercises for the affected arm should be prescribed. Physical therapy should be designed to bring the injured arm back to the level of the uninjured arm.

Exercise Phase

Prior to the exercise phase, subjects should have an aerobic work capacity test and strength, balance, and gait evaluations. Once physical status has been determined, the person should be assigned to one of the following programs:

1. Small-group (four to six) pool or chair exercises supervised by exercise specialists or physical therapists
2. Small-group exercise including weight-bearing activities supervised by exercise specialists
3. Large-group (10 to 20) exercise supervised by exercise specialists
4. Individual unsupervised exercise or community programs

As the subject's total fitness improves, she or he increases the intensity and progresses to the next program, where more strenuous and complex movement patterns are encouraged. Each exercise program, to the extent possible, follows the guidelines for prevention of osteoporosis.

In programming for subjects with severe osteopenia or fractures, a particularly difficult problem is determining what can be done without endangering the subject. Questions to be asked should include:

1. Which movements or events, if any, cause a fragile vertebra to collapse?
2. Which exercises can be used to strengthen the bone without damage?
3. Which muscle groups surrounding a hip fracture should be trained to enhance strength, gait, and balance, and how can the involved muscles be trained without loosening the prosthesis?
4. How can the possibilities of falls be minimized during weight-bearing exercise?

A careful evaluation of the individual subject's abilities and risks of falls and fractures is a must in planning an exercise program. The patient's program should then be based on avoiding high-risk activities, both in the exercise program and ADL, and addressing areas of limitation. Fitness considerations should not outweigh safety.

General principles in programming for subjects with severe osteopenia or osteoporosis include the following:

1. Avoid high-impact activities or activities that carry a high risk of falls (e.g., ice skating).
2. Progress very gradually in intensity and movement complexity. Older, sedentary subjects are often uncomfortable with exercise and find it difficult to learn exercise routines or maintain correct exercise posture and coordinated movement.

3. Use with caution complex movement patterns that may cause subjects to trip or lose their balance. Weight-bearing activities should be adapted to the subject's movement capacity.

PROGNOSIS AND FOLLOW-UP

General Prognosis

Hip fractures are associated with 12% to 20% excess mortality.[45] Only one quarter of hip fracture patients regain full independence,[19] while half require some assistance with ADL and the final quarter are totally disabled.[59] Vertebral fractures cannot be repaired and 95% of women who sustain a vertebral fracture will suffer six or more additional vertebral fractures within the following 10 years.[94]

Prognosis With Physical Therapy and Exercise

The benefits of physical therapy and exercise for strength, flexibility, and aerobic capacity are well established. Increased strength, flexibility, and aerobic capacity are important factors in maintaining independence, performing ADL, and the quality of life. Few studies have addressed the effects of these interventions on balance, gait, or reaction time. Exercise programs have been shown to increase bone mass or decrease loss in a wide variety of subjects, including subjects with osteoporosis. Although no intervention studies have addressed the effects of exercise on falls or fractures, cross-sectional and longitudinal studies indicate that risk is smaller in subjects with greater activity levels.

Follow-up

It is important to encourage patients to continue with their exercises, either at home or in an organized program, by providing routine follow-up visits after the initial intensive physical therapy phase. Patients should continue to exercise at least 3 days per week in order to sustain or improve their condition. Without encouragement, many patients will discontinue exercise and lose the progress they have made in combating osteoporosis. A suggested follow-up schedule is quarterly the first year, every 6 months the following 2 years, and annually in the fourth and fifth years.

A problem with evaluating a person's change or rate of change in bone mineral density or the other parameters described is that the coefficient of variation for the measurement techniques is relatively large compared to the expected change. It is therefore difficult to determine whether a change has occurred, or its extent, on an individual basis.[20] Further precision can be gained by taking multiple measures at each time point, over a longer period of time or more frequently, or a combination of these. Follow-up measures can provide a feeling of accomplishment and motivate patients. These are important aspects of a successful treatment program.

REFERENCES

1. Agre JC, Pierce LE, Raab DM, et al: Light resistance and stretching exercise in elderly women: Effect upon strength. *Arch Phys Med Rehabil* 1988; 69:273–276.
2. Aloia JF, Cohn SH, Ostuni J, et al: Prevention of involutional bone loss by exercise. *Ann Intern Med* 1978; 89:356–358.
3. American Academy of Orthopedic Surgeons: *Joint Motion. Method of Measuring and Recording*. Edinburgh, Churchill Livingstone, 1966.
4. American College of Sports Medicine: *Guidelines for Exercise Testing and Prescription*, ed 3. Philadelphia, Lea & Fabiger, 1986.
5. Aniansson A, Gustafsson E: Physical training in elderly men with special reference to quadriceps muscle strength and morphology. *Clin Physiol* 1981; 1:87–98.
6. Aniansson A, Ljungberg P, Rundgren A, et al: Effect of a training programme for pensioners on condition and muscular strength. *Arch Gerontol Geriatr* 1984; 3:229–241.
7. Astrom J, Ahnqvist S, Beertema J, et al: Physical activity in women sustaining fracture of the neck of the femur. *J Bone Joint Surg (Br)* 1987; 69B:381–383.
8. Baylor AM, Spirduso WW: Systematic aerobic exercise and components of reaction time in older women. *J Gerontol* 1988; 43:121–126.
9. Beverly MC, Rider TA, Evans MJ, et al: Local bone mineral response to brief exercise that stresses the skeleton. *Br Med J* 1989; 299:233–235.
10. Block JE, Friedlander AL, Brooks GA, et al: Determinants of bone density among athletes engaged in weight-bearing and non–weight-bearing activity. *J Appl Physiol* 1989; 67:1100–1105.
11. Boyce WJ, Vessey MP: Habitual physical inertia and other factors in relation to risk of fracture of the proximal femur. *Age Ageing* 1988; 17:319–327.
12. Buccola VA, Stone WJ: Effects of jogging and cycling programs on physiological and personality variables in aged men. *Res Q* 1975; 46:134–139.
13. Campbell AJ, Borrie MJ, Spears GF: Risk factors for falls in a community-based prospective study of people 70 years and older. *J Gerontol* 1989; 44:M112–117.
14. Canalis E: Regulation of bone remodeling, in Favus

MJ (ed): *Primer on the Metabolic Bone Diseases and Disorders of Mineral Metabolism*. Kelseyville, Calif, American Society for Bone and Mineral Research, 1990, pp 23–26.

15. Chapman EA, deVries HA, Swezey R: Joint stiffness: Effects of exercise on young and old men. *J Gerontol* 1972; 27:218–221.

16. Chow RK, Harrison JE, Notarius C: Effect of two randomised exercise programmes on bone mass of healthy postmenopausal women. *Br Med J* 1987; 292:607–610.

17. Chow RK, Harrison JE, Sturtbridge W, et al: The effect of exercise on bone mass of osteoporotic patients on fluoride treatment. *Clin Invest Med* 1987, 10:59–63.

18. Clarkson PM: The effect of age and activity level on simple and choice fractionated response time. *Eur J Appl Physiol* 1978; 40:17–25.

19. Cummings SR: Epidemiology of osteoporotic fractures, in Genant HK (ed). *Osteoporosis Update 1987*, San Francisco, Radiology Research and Education Foundation, 1987, pp 7–12.

20. Cummings SR: Use of bone density measurements, in Genant HK (ed): *Osteoporosis Update 1987*, San Francisco, Radiology Research and Education Foundation, 1987, pp 115–121.

21. Cummings SR, Nevitt MC: A hypothesis: The causes of hip fractures. *J Gerontol* 1989; 44:M107–M111.

22. Dalsky GP, Stocke KS, Ehsani AA, et al: Weight-bearing exercise training and lumbar bone mineral content in postmenopausal women. *Ann Intern Med* 1988; 108:824–828.

23. Daniell HW: Osteoporosis and the slender smoker. *Arch Intern Med* 1976; 136:298–304.

24. Danneskiold-Samsoe B, Lyngberg K, Risum T, et al: The effect of water exercise therapy given to patients with rheumatoid arthritis. *Scand J Rehab Med* 1987; 19:31–35.

25. deVries HA: Physiological effects of an exercise training regimen upon men aged 52 to 88. *J Gerontol* 1970; 25:325–336.

26. Dustman RE, Ruhling RO, Russell EM, et al: Aerobic exercise training and improved neuropsychological function of older adults. *Neurobiol Aging* 1984; 5:35–42.

27. Era P, Heikkinen E: Postural sway during standing and unexpected disturbance of balance in random samples of men of different ages, *J Gerontology* 1985; 40:287–295.

28. Exton-Smith AN: Clinical manifestations, in Exton-Smith AN, Evans G (eds): *Care of the Elderly: Meeting the Challenge of Dependency*. London, Academic Press, 1977, pp 41–53.

29. Farley SMG, Perkel V, Tudtud-Hans LA, et al: Fluoride and calcium therapy for osteoporosis increases trabecular vertebral bone density above the fracture threshold, in DeLuca HF, Mazess R (eds): *Osteoporosis: Physiological Basis, Assessment, and Treatment*. Amsterdam, Elsevier, 1990, pp 7–16.

30. Fiatarone MA, Marks EC, Ryan ND, et al: High-intensity strength training in nonagenarians, *JAMA* 1990; 263:3029–3034.

31. Frekany GA, Leslie DK: Effects of an exercise program on selected flexibility measurements of senior citizens. *Gerontologist* 1975; 4:182–183.

32. Frontera WR, Meredith CN, O'Reilly KP, et al: Strength conditioning in older men: Skeletal muscle hypertrophy and improved function. *J Appl Physiol* 1988; 64:1038–1044.

33. Frost HM: A new direction for osteoporosis research: A review and proposal. *Bone* 1991; 12:429–437.

34. Gehlsen GM, Grigsby SA, Winant DM: Effects of an aquatic fitness program on the muscular strength and endurance of patients with multiple sclerosis. *Phys Ther* 1984; 64:653–657.

35. Gehlsen GM, Whaley MH: Falls in the elderly. II. Balance, strength, and flexibility. *Arch Phys Med Rehabil* 1990; 71:739–741.

36. Gleeson PB, Protas EJ, LeBlanc AD, et al: Effects of weight lifting on bone mineral density in premenopausal women. *J Bone Min Res* 1990; 5:153–158.

37. Grimby G: Muscle changes and trainability in the elderly. *Top Geriatr Rehabil* 1990; 5:54–62.

38. Guesens P, Dequeker J, Verstraeten A, et al: Age, sex and menopause-related changes of vertebral and peripheral bone: Population study with dual and single photon absorptiometry and radiogrammetry. *J Nucl Med* 1987; 27:1540–1549.

39. Gutman GM, Herbert CP, Brown SR: Feldenkrais versus conventional exercises for the elderly. *J Gerontol* 1977; 32:562–572.

40. Heaney RP: Management of osteoporosis: Nutritional considerations. *Clin Invest Med* 1982; 5:185–187.

41. Heaney RP, Recker RR: Effects of nitrogen, phosphorus and caffeine on calcium balance in women. *J Lab Clin Med* 1982; 99:46–55.

42. Heaney RP, Recker RR, Saville PD: Menopausal changes in calcium balance performance *J Lab Clin Med* 1978; 92:953–963.

43. Heinrich CH, Going SB, Pamenter RW, et al: Bone mineral content of cyclically menstruating female resistance and endurance trained athletes *Med Sci Sports Exerc* 1990; 22:558–563.

44. Himann JE, Cunningham DA, Rechnitzer PA, et al: Age-related changes in speed of walking. *Med Sci Sports Exerc* 1988; 20:161–166.

45. Holbrook TL, Grazier K, Kelsey JL, et al: *The Frequency of Occurrence, Impact and Cost of Musculoskeletal Conditions in the United States*. Chicago, American Academy of Orthopedic Surgeons, 1984.

46. Holtrop ME: Light and electron microscopic structure of bone-forming cells, in Hall BK (ed): *Bone. The Osteoblast and Osteocyte*, vol 1. Caldwell, NJ, Telford Press, 1990, pp 1–39.

47. Huddleston AL, Rockwell D, Kulund DN, et al: Bone mass in lifetime tennis athletes. *JAMA* 1980; 244:1107–1109.

48. Ismail F, Epstein S, Gorman K, et al: The influence of exercise on bone mineral metabolism in the elderly (abstract). *J Bone Min Res* 1989; 4:S231.

49. Jacobson PC, Beaver W, Grubb SA, et al: Bone density in women: College athletes and older athletic women. *J Orthoped Res* 1984; 2:328–332.

50. Johnell O, Nilsson B, Obrant K, et al: Age and sex

patterns of hip fracture—changes in 30 years. *Acta Orthop Scand* 1984; 55:290–292.

51. Jones HH, Priest JD, Hayes WC: Humeral hypertrophy in response to exercise. *J Bone Joint Surg (Am)* 1977; 59A:204–208.
52. Jones PRM, Hardman AE, Hudson A, et al: Influence of brisk walking on the broadband ultrasonic attenuation of the calcaneus in previously sedentary women aged 30–61 years. *Calcif Tissue Int* 1991; 49:112–115.
53. Krolner B, Toft B, Nielson SP, et al: Physical exercise as prophylaxis against involutional vertebral bone loss: A controlled trial. *Clin Sci* 1983; 64:541–546.
54. Lanyon LE: Strain-related bone modeling and remodeling. *Top Geriatr Rehabil* 1989; 4:13–24.
55. Lesser M: The effects of rhythmic exercise on the range of motion in older adults, *Am Correct Ther J* 1978; 32:118–122.
56. Lichtenstein MJ, Shields SL, Shiavi RG, et al: Exercise and balance in aged women: A pilot controlled clinical trial. *Arch Phys Med Rehabil* 1989; 70:138–143.
57. Lucht U: Prospective study of accidental falls and resulting injuries in the homes of elderly people *Acta Sociomed Scand* 1971; 2:105–120.
58. Margulies JY, Simkin A, Leichter I, et al: Effect of intense physical activity on the bone-mineral content in the lower limbs of young adults. *J Bone Joint Surg (Am)* 1986; 68A:1090–1093.
59. Martin AD, Houston CS: Osteoporosis, calcium and physical activity. *Can Med Assoc J* 1987; 136:587–593.
60. Martin AD, Silverthorn KG, Houston CS, et al: Trends in fracture of the proximal femur in two million Canadians, 1972 to 1984. *Clin Orthop Rel Res* 1991; 266:111–118.
61. Mazess R, Collick B, Trempe J, et al: Performance evaluation of a dual energy x-ray bone densitometer. *Calcif Tissue Int* 1989; 44:228–232.
62. Mazess RB: Bone densitometry for clinical diagnosis and monitoring, in DeLuca HF, Mazess R (eds): *Osteoporosis: Physiological Basis, Assessment and Treatment*. Amsterdam, Elsevier, 1990, pp 63–85.
63. Melton LJ: Fracture patterns, in DeLuca HF, Mazess R (eds): *Osteoporosis: Physiological Basis, Assessment, and Treatment*. New York, Elsevier, 1990, pp 39–44.
64. Melton LJ, Kan SH, Frye MA, et al: Epidemiology of vertebral fractures in women. *Am J Epidemiol* 1989; 129:1000–1011.
65. Melton LJ, Wahner HW, Richelson LS, et al: Osteoporosis and the risk of hip fracture. *Am J Epidemiol* 1986; 124:254–261.
66. Moroz D, Sale D, Webber C: The effect of intensive training on axial and appendicular bone mineral in normal postmenopausal women (abstract). *J Bone Mineral Res* 1989; 4:S233.
67. Montoye HJ, Smith EL, Fardon DF, et al: Bone mineral in senior tennis players. *Scand J Sports Sci* 1980; 2:26–32.
68. Mosekilde L: Age-related changes in vertebral trabecular bone architecture—assessed by a new method. *Bone* 1988; 9:247–250.
69. Mundy GR: Bone resorbing cells, in Favus MJ (ed): *Primer on the Metabolic Bone Diseases and Disorders of Mineral Metabolism*. Kelseyville, Calif, American Society for Bone and Mineral Research, 1990, pp 18–22.

70. Munns K: Effect of exercise on range of joint motion in elderly subjects, in Smith EL, Serfass RC (eds): *Exercise and Aging: The Scientific Basis*. Hillside, NJ, Enslow, 1981, pp 167–178.
71. Nelson ME, Fisher EC, Dilmanian FA, et al: A 1-y walking program and increased dietary calcium in postmenopausal women: Effects on bone. *Am J Clin Nutr* 1991; 53:1304–1311.
72. Nevitt MC, Cummings SR, Kidd S, et al: Risk factors for recurrent nonsyncopal falls: A prospective study. *JAMA* 1989; 261:2663–2668.
73. Nilsson BE, Westlin NE: Bone density in athletes. *Clin Orthop* 1971; 77:179–182.
74. Notelovitz M, Martin D, Tesar R, et al: Estrogen therapy and variable-resistance weight training increase bone mineral in surgically menopausal women. *J Bone Mineral Res* 1991; 6:583–590.
75. Osness WH: Assessment of physical function among older adults, in Leslie DK (ed): *Mature Stuff: Physical Activity for the Older Adult*. Reston, Va, American Alliance for Health, Physical Education, Recreation and Dance, 1989, pp 93–115.
76. Panton LB, Graves JE, Pollock ML, et al: Effect of aerobic and resistance training on fractionated reaction time and speed of movement. *J Gerontol* 1990; 45:M26–M31.
77. Parfitt AM: The physiologic and clinical significance of bone histomorphometric data, in Recker RR (ed): *Bone Histomorphometry: Techniques and Interpretation*. Boca Raton, Fla, CRC, 1983, pp 143–223.
78. Priest JD, Jones HH, Tichenor CJC, et al: Arm and elbow changes in expert tennis players. *Minn Med* 1977; 60:399–404.
79. Prince RL, Smith M, Dick IM, et al: Prevention of postmenopausal osteoporosis. *N Engl J Med* 1991; 325:1189–1195.
80. Raab DM, Agre JC, Smith EL: Light resistance and stretching exercise in elderly women: Effect upon flexibility. *Arch Phys Med Rehabil* 1988; 69:268–272.
81. Ray WA, Griffin MR: Prescribed medications and the risk of falling. *Top Geriatr Rehabil* 1990; 5:12–20.
82. Riggs BL: Causes of age-related bone loss and fractures, in DeLuca HF, Mazess R (eds): *Osteoporosis: Physiological Basis, Assessment, and Treatment*. Amsterdam, Elsevier, 1990, pp 7–16.
83. Rikli R, Busch S: Motor performance of women as a function of age and physical activity level. *J Gerontol* 1986; 41:645–649.
84. Rikli RE, Edwards DJ: Effects of a three-year exercise program on motor function and cognitive processing speed in older women. *Res Q Exerc Sport* 1991; 62:61–67.
85. Rikli RE, McManis BG: Effects of exercise on bone mineral content in postmenopausal women. *Res Q Exerc Sport* 1990; 61:243–249.
86. Roberts BL: Effects of walking on balance among elders. *Nurs Res* 1989; 38:180–182.
87. Rockwell JC, Sorenson AM, Baker S, et al: Weight training decreases vertebral bone density in premenopausal women: A prospective study. *J Clin Endocrinol Metab* 1990; 71:988–993.

88. Rodan GA: Introduction to bone biology. *Bone* 1992; 13:S3–S6.

89. Rubin CT, Lanyon LE: Regulation of bone formation by applied dynamic loads. *J Bone Joint Surg (Am)* 1984; 66A:397–402.

90. Rubin CT, Lanyon LE: Regulation of bone mass by mechanical strain magnitude. *Calcif Tissue Int* 1985; 37:411–417.

91. Rundgren A, Aniansson A, Ljungberg P, et al: Effects of a training programme for elderly people on mineral content of the heel bone. *Arch Gerontol Geriatr* 1984; 3:243–248.

92. Sandler RB, Cauley JA, Hom DL, et al: The effects of walking on the cross-sectional dimensions of the radius in postmenopausal women. *Calcif Tissue Int* 1987; 41:65–69.

93. Saville PD: Changes in bone mass with age and alcoholism. *J Bone Joint Surg (Am)* 1965; 47A:492–499.

94. Scott WW: Osteoporosis-related fracture syndromes, in *Osteoporosis: National Institutes of Health Consensus Development Conference, April 2–4, 1984. Program and Abstracts.* Washington, DC, National Institutes of Health, 1984, pp 20–24.

95. Simkin A, Ayalon J, Leichter I: Increased trabecular bone density due to bone-loading exercises in postmenopausal osteoporotic women. *Calcif Tissue Int* 1986; 40:59–63.

96. Sinaki M, Wahner HW, Offord KP, et al: Efficacy of nonloading exercises in prevention of vertebral bone loss in postmenopausal women: A controlled trial. *Clin Proc* 1989; 64:762–769.

97. Slemenda CW, Hui SL Longcope C, et al: Cigarette smoking, obesity and bone mass. *J Bone Mineral Res* 1989; 4:737–741.

98. Smith EL: Special considerations in developing exercise programs for the older adult, in Matarazzo JD, Weiss SM, Herd JA, et al (eds): *Behavioral Health: A Handbook of Health Enhancement and Disease Prevention.* New York, Wiley & Sons, 1984, pp 525–546.

99. Smith EL, Gilligan C: Fitness declines and assessment in the older adult, in Drury TF (ed): *Assessing Physical Fitness and Physical Activity in Population Based Surveys.* Washington, DC, US Public Health Service, National Center for Health Statistics, DHHS Publication No. 89-1253, pp 293–345.

100. Smith EL, Gilligan C: Mechanical forces and bone, in Peck WA (ed): *Bone and Mineral Research 6.* New York, Elsevier, 1989, pp 139–173.

101. Smith EL, Gilligan C: Physical activity prescription for the older adult. *Physician Sportsmed* 1983; 11:91.

102. Smith EL, Gilligan C, Shea MM, et al: Exercise reduces bone involution in middle-aged women. *Calcif Tissue Int* 1989; 44:312–321.

103. Smith EL, Reddan W, Smith PE: Physical activity and calcium modalities for bone mineral increase in aged women. *Med Sci Sports Exerc* 1981; 13:60–64.

104. Spirduso WW: Physical fitness, aging and psychomotor speed: A review. *J Gerontol* 1980; 35:850–865.

105. Spirduso WW: Reaction and movement time as a function of age and physical activity level. *J Gerontol* 1975; 30:435–440.

106. Spirduso WW, Clifford P: Replication of age and physical activity effects on reaction and movement time. *J Gerontol* 1978; 33:26–30.

107. Spitzer TA, Moore JR, Hopkins DR, et al: Aquatic exercise research: A comparison of selected training responses to water aerobics and low-impact aerobics, *AKWA Lett* 1991; 4:5.

108. Tinetti ME, Speechley M, Ginter SF: Risk factors for falls among elderly persons living in the community. *N Engl J Med* 1988; 319:1701–1707.

109. Tinetti ME: Performance-oriented assessment of mobility problems in elderly patients. *J Am Geriatr Soc* 1986; 34:119–126.

110. Wahner HW, Dunn WL, Riggs BL: Assessment of bone mineral, part 2. *J Nucl Med* 1984; 25:1241–1253.

111. Watson RC: Bone growth and physical activity in young males, in Mazess RB (ed): *International Conference on Bone Mineral Measurements.* Washington, DC, National Institutes of Health, NIH Publication No 75-683, pp 380–385.

112. Whipple RH, Wolfson LI, Amerman PM: The relationship of knee and ankle weakness to falls in nursing home residents: An isokinetic study. *J Am Geriatr Soc* 1987; 35:13–20.

113. White MK, Martin RB, Yeater RA, et al: The effects of exercise on the bones of postmenopausal women. *Int Orthop* 1984; 7:209–214.

114. Wickham CAC, Walsh K, Cooper C, et al: Dietary calcium, physical activity, and risk of hip fracture: A prospective study. *Br Med J* 1989; 299:889–892.

115. Wong G: Isolation and behavior of isolated bone-forming cells, in Hall BK (ed): *Bone. The Osteoblast and Osteocyte,* vol 1. Caldwell, NJ, Telford Press, 1990, pp 171–192.

116. Woollacott MH: Change in posture and voluntary control in the elderly: Research findings and rehabilitation. *Topics Geriatr Rehabil* 1990; 5:1–11.

Index

411